Anesthesia and neurosurgery

ANESTHESIA AND NEUROSURGERY

JAMES E. COTTRELL, M.D.

Professor and Chairman, Department of Anesthesiology,
State University of New York,
Downstate Medical Center,
Brooklyn, New York

HERMAN TURNDORF, M.D.

Professor and Chairman, Department of Anesthesiology,
New York University Medical Center,
New York, New York

with 131 illustrations

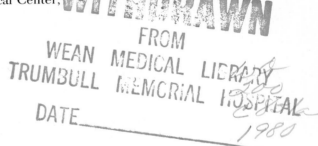
The C. V. Mosby Company

ST. LOUIS • TORONTO • LONDON   1980

The C. V. Mosby Company
11830 Westline Industrial Drive, St. Louis, Missouri 63141

Library of Congress Cataloging in Publication Data

Main entry under title:

Anesthesia and neurosurgery.

    Bibliography: p.
    Includes index.
    1. Nervous system—Surgery. 2. Anesthesia in
neurology. I. Cottrell, James E. II. Turndorf, Herman.
[DNLM: 1. Anesthesia. 2. Neurosurgery. WO200.3 A578]
RD593.A5 617′.967′48   79-24676
ISBN 0-8016-1036-2

GW/CB/B 9 8 7 6 5 4 3 2   01/D/079

Contributors

DONALD P. BECKER, M.D.

Professor and Chairman, Division of Neurological Surgery, Virginia Commonwealth University; Attending Neurosurgeon, Medical College of Virginia Hospitals, Medical College of Virginia, Richmond, Virginia

DEREK A. BRUCE, M.B., Ch.B.

Associate Neurosurgeon, Children's Hospital of Philadelphia; Assistant Professor of Neurosurgery, University of Pennsylvania School of Medicine, Philadelphia, Pennsylvania

JAMES E. COTTRELL, M.D.

Professor and Chairman, Department of Anesthesiology, State University of New York, Downstate Medical Center, Brooklyn, New York

HARRY B. DEMOPOULOS, M.D.

Associate Professor, Department of Pathology, New York University Medical Center, New York, New York

EUGENE S. FLAMM, M.D.

Associate Professor, Department of Neurosurgery, New York University Medical Center, New York, New York

RICHARD P. GREENBERG, M.D.

Assistant Professor of Neurosurgery, Division of Neurological Surgery, Medical College of Virginia—Virginia Commonwealth University, Richmond, Virginia

AKE GRENVIK, M.D.

Professor of Anesthesiology, Division of Critical Care Medicine, Department of Anesthesiology/ CCM, University Health Center of Pittsburgh, University of Pittsburgh, Pittsburgh, Pennsylvania

RICHARD L. GRIFFITH, M.D., Ph.D.

Assistant Professor, Department of Anesthesiology and Surgery, Medical College of Virginia, Richmond, Virginia

BHAGWANDAS GUPTA, M.D.

Resident, Department of Anesthesiology, New York University School of Medicine, New York, New York

MAGNUS HAGERDAL, M.D.

Assistant Professor, Department of Anesthesiology, University of Lund, Lund, Sweden

JAMES R. HARP, M.D.

Professor and Chairman, Department of Anesthesiology, Temple University, Philadelphia, Pennsylvania

WILLIAM D. HETRICK, M.D.

Anesthesia Staff, Mercy Hospital, Pittsburgh, Pennsylvania

GERALD HOCHWALD, M.D.

Professor, Departments of Neurology and of Physiology and Biophysics, New York University Medical Center, New York, New York

BRYAN JENNETT, M.D.

Professor of Neurosurgery, Institute of Neurological Sciences, The Southern General Hospital, University of Glasgow, Glasgow, Scotland

JULIUS KOREIN, M.D.

Professor of Neurology, New York University Medical Center; Chief of Electroencephalography, Bellevue Hospital Center, New York, New York

IRVIN I. KRICHEFF, M.D.

Professor of Radiology, Department of Radiology (Neuroradiology Section), New York University Medical Center, New York, New York

NIELS A. LASSEN, M.D.

Chairman, Department of Clinical Physiology, Bispebjerg Hospital, Copenhagen, Denmark

JOSEPH P. LIN, M.D.

Professor of Radiology, Department of Radiology (Neuroradiology Section), New York University Medical Center, New York, New York

MARTHA JANE MATJASKO, M.D.

Associate Professor, Department of Anesthesiology, University of Maryland Hospital, University of Maryland School of Medicine, Baltimore, Maryland

PHILIPPA NEWFIELD, M.D.

Assistant Clinical Professor, Anesthesia and Neurosurgery, University of California, San Francisco, San Francisco, California

JEROME B. POSNER, M.D.

Department of Neurology, Memorial Sloan-Kettering Cancer Center and Cornell University Medical College, New York, New York

DAVID J. POWNER, M.D.

Assistant Professor of Anesthesiology, Division of Critical Care Medicine, Department of Anesthesiology/CCM, University Health Center of Pittsburgh, University of Pittsburgh, Pittsburgh, Pennsylvania

JOSEPH RANSOHOFF, M.D.

Professor and Chairman, Department of Neurosurgery, New York University Medical Center, New York, New York

DAVID A. ROTTENBERG, M.D.

Department of Neurology, Memorial Sloan-Kettering Cancer Center and Cornell University Medical College, New York, New York

STANLEY I. SAMUELS, M.D., B.Ch.

Assistant Professor of Anesthesia, Department of Anesthesia, Stanford University School of Medicine, Stanford, California

MYRON L. SELIGMAN, Ph.D.

Research Assistant Professor, Departments of Pathology and Neurosurgery, New York University Medical Center, New York, New York

JAMES V. SNYDER, M.D.

Associate Professor of Anesthesiology, Division of Critical Care Medicine, Department of Anesthesiology/CCM, University Health Center of Pittsburgh, University of Pittsburgh, Pittsburgh, Pennsylvania

HUMBERT G. SULLIVAN, M.D.

Associate Professor and Attending Neurosurgeon, Section of Neurological Surgery, Medical College of Georgia; Chief of Neurosurgery, Veterans Hospital, Augusta, Georgia

HERMAN TURNDORF, M.D.

Professor and Chairman, Department of Anesthesiology, New York University Medical Center, New York, New York

BERNARD WOLFSON, M.B., Ch.B., F.F.A.R.C.S.

Clinical Professor, Department of Anesthesia, University of Pittsburgh; Director of Anesthesiology Research Lab, Mercy Hospital, Pittsburgh, Pennsylvania

Foreword

What is neuroanesthesia? The term "neuroanesthesia" often carries with it the connotation of a medical subspecialty from which others are excluded. When faced with occasional patients with acute neurosurgical disease, many practicing anesthesiologists have developed an unnecessary sense of professional inadequacy. This feeling is not justified, since neuroanesthesia is simply the application of basic information concerning the pathophysiology of acute central nervous system disease in a context of understanding the intracranial effects of drugs and anesthetic techniques. Since "neuroanesthesia" is not defined in standard medical dictionaries, the meaning given to it in the foregoing sentence is suggested as a working definition. This book provides much of this prerequisite information; it represents neuroanesthetic practice as an amalgam of neurology, neurosurgery, and anesthesiology. The chapters have been drawn from the experience of investigative and academic anesthesiologists and neurosurgeons working in centers with large numbers of neurosurgical cases.

A better appreciation of what is meant by the term "neuroanesthesia" can be gained through a historical perspective of its development. Neuroanesthetic evolution is based on separate and combined progress in neurosurgery and anesthesia. While each of these fields has a rich history of its own, the present narrative focuses on the major events that impinge on the development of neuroanesthesia.

The oldest neurosurgical procedure, trephination, dates back to the ancient Greeks and Romans and was probably performed without narcosis or sedation. Accelerated progress in neurosurgery occurred at the end of the nineteenth century when the discovery of antisepsis and anesthesia was merged with neurologic diagnostic techniques, leading to the localization of lesions in the central nervous system.[1]

About 40 years following the introduction of general anesthesia in 1844-1846, Sir Victor Horsley, the British neurosurgeon, experimented with chloroform and ether in order to find the best general anesthetic agent for neurosurgery. Horsley chose chloroform, while Harvey Cushing selected ether as the best neuroanesthetic. Cushing, who also introduced record keeping and blood pressure measurement into anesthetic practice in the United States, felt that blood pressure control with chloroform was poor when compared with the control provided by ether. The early twentieth century neurosurgeons also seemed to appreciate that the anesthetic agent could affect intracranial conditions in terms of brain congestion or tension.[2] Because of a possible adverse effect of general anesthesia on systemic and intracranial conditions, DeMartel (1913) and then Cushing (1917) advocated that local anesthesia be used for all neurosurgical procedures. By 1923 Davidoff had suggested that a combination of tribromoethanol and local anesthesia actually lowered intracranial pressure. Thiopental was first employed in clinical anesthesia by Lundy and Waters in 1934. It became widely used for neuroanesthesia in combination with nitrous oxide and oxygen following

World War II. Trichloroethylene was employed during the same period, and halothane found its way into neuroanesthesia in the late 1950's. Generally, most anesthetic drugs, when introduced into anesthesia for neurosurgery, were initially employed because of their overall safety and ease of administration rather than because of any special advantage to the neurosurgical patient.

Introduction of the more versatile and potent general anesthetics created the need for improved airway and ventilation control. Around 1928 endotracheal intubation was employed, and this facilitated the use of controlled ventilation in neuroanesthesia. Lundy stated in 1942 that it is "difficult to reduce intracranial pressure unless resort is made to artificial respiration. . . ."[3] From this early observation, controlled ventilation or hyperventilation has become a central element in neuroanesthetics performed in patients with intracranial hypertension. Much later Adams found that hyperventilation can ameliorate ICP increases caused by volatile anesthetics.[4]

The modern scientific bases for neuroanesthetic practice dates from the introduction of cerebral blood flow and metabolism measurement in man by Kety and Schmidt in 1945 and from the continuous measurement of intracranial pressure monitoring in neurosurgical patients by Lundberg in 1960.[5,6] Application of these techniques has led to our understanding of the powerful actions of anesthetic drugs, blood pressures, intracranial pressure, carbon dioxide, and oxygen tension on the intracranial and spinal compartments. This is the central core of neuroanesthesia.

Continuous direct measurement of intracranial pressure provided the first detailed description of the intracranial pressure–elevating effects of modern volatile anesthetic agents.[7] During the 1960's, groups at the Universities of Pennsylvania and Glasgow found that halothane as well as certain other anesthetics increased cerebral blood flow by reducing cerebrovascular resistance.[8,9] From this information they deduced that the increase in intracranial tension associated with halothane was caused by an increase in cerebral blood volume related to the pharmacologically induced cerebral vascular dilation.[10] These investigations established a fundamental neuroanesthetic principle: drugs and physiologic changes that elevate cerebral blood flow have the potential to increase intracranial pressure and vice versa.

Although thiopental had earlier been shown to reduce cerebral blood flow and metabolism, it was not until 1972 that Hunter's observations on dural tension suggested that barbiturate anesthesia might actually improve operating conditions.[11] Later Shapiro found that thiopental actually reduced elevated intracranial pressure while simultaneously increasing cerebral perfusion pressure.[12] Thus the old neurosurgical fear that all general anesthetics put their patients at greater risk by increasing brain tension and congestion had been eliminated. In fact, as discussed in the present book, barbiturates may have broader applications in neuroresuscitation. The intracranial pressure–reducing actions of barbiturates have received application in neurologic intensive care of head-injured and encephalitic patients. In stroke models, barbiturates reduce the area of infarction for unknown reasons, and they may soon be applied in patients. It is possible that they may be useful in reducing brain damage caused by circulatory arrest. The use of barbiturates first in the operating room and then in the intensive care unit represents the coming of a mature status of neuroanesthesia. A measure of this maturity is the subspecialty's transference of expertise and knowledge into other areas of medicine.

Although increased intracranial pressure and brain compression had long been recognized by neurosurgeons, it was not until the 1960's that their relationship to neurologic dysfunction and death was understood. Prior to that time our understanding of intracranial pressure dynamics was based on modifications of the Morris-Kellie doctrine by Burrows and Weed. Langfitt summarizes this by stating that "the craniospinal intradural space is nearly constant in volume and that its contents are nearly incompressible."[13] Further modifications in understanding intracranial volume pressure relationships emerged from Langfitt's laboratory. His experimental team established the concept of intracranial compliance to explain ICP changes during expansion of an intracranial mass. Langfitt also defined a state of cerebral "vasomotor paralysis" wherein cerebral blood flow regulation is disturbed by intracranial hypertension. Taken together, reduced intracranial compliance and dysfunctional cerebral blood flow regulation provide a basis for understanding the large spontaneous ICP increases (plateau waves) that may be accompanied by neurologic deterioration as described by Lundberg. Later work by Risberg and Lundbery showed that cerebral blood volume increases were associated with the plateau waves.[14]

With the foregoing fund of knowledge at hand the neuroanesthesiologist selects from drugs and techniques that will provide an optimal environment for the brain. Aside from anesthetic choice and controlled ventilation, these selections may include elective hypotension, hypothermia steroids, osmotic and tubular diuretics. None of these methods is foreign to the general practice of anesthesia. What classifies these techniques as neuroanesthetic methods is the rationale and timing of their administration in the neurosurgical patient.

Harvey M. Shapiro, M.D.

*Assistant Professor of
Anesthesiology and Neurosurgery,
University of California, San Diego,
La Jolla, California*

REFERENCES

1. Wilkins, R. H., editor: Neurosurgical classics, New York, 1965, Johnson Reprint Corp., p. 15.
2. Schapira, M.: Evolution of anesthesia for neurosurgery, N.Y. State J. Med. **64**:1301, 1964.
3. Lundy, J. S.: Clinical anesthesia, Philadelphia, 1942, W. B. Saunders Co., p. 3.
4. Adams, R. W., Gronert, G. A., Sundt, T. M., and others: Halothane, hypocapnia and cerebrospinal fluid pressure in neurosurgery, Anesthesiology **37**:510, 1972.
5. Kety, S. S., and Schmidt, C. F.: The determination of cerebral blood flow in man by the use of nitrous oxide in low concentrations, Am. J. Physiol. **143**:53, 1945.
6. Lundberg, N.: Continuous recording and control of ventricular fluid pressure in neurosurgical practice, Acta Psychiatr. Neurol. Scand. **36**(Suppl. 149):1, 1960.
7. Marx, G. F., Andrews, I. C., and Orkin, L. R.: Cerebrospinal fluid pressures during halothane anesthesia, Can. Anaesth. Soc. J. **9**:239, 1962.
8. Wollman, H., Alexander, S. C., Cohen, P. J., and others: Cerebral circulation of man during halothane anesthesia, Anesthesiology **25**:180, 1964.
9. McDowall, D. G.: The effects of clinical concentrations of halothane on the blood flow and oxygen uptake of the cerebral cortex, Br. J. Anaesth. **39**:186, 1967.
10. Jennett, W. B., and McDowall, D. G.: Effect of anaesthesia on intracranial pressure, J. Neurol. Neurosurg. Psychiatry **27**:582, 1964.
11. Hunter, A. R.: Thiopentone supplemented anaesthesia for neurosurgery, Br. J. Anaesth. **44**:506, 1972.
12. Shapiro, H. M., Galindo, A., Wyte, S. R., and others: Rapid intraoperative reduction of intracranial pressure with thiopentone, Br. J. Anaesth. **45**:1057, 1974.
13. Langfitt, T. W.: Increased intracranial pressure, Clin. Neurosurg. **16**:436, 1968.
14. Risberg, J., Lundberg, N., and Ingvar, D. H.: Regional cerebral blood volumes during acute transient rises of the intracranial pressure (plateau waves), J. Neurosurg. **31**:303, 1967.

Preface

During the early days of my anesthesia career I was frequently challenged to manage patients with surgically amenable neurologic disease processes. Later my attention was focused on their intensive care management as well. Because of my concern and interest in this topic and after frequent visits to the library, I became frustrated to learn that there was no good reference source for theoretical and clinical management of these patients.

After residency training while practicing at New York University, I began to consider writing or editing a textbook that would incorporate an organized basic science curriculum with the clinical practice of neuroanesthesia. My interest in neurology allied me with Joe Ransohoff's dynamic team. His enthusiasm for the "best" neurosurgery continued my thoughts in this direction.

This book was further stimulated by my activities in the Society of Neurosurgical Anesthesia and Neurologic Supportive Care (SNANSC) and by my association with its founding members—Jack Michenfelder, Harvey Shapiro, Maurice Albin, Jim Harp, and Brian Marshall.

I believe that my earlier desire to combine an organized clinical approach with basic scientific knowledge has been accomplished in *Anesthesia and Neurosurgery*. The opening chapters review the physiology of cerebral and spinal cord blood flow, brain oxygen consumption, and cerebrospinal fluid dynamics. The text then proceeds with a review of the mechanics and mathematics of intracranial pressure (ICP) monitoring, followed by clinical aspects of ICP control. A description of neuroradiologic diagnostic tools that essentially involve positioning leads the way to a discussion of the anesthetic agents and techniques applied during these procedures. The anesthetic management of supratentorial tumors has been separated from that of posterior fossa procedures because of the special monitoring problems of the latter. The management of severe head injury, its resultant peripheral sequelae, barbiturate protection of the ischemic brain, and neurointensive care are covered in depth. Altered consciousness and coma states are reviewed before brain death criteria are presented. Mechanisms of injury and treatment of acute spinal cord trauma by mechanical, pharmacologic, surgical, and anesthetic techniques are brilliantly discussed. Neurophysiologic brain monitoring using evoked potentials should stimulate wider clinical application to patient management. Physiologic and pharmacologic aspects of induced hypotension are discussed with emphasis on the patient with intracranial mass lesions.

The authors of this text are physicians of considerable expertise and dedication who have contributed their many years of experience toward making *Anesthesia and Neurosurgery* a valuable reference source for clinicians who actively manage patients with neurologic disease. Teachers should benefit from this text because of its completeness. Most of all, it is hoped that patients will directly benefit from the improved clinical care that this text promotes.

I am indebted and grateful to Herman Turndorf, M.D., for allowing me to pursue my interests while a member of his department at New York University and for his guidance as coeditor.

James E. Cottrell

xii

Contents

xiii

1

Cerebral and spinal cord blood flow

NIELS A. LASSEN

Knowledge of cerebral blood flow (CBF) is essential for the proper treatment of patients with major intracranial disease and for neuroanesthesia in particular. Before going into details regarding CBF and its regulation, it may be useful to stress some general relations: *cerebral vasodilators tend to increase intracranial blood volume and hence to raise intracranial pressure (ICP)*. These effects are much enhanced in patients with a space-occupying intracranial mass in whom the induced ICP increase may result in generalized cerebral ischemia. Even more important is, perhaps, that the increase in blood volume may aggravate mass displacement and cause localized compression and ischemia.

Spinal cord blood flow (SCBF) will also be discussed. As might be expected, SCBF is basically similar in all aspects to CBF. It would therefore appear reasonable to also apply the therapeutic principles proposed for brain-injured patients to patients with spinal cord lesions. This is attempted in the section on clinical inferences concluding this chapter.

MEASUREMENT OF BLOOD FLOW

Freely diffusible indicators, mainly inert gases and nondiffusible indicators in the form of labeled microspheres, constitute the two main approaches to measuring blood flow. In both cases the indicator reaches the tissue via the arterial blood, and in both cases it is assumed that there is complete mixing of indicator and blood. This is called equivalent entry of indicator and blood or the bolus fractionation principle. It is by virtue of this equivalence that one can, by observing the indicator, calculate blood flow.

Inert gas inhalation method

The Kety-Schmidt method is based on measuring the mean transit time ($\bar{t}$) for tracer molecules traversing the brain. The technique requires 10 to 15 minutes of inhalation of an inert gas suitable for analysis in the series of arterial and cerebral venous blood samples that are collected over 10 to 15 minutes. Gases used are nitrous oxide (N_2O), argon (Ar), [85]Kr, and ^{133}Xe, the latter two being radioactive.[79,144,131,162] The method yields a value for the average CBF/100 g of tissue and per minute. This flow is obtained without it being necessary—indeed without it being possible—first to measure total brain flow and total brain weight.

Applied to humans the Kety-Schmidt method is practically atraumatic in that the internal jugular vein can be either punctured directly on the neck or be catheterized from the cubital or femoral vein. This method, which has the advantage of allowing simultaneous measurement of the cerebral meta-

1

bolic rate of oxygen and glucose, has been widely applied to the study of anesthetic drugs in humans. It can also be applied to animals, in which cerebral venous blood is usually sampled from the superior sagittal sinus exposed by a small craniotomy. With ^{133}Xe as indicator and using 50 μl blood samples the method can be used in rats,[28] but the method cannot readily be used for measuring spinal cord flow because of the difficulty of obtaining representative venous blood samples.

Inert gas injection method

The inert gas injection method was developed by Lassen and Ingvar[77] for obtaining regional flow values. It is also based on measuring the mean transit time ($\bar{t}$) of the tracer molecules. The commercially available ^{133}Xe now is most widely used, since it allows external recording of the tracer over the head and has a suitably long half-life of 5.5 days.[54,78,97] The radioactive gas is dissolved in physiologic saline injected as a bolus via the internal or vertebral artery. The washout is usually followed over 10 to 15 minutes. But it is the initial, steepest part of the curves that contains the most valuable information, because the initial slope is dominated by the washout from the fastest flow component: the cerebral cortex. Despite the technical differences, the method may be considered merely as a modification of the Kety-Schmidt technique. The two methods also have practically the same normal values for CBF of about 50 ml/100 g/min.

Applied to humans, the intra-arterial [133]xenon method is usually performed in patients in whom cerebral angiography is indicated. Thus the risk of the arterial puncture is eliminated, and the injection itself, of sterile saline with its physically dissolved small amount of inert gas, can be considered quite innocuous provided care is taken to avoid injecting gas bubbles or small clots. We use a thin and soft heparinized catheter, frequent rinsing with dilute heparin-saline, and tight stopcocks (to avoid reflux of blood at the catheter tip). With this approach no complications have occurred in our current series of 320 cases studied over 5 years (see also reference 55). The number of detectors has been gradually increased. The most recently developed instrument has 254 individual crystals and photomultipliers,[135] an approach that allows a much higher total counting rate to be recorded than with the conventional single-crystal Anger gamma camera.[48]

In animal studies, common carotid artery ^{133}Xe injection via the lingual artery is often employed. In this case it is necessary to surgically remove the soft tissues over the calvaria as well as very narrow collimation of the detector to avoid contamination by ^{133}Xe reaching extracerebral tissues.[46] The risk of incurring traumatic spasms of the arteries to the brain should be remembered[47] and it is therefore best, if possible, to avoid more extensive surgical exposure of the vessels on the neck. The method has recently been adapted for the study of CBF in rats.[50] In such small animals one cannot gainfully employ multiple probes, and the flow value obtained is therefore to be considered an average value that multiplied by the simultaneously measured cerebral arteriovenous oxygen difference also yields a value for the oxygen uptake—just as in the Kety-Schmidt method. In comparing the two methods as adapted to rat studies, the greater ease with which multiple studies are made by the ^{133}Xe injection method and its higher time resolution (the initial slope can be adequately defined in just 15 seconds or even less) may be mentioned.

Spinal cord blood flow cannot be measured with ^{133}Xe and external recording because it is not possible to secure selective labeling and/or selective recording of the cord.

Hydrogen clearance

Tissue can be labeled by injection via an artery or by just inhaling hydrogen gas at low concentration. The tissue concentration is monitored by tiny polarographic platinum wire electrodes such as those for oxygen tension measurements.[104] This method can be used both in brain and spinal cord tissue.

The blood flow is calculated from the initial slope. The hydrogen clearance must be characterized as an invasive technique because it demands exposure and insertion of the electrode. But the trauma to the tissue is seemingly not a major problem, since the results agree quite well with those found by other methods.

Microspheres and autoradiography of diffusible tracers

Of the many other methods available only a few have gained wider application than those using labeled microspheres[4,84,103] and autoradiographic analysis of tissue distribution of diffusible tracers.[112] The trauma resulting from these methods (tissue sampling) limits their use to animal studies. Their advantage lies in yielding simultaneous flow measurements in many small anatomically well-defined tissue elements: this permits mapping the blood flow distribution in the entire central nervous system.

METABOLIC REGULATION OF CEREBRAL BLOOD FLOW

The normal brain has a high and rather stable overall (global) metabolic rate of oxygen both in sleep and resting wakefulness, as well as in various types of brain work and also has a relatively high and stable overall CBF.[72] This picture of constancy of energy production and delivery to the brain is, however, somewhat misleading, because at a *regional* level such physiologic variations in brain activity produce the same pattern as found in other organs: more work results in a higher level of oxidative metabolism and higher blood flow. To give an example, during voluntary movements of the hand, both CBF and oxygen uptake increase within seconds by about 30% in the contralateral primary (rolandic) hand area.[94,109] Many other regional patterns of CBF increase have been defined. Reading a text aloud, to take another example, activates at least 14 discrete cortical areas—7 in each hemisphere.[71] It would appear that the observed stability of the overall values mainly reflects the smallness of the cortical areas engaged in the types of brain work studied.

These findings have established the general pattern of metabolic regulation of CBF. It means that when a given cortical region is active in a given task, more ions are pumped across membranes and more transmitter substance extruded, uptaken again, or resynthesized. In disease states such as epileptic seizure or coma of various types this regulation is well known: high metabolism and flow in epilepsy, low values in coma (Fig. 1-1). Because the changes in metabolism are met by parallel changes in flow, the jugular venous oxygen tension and that of the tissue are expected to remain fairly constant. This is indeed the case. If anything, increased activity in a tissue area tends to increase both Po_2 values slightly.

Since the Po_2 values normally are stable or even increase during brain tissue activity, it is unlikely that oxygen lack constitutes the feedback message that adjusts flow to match metabolism. What is it, then, that couples flow to metabolism? This fundamental question cannot be answered. At present two main possibilities are being considered, namely H^+ and K^+ concentration changes (increases) in the extracellular fluid surrounding the brain arterioles. Ca^{++} concentration variations (decreases) may also play a role.

Barbiturates and Althesin

A depression in cortical functional activity and an associated reduction in metabolism and flow to about 60% of the normal value is seen during barbiturate intoxication. This is conventionally taken to exemplify the metabolic regulation of CBF. Why flow decreases in this case is perhaps even more mysterious than why it increases during activation, because no strong vasoconstrictor stimulus is known to accumulate in the brain during barbiturate intoxication. Several other drugs show the same pattern. A striking example is that of althesin, a steroid with anesthetic properties that has been studied by McDowall and co-workers.[81] They found that the cerebrovascular resistance increased less than four seconds after the electroencephalogram started to show changes. Thus the coupling of metabolism and flow is tight even in the time domain, and yet we have no solid information as to its mechanism.

Pain and anxiety

In normal humans painful stimuli cause a large rise in oxygen uptake and in CBF.[57] Anxiety may elicit the same type of response.[61] Both produce arousal responses that probably involve intracerebral noradrenergic fiber tracts arising from the brain stem. The phenomenon has also been observed in patients with severe brain injuries.[56]

As already stated, cerebral vasodilatation increases cerebral blood volume and ICP. In critical cases this may precipitate incarceration at the tentorium. Hence it follows that noxious stimuli should be avoided in patients with space-occupying lesions even if they are semicomatose. With fully controlled mechanical ventilation in neurologic intensive care, the liberal use of analgesics to avoid pain, even in apparently nonresponding patients, has become a widely accepted practice. Conversely, it would seem contraindicated to try to assess the coma level in patients with a large intracranial mass by using a strongly painful stimulus. In the spontaneously respiring patient the associated tendency to acute hyperventilation may largely offset the noxious effect. But the procedure is, nevertheless, not recommended. Such painful stimulation tends to increase CBF, ICP, and to aggravate brain stem in-

carceration as detected clinically in the form of an attack of decerebrate rigidity.

AUTOREGULATION OF CEREBRAL BLOOD FLOW

At a given stable level of brain function, as in the resting awake state in normal humans and in maintained normocapnia, CBF does not vary much. In particular, CBF remains practically constant even if the cerebral perfusion pressure is varied over quite a wide range (Fig. 1-1). This so-called autoregulation of CBF is usually tested by varying the arterial blood pressure. It has the nature of an active vascular response in that arteriolar constriction results when the distending pressure is increased and dilatation results when it is decreased.

Autoregulation of blood flow occurs in many other tissues, which suggests a common mechanism. The perivascular sympathetic nerves on the brain arteries are not necessary for the response,[27,110,145] yet their activation modifies the autoregulation curve in that a shift toward higher pressure levels occurs (see discussion of neurogenic control on p. 9). Because the metabolic pattern is different in the different tissues, it appears most likely that the autoregulation results from a myogenic response of the smooth muscle cells of the arteriolar wall, which constricts when the stretch force is increased. The autoregulation of CBF is easily abolished

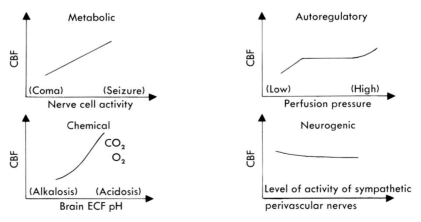

Fig. 1-1. Control of CBF.

by trauma or other noxious stimuli, in particular following hypoxia. Apparently, the vasodilatation chemically induced by lactic acid and other factors can readily overrule the autoregulatory vasoconstrictor response to a pressure increase.

Autoregulation can be tested by using angiotensin to increase blood pressure and trimethaphan camphorsulfonate (Arfonad) to decrease it. There is evidence that these two drugs do not have direct effects on the cerebral vessels, presumably because they do not readily cross the vascular endothelium of the brain vessels—the blood-brain barrier. Thus the drugs only influence the tone of the cerebral resistance vessels through their effect on systemic arterial pressure. In most patients, ICP and cerebral venous pressure are low and practically uninfluenced by the induced blood pressure variations. Hence the systemic blood pressure equals almost the cerebral perfusion pressure (in the recumbent position). However, in patients with increased ICP, variations in this parameter must be taken into account.

Autoregulation of CBF explains the constancy of CBF normally found with moderate elevations of ICP. As with arterial hypotension this decreases the transmural distending pressure and results in a cerebral vasodilatation so that CBF remains constant.[53,136]

Autoregulation has a lower limit—in normotensives a mean arterial blood pressure (MABP) of about 60 mm Hg (Fig. 1-1). Below this limit, CBF decreases, and the cerebral arteriovenous oxygen difference increases. At an even lower MABP (in normotensives about 40 mm Hg) symptoms of cerebral ischemia in the form of mild hyperventilation, dizziness, "slow cerebration" (and eventually syncope) appear. Autoregulation has also an upper limit—in normotensives a MABP of about 130 mm Hg. Above this limit the pressure breaks through the constrictor response. The forced dilatation of the brain arterioles usually occurs at many discrete sites (multifocally). It is associated with a disruption of the blood-brain barrier and is presumably related to stimulation of the micropinocytotic vesicles and with edema. It has

repeatedly been found that vasodilator stimuli (such as tissue acidosis or papaverine) enhance the barrier damage and edema formation caused by severe induced hypertension. Many patients with acute brain injuries have brain tissue regions with vasodilatation and high CBF (luxury perfusion). Such patients *cannot tolerate even moderate hypertension*, as is evident from the previous discussion and from much clinical and experimental evidence.

In chronic arterial hypertension, the autoregulatory curve is displaced to the right, the cerebral vessels having adapted to the higher pressure level by hypertrophy of the vessel wall. Thus chronic hypertensives tolerate a high arterial blood pressure much better than do normotensives (the breakthrough point or upper limit of autoregulation is increased). However, it should be noted that the adaptation of the vessels takes some time (probably one to two months). It is well known that in subacute hypertension, as seen in children with glomerulonephritis or in hypertensive toxemia of pregnancy, arterial pressure values that do not cause symptoms in elderly hypertensives are not tolerated. In such subacute cases with encephalopathic symptoms one must strive to completely normalize the blood pressure.

Of even greater clinical significance is the displacement to the right of the lower limit of autoregulation of CBF and of the ischemic threshold as well. Chronic hypertensives do not tolerate an acute pressure reduction to the same low levels as do normotensives. This is well known. But because it is difficult to know the habitual systemic blood pressure of a given patient, it is difficult to properly classify patients in everyday clinical practice. It can be added that following a gradual pressure reduction in a chronic hypertensive, the brain's tolerance to hypotension may improve—the autoregulation curve may in some cases shift back toward its normotensive position.[132, 133]

Induced hypotension

This procedure is widely used in special neuroanesthetic situations, especially during aneurysm surgery. If the skull is open, the intracranial pressure is zero, which may partially explain the observed tolerance to very low mean arterial pressures, which go as low as the ischemic pressure threshold of about 40 mm Hg. I do not intend to review the subject but merely to stress that chronic hypertensive patients cannot tolerate pressures as low as normotensives. It should also be noted that in patients in whom the disease or the surgical intervention has impaired tissue circulation (due to tissue compression or clipping of an artery), hypotension is the most effective means of severely compromising tissue perfusion!

During temporary clamping of the internal carotid artery, which is necessary in order to perform endarterectomy at the carotid bifurcation, a special form of regional induced arterial hypotension is produced by the vascular surgeon as the distal arterial "stump" pressure decreases. It has been claimed that during this procedure a stump pressure of 50 mm Hg suffices to assure that the ipsilateral hemisphere is adequately perfused. But according to the above-mentioned facts, hypertensives need a higher pressure than normotensives, a finding that agrees with the clinical experience of Sundt and co-workers[134] in a large number of patients undergoing endarterectomy in whom the adequacy of hemispheric perfusion was measured directly using the intra-arterial [133]xenon injection method. It would appear more reasonable, therefore, to rely on EEG and on [133]xenon washout to monitor the adequacy of cerebral perfusion during carotid surgery and thus to determine in which cases a temporary bypass shunt must be employed.

Hypovolemic hypotension

Hemorrhagic shock differs from drug-induced hypotension in that the reduced blood volume causes a marked increase in the activity in the sympathetic nervous system, including the sympathetic vasoconstrictor fibers going to the brain. The resultant increase in cerebrovascular tone means a displacement of the autoregulatory curve to the right, that is, the lower limit of CBF autoregulation as well as the lowest tolerated ischemia-producing pressure level are both *increased* (see the discussion of neurogenic control of CBF, p. 9). Therefore, in hemorrhagic hypotension, signs of brain ischemia develop at a higher pressure level than during induced hypotension. This is a well-known clinical fact that may be explained as just outlined *and* by the fact that if anxiety supervenes, the metabolic demand and hence the lowest level of adequate blood supply are augmented. The value of strong analgesics or of alpha blocking drugs in curtailing both sympathetic discharge and relieving anxiety in such cases should be borne in mind. This may explain why such drugs may be of considerable symptomatic value in hemorrhagic shock even if the arterial blood pressure remains at the same low level.[130]

Ischemia

Brain tissue ischemia is meant to indicate a blood flow *so low that it compromises tissue oxygenation*. With this definition the very low CBF during severe barbiturate intoxication combined with hypothermia is not classified as ischemia because the low flow suffices to sustain the very low metabolic rate.

In the section on induced hypotension, signs of ischemia of the whole brain were listed; they probably can be attributed mainly to brain stem ischemia and appear at an average CBF of approximately 30 ml/100 g/min. But since this flow value refers mainly to the flow in the hemispheres—the bulk of the brain—it is not justified to take this value to indicate the critical flow of the most sensitive structure, which is presumably the brain stem.

On the regional level it is, however, possible quite accurately to define critical thresholds of flow: in normothermic, lightly anesthetized humans, the EEG over a hemisphere (studied during temporary carotic clamping for endarterectomy) starts to diminish in amplitude when CBF drops below 20 ml/100 g/min.[134,141] This threshold agrees remarkably well with that of the 18 to

20 ml/100 g/min obtained by Branston and coworkers in baboons lightly anesthetized with chloralose.[14] Using hydrogen electrodes implanted into the cortex these authors found that below this threshold—the flow reduction being induced by clamping the middle cerebral artery transorbitally—the evoked cortical response as well as the spontaneous electrical activity started to diminish. Thus, both clinical and experimental studies concur and show that the *ischemic threshold of beginning cortical failure* lies at about 20 ml/100 g/min.

In baboon studies a lower CBF level of about 15 ml/100 g/min was observed, below which both spontaneous and evoked electrical activity fail in the cortex.[14] Below this *ischemic threshold of electrical silence* is a further ischemic threshold of metabolic failure at about 8 to 10 ml/100 g/min, below which massive release of K^+ occurs from the intracellular compartment.[6] A marked decrease in tissue ATP occurs at about the same low threshold. It is as yet not quite clear if a sustained flow in the interval 10 to 15 would suffice to supply enough energy to keep the Na^+-K^+ pumps from failing due to ATP lack. (Recent results from Morawetz and co-workers[89] suggest that two to three hours of ischemia below a CBF threshold of 12 ml leads to cell death.)

If the above-mentioned relations are confirmed by more data, it would appear that for prolonged ischemia there exists a *penumbral CBF zone* between 15 and 20 ml/100 g/min—perhaps even between 10 and 20 ml/100 g/min—in which tissue oxygenation is inadequate to sustain normal neuronal function but yet is sufficient for the cells to survive. It is not yet known how often such a penumbral—"between life and death"—state arises with a reversible ischemic paralysis of the nerve cells. That the state does exist is, however, suggested by the numerous cases of completely reversible focal ischemic attacks, which may last hours and produce hemiparesis and/or aphasia.

Arterial occlusion and tissue compression by a space-occupying lesion or by a surgeon's spatula appear to be the two most frequent states in which cerebral ischemia can be expected. If it is penumbral, then therapeutic measures may determine if symptom remission or cell death will occur. In an acute vascular occlusion an *elevation* of the systemic blood pressure enhances collateral flow; in increased ICP situations this pressure must be lowered. If we could accurately measure in the clinical setting the reduced regional flows before and after attempted therapy, then rational institution of therapy would be vastly facilitated. The positron-emission CT scanners currently being developed may make possible precisely such measurements.

In mentioning ischemia due to tissue compression it should be stressed that because the brain is a *semisolid* object, the strain and stresses that locally increase tissue pressure beyond the blood pressure can readily occur when quite small overall pressures are applied. To gently and lightly compress the brain with retractors is perhaps the single most significant technical advance made over the last some 20 years by the joint efforts of neurosurgeons and neuroanesthetists.

CHEMICAL CONTROL OF CEREBRAL BLOOD FLOW: EFFECTS OF CO_2 AND O_2

Variations in arterial P_{CO_2} exert a profound influence on CBF (Fig. 1-1). Hypercapnia causes intense cerebral vasodilatation, and hypocapnia causes a vasoconstriction so intense that the limit of brain hypoxia is reached. Around the normal arterial P_{CO_2}, CBF changes about 4% for each millimeter of mercury change in arterial P_{CO_2}. Since the reproducibility of the intra-arterial ^{133}Xe method for measuring CBF is about the same, the effects of 1 mm Hg variations in arterial P_{CO_2} can, practically, be measured. Very accurate arterial P_{CO_2} determinations are consequently indispensable for evaluating CBF data.

In humans one can readily vary P_{CO_2} between, say, 30 to 45 mm Hg without measurably changing the steady state with regard to overall cerebral function and oxygen uptake. In this range the effect of CO_2 is presumably solely a function of the local chemical milieu. In very lightly anesthetized animals larger increases in P_{CO_2} may cause arousal (awakening, probably combined with pain and/or anxiety and fear). This mechanism, which seems to involve noradrenergic neurones arising from the brain stem, may increase the oxygen uptake of the entire brain.[18] In such animals the CO_2 effect on CBF is much enhanced. This brain stem mechanism is, however, most likely to be of secondary nature due to the brain stem's role in the CO_2-induced activation of neuronal function and metabolism in the hemispheres. (In my opinion, no completely convincing evidence has yet been put forward to prove the existence of a primary "brain stem center for the regulation of CBF" [see reference 7].) Space does not allow this topic to be further discussed, but it should be recalled that both the functionally isolated middle cerebral artery territory and the completely isolated spinal cord show a preserved CO_2 responsiveness.[63,124]

The carbon dioxide reactivity is mediated by pH variations in the cerebrospinal fluid around and inside the wall of the arterioles.[29,39,75] The pH at this site depends on the tension of the freely diffusible CO_2 gas *and* on the local cerebrospinal fluid and bicarbonate concentration, bicarbonate being practically unable to cross the vascular endothelium (the blood-brain barrier). This dual nature of the chemical control, by arterial P_{CO_2} and by local CSF bicarbonate, is of importance for understanding the vasoparalysis seen in both severe hypercapnia and in deeper levels of halothane anesthesia.[90] It is unclear precisely how the pH variations influence the tone of the smooth muscle cells in the arteriolar wall. It appears most likely that it is the pH *inside* those cells that matters and that the effect involves changes in the concentration of ionized calcium.

The arterial P_{CO_2}-induced changes in CBF appear to subserve the pH regulation of the brain. With an increase in arterial P_{CO_2}, flow increases, which allows a more efficient washout of the metabolically produced CO_2. As a consequence, the change in tissue P_{CO_2} and therefore also in tissue pH is dampened.

The converse holds true for a decrease in arterial P_{CO_2}. Of even greater importance for the homeostasis of tissue P_{CO_2} and pH are the changes in pulmonary ventilation caused by the CO_2-induced pH changes in the CSF at the brain stem, where the central chemoreceptors are located. Due to the changes in both CBF and pulmonary ventilation, both of which are coupled to and monitor local CSF pH, this value is kept rather constant; this combined system will normally dampen approximately 95% of the brain tissue pH change, which a step increase in inspired P_{CO_2} would otherwise have produced. Adding to this the buffering capacity of the brain *and* the metabolically induced bicarbonate changes in brain tissue, it must be concluded that brain tissue pH is safeguarded in a truly remarkable way against acute respiratory acidosis and alkalosis.

The compensation for chronic changes in arterial P_{CO_2} involves alterations in CSF bicarbonate that practically normalize CSF pH. In this case CBF is also practically normal, since the CSF pH adaptation parallels (and causes) CBF adaptation.[31,103,119] These adaptive changes (in contrast to those mentioned in the previous section) take 24 to 36 hours to develop fully.[19] As a clinical implication of the slowness of these adaptive CSF bicarbonate changes it follows that a chronically elevated arterial P_{CO_2} should usually *not be acutely normalized*. If this is nevertheless done, the patient will for some hours suffer clinical signs as in acute hypocapnia, including dizziness and somnolence with subnormal CBF. This situation can be avoided by normalizing arterial P_{CO_2} gradually over one to two days.

Oxygen

Moderate changes in oxygen tension around the normal level (100 mm Hg or so) do not measurably influence CBF. Thus, in moderate arterial hypoxia and hyperoxia, the unchanged CBF and oxygen uptake means that tissue and cerebral venous P_{O_2} tend to vary with (but much less than) the arterial P_{O_2}. This means that tissue P_{O_2} cannot be considered a controlled factor in the same strict sense as tissue pH. Or, in other words, at normal arterial gas tension levels pH control overrides—is more sensitive than —PO_2 control. With a more marked degree of arterial hypoxia, CBF increases. This increase appears to be a threshold phenomenon, since a measurable flow increase is not seen until arterial PO_2 decreases below about 50 mm Hg[69,81]—at a level below which hypoxia causes progressive brain tissue lactic acidosis.[121] This topic is not clarified yet because moderate hypoxia tends to cause alkalotic shifts around pial arterioles. Yet before accurate pH measurements have been made inside the brain tissue (where the main resistance vessels are located), one cannot exclude an acid shift here. If found, chemical control by high CO_2 and low O_2 is basically the same (at very low PO_2 values other chemical factors probably also play a role).

Variations in the oxygen-carrying capacity of the blood as seen in anemia and polycythemia cause compensatory flow changes that keep cerebral venous gas tensions normal. Therefore, no stimulus for chemical control is detectable. The percentage changes in blood viscosity assessed in vivo are approximately equal to those in CBF.[8,80,114] Therefore, changes in diameter of the arterioles may not take place. If this is so, then the flow changes are not caused by any alteration in cerebrovascular control but merely by the viscosity changes. This fact does not mean that viscosity is a limiting factor, for even in the case of polycythemia, carbon dioxide inhalation produces a sharp increase of CBF, and in anemia, hyperventilation decreases CBF.

CO_2 and O_2 in neuroanesthesia

Only a few comments on this topic need be made. The importance of avoiding hypercapnia as well as anoxia or anoxia combined with hypercapnia (asphyxia) is obvious. They constitute vasodilator stimuli, which in patients with space-occupying intracranial lesions may fatally increase ICP and increase mass displacement. A specific example of utmost clinical importance is that of the patient with a head injury in whom adequate ventilation must be assured from the earliest stage.

Moderate hypocapnia

The value of inducing cerebral vasoconstriction by hyperventilation during a neurosurgical procedure is well established. Long-term treatment (days or even weeks) with controlled ventilation is used in several clinics. This usually implies a state of moderate hypocapnia but, as a result of the *adaptation* (normalization) of CSF pH and consequently of CBF at the lower PCO_2 value, this procedure cannot be expected to yield prolonged vasoconstriction. It is likely therefore, as stated by Rossanda and colleagues,[115] that the main beneficial effect of this type of intensive care is the result of avoidance of any episodes of anoxia or asphyxia and the ability to safely use effective doses of analgesic and sedative drugs.

Severe hypocapnia

There is evidence that at an arterial PCO_2 below 20 mm Hg, CBF is so low that the ischemic threshold for sustaining normal neuronal function (20 ml/100 g/min) is practically reached. This has aroused an intense discussion of whether the beneficial effect of hyperventilation (lower CSF pressure) is not offset by the noxious effect of tissue hypoxia. This topic has been reviewed by Harp and Wollman,[45] who concluded that the evidence for such a noxious effect with even marked hypocapnia (decreased to 10 mm Hg) was not at hand. Nevertheless, because of the scarcity of clinical observations in various age groups, especially in patients with intracranial disease, they recommended that for prolonged treatment the arterial PCO_2 should perhaps not be set at less than 25 mm Hg. This must be considered a conservative attitude, but it is reasonable, since at present there are no known therapeutic gains at excessively low PCO_2 values.

NEUROGENIC CONTROL OF CEREBRAL BLOOD FLOW

The arteries on the brain surface and even the larger arterioles inside the brain tissue are supplied by a network of sympathetic and parasympathetic nerve fibers that run in the same nerve strands.[91] The sympathetic fibers stem from the superior cervical ganglion and the parasympathetic from the facial nerve.

The pial arteries respond to topical (local) application of norepinephrine and acetylcholine with constriction and dilatation, respectively.[70,143] The responses are blocked by the corresponding specific antagonists, but these antagonists themselves do not influence the vessel diameter when they are applied in the same low concentrations that counteract the agonists. Thus, under the conditions studied, *no evidence of a tonic autonomic control over pial arterial tone has been adduced.*

A truly colossal experimental effort from numerous laboratories has been made to elucidate the physiologic role of the perivascular nerves. Without even attempting to review this literature and the presumed reasons for the often conflicting results, it shall be stated *that maximal stimulation of the sympathetic nerves reduces CBF by 5% to 10%*[4,66,84] *and that a similarly moderate vasodilator response to parasympathetic stimulation has also been shown.*[116]

This shows that the blood flow changes in response to sustained maximal neurogenic stimulation are quite small (Fig. 1-1). They correspond to the effect of changes in arterial P_{CO_2} of 1 to 2 mm Hg and cannot, thus, be of any great importance for regulating CBF. What then can be the functional role of the nervous control of blood flow to the brain, which certainly is much less intense than in other organs? Since the nerves supply mainly the somewhat larger arteries and arterioles, it has been suggested that the nerves may be of importance in regulating cerebral vascular volume and hence, indirectly, intracranial pressure, as suggested independently by Edvinsson and colleagues[26] and by Deshmukh and colleagues.[25]

Resetting of the autoregulatory curve to the right by sympathetic stimulation

Recent studies, in part published only in preliminary fashion, elucidate the role of the sympathetic innervation of the brain arteries in a little more detail. Fitch, MacKenzie, and Harper[33] found that during sympathetic stimulation the lower part of the autoregula-

tion curve was altered and that, at any given arterial pressure, CBF was less during hemorrhagic hypotension than during pharmacologically produced hypotension, an effect that was traced to the increased sympathetic nervous activity during hemorrhagic shock. This shows that the autoregulatory response to bleeding is less "perfect" than the response to similar reductions of the perfusion pressure following drugs or an increased ICP. The sympathetic nerves thus counteract the autoregulatory CBF response to a decrease of arterial pressure. Precisely the same is well known from kidney physiology, where autoregulation cannot be seen at all if hypotension is produced by bleeding. This phenomenon, that drug-induced hypotension is better "tolerated" than hemorrhagic shock, is, moreover, well known clinically, and it has been referred to already in the discussion of the clinical corollaries of autoregulation.

What about the upper end of the autoregulatory curve? Even this curve segment appears to be displaced to the right by sympathetic stimulation.[11] This means that acute hypertension is better tolerated if the sympathetic nerves are stimulated simultaneously: the upper limit of the autoregulatory plateau—the breakthrough point—is displaced to the right just as in chronic hypertension.

The fact that intense sympathetic stimulation is associated with spontaneous increases in systemic arterial pressure makes very good sense indeed. The sympathetic nerves, by enhancing arterial and arteriolar tone during states of arousal, effort, anger, and so forth, enable the brain to tolerate increased arterial pressure without initiating the noxious sequence of arterial overstretching, blood-brain barrier leakage, and fluid extravasation.[44]

Animal experiments have clearly shown that during cervical sympathetic stimulation, the initial response is a much more pronounced degree of CBF reduction than that seen when the stimulation is continued (an "escape" phenomenon). This is of particular importance because the autoregulatory vasoconstrictor response to a blood pressure rise takes several seconds to become effective.

The effect of the sympathetic nerves on brain vessels is to acutely enhance their tonus so that the response curve is reset, as in chronic hypertension, in accordance with the effect of the sympathetic nerves on the heart where also a resetting to a new functional level results from such stimulation.

CEREBRAL BLOOD FLOW IN SOME DISEASE STATES
Brain tissue acidosis (lactic acidosis)

Even a brief period of inadequate perfusion of brain tissue leads to an intense production of lactic acid. Brain lactic acidosis is a more common and more dangerous disorder than well-known systemic acidosis such as uremic acidosis, diabetic ketoacidosis, and systemic lactic acidosis.

Brain lactic acidosis is marked in patients resuscitated after cardiac arrest. It is present in areas of focal ischemia resulting from cerebrovascular disease and often develops in severe traumatic brain injury or in cases of brain tumor.[93] In the latter two tumor cases, the ischemia is presumably caused by severe, often transitory, increases in ICP. Perhaps even the concept of a local increase in brain tissue pressure can be invoked. For example, it would be reasonable to believe that the brain tissue around an acute hematoma is locally under an increased pressure that limits circulation.

With the conditions mentioned, brain hypoxia, ischemic infarction, trauma, tumor, hematoma (which could be called an "acute tumor"), the list is still not complete. Brain lactic acidosis is probably also present in severe cases of meningitis and subarachnoid bleeding, and it reaches extreme degrees in so-called brain death. It is on this basis that brain tissue lactic acidosis claims far more clinical importance than does classic systemic acidosis. Brain tissue acidosis is characterized by a state of cerebral vasomotor paralysis, particularly abolition of CBF autoregulation. This so-called luxury perfusion syndrome[73] is a pathophysiologic consequence of the chemical control: the local acidosis causes a dilatation of the brain arteries. The blood flow sometimes exceeds the normal flow but more often the hyperemia is only relative, that is, in excess of local metabolic demands. Paradoxical flow responses frequently occur as when strong vasodilator stimuli such as carbon dioxide or papaverine lead to a flow decrease (intracerebral steal) or vasoconstrictor stimuli such as hypocapnia or aminophylline cause a flow increase in acidotic brain tissue (inverse intracerebral steal). Variations in intracranial pressure appear to underlie many of these paradoxical reactions.

Brain edema is often associated with lactic acidosis. The edema is, in part at least, related to the vasomotor paralysis that tends to increase the capillary hydrostatic pressure. Blood-brain barrier damage is also commonly involved, as shown by the radioisotope scanning technique used clinically. The edema causes distortion of brain tissue and an increase in intracranial pressure; both these factors tend to induce further tissue hypoxia and hence further tissue lactic acidosis. A most dangerous vicious circle is thus operating.

It is therefore important to combat the acidosis by securing adequate oxygenation of the arterial blood and by reducing the arterial P_{CO_2}. Controlled, moderate hyperventilation by intubation and respirator assistance is now widely used in the intensive therapy of brain-injured patients, in particular patients with traumatic brain injury. Another therapeutic aim is to avoid cerebral vasodilator drugs. To give a specific example, drugs that depress respiration (morphine, meperidine, and so on) are most emphatically contraindicated in a brain-injured patient with spontaneous respiration. This contraindication also holds for volatile anesthetic agents such as halothane, which can induce a most dangerous triad of hypotension, hypercapnia, and cerebral vasodilatation beyond that caused by carbon dioxide. Administration of such drugs is only permissible when ventilation and arterial pressure are controlled.

Recognition of these facts is not based on

CBF measurements alone. Indeed, ICP measurements have been more important. Yet, it is the combined pressure and flow data that constitute the conceptual basis for the intensive care (including neuroanesthesia) of the brain-injured patient.

Cerebral blood flow in brain tumors

The general reaction of the cerebral circulation to a space-occupying lesion was given in the previous section. With regard to brain tumors it may be added that some tumors, in particular glioblastomas, are highly vascular and have a CBF characterized by fast, shunt-like pathways as well as slower flow components (heterogeneity is evidenced by a bending shape of the two-minute semilogarithmic ^{133}Xe wash-out curves). Other tumors have a lower flow than the intact brain. Yet, probably because of acidosis in peritumoral brain tissue, even such tumors (e.g., a meningioma or a metastasis) may yet show up as hyperemic.

The loss of autoregulation of CBF in the tumor-peritumor area has been mentioned repeatedly. More interesting is the fact that sometimes, usually with fairly large tumors, an elevation of the systemic blood pressure does not change but may even cause a *decrease* in the CBF over the tumor site.[101] This paradoxical finding contrasting with the lost autoregulation usually found has been termed "false autoregulation." It is also seen in severe traumatic brain injury (contusion). Most likely the elevation in blood pressure causes a local elevation in tissue pressure so that the local perfusion pressure is unchanged or even decreases.

In solitary brain tumors one often finds lost autoregulation in tissue regions that lie *remote* from the tumor.[30] This appears to correspond to zones of tissue compression due to mass displacement. It is typically found close to the tentorium, that is, in the posterior part of the temporal lobe. Probably these tissue areas have (intermittently?) been rendered ischemic by compression, and the findings may correspond to a clinical state of imminent tentorial herniation.

The therapeutic inferences of these various findings differ only on one significant point from those above outlined under the heading of brain tissue acidosis: in brain tumors the value of steroids is firmly established.

Cerebral blood flow in cerebrovascular disease and in senile dementia

In apoplexy (stroke), the patient acutely develops focal neurologic symptoms. Arterial pathology, either thromboembolic or hemorrhagic, is usually suspected. But surprisingly often (in about 50% of the ischemic cases in many investigations) the arteriographic study obtained by intra-arterial injection of x-ray contrast material is negative in that no relevant lesions can be seen.

CBF studies have contributed to what appears to be the solution of this riddle by demonstrating that even angiographically negative stroke cases often have widespread changes in flow: regions with low or high CBF occur, and vasomotor responses are abolished.[106] This finding supports the theory that lysis of a thromboembolic occlusion often takes place.

Two studies of experimental infarction produced by clipping the middle cerebral artery are of particular interest because the size of the infarct diminished markedly when the animals were hyperventilated[129] but increased when acetazolamide (Diamox) was given.[111] In the normal brain, hypocapnia resulting from hyperventilation reduces CBF, and carbonic anhydrase inhibition caused by acetazolamide increases CBF. In the vasoparalytic focal area, the flow changes go in the opposite direction (paradoxical reactions). Christensen, Paulson, and colleagues have recently tried to employ hyperventilation as a treatment in a series of patients with apoplexy, but no convincing clinical improvement was seen. A likely explanation is that the treatment was not started until some hours after the onset of symptoms.[21]

Many people, lay as well as medical, think that common senile or presenile atrophic brain disease (senile dementia, or senility) is caused by cerebrovascular disease in the form of a chronic, relentlessly stenosing arteriosclerotic process. Dementia in the old is often simply called "cerebral arteriosclerosis," a term expressing this thought. However, this thought is erroneous, for there is no relationship between the location of the pathologic changes in the brain and the vascular anatomy. Patients with senile dementia have a reduced CBF, but it is only reduced in proportion to the decrease in cerebral oxygen uptake, that is, the blood supply relative to demand is normal.[76] The control of cerebral circulation, including its autoregulation, is normal—in sharp contrast to what would be predicted by the chronic, progressive stenosis concept.[122]

Cerebral blood flow in arterial hypertension

Many years ago it was established that hypertensive subjects without brain symptoms have a perfectly normal CBF.[72] In other words, the cerebrovascular resistance is increased in proportion to the increase in pressure. As already mentioned, an autoregulation of CBF is preserved, but it is reset at a higher pressure.

The observations made during induced hypertension are of particular interest. As already mentioned, in normotensive as well as in chronic hypertensive subjects, an upper limit of autoregulation has been found (at a higher level in hypertensives) beyond which CBF suddenly increases.[125,133] The clinical syndrome termed acute hypertensive encephalopathy is presumably initiated by this so-called breakthrough of autoregulation, that is, the symptoms are caused by overdistension of vessel walls, multifocal damage of the blood-brain barrier, and by outfiltration of edema fluids—*not* to vascular spasms, as was widely assumed previously.[75]

Cerebral blood flow in epileptic seizures

The marked flow increase in the brain during seizure activity has long been recognized. In spontaneously breathing animals

and humans, a temporary asphyxia supervenes. But CBF increases by about 100% even if normoxia and normocapnia are maintained throughout by artificial ventilation combined with curarization.[17,108]

The mechanism of the flow increase has recently been debated. In spontaneously breathing animals, a pronounced brain tissue lactic acidosis develops during the seizures.[42,64,65] In animals kept normoxic and normocapnic, it is more difficult to demonstrate the acidosis.[10,22,108] Now this problem has been solved: animal experiments involving rapid freezing of the brain tissue show about a six-fold increase in tissue lactate (from 1.1 to 6.7 mmol/l) after only five seconds of seizure activity.[13] Supportive evidence is available from the observation of a temporary increase in the respiratory quotient of the brain (from just below 1.0 to about 1.3) during induced seizures.[17,108] The simultaneous increase in cerebral venous P_{O_2} indicates that tissue hypoxia probably is not involved in producing the lactic acidosis. Perhaps the accelerated utilization and production of adenosine triphosphate (ATP) change the balance between the initial (glycolytic) and the final (oxidative) breakdown of glucose without oxygen lack being involved.

Secondary factors might, however, also play a role. The autoregulation of CBF is not upheld during seizures,[15,108] presumably because of the acidosis. The increase in arterial pressure during seizure will therefore contribute to the increase in CBF. Other flow-increasing factors such as an increase in brain extracellular fluid potassium concentration or osmolality could also be involved.

A special form of epileptic seizures sometimes occurs in patients with subacute hypertension, as in nephritis or hypertensive toxemia of pregnancy. Often the patient already has signs of incipient hypertensive encephalopathy with headache, vomiting, and so on, suggesting that the state of (multifocal) blood-brain barrier damage and edema mentioned above is developing. The massive acceleration of this process, caused by the combined effect of the vasodilatation by the seizure activity and the associated further rise in blood pressure, often proves fatal. To avoid manifest eclampsia is essential.

GENERAL OUTLINE OF PHARMACOLOGY OF CEREBRAL BLOOD FLOW

Even a brief discussion of drug effects on CBF would necessitate the reviewing of a great number of studies involving many different methodologic approaches. Furthermore, because most of the studies concern effects in normal animals or normal humans, it would be difficult to illustrate adequately that cerebral circulatory responses to drugs are often totally different in brain diseases. This fact was stressed in the section on brain tissue acidosis where the paradoxical CBF changes—steal or inverse steal—were presented. This fact is important for the clinical application of CBF data, since it is in such states that flow changes really matter. With this consideration in mind, a summary of drug effects on CBF in the normal brain will be given.

Drugs with no effect on cerebral blood flow

Many substances, such as norepinephrine, angiotensin, or trimethaphan, that influence vascular tone markedly in other organs are without direct influence on CBF even if they are infused directly into the internal carotid artery.[95,96] In the doses used these drugs influence CBF only secondarily, that is, as a result of their effect on systemic arterial pressure. However, epinephrine appears to increase CBF,[128] but this effect is probably a flow response secondary to anxiety and arousal, not a direct vasomotor response. Alpha-receptor blocking agents such as phenoxybenzamine, phentolamine or hydergine, are in the doses usually given to humans without influence on CBF.[51,98,123]

Mineralocorticoids, usually in the form of dexamethasone, are widely used in neurologic intensive care. The fact that no rapid effects are seen either on mental state or ICP suggests absence of acute effects on CBF. The available reports concern the effect over

two to five days in brain tumor cases.[43,113] Increase in CBF and restoration of CBF autoregulation were found. These effects are most likely secondary to a decrease of tissue edema and of ICP and on tissue displacement.

Without attempting to review the use of steroids, a controversial field, it may be mentioned that while the beneficial effect of such steroids in brain tumor cases is well established, the value of their use in brain trauma and stroke cases is much less firmly proven. Perhaps, as compared to trauma cases, in tumors the edema is in a more nearly steady state, with production balancing (almost) removal, and that, therefore, the steroids' fairly minor antiedema influence can more readily be discerned over the course of some days.

Cerebral vasodilators

The list of vasodilators comprises acetazolamide, papaverine, volatile anesthetic agents, and drugs that cause high arterial PCO_2 or hyperosmolality.[3,128] To this list must also be added the drugs that appear to increase brain flow secondary to enhancement of neuronal function: analeptic drugs, ketamine, nicotine, and epinephrine belong to this group.

Recently it has been shown that the strong vasodilator drug hydralazine (Neprezol) is a cerebral vasodilator. This was evidenced by a moderate increase in CBF despite systemic hypotension and by an increase in intracranial pressure.[100] It is possible that sodium nitroprusside also influences the cerebral resistance vessels directly.[58]

Cerebral vasoconstrictors

A direct vasoconstrictor action is found with drugs that cause reduced arterial PCO_2 or hypo-osmolality and with xanthine derivatives such as theophylline (a component of many pharmaceutical preparations, for example, aminophylline, Euphyllin, Cordalin and xanthinol niacinate).[40] Drugs that depress cerebral function also tend to decrease CBF (if an independent vasodilator effect is absent)—the barbiturates belong to this group. Hypothermia also causes vasoconstriction.

PHARMACOLOGIC EFFECTS OF SPECIFIC ANESTHETIC DRUGS ON CEREBRAL BLOOD FLOW

Until recently, general anesthetic agents were considered to produce unconsciousness and analgesia by depressing cerebral functional activity, metabolism, and blood flow. Barbiturates have this effect and were taken to represent all anesthetic drugs. However, recent studies have completely changed this simplistic concept, and excitation in some brain regions by some drugs has been shown by many authors. A notable example is that of ketamine, which produces enhanced electrical activity in many structures and produces an unresponsive state resembling catalepsia. Here also it seems that the CBF change (an increase) is related, directionally at least, to that of brain metabolism (an increase).

With regard to effect on CBF, anesthetic drugs may be classified as follows: all gaseous anesthetic agents, even nitrous oxide, are cerebral vasodilators; IV anesthetic drugs are cerebral vasoconstrictors, ketamine constituting the only exception so far known.

Halothane

Halothane has repeatedly been shown to be a cerebral vasodilator. In clinical studies with 1.2% halothane in oxygen, normocapnia, and hypotension, Wollman and colleagues[146] found a CBF increase of 14% associated with a decrease of 9% in the cerebral metabolic rate of oxygen ($CMRO_2$), whereas Christensen and colleagues,[20] with 1.0% halothane in oxygen, normocapnia, and a maintained arterial pressure, found CBF increase of 27% and a $CMRO_2$ decrease of 26% in young men. Experimental studies by Smith[126] showed a good correlation of $CMRO_2$ and cerebral arteriovenous oxygen difference with depth of halothane anesthesia.

Studies in which halothane was given to patients with moderate intracranial hypertension always showed a further increase of ICP, which might occur quite suddenly, probably leading to local compressions resulting from brain mass displacement.[34] Under clinical conditions, these marked ICP increases are transient (10 to 30 min) and may be minimized or even abolished by prior induction of hypocapnia (10 min) in the majority of cases but not in all.[1] The recovery from a hypocapnic halothane anesthesia deserves special attention to adequacy of ventilation.[60]

Methoxyflurane

Methoxyflurane resembles halothane in its cerebral metabolic effects (dose-dependent $CMRO_2$ decrease), and it also increases CBF.[87] Administration of 1.5% methoxyflurane to patients with space-occupying lesions induces an ICP increase that cannot be completely counteracted by moderate hyperventilation.[35]

Isoflurane and enflurane

Isoflurane and enflurane both cause a significant cerebral metabolic depression associated with cerebral vasodilatation in dogs.[24,86] During enflurane anesthesia induced hypocapnia seizure activity was sometimes elicited, and was associated with an increase of $CMRO_2$.

Nitrous oxide

Nitrous oxide, administered in a concentration of 70% in humans, causes a decrease in $CMRO_2$ of about 25% without significantly affecting the CBF during normocapnia.[147] Besides the unaffected CBF, Smith and coworkers[127] demonstrated that the cerebral autoregulation is well preserved during nitrous oxide anesthesia in humans. In the face of reduced $CMRO_2$, the unchanged CBF may be considered a state of relative increase in flow. In agreement with this concept Henriksen and Jørgensen[49] found ICP increases associated with 66% nitrous oxide administration in patients with intracranial disorders and concluded that nitrous oxide was a significant cerebral vasodilator.

When evaluating the effects of nitrous oxide, the previously mentioned arousal reactions (increase in CBF and ICP) associated with painful stimuli and anxiety in patients subjected to incomplete anesthesia should be recalled. The excitation phase during nitrous oxide induction represents a phenomenon influencing CBF and ICP in the same manner.[16]

Cyclopropane

Cyclopropane used clinically, in concentrations ranging from 5% to 37%, causes a depression of $CMRO_2$, without correlation with the depth of anesthesia.[2] Furthermore, increased cerebral lactate production was found following 5% cyclopropane. Twenty percent cyclopropane increases the CBF by about 50% during normocapnia in humans.[128] These rather unusual and variable cerebral effects of increasing concentrations of cyclopropane have been found experimentally to be secondary to an increase in the concentration of circulating catecholamines associated with this anesthetic agent.[88]

All the above-mentioned anesthetic agents reduce the ventilatory carbon dioxide response, and consequently arterial PCO_2 is increased during spontaneous respiration. Thus, during spontaneous respiration, an additional cerebral vasodilatation is provoked by these anesthetic agents.

Barbiturates

Pierce and colleagues[107] demonstrated thiopental to be a pronounced and dose-dependent cerebral vasoconstrictor in humans. During normocapnia, deep thiopental anesthesia causes a parallel reduction of about 50% of $CMRO_2$ and CBF, the latter being further reduced when hypocapneic vasoconstriction is added. Interpretation of the cerebral metabolic depression induced by thiopental may be difficult, as experimental studies have disclosed an acute tolerance to thiopental.[5] The same dose-dependent and parallel reductions of CBF and $CMRO_2$ following phenobarbital have been demonstrated experimentally.[92]

The mechanism by which barbiturates influence the brain is still a matter of discussion. Most likely the anesthetic effects are due to functional effects on membranes (perhaps in the synapses) in contrast to the cerebral effect of hypothermia, which also can be assumed to influence the cellular enzymes directly.

With regard to the protective effect of barbiturates in experimental focal cerebral ischemia it is possible that the main effect is on the nonischemic areas. The flow decrease in such areas might increase pressure and flow through the collaterals to the ischemic area, the "inverse steal" effect.[85]

Narcotic analgesics and neuroleptic drugs

Incremental doses of morphine cause progressive and parallel decreases of $CMRO_2$ and CBF of about 15% in dogs with maintained normocapnia.[138] This effect could be reversed by N-allynormorphine. However, when N-allynormorphine was given alone it had cerebral effects similar to but less pronounced than morphine. Meperidine (Demerol) causes a $CMRO_2$ reduction of the same order as morphine.[83] Although morphine is a cerebral vasoconstrictor, this effect is completely abolished by hypercapnic vasodilatation. It has recently been demonstrated during normocapnia that morphine-nitrous oxide anesthesia does not significantly affect CBF or cerebral autoregulation in normal humans.[59]

Fentanyl (Sublimaze) has been shown in normal humans not to influence either CBF or $CMRO_2$ significantly under normocapnia.[118] In dogs, fentanyl causes a marked and short-lasting decrease of both CBF and $CMRO_2$, whereas droperidol (Inapsine) was found to be a more potent and long-acting cerebral vasoconstrictor that does not influence $CMRO_2$.[87] To produce neuroleptanesthesia, a combination of fentanyl and droperidol is administered. In animal studies, this combination causes a long-lasting CBF decrease, combined with an initial $CMRO_2$ reduction. A significant ICP decrease in patients with normal CSF pathways as well as with intracranial space-occupying lesions is associated with neuroleptanesthesia.[32]

The benzodiazepine derivative diazepam

(Valium) has recently been shown to cause a parallel depression of both $CMRO_2$ and CBF in comatose patients with diffuse brain damage.[23]

Ketamine

Clinical studies have proved ketamine to be a pronounced cerebral vasodilator, as it increases CBF by 62% and $CMRO_2$ by 12% during normocapnia.[139] The vasodilatation is so pronounced in normal humans that a marked ICP increase results.[37] Although ketamine has anesthetic properties, it has been shown to be a cerebral stimulant that is able to induce seizure activity in epileptics.[9] Hougaard, Hansen, and Brodersen[52] have suggested that ketamine is not a direct cerebrovasodilator but that it affects regional blood flow secondary to drug-induced changes in regional neuronal activity.

Ketamine has repeatedly been shown to provoke substantial increases of ICP in patients with intracranial pathology.[38,120] This increase might be reversed with thiopental given after the administration of ketamine.[148]

Althesin

Althesin is a steroid compound with short-lasting anesthetic properties. Experimentally it has been found to cause a marked $CMRO_2$ reduction and a concomitant clear-cut vasoconstriction.[106] A further increase of the dose causes a further CBF decrease, but simultaneously a marked hypotension is induced. In normal humans the short-lasting vasoconstriction is so pronounced that a marked ICP reduction has been demonstrated during normocapnia.[138] Althesin has also been found to be a valuable drug in the presence of intracranial hypertension.[143]

Curare

Previously it has been claimed that IV administration of tubocurarine was without any influence on the brain. In neurosurgical patients with normal ICP, Tarkkanen and co-workers[140] found a significant ICP increase associated with curare medication during maintained normocapnia. They suggested from their data that the pressure increase was caused by increased pulsatile blood flow in the brain, associated with histamine release. If so, pancuronium might be preferable as a relaxant drug. Another explanation of the ICP increase would be an arousal effect during incomplete anesthesia, and in this case the type of muscle relaxant is immaterial.

REGULATION OF SPINAL CORD BLOOD FLOW

Hydrogen clearance has shown that the blood flow in the lateral funiculus of the spinal cord is normally about 15 to 20 ml/100 g/min.[36,68] This is about the same level as found in cerebral white matter. The flow reacts to CO_2[36,63] and shows the typical autoregulation curve with a break-through point of flow increase for blood pressures above 130 mm Hg.[68] It is of particular interest that both responses are preserved after severing the cord high in the neck.[63] This shows that these vasomotor responses are locally controlled and in particular that brain stem mechanisms are not obligatorily involved. More specifically, by cord sectioning, the central control of the sympathetic nervous system is disconnected and this in the acute phase would be expected to reduce the activity in the sympathetic nervous system to a very low level. Hence the experiments speak against the perivascular sympathetic nerves being important for the two control mechanisms mentioned.

In the spinal cord gray matter it is more difficult to measure flow with the hydrogen clearance because the tissue mass is so small. The most reliable data are probably those obtained by the autoradiographic technique showing normal values of about 60 ml/100 g/min.[117] No details of spinal cord gray matter flow regulation similar to those of gray matter in the brain are available. There is, however, no reason to suspect that they would differ from those of the brain cortex.

Experimental spinal cord trauma has been studied with the hydrogen clearance method by two groups, who report conflicting results. Kobrine and Doyle[67] found that spinal cord white matter flow doubled and that this flow increase was prevented by giving an antihistaminic drug. Griffiths[41] found mostly a reduction in flow, hyperemia only being present in two of eight dogs. Small details in modes of producing the mechanical trauma and care of the animal in general probably explain the differences as suggested by the study of Bingham and co-workers.[12] Griffiths also could demonstrate a reduction or even abolition of the vasodilatation to CO_2 inhalation (in some cases flow actually dropped—a steal effect), while the vasoconstriction to a lowering of Pco_2 was better preserved.[41] These findings are thus quite similar to those found in traumatically injured brain tissue. Yet this reduced flow does not in itself constitute certain evidence of tissue hypoxia reaching levels low enough to make this factor important to the viability of the cord. In addition, blood flow in the brain is often reduced to about 50% of the normal level after trauma, without this being considered indicative of a noxious hypoxic state. Rather the finding may be interpreted to indicate the "metabolic control"—inactivity of the tissue leading to a reduced metabolic demand and to a reduced oxygen delivery, a reduced flow.

CONCLUDING CLINICAL COMMENTS RELATING TO NEUROANESTHESIA AND NEUROLOGIC INTENSIVE CARE

As repeatedly pointed out in the above text, we can influence flow and metabolism in the brain in several ways, depending on the choice of anesthetic drugs and technique.

We may therefore ask what level of cerebral blood flow is the most appropriate in patients with acute traumatic brain injury or with a brain tumor? Induction of cerebral hyperemia in a patient with a space-occupying intracranial lesion should always be avoided, as it increases blood volume and edema and thus tends to augment intracranial pressure and mass displacement of brain tissue (often blood flow decreases—a steal effect). Consequently, cerebral vasodilators, for example, inhalation anesthetic agents and hypercapnia, are contraindicated. Arousal, pain, or seizure activity must also be considered noxious stimuli, as can be ascertained by continuous intracranial pressure recordings.

Conversely, induction of vasoconstriction —mainly in the more intact parts of the brain —tends to decrease and stabilize the intracranial pressure and counteract edema formation. Thus the perfusion pressure and blood flow to marginally perfused lesioned areas may improve (inverse steal). The anesthetic technique should involve hypocapnia, and the drugs of choice should be potent depressors of cerebral metabolism, preferably with a potent associated vasoconstrictor effect as seen with barbiturates, neuroleptanesthetics, and Althesin. It is important to avoid marked hypotension, as a crucial decrease in perfusion pressure may be expected to occur in areas with edema. However, provided no acute vascular occlusions are suspected, there are reasons to favor moderate hypotension because this is known to reduce edema production in damaged regions with high flow (luxury perfusion). The use of steroids is of established value in brain tumor cases, whereas its value in other acute disorders such as ischemic or hemorrhagic stroke or following head injury or hypoxic brain insult, is not yet clarified.

These comments have been made without much regard for the difficulties inherent in their implementation. Many finer points have been omitted. The clinical chapters will supply them and thus moderate the idealized "principles." Yet they constitute the basis for the rational therapy and are widely accepted in the field today, so widely that the editors of this volume invited me to attempt to outline them in this chapter.

The final comments relate to traumatic injury of the spinal cord. In this situation a primary factor is obviously whether or not local tissue compression persists. But, there are reasons to believe, secondary factors in form of tissue edema and/or hemorrhage also influence the local functional deficit. Hence, according to the principles already discussed in case of the brain, a regimen involving moderate hypotension, hypocapnia, barbiturate anesthesia, and (possibly) steroids— and avoidance of all nervous tissue vasodilator stimuli, for example, volatile anesthetics. Perhaps alpha adrenolytic drugs may be of special value (beyond their effect on blood pressure) in blocking adverse noradrenergic effects on the microcirculation of the cord.[99]

In high and complete cord lesion the distal stump develops a certain automaticity after a transition phase of virtually abolished function (spinal shock). No aspect of the text discussed these parameters and their modification by therapeutic measures would seem likely to be able to shorten the transition phase or influence the final functional state of the severed cord. Hence, from the point of view of the present review, therapy must be directed to minimizing the local effects of the injury. That this *can* be done has been shown in animal models,[99] but a generally accepted clinical intensive care regimen for spinal cord trauma has not yet emerged. This contrasts to the situation for brain trauma, in which prolonged controlled ventilation analgesia, sedation, and control of intracranial hypertension is widely implemented and has been shown to be of value. The rarity of the cord lesions is a serious impediment in obtaining clinical documentation of the value of various forms of treatment. It is tempting, as has been done in this chapter, to transfer the experience from brain to cord. After all the cord is simply an extension of the brain.

REFERENCES

1. Adams, R. W., Gronert, G. A., Sundt, T. M., and Michenfelder, J. D.: Halothane, hypocapnia, and cerebrospinal fluid pressure in neurosurgery, Anesthesiology 37:510, 1972.
2. Alexander, S. C., Colton, E. T., Smith, A. L., and Wollman, H.: The effects of cyclopropane on cerebral and systemic carbohydrate metabolism, Anesthesiology 32:236, 1970.
3. Alexander, S. C., and Lassen, N. A.: Cerebral circulatory response to acute brain disease: implications for anesthetic practice, Anesthesiology 32: 60, 1970.
4. Alm, A., and Bill, A.: The effect of stimulation of the cervical sympathetic chain on retinal oxygen tension and on uveal, retinal and cerebral blood flow in cats, Acta Physiol. Scand. 88:84, 1973.
5. Altenburg, B. M., Michenfelder, J. D., and Theye, R. A.: Acute tolerance to thiopental in ca-

nine cerebral oxygen consumption studies, Anesthesiology 31:443, 1969.
6. Astrup, J., Symon, L., Branston, N. M., and Lassen, N. A.: Cortical evoked potentials and extracellular K^+ and H^+ at critical levels of brain ischemia, Stroke 8:51, 1977.
7. Bates, D., Weinshilboum, R. M., Campbell, R. J., and Sundt, Th.: The effect of lesions in the locus coeruleus on the physiological responses of the cerebral blood vessels in cats, Brain Res. 136: 431, 1977.
8. Benis, A. M., Usami, S., and Chien, S.: Effect of hematocrit and inertial losses on pressure-flow relations in the isolated hindpaw of the dog, Circ. Res. 27:1047, 1970.
9. Bennett, D. R., Madsen, J. A., Jordan, W. S., and Wiser, W. C.: Ketamine anesthesia in brain-damaged epileptics: electroencephalographic and clinical observations, Neurology (Minneap.) 23:449, 1973.
10. Beresford, H. R., Posner, J. B., and Plum, F.: Changes in brain lactate during induced cerebral seizures, Arch. Neurol. 20:243, 1969.
11. Bill, A., Linder, J., and Linder, M.: Sympathetic effect on cerebral blood vessels in acute arterial hypertension, Acta Physiol. Scand. 96:27A, 1976.
12. Bingham, W. G., Sirinek, L., Crutcher, K., and Hohanacky, C.: Effect of spinal cord injury on cord and cerebral blood in monkey, Acta Neurol. Scand. 56(suppl.):64, 238, 1977.
13. Bolwig, T. G., and Quistorff, B.: In vivo concentration of lactate in the brain of conscious rats before and during seizures: new ultra-rapid technique for the freeze-sampling of brain tissue, J. Neurochem. 21: 1345, 1973.
14. Branston, N. M., Symon, L., Crockard, H. A., and Pasztor, E.: Relationship between the cortical evoked potential and local cortical blood flow following acute middle cerebral artery occlusion in the baboon, Exp. Neurol. 45:195, 1974.
15. Brennan, R. W., and Plum, F.: Dissociation of autoregulation and chemical regulation in cerebral circulation following seizures. In Russell, R. W. R., editor: Brain and blood flow, London, 1971, Pitman Publishing, p. 218.
16. Brodersen, P.: Discussion on psychoactive drugs and anxiety; their influence on cerebral circulation and metabolism. In Ingvar, D. H., and Lassen, N. A., editors: Brain work: the coupling of function, metabolism and blood flow in the brain, Copenhagen, 1975, Munksgaard, p. 464.
17. Brodersen, P., Paulson, O. B., Bolwig, T. G., Rogon, Z. E., Rafaelsen, O. J., and Lassen, N. A.: Cerebral hyperemia in electrically induced epileptic seizures, Arch. Neurol. 28:334, 1973.
18. Carlsson, Ch., Hägerdal, M., and Siesjö, B. K.: Increase in cerebral oxygen uptake and blood flow in immobilization stress, Acta Physiol. Scand. 95: 206, 1975.
19. Christensen, M. S., Brodersen, P., Olesen, J., and

Paulson, O. B.: Cerebral apoplexy (stroke) treated with or without prolonged artificial hyperventilation. II. Cerebrospinal fluid acid-base balance and intracranial pressure, Stroke 4:620, 1973.

20. Christensen, M. S., Høedt-Rasmussen, K., and Lassen, N. A.: Cerebral vasodilatation by halothane anaesthesia in man and its potentiation by hypotension and hypercapnia, Br. J. Anaesth. **39:** 927, 1967.

21. Christensen, M. S., Paulson, O. B., Olesen, J., Alexander, S. C., Skinhøj, E., Dam, W. H., and Lassen, N. A.: Cerebral apoplexy (stroke) treated with or without prolonged, artificial hyperventilation. I. Cerebral circulation, clinical course, and cause of death, Stroke 4:568, 1973.

22. Collins, R. C., Posner, J. B., and Plum, F.: Cerebral energy metabolism during electroshock seizures in mice, Am. J. Physiol. **218:**943, 1970.

23. Cotev, S., and Shalit, M. N.: Effects of diazepam on cerebral blood flow and oxygen uptake after head injury, Anesthesiology **43:**117, 1975.

24. Cucchiara, R. F., Theye, R. A., and Michenfelder, J. D.: The effects of isoflurane on canine cerebral metabolism and blood flow, Anesthesiology **40:** 571, 1974.

25. Deshmukh, V. D., Harper, A. M., Rowan, J. O., and Jennett, W. B.: Studies on neurogenic control of the cerebral circulation, Eur. Neurol. **6:**166, 1971/72.

26. Edvinsson, L., Nielsen, K. C., Owman, C., and West, K. A.: Sympathetic adrenergic influence on brain vessels as studies by changes in cerebral blood volume of mice, Eur. Neurol. **6:**193, 1971/72.

27. Eklöf, B., Ingvar, D. H., Kågström, E., and Olin, T.: Persistence of cerebral blood flow autoregulation following chronic bilateral cervical sympathectomy in the monkey, Acta Physiol. Scand. **82:**172, 1971.

28. Eklöf, B., Lassen, N. A., Nilsson, L., Norberg, K., and Siesjö, B. K.: Blood flow and metabolic rate for oxygen in the cerebral cortex of the rat, Acta Physiol. Scand. **88:**587, 1973.

29. Elliott, K. A. C., and Jasper, H. H.: Physiological salt solutions for brain surgery; studies of local pH and pial vessel reactions to buffered and unbuffered isotonic solutions, J. Neurosurg. **6:**140, 1949.

30. Endo, H., Larsen, B., and Lassen, N. A.: Regional cerebral blood flow alterations remote from the site of intracranial tumors, J. Neurosurg. **46:**271, 1977.

31. Fencl, V., Vale, J. R., and Broch, J. A.: Respiration and cerebral blood flow in metabolic acidosis and alkalosis in humans, J. Appl. Physiol. **27:**67, 1969.

32. Fitch, W., Barker, J., Jennett, W. B., and McDowall, D. G.: The influence of neuroleptanalgesic drugs on cerebrospinal fluid pressure, Br. J. Anaesth. **41:**800, 1969a.

33. Fitch, W., MacKenzie, E. T., and Harper, A. M.: Effects of decreasing arterial blood pressure on cerebral blood flow in the baboon; influence of the sympathetic nervous system, Circ. Res. **37:**550, 1975.

34. Fitch, W., and McDowall, D. G.: Effect of halothane on intracranial pressure gradients in the presence of intra-cranial space-occupying lesions, Br. J. Anaesth. **43:**904, 1971.

35. Fitch, W., McDowall, D. G., and Jennett, W. B.: The effect of methoxyflurane on cerebrospinal fluid pressure in patients with and without intracranial space-occupying lesions, Br. J. Anaesth. **41:**564, 1969b.

36. Flohr, H., Pöll, W., and Brock, M.: Regulation of spinal cord blood flow. In Russell, R. W. R., editor: Brain and blood flow, Pitman Publ., London, 1970, p. 406.

37. Gardner, A. E., Olson, B. E., and Lichtiger, M.: Cerebrospinal fluid pressure during dissociative anesthesia with ketamine, Anesthesiology **35:**226, 1971.

38. Gibbs, J. M.: The effect of intravenous ketamine on cerebrospinal fluid pressure, Br. J. Anaesth. **44:** 1298, 1972.

39. Gotoh, F., Tazaki, Y., and Meyer, J. S.: Transport of gases through brain and their extravascular vasomotor action, Exp. Neurol. 4:48, 1961.

40. Gottstein, U., and Paulson, O. B.: Effect of intra-carotid aminophylline infusion on the cerebral circulation, Stroke 3:560, 1972.

41. Griffiths, I. R.: Spinal cord blood flow after acute impact injury. In Harper, A. M., and others, editors: Blood flow and metabolism of the brain, Edinburgh, London, New York, 1975, Churchill Livingstone Publ., p. 427.

42. Gurdjian, E. S., Webster, J. E., and Stone, W. E.: Cerebral metabolism in metrazol convulsions in the dog, Res. Publ. Assoc. Res. Nerv. Ment. Dis. **26:**184, 1947.

43. Hadjidimos, A., Steingrass, U., Fischer, F., Reulen, H. J., Weirauch, D., and Schürmann, K.: RCBF and cerebral vasomotor response in brain tumors following dexamethasone treatment. In Langfitt, Th. W., and others, editors: Cerebral circulation and metabolism, New York-Heidelberg-Berlin, 1975, Springer-Verlag, p. 318.

44. Hardebo, J. E., Edvinsson, L., and Owman, Ch.: Influence of the cerebrovascular sympathetic innervation on blood-brain barrier function, Acta Physiol. Scand. **452**(suppl.):65, 1977.

45. Harp, J. R., and Wollman, H.: Cerebral metabolic effects of hyperventilation and deliberate hypotension, Br. J. Anaesth. **45:**256, 1973.

46. Harper, A. M., and Jennett, W. B.: Simultaneous measurement of beta and gamma clearance curves of radioactive inert gases from the monkey brain. In Bain, W. H., and Harper, A. M., editors: Blood flow through organs and tissues, Edinburgh and London, 1968, E. & S. Livingstone Ltd., p. 214.

47. Harper, A. M., Deshmukh, D., Sengupta, J. O.,

and Jennett, W. B.: The effect of experimental spasm on the CO_2 response of cerebral blood flow in primates, Neuroradiology **3**:134, 1972.

48. Heiss, W. D., Prosenz, P., and Roszuczky, A.: Technical considerations in the use of a gamma camera 1,600-channel analyzer system for the measurement of regional cerebral blood flow, J. Nucl. Med. **13**:534, 1972.

49. Henriksen, H. T., and Jørgensen, P. B.: The effect of nitrous oxide on intracranial pressure in patients with intracranial disorders, Br. J. Anaesth. **45**:486, 1973.

50. Hertz, M. M., Hemmingsen, R., and Bolwig, T. G.: Rapid and repetitive measurements of blood flow and oxygen consumption in the rat brain using intraarterial Xenon injection, Acta Physiol. Scand. **101**:501, 1977.

51. Hoff, J. T., Sengupta, D., Harper, M., and Jennett, B.: Effect of alpha-adrenergic blockade on response of cerebral circulation of hypocapnia in the baboon, Lancet **2**:1337, 1972.

52. Hougaard, K., Hansen, A., and Brodersen, P.: The effect of ketamine on regional cerebral blood flow in man, Anesthesiology **41**:562, 1974.

53. Häggendal, E., Löfgren, J., Nilsson, N. J., and Zwetnow, N. N.: Effects of varied cerebrospinal fluid pressure on cerebral blood flow in dogs, Acta Physiol. Scand. **79**:262, 1970.

54. Høedt-Rasmussen, K., Sveinsdottir, E., and Lassen, N. A.: Regional cerebral blood flow in man determined by intraarterial injection of radioactive inert gas, Circ. Res. **16**:309, 1965.

55. Ingvar, D. H., and Lassen, N. A.: Cerebral complications following measurements of regional cerebral blood flow (rCBF) with the intra-arterial ^{133}Xenon injection method, Stroke **4**:658, 1973.

56. Ingvar, D. H., and Risberg, J.: Increase of regional cerebral blood flow during mental effort in normals and in patients with focal brain disorders, Exp. Brain Res. **3**:195, 1967.

57. Ingvar, D. H., Rosen, I., Eriksson, M., and Elmquist, D.: Activation patterns induced in the dominant hemisphere by skin stimulation. In Zotterman, Y., editor: Sensory functions of the skin, Elmsford, N.Y., 1976, Pergamon Press, Inc., p. 549.

58. Ivankovich, A. D., Miletich, D. J., Albrecht, R. F., and Zahed, B.: Sodium nitroprusside and cerebral blood flow in the anesthetized and unanesthetized goat, Anesthesiology **44**:21, 1976.

59. Jobes, D. R., Kennell, E., Bitner, R., Swenson, E., and Wollman, H.: Effects of morphine-nitrous oxide anesthesia on cerebral autoregulation, Anesthesiology **42**:30, 1975.

60. Jørgensen, P. B., and Misfeldt, B. B.: Intracranial pressure during recovery from nitrous oxide and halothane anaesthesia in neurosurgical patients, Br. J. Anaesth. **47**:977, 1975.

61. Kety, S. S.: Round table discussion of psychoactive drugs and anxiety, their influence on cerebral circulation and metabolism. In Ingvar, D. D. and Lassen, N. A., editors: Brain work: the coupling of function, metabolism and blood flow in the brain," Copenhagen, 1975, Munksgaard, p. 472.

62. Kety, S. S., and Schmidt, C. F.: The nitrous oxide method for the quantitative determination of cerebral blood flow in man: theory, procedure and normal values, J. Clin. Invest. **27**:476, 1948.

63. Kindt, G. W., Ducker, T. B., and Huddlestone, J.: Regulation of spinal cord blood flow. In Ross Russell, R. W., editor: Brain and blood flow, London, 1970, Pitman Publ., p. 401.

64. King, L. J., Lowry, O. H., Passoneau, J. V., and Venson, V.: Effects of convulsants on energy reserves in the cerebral cortex, J. Neurochem. **14**: 599, 1967.

65. Klein, J. R., and Olsen, N. S.: Effect of convulsive activity upon the concentration of brain glucose, glycogen, lactate and phosphates, J. Biol. Chem. **167**:747, 1947.

66. Kobayashi, S., Waltz, A. G., and Rhoton, A. L.: Effects of stimulation of cervical sympathetic nerves on cortical blood flow and vascular reactivity, Neurology (Minneap.) **21**:297, 1971.

67. Kobrine, A. I., and Doyle, T. F.: Histamine in spinal cord injury. In Harper, A. M., and others, editors: Blood flow and metabolism of the brain, Edinburgh, London, New York, 1975, Churchill Livingstone Publ., p. 430.

68. Kobrine, A. I., and Doyle, T. F.: Physiology of spinal cord blood flow. In Harper, A. M., and others, editors: Blood flow and metabolism of the brain, Edinburgh, London, New York, 1975, Churchill Livingstone Publ., p. 416.

69. Kogure, K., Scheinberg, P., Reinmuth, O. M., Fujishima, M., and Busto, R.: Mechanisms of cerebral vasodilatation in hypoxia, J. Appl. Physiol. **29**:223, 1970.

70. Kuschinsky, W., and Wahl, M.: The functional significance of β-adrenergic and cholinergic receptors at pial arteries: a microapplication study. In Langfitt, Th. W., and others, editors: Cerebral circulation and metabolism, New York-Heidelberg-Berlin, 1975, Springer-Verlag, p. 470.

71. Larsen, B., Skinhøj, E., Soh, K., Endo, H., and Lassen, N. A.: The pattern of cortical activity provoked by listening and speech revealed by rCBF measurements, Acta Neurol. Scand. **56**(suppl.):64, 268, 1977.

72. Lassen, N. A.: Cerebral blood flow and oxygen consumption in man, Physiol. Rev. **39**:183, 1959.

73. Lassen, N. A.: The luxury-perfusion syndrome and its possible relation to acute metabolic acidosis localized within the brain, Lancet **2**:1113, 1966.

74. Lassen, N. A.: Brain extracellular pH: The main factor controlling cerebral blood flow, Scand. J. Clin. Lab. Invest. **22**:247, 1968.

75. Lassen, N. A., and Agnoli, A.: Upper limit of autoregulation of cerebral blood flow: on the pathogenesis of hypertensive encephalopathy, Scand. J. Clin. Lab. Invest. **30**:113, 1972.

76. Lassen, N. A., Feinberg, I., and Lane, M. H.: Bilateral studies of cerebral oxygen uptake in young and aged normal subjects and in patients with organic dementia, J. Clin. Invest. **39**:491, 1960.

77. Lassen, N. A., and Ingvar, D. H.: The blood flow of the cerebral cortex determined by radioactive Krypton-85, Experientia **17**:42, 1961.

78. Lassen, N. A., and Ingvar, D. H.: Regional cerebral blood flow measurement in man; a review, Arch. Neurol. **9**:615, 1963.

79. Lassen, N. A., and Munck, O.: The cerebral blood flow in man determined by the use of radioactive Krypton, Acta Physiol. Scand. **33**:30, 1955.

80. Marc-Vergnes, J. P., Blavo, M. C., Coudert, J., Antezana, G. Dedieu, P., and Durand, J.: Cerebral blood flow and metabolism in high altitude residents (abstract), Stroke **4**:345, 1973.

81. McDowall, D. G.: In Payne, J. P., and Hill, D. W., editors: Oxygen measurements in blood and tissues, London, 1966, Churchill Livingstone, p. 205.

82. McDowall, D. G., Okuda, Y., Jones, G. M., Ali, M. D., and Norton, P. M.: Changes in cerebral venous oxygen tension with anaesthetic drugs. In Inguar, D. H., and Lassen, N. A., editors: Brain work: the coupling of function, metabolism and blood flow in the brain, Copenhagen, 1975, Munksgaard Publ., p. 253.

83. Messick, J. M., and Theye, R. A.: Effects of pentobarbital and meperidine on canine cerebral and total oxygen consumption rates, Can. Anaesth. Soc. J. **16**:321, 1969.

84. Meyer, N. W., and Klassen, A. C.: Regional brain blood flow during sympathetic stimulation. In Langfitt, Th. W., and others: Cerebral circulation and metabolism, New York-Heidelberg-Berlin, 1975, Springer-Verlag, p. 459.

85. Michenfelder, J. D.: The interdependency of cerebral functional and metabolic effects following massive doses of thiopental in the dog, Anesthesiology **41**:231, 1974.

86. Michenfelder, J. D., and Cucchiara, R. F.: Canine cerebral oxygen consumption during enflurane anesthesia and its modification during induced seizures, Anesthesiology **40**:575, 1974.

87. Michenfelder, J. D., and Theye, R. A.: Effects of fentanyl, droperidol, and innovar on canine cerebral metabolism and blood flow, Br. J. Anaesth. **43**:630, 1971.

88. Michenfelder, J. D., and Theye, R. A.: Effects of cyclopropane on canine cerebral blood flow and metabolism: modification by catecholamine suppression, Anesthesiology **37**:32, 1972.

89. Morawetz, R. B., Jones, T. H., Ojemann, R. G., Marcoux, F. W., DeGirolami, U., and Crowell, R. M.: Regional cerebral blood flow during temporary middle cerebral occlusion in waking monkeys, Acta Neurol. Scand. **56**(suppl.):64, 114, 1977.

90. Morita, H., Nemoto, E. M., Leyaert, A. L., and Stezoski, S. W.: Brain blood flow autoregulation and metabolism during halothane anesthesia in monkeys, Am. J. Physiol. **233**:H-670, 1977.

91. Nielsen, K. C., Edvinsson, L., and Owman, C.: Cholinergic innervation and vasomotor response of brain vessels. In Langfitt, Th. W., and others, editors: Cerebral circulation and metabolism, New York-Heidelberg-Berlin, 1975, Springer-Verlag, p. 473.

92. Nilsson, L., and Siesjö, B. K.: The effect of phenobarbitone anaesthesia on blood flow and oxygen consumption in the rat brain, Acta Anaesthesiol. Scand. **57**(suppl.):18, 1975.

93. Olesen, J.: Total CO_2, lactate, and pyruvate in brain biopsies taken after freezing and tissue in situ, Acta Neurol. Scand. **46**, 141, 1970.

94. Olesen, J.: Contralateral focal increase of cerebral blood flow in man during arm work, Brain **94**:635, 1971.

95. Olesen, J.: Effect of intracarotid epinephrine, norepinephrine and angiotensin on the regional cerebral blood flow in man, Neurology (Minneap.) **22**:978, 1972.

96. Olesen, J.: Quantitative evaluation of normal and pathologic cerebral blood flow regulation to perfusion pressure: changes in man, Arch. Neurol. **28**, 143, 1973.

97. Olesen, J., Paulson, O. B., and Lassen, N. A.: Regional cerebral blood flow in man determined by the initial slope of the clearance of intra-arterially injected ^{133}Xe, Stroke **2**:519, 1971.

98. Olesen, J., and Skinhøj, E.: Effects of ergot alkaloids (Hydergine) on cerebral haemodynamics in man, Acta Pharmacol. Toxicol. (Copenhagen) **31**: 75, 1972.

99. Osterholm, J. L.: The pathophysiological response to spinal cord injury, J. Neurosurg. **40**:1, 1974.

100. Overgaard, J., and Skinhøj, E.: The effect of hydralazine on intracranial pressure and cerebral blood flow. In Harper, A. M., and others, editors: Blood flow and metabolism of the brain, Edinburgh, London, New York, 1975, Churchill Livingstone, p. 11.16.

101. Palvölgyi, R.: Regional cerebral blood flow in patients with intracranial tumors, J. Neurosurg. **31**: 149, 1969.

102. Pannier, J. L., and Leusen, I.: Circulation to the brain of the rat during acute and prolonged respiratory changes in the acid-base balance, Pflüg Arch. **338**:347, 1973.

103. Pannier, J. L., Weyne, J., Demeester, G., and Leusen, I.: Influence of changes in the acid-base composition of the ventricular system on cerebral blood flow in cats, Pflüg. Arch. **333**:337, 1972.

104. Pasztor, E., Symon, L., Dorsch, N. W. C., and Branston, N. M.: The hydrogen clearance method in assessment of blood flow in cortex, white matter and deep nuclei of baboons, Stroke **4**:556, 1973.

105. Paulson, O. B., Lassen, N. A., and Skinhøj, E.: Regional cerebral blood flow in apoplexy without

arterial occlusion, Neurology (Minneap.) **21**:125, 1970.

106. Pickerodt, V. W. A., McDowall, D. G., Coroneos, N. J., and Keany, N. P.: Effect of Althesin on cerebral perfusion, cerebral metabolism and intracranial pressure in the anaesthetized baboon, Br. J. Anaesth. **44**:751, 1972.

107. Pierce, E. C., Lambertsen, C. J., Deutsch, S., Chase, P. E., Linde, H. W., Dripps, R. D., and Price, H. L.: Cerebral circulation and metabolism during thiopental anesthesia and hyperventilation in man, J. Clin. Invest. **41**:1964.

108. Plum, F., Posner, J. B., and Troy, B.: Cerebral metabolic and circulatory responses to induced convulsions in animals, Arch. Neurol. **18**:1, 1968.

109. Raichle, M. E., Grubb, R. L., Mokhtar, H. G., Eichling, J. O., and Ter-Pogossian, M. M.: Correlation between regional cerebral blood flow and oxidative metabolism, Acta Neurol. **33**:523, 1976.

110. Rapela, C. E., Green, H. D., and Denison, A. B., Jr.: Baroreceptor reflexes and autoregulation of cerebral blood flow in the dog, Circ. Res. **21**:559, 1967.

111. Regli, F., Yamaguchi, T., and Waltz, A. G.: Effects of acetazolamide on cerebral ischemia and infarction after experimental occlusion of middle cerebral artery, Stroke **2**:456, 1971.

112. Reivich, M., Jehle, J., Sokoloff, L., and Kety, S. S.: Measurement of regional cerebral blood flow with antipyrine-^{14}C in awake cats, J. Appl. Physiol. **27**:296, 1969.

113. Reulen, H. J., Hadjidimos, A., and Schürmann, K.: The effect of dexamethasone on water and electrolyte content and on rCBF in perifocal brain oedema in man. In Reulen, H. J., and Schürmann, K., editors: Berlin, Heidelberg, New York, 1972, Springer-Verlag, p. 239.

114. Rosenblum, W. I.: Effects of reduced hematocrit on erythrocyte velocity and fluorescein transit time in the cerebral microcirculation of the mouse, Circ. Res. **29**:96, 1971.

115. Rossanda, M., Collice, M., Porta, M., and Beselli, L.: Intracranial hypertension in head injury: clinical significance and relation to respiration. In Lundberg, N., Pontén, U., and Brock, M., Intracranial pressure II; Berlin, Heidelberg, New York, 1975, Springer Verlag, p. 475.

116. Salanga, V. D., and Waltz, A. G.: Regional cerebral blood flow during stimulation of tenth cranial nerve, Stroke **4**:213, 1973.

117. Sandler, A. N., and Tator, C. H.: The effect of spinal cord trauma on spinal cord blood flow in primates. In Harper, A. M., and others, editors: Blood flow and metabolism of the brain, Edinburgh, London, New York, 1975, Churchill-Livingstone, p. 422.

118. Sari, A., Okuda, Y., and Takeshita, H.: The effects of thalamonal on cerebral circulation and oxygen consumption in man, Br. J. Anaesth. **44**:330, 1972.

119. Severinghaus, J. W., Chiodi, H., Eger, E. I., II,

Brandstater, B., and Hornbein, T. F.: Cerebral blood flow in man at high altitude; role of cerebrospinal fluid pH in normalization of flow in chronic hypocapnia, Circ. Res. **19**:274, 1966.

120. Shapiro, H. M., Wyte, S. R., and Harris, A. B.: Ketamine anaesthesia in patients with intracranial pathology, Br. J. Anaesth. **44**:1200, 1972.

121. Siesjö, B. K., and Nielsen, L.: The influence of arterial hypoxemia upon labile phosphates and upon extracellular and intracellular lactate and pyruvate concentration in the rat brain, Scand. J. Clin. Lab. Invest. **27**:83, 1971.

122. Simard, D., Olesen, J., Paulson, O. B., Lassen, N. A., and Skinhøj, E.: Regional cerebral blood flow and its regulation in dementia, Brain **94**:273, 1971.

123. Skinhøj, E.: The sympathetic nervous system and the regulation of cerebral blood flow in man, Stroke **3**:711, 1972.

124. Skinhøj, E., and Paulson, O. B.: Carbon dioxide and cerebral circulatory control; evidence of a non focal site of action of carbon dioxide on cerebral circulation, Arch. Neurol. (Chic.) **20**:249, 1969.

125. Skinhøj, E., and Strandgaard, S.: Pathogenesis of hypertensive encephalopathy, Lancet **1**:461, 1973.

126. Smith, A. L.: Dependence of cerebral venous oxygen tension on anesthetic depth, Anesthesiology **39**:291, 1973.

127. Smith, A. L., Neigh, J. L., Hoffman, J. C., and Wollman, H.: Effects of general anesthesia on autoregulation of cerebral blood flow in man, J. Appl. Physiol. **29**:665, 1970.

128. Sokoloff, L.: The action of drugs on the cerebral circulation. Pharmacol. Rev. **11**:1, 1959.

129. Soloway, M., Nadel, W., Albin, M. S., and White, R. J.: The effect of hyperventilation on subsequent cerebral infarction, Anesthesiology **29**:975, 1968.

130. Stone, H. H., MacKrell, T. N., Brandstater, B. J., Haidak, G. L., and Nemir, P., Jr.: The effect of induced hemorrhagic shock on the cerebral circulation and metabolism of man, Surg. Forum **5**:68, 1955.

131. Strandell, T., and Lundbergh, P.: Measurements of ^{133}Xe activity in blood sampled in plastic and glass syringes, Scand. J. Clin. Lab. Invest. **32**:89, 1973.

132. Strandgaard, S.: Autoregulation of cerebral blood flow in hypertensive patients; the modifying influence of prolonged antihypertensive treatment on the tolerance to acute, drug-induced hypotension, Circulation **53**:720, 1976.

133. Strandgaard, S., Olesen, J., Skinhøj, E., and Lassen, N. A.: Autoregulation of brain circulation in severe arterial hypertension, Br. Med. J. **1**:507, 1973.

134. Sundt, T. M., Sharbrough, F. W., Anderson, R. E., and Michenfelder, J. D.: Cerebral blood flow measurements and electroencephalograms during carotid endarterectomy, J. Neurosurg. **41**:310, 1974.

135. Sveinsdottir, E., Larsen, B., Rommer, P., and Lassen, N. A.: A multidetector scintillation camera with 254 channels, J. Nucl. Med. **18:**168, 1977.

136. Symon, L., Pasztor, E., Dorsch, N. W. C., and Branston, N. M.: Physiological responses of local areas of the cerebral circulation in experimental primates determined by the method of hydrogen clearance, Stroke **4:**632, 1973.

137. Takahashi, T., Takasaki, M., Namiki, A., and Dohi, S.: Effects of Althesin on cerebrospinal fluid pressure, Br. J. Anaesth. **45:**179, 1973.

138. Takeshita, H., Michenfelder, J. D., and Theye, R. A.: The effects of morphine and N-allylnormorphine on canine cerebral metabolism and circulation, Anesthesiology **37:**605, 1972.

139. Takeshita, H., Okuda, Y., and Sari, A.: The effects of ketamine on cerebral circulation and metabolism in man, Anesthesiology **36:**69, 1972.

140. Tarkkanen, L., Laitinen, L., and Johansson, G.: Effects of d-tubocurarine on intracranial pressure and thalamic electrical impedance, Anesthesiology **40:**247, 1974.

141. Trojaborg, W., and Boysen, G.: Relation between EEG, regional cerebral blood flow and internal carotid artery pressure during carotid endarterectomy, Electroenceph. Clin. Neurophysiol. **34:** 61, 1973.

142. Turner, J. M., Coroneos, N. J., Gibson, R. M., Powell, D., Ness, M. A., and McDowall, D. G.: The effect of Althesin on intracranial pressure in man, Br. J. Anaesth. **45:**168, 1973.

143. Wahl, M., Kuschinsky, W., Bosse, O., Olesen, J., Lassen, N. A., Michaelis, J., and Thurau, K.: Effect of l-norepinephrine on the diameter of pial arterioles and arteries in the cat, Circ. Res. **31:** 243, 1973.

144. Wald, A., Hass, W. K., and Ransohoff, J.: Totorial: Experience with a mass spectrometer system for blood gas analysis in humans, J. Assoc. Advan. Instrum. **5:**325, 1971.

145. Waltz, A. G., Yamaguchi, T., and Regli, F.: Regulatory responses of cerebral vasculature after sympathetic denervation, Am. J. Physiol. **221:**298, 1971.

146. Wollman, H., Alexander, S. C., Cohen, P. J., Chase, P. E., Melman, E., and Behar, M. G.: Cerebral circulation of man during halothane anesthesia: effects of hypocarbia and of d-tubocurarine, Anesthesiology **25:**180, 1964.

147. Wollman, H., Smith, T. C., Chase, P. E., and Molen, R. A.: Cerebral circulation during general anesthesia and hyperventilation in man: thiopental induction to nitrous oxide and d-tubodurarine, Anesthesiology **26:**329, 1965.

148. Wyte, S. R., Shapiro, H. M., Turner, P., and Harris, A. B.: Ketamine-induced intracranial hypertension, Anesthesiology **36:**174, 1972.

2

Brain oxygen consumption

JAMES R. HARP
MAGNUS HAGERDAL

This chapter concerns the effect of a variety of anesthetic drugs and techniques upon brain work and upon the relationship between brain work and brain energy supply. Cerebral blood flow is discussed in terms of substrate availability relative to energy consumption. Finally, we review at length the possibility of brain protection in hypoxia and ischemia by various anesthetic agents and techniques.

Knowledge of the principles to be outlined should make it possible for neuroanesthesiologists to more rationally plan patient management. In particular, the principle of brain protection may be always applicable in neuroanesthesia since the central nervous system is nearly always subject to stress during neurosurgery. Specific details presented are factual and current at writing but by no means represent a complete state of knowledge, for the answers to many important questions remain to be gleaned from laboratory and clinical research.

CEREBRAL METABOLIC RATE FOR OXYGEN (CMRO$_2$)

The central nervous system comprises less than 2% of body mass, yet it consumes 20% of resting body oxygen uptake.[54] While there are demonstrable regional variations in oxygen use during mental activity, the overall average CMRO$_2$ varies only slightly across a wide range of mental activity with no de-monstrable difference in CMRO$_2$ between sleep and mental concentration.[33,55] Metabolic or pharmacologic coma may markedly lower CMRO$_2$,[24,30,53] and seizure activity may produce a great increase in CMRO$_2$.[48]

Brain tissue may consume oxygen through three processes.[11] Most important is the process of reduction of molecular oxygen by the electron-transfer oxidases producing H$_2$O. This process is the energy provider, and 99% of CMRO$_2$ is destined for the electron-transfer oxidases. Energy of oxidation is captured in the form of high-energy phosphate bonds. The other oxygen consuming processes, oxygen transferase systems, and mixed function oxidase systems are involved in synthetic and detoxification reactions. Mixed function oxidase systems are needed for neurotransmitter synthesis, for example.

In humans, under normal circumstances, virtually all brain energy is received from aerobic combustion of glucose, and virtually all of CMRO$_2$ is used in this manner. A small fraction (5%) of glucose consumption occurs anaerobically, producing lactic acid.[1] Complete oxidation of 1 mol of glucose through the electron transfer system produces 38 mol of adenosine triphosphate (ATP). Glycolytic metabolism of 1 mol of glucose to lactate produces 2 mol of ATP. In hypoxia the electron transfer system cannot function, and glycolytic consumption of glucose may increase five- to six-fold. The maximal increase

25

in glycolysis yields only about 2.5% of resting brain tissue energy requirements. Since brain tissue has scant energy stores (see below), hypoxic conditions that might be tolerated for hours in an extremity produce brain injury in minutes.

That 5% of brain glucose consumption normally is glycolytic should not be taken to signify marginal brain oxygen supply. More probably, it reflects out-leaking of lactic acid along a concentration gradient.[41] When blood lactate level is elevated artificially, brain tissue takes up lactate and consumes it. In addition, as will be discussed subsequently, production and pool size of lactate and other acid metabolic intermediates fluctuate to compensate for changes in brain intracellular hydrogen ion concentration.[49]

While virtually all glucose taken up by the brain eventually ends as lactate or carbon dioxide, this does not happen at once. Labeled glucose carbon has a half-life in brain of several hours. This indicates that glucose enters amino acid pools and participates in other synthetic processes. Anesthesia with a variety of agents appears to markedly limit the number of choices presented to glucose molecules,[16] thus most anesthetics reduce the half-life of glucose in brain. This may indicate that the synthetic and other processes are more inhibited than the energy-producing processes.

Following prolonged starvation, ketone bodies, acetoacetate and beta-hydroxybuterate replace glucose as the predominant fuel for brain metabolism, supplying approximately two thirds of the caloric needs.[43] This is necessary, since if adult brain continued to oxidize glucose during starvation at the normal rate (110 to 145 g/24 hr in adults) total body protein store would shortly be given up to gluconeogenesis. As with lactic acid, brain consumption of ketone bodies relates to the blood level of these substances. It is important to realize that even when ketone bodies provide the predominant source of brain energy substrate, hypoglycemia cannot be tolerated. Glucose may be needed as a four-carbon fragment source to permit regeneration of oxaloacetate for the tricarboxylic acid cycle.

Table 2-1. Dimensions of cerebral metabolism

	Rates of consumption or production in humans (whole brain)
Oxygen (CMRO$_2$)	3.3 ml/100 g/min
	1.5 μmol/g/min
Glucose (CMR gl)	4.5 mg/100 g/min
	0.25 μmol/g/min
Lactate (CMR lac)	0.56 mg/100 g/min
	9 μmol/g/min
ATP	9 μmol/g/min

Since brain tissue contains considerable glucose and some glycogen (possibly as astrocytic rather than neuronal deposits) and since the brain is capable of generating carbon skeletons for the tricarboxylic cycle through anaplerotic reactions,[17] the critical element in maintenance of adequate brain energy supply is oxygen. Thus whether the stress experienced be "ischemic" or "hypoxic," the final common element of stress is hypoxia. Only in iatrogenic or pathologic insulin excess does dearth of glucose become critical.

Tables 2-1 and 2-2 present the dimensions of cerebral metabolism as used in the context of this review. The values for metabolic rate are often reported in terms of milliliters or milligrams per 100 g brain tissue per minute in anesthesia literature, while neurochemists generally refer to micromoles per gram per minute. The values given are for whole brain; metabolic rate in cortical tissue may be half again larger.[50] Smaller animals having less elegant cortical cytoarchitecture and hence greater neuronal density have higher values for CMRO$_2$. Normal cortical CMRO$_2$ in the dog is 5.6 ml 100 g^{-1} min^{-1}, and in the rat, 10.9 ml 100 g^{-1} min^{-1}.[50]

Brain cortical tissue metabolite levels given in Table 2-2 point out preservation of ATP levels until hypoxic stress is severe. Glucose levels are well maintained even during maximum hypoxic activation of glycoly-

Table 2-2. Dimensions of cerebral metabolism*

Representative cortical energy metabolite levels, wistar rat, wet weight*	Glycogen	Glucose	Lactate	Phospho-creatine	ATP	NADH
Normoxia	2	3	1.5	5	3.0	0.015
Moderate Hypoxia EEG slowing	—	6	10	3.5	3.0	0.025
Lethal Hypoxia EEG isoelectric	—	4.5	30	1.0	1.5	0.040

*Dimensions are given in micromoles/gram.

sis, provided cerebral circulation is upheld. The objective in neuroanesthesia is to avoid the lethal hypoxic condition in which ATP levels are lowered. Those of us who have monitored electroencephalogram (EEG) during hypotensive anesthesia have doubtless seen periods of EEG isoelectricity during hypotensive overshoot. This condition cannot be permitted to persist for more than three or four minutes and is best avoided altogether.

Anesthesia and cerebral metabolic rate for oxygen

With this background, we turn to review available information describing effects of anesthesia upon $CMRO_2$. Three basic methods of measurement have been used, the Kety and Schmidt technique, the Rapella technique, and the *d*-oxyglucose technique of Sokoloff and Reivich. Each of these gives nearly quantitative data. An additional, less reliable method, the closed box technique of Lowry produces semiquantitative results. (See reference 23 for general discussion.)

Kety and Schmidt technique

This method of cerebral blood flow measurement is described in Chapter 1. It is based upon the law of conservation of matter and can provide absolutely quantitative data. By knowing the solubility of an indicator in brain tissue and the concentration of the indicator in arterial (capillary) blood after an appropriate equilibration period, one can calculate the concentration of indicator in brain tissue. Determination of arterial to cerebral venous content difference during the saturation period makes possible calculation of cerebral blood flow according to the Fick principle.

Having determined cerebral blood flow, one can then measure arterial to cerebral venous content differences for oxygen, glucose, lactate, and so on and determine cerebral uptake or production rates. The values represent average rates for the average tissue served by the sampled venous drainage. All of the data in humans are based on jugular bulb venous samples and are therefore representative of whole brain. Limitations of this method include requirement for steady state conditions and inability to measure regional changes.

Barbiturates

Table 2-3 presents representative data from Kety-Schmidt studies in humans. Thiobarbiturates in dosages producing marked sedation, so called "twilight sleep," do not alter $CMRO_2$.[31] In light plane anesthesia, where skin incision causes some movement, $CMRO_2$ is reduced by one-third.[62] When deep coma is induced so that electroencephalogram (EEG) becomes isoelectric, $CMRO_2$ is reduced by one-half.[44] Michenfelder, using the Rapella sagittal sinus outflow method in dogs having cardiopulmonary bypass, deter-

Table 2-3. Effect of anesthetic agents upon cerebral metabolic rate for oxygen in humans

Agent	Technique	Condition	$CMRO_2$ (ml² × 100 g⁻¹ × min⁻¹)	From control (%)
Thiopental	Kety and Schmidt	Awake	3.3	—
	N_2O; whole brain	Sedated	3.3	0
		Light (0.5-1.6 g IV)	2.1	36
		Isoelectric (0.2-3.8 g IV)	1.5	54
Nitrous oxide	Kety and Schmidt	Awake	3.09	—
	⁸⁵Kr; whole brain	70% N_2O	2.45	20
Morphine	Kety and Schmidt	Awake	3.09	10
Nitrous oxide	⁸⁵Kr; whole brain	70% N_2O	2.70	
		2 mg/kg morphine		
Halothane	Kety and Schmidt	Awake	2.98	26
	⁸⁵Kr; whole brain	1% in O_2	2.19	

mined that greater than 50% reduction in $CMRO_2$ could not be produced, even with massive doses of barbiturates.[37] He interprets this to indicate that barbiturates affect primarily energy-consuming processes related to neurophysiologic activity, which ceases at EEG isoelectricity. This phenomenon might, however, be explained by the logarhythmic nature of dose response, with increment of effect remaining linear when dose increment is in multiples. More recent studies from that laboratory have demonstrated alinear $CMRO_2$ dose response to several volatile anesthetics, with greatest decline in $CMRO_2$ in light planes.[57] Oxybarbiturates have comparable effects upon $CMRO_2$ as thiobarbiturates, and very low levels of $CMRO_2$ have been measured in barbiturate overdosage.

Very importantly, barbiturates reduce cerebral blood flow (CBF) at least as much as $CMRO_2$. Indeed, Lübbers found reduction in tissue oxygen tension during barbiturate anesthesia indicating reduction of CBF greater than reduction of $CMRO_2$. As discussed in the chapters on intracranial hypertension and on intensive care, this tendency to reduction of CBF is of great value for patients having intracranial hypertension. One must remember the cardiac depressant effect of barbiturates. We know of one instance in which brain extruding from an ax wound gave

ample evidence of intracranial hypertension, and barbiturate induction was promptly followed by cardiac collapse because there had been much bleeding from the scalp.

Nitrous narcotic

The nitrous oxide, narcotic, relaxant technique has become very popular in neuroanesthesia. Careful studies in humans show that $CMRO_2$ is only minimally reduced by nitrous oxide.[1,52,63] Animal studies have shown modest elevation of $CMRO_2$ in association with nitrous oxide.[47,60] Data describing $CMRO_2$ changes following morphine are in conflict. Seven male volunteers given 60 mg morphine sulphate intravenously over 10 minutes had $CMRO_2$ measured 10 to 35 minutes following completion of injection. No volunteer lost consciousness, though they were "somnolent," and no respiratory support was needed. $CMRO_2$ was reduced 41% and administration of nalorphine increased $CMRO_2$ toward control, with 17% depression of $CMRO_2$ remaining after 25 mg nalorphine intravenously.[40] In another carefully controlled study in humans, Jobes, Kennel and co-workers[27] found that a similar IV dose of morphine (1 mg/kg) produced only a 10% reduction in $CMRO_2$, and increasing the dose to 2 mg/kg caused no additional depression. Animal studies support the 10% figure, showing, in the dog, 17% reduction of $CMRO_2$ after 2 mg/kg morphine sulfate, 24% reduction of $CMRO_2$ after fentanyl (Sublimaze) and 14% reduction of $CMRO_2$ after meperidine (Demerol).[36,58]

As with barbiturates, narcotics have no tendency to produce cerebral hyperemia. CBF is reduced in parallel with $CMRO_2$. Because of their respiratory depressant effects, all narcotics tend to produce hypercapnia, and increased $Paco_2$ can produce increased intracranial pressure of such severity as to produce herniation of the brain at the tentorium or foramen magnum. Therefore, *narcotics should be omitted in preoperative medication for the patient having intracranial hypertension.*

Other intravenous agents

Ketamine produces a transient increase in cerebral oxygen consumption (16% following 2 mg/kg in the dog)[13] with simultaneous marked increase in CBF. By 30 minutes, both CBF and $CMRO_2$ return to control levels. In humans, ketamine, 3 mg/kg, intravenously produced a 60% increase in CBF but no measurable increase in $CMRO_2$.[59] Studies of effects of ketamine upon regional cerebral blood flow in humans show marked increases in frontal and parietal-occipital regions. As described in Chapter 8 on intracranial pressure, increased intracranial pressure occurs during ketamine anesthesia and may contraindicate use of the agent in patients with intracranial hypertension.

While althesin is not available in the United States, it has become a popular choice for neuroanesthesia in Europe. Its effects upon CBF and $CMRO_2$ appear to be identical to those of thiobarbiturates.[28]

Volatile agents

Halothane (Fluothane) and enflurane (Ethrane) have similar effects upon CBF and $CMRO_2$, each producing dose-related reduction of $CMRO_2$ accompanied by a state of relative hyperemia.[10,11,35,64] These drugs appear capable of depressing $CMRO_2$ more markedly than do thiobarbiturates. Michenfelder has shown that halothane can produce profound (10% of control) reduction in $CMRO_2$, which may be accompanied by abnormal tissue energy metabolite levels and which may be irreversible.[38] Fink observed similar effects of halothane upon liver slices. In light anesthesia, halothane and enflurane may reduce $CMRO_2$ 15% to 20%, while levels used to produce hypotensive anesthesia may lower $CMRO_2$ 50%. Enflurane may produce seizures, especially during deep enflurane combined with hypocapnia. During seizure, there is a sudden increase in cerebral arterial-to-venous oxygen content difference, probably indicating sudden increase in $CMRO_2$ as seen with other types of seizure.

The hyperemic effect of halothane and enflurane probably results from direct arteriolar dilatation. However, the time course indicates that the effect upon arteriolar muscle is not instantaneous, and the mechanism may involve alteration of the interrelationship between cerebral blood flow and local cerebral metabolism.[51] When arterial blood pressure is maintained with vasopressors during deep anesthesia, CBF is greatly increased. As discussed in Chapter 8 on intracranial pressure, this cerebral vasodilation can increase intracranial pressure to dangerous levels.

Other inhalation agents

Cyclopropane and diethylether have been found to have a biphasic effect upon cerebral oxygen consumption with greater degrees of reduction of $CMRO_2$ at low than at high dose levels.[2,65] These results are somewhat uncertain. In the case of cyclopropane, one of six volunteers studied had excessive reduction (10% of control) of $CMRO_2$ during 5% cyclopropane. Furthermore, a later study from the same laboratory found $CMRO_2$ reduced 23% during 20% cyclopropane rather than 11% reported in the study evidencing the biphasic effect.[52] We feel that evidence for the phenomenon is unconvincing.

Hypothermia

Hypothermia depresses $CMRO_2$ by about 5% per degree centigrade reduction in body temperature. This response is linear to 22° C in the rat, with $CMRO_2$ at 22° C being 25%

of normal.[21] Traditionally the effect of hypothermia upon metabolic rate is expressed as the factor by which metabolism is altered following a 10° C change in temperature (Q10). In humans, Q10 is probably about 2. If hypothermia is to be used clinically as a means for lowering $CMRO_2$, steps must be taken to prevent the stress response to cold. Whole body and probably cerebral oxygen consumption may be greater than normal during shivering.

EFFECT OF ANESTHETIC DRUGS UPON THE BALANCE BETWEEN ENERGY PRODUCTION AND ENERGY CONSUMPTION

Knowing the effect of anesthetic drugs upon brain oxygen consumption tells nothing of the adequacy of brain energy production relative to brain energy need. Early studies of Quastel and Wheatley were interpreted to show a "hypoxic" effect of anesthetic drugs, with energy production being inhibited. If this is so, an anesthetic state should produce the opposite of a protective effect; that is, one should detect some change in brain energy metabolite pattern toward that seen in hypoxia-ischemia as previously outlined in Table 2-2. If, on the other hand, anesthetics affect primarily energy-consuming processes, an opposite and more hopeful situation would exist. How does one evaluate "energy balance"? This will be considered in the following section.

Techniques for measuring energy metabolites

All of the intermediary energy metabolites have rapid turnover in brain tissue, and great care is required to avoid autolytic artifact in sampled tissue. Lactate level begins to increase and phosphocreatine to decrease in seconds when oxygen supply is interrupted. Some method for quick stopping metabolism is required, such as heat denaturation of enzyme systems by microwave irradiation or near-instantaneous freezing. Beginning with Kerr in 1935[29] many techniques have been developed, for example, superfusing exposed brain with liquid nitrogen or scooping out

brain tissue with cold curettes or application of cold probes to exposed cortex. Techniques for freezing unanesthetized animals have relied upon use of very small animals, such as mice, which can be totally immersed in liquid nitrogen.[9,15,19] A recently developed technique used in anesthesia research by Biebeck uses compressed CO_2 to blow the cranial contents through a small puncture hole, out against a plate cooled in liquid nitrogen (freeze blowing).[61] Techniques using animal immersion are not completely free from postmortem autolysis. The freeze-blowing technique does not permit separate sampling of different brain anatomic components and chiefly for this reason, we have preferred the technique of funnel freezing developed by Siesjo and Ponten, wherein a plastic funnel is affixed to the skull of a lightly anesthetized rat, and liquid nitrogen is poured into the funnel.[45,46] Brain tissue freezes in layers, with circulation being well maintained in advance of the freezing front. The entire brain can be examined, and numerous studies have shown that 70% nitrous oxide anesthesia has no measurable effect upon brain energy metabolism.

Defining energy state

As pointed out in the discussion of Table 2-2, ATP is preserved at the expense of phosphocreatine and ADP through the creatine phosphokinase and adenylate kinase reactions.

$$ATP \rightleftharpoons ADP + Pi \qquad (1)$$

$$PCr + ADP + H^+ \rightleftharpoons Cr + ATP \qquad (2)$$

$$ADP + ADP \rightleftharpoons ATP + AMP \qquad (3)$$

Because of this, ATP level is not a perfect indicator of tissue energy state. Phosphocreatine might serve as an early warning of energy imbalance (i.e., production of energy lower than consumption of energy). However, as seen in equation (2) above, the creatine phosphokinase reaction is pH sensitive, and alkalosis alone will produce an increase in phosphocreatine level, while acidosis will produce the opposite effect.[32] Lactate level, which may reflect relative increase in glycolysis in hypoxia-ischemia, is equally affected by pH in a complex manner.

$$Pyruvate + NADH + H^+ \rightleftharpoons lactate + NAD \quad (4)$$

Increase in hydrogen ion concentration tends to increase the ratio of lactate to pyruvate (equation 4); however, because of the hydrogen ion sensitivity of phosphofructokinase, the primary regulatory enzyme in glycolysis, the absolute level of lactate, and all other acidic metabolic intermediates change out of phase with hydrogen ion. Alkalosis increases brain tissue levels of lactate, pyruvate, glutamate, and many other organic acids, while acidosis has the opposite effect. Because of these considerations, a more desirable way to evaluate brain energy state is by means of the energy charge potential of Atkinson.[6]

EC (energy charge) =

$$\frac{(ATP) + 0.5 (ADP)}{(ATP) + (ADP) + (AMP)} \quad (5)$$

As seen in equation 5, this ratio indicates the degree to which brain adenosine is "charged" with high energy phosphates.

Effect of anesthetics upon energy state

While the observations of inhibition of in vivo brain tissue metabolism by anesthetics suggested an energy production block during anesthesia, early studies by Stone,[56] Mayman,[34] Gatfield,[18] Brunner,[9] and others showed an actual increase in brain tissue levels of glycogen and phosphocreatine and a decline in lactic acid levels. These findings

seem to suggest that anesthesia is a high energy state. However, the technique of tissue preparation in many of these studies permitted postmortem autolysis. This may have lowered glycogen and phosphocreatine and elevated lactate in control animals. Thus by preventing this energy run down, anesthetic reduction of brain energy use would appear to create a high energy state.

We have mentioned the effect of intracellular alkalosis upon lactate and phosphocreatine. Barbiturate anesthesia produces intracellular alkalosis. One should expect corresponding elevation of both phosphocreatine and lactate (equation 2 and equation 4). Phosphocreatine is slightly increased. Lactate, however, is considerably reduced. This is because glycolysis is slowed during barbiturate anesthesia by inhibition of phosphofructokinase. It is this inhibition of glycolysis that leads to reduction in metabolites subsequent to glucose 6 phosphate and causes the alkalosis.

As shown in Table 2-4, anesthesia with N_2O, halothane, and pentobarbital has no effect upon brain energy balance as reflected in energy charge potential.[42] This should indicate a potential protective effect in anesthetic reduction of brain energy consumption.

CEREBRAL PROTECTION WITH BARBITURATES

Arnfred and Secher in 1962 reported that pentobarbital prolonged the survival time in mice exposed to a hypoxic gas mixture.[5]

Table 2-4. Effect of anesthetic agents upon cerebral energy state*†

Agent and dose	PCr (mmol/kg)	Cr (mmol/kg)	ATP (mmol/kg)	ADP (mmol/kg)	AMP (mmol/kg)	ECP
Fentanyl (0.026 mg/kg subcutaneously)	4.96	6.28	3.08	0.287	0.022	0.951
N_2O (70% in O_2)	4.83	5.95	3.04	0.287	0.020	0.951
Halothane (1% in O_2)	4.97	5.93	3.05	0.284	0.022	0.951
Pentobarbital (60 mg/kg)	5.21	5.78	3.09	0.276	0.019	0.954

*From Nilsson, L., and Seisjo, B. K.: Influence of anaesthetics on the balance between production and utilization of energy in the brain, J. Neurochem. **23:**29, 1974.

†PCr, Phosphocreatine; Cr, creatine; ECP $= \dfrac{ATP + 0.5 (ADP)}{ATP + ADP + AMP}$

Their study was not conclusive, mainly because they did not control body temperature in the animal; this was the first suggestion that barbiturates might protect the brain during insufficient oxygen supply. Four years later, Goldstein and co-workers reported that pretreatment with pentobarbital in dogs prolonged the time of complete cerebral ischemia, after which recovery was possible.[20]

The mechanism for this protective effect was thought to be the decrease in cerebral metabolic rate that follows a decrease in body temperature. At this time, however, it was generally accepted that brain cells are extremely sensitive to lack of oxygen and that the cells die after three to five minutes of anoxia. Cerebral protection could, therefore, only be achieved with pretreatment, but once the damage had occurred, the brain cells were supposed to be dead and no therapy was possible. During the last ten years, however, several reports have been published indicating that the brain cells are more resistant to hypoxia and ischemia than was previously anticipated.

In 1968, Ames described what he called the "no reflow phenomenon."[4] Ames produced complete cerebral ischemia in rabbits by sectioning the basilar artery and inflating a pneumatic cuff around the neck of the animal. After the ischemic period, the cuff was released, carbon black was injected into the circulation, the animals were sacrificed, and the brains sectioned. Ames noticed that if the ischemic period had been five minutes or longer, there were areas of the brain that had not been reperfused. Ames suggested that perhaps brain cells, per se, are not extremely sensitive to lack of oxygen, but rather that secondary factors, that is, circulation, influence the pertinent brain damage.

Hossman and co-workers in 1973 reported, from work in cats and monkeys, that they could record a spontaneously returning EEG activity when the animals were allowed to recover after 60 minutes of complete ischemia.[26] This finding indicated that at least some brain cells had survived this severe insult. It is important to notice, however, that the Hossman group used pentobarbital sodium (Nembutal) anesthesia for their animals. Furthermore, as there was no circulation to the brain, the temperature dropped with time in the brain tissue. There are other reports, however, supporting the idea that brain cells can survive prolonged periods of hypoxia or ischemia.

Ljündgren in 1974 and Nordstrom in 1978 showed that brain cells can recover metabolically after up to 30 minutes of complete ischemia. These findings have revived the question as to whether or not it is possible to institute therapy to ameliorate brain damage after a lesion has occurred, that is, after a stroke or cardiac standstill. That barbiturates can be protective when given after a cerebral lesion was first demonstrated by Hoff and co-workers[25] in a stroke model using thiopental, 40 mg/kg, given 15 minutes after clamping of the middle cerebral artery in dogs. This significantly improved the neurologic outcome and also caused a smaller size infarction when compared to control animals. One year later, the same research group published a study in primates.[25] Baboons were anesthetized with halothane or pentobarbital prior to middle cerebral artery occlusion. Significantly less infarction was found in animals treated with pentobarbital 90 mg/kg or more. Although 60 mg/kg pentobarbital is a dose large enough to cause a flat EEG, it did not improve the neurologic outcome or decrease the size of the infarction. With pentobarbital, 90 mg/kg, and larger doses, there were severe circulatory side effects.

To minimize the barbiturate effects on the circulation, Michenfelder and co-workers[39] tried to divide the dose and give the drug over a longer period of time. They were able to show, in Java monkeys, that pentobarbital, 14 mg/kg, given 30 minutes after occlusion of the middle cerebral artery, followed by pentobarbital, 7 mg/kg, every 2 hours for 48 hours, significantly improved the neurologic outcome and decreased the size of the infarction compared to control animals.

In regional ischemia (stroke) there is good experimental evidence that barbiturates, both when given before and after the lesion, decrease the size of the infarction and improve the neurologic outcome. Pentobarbital, as well as thiopental, has been used with good results. The doses required to achieve protection in experimental animals have been large, but it has also been shown that the dose can be divided and given over a longer period of time. Barbiturate protection in regional ischemia appears to be an all-or-nothing response, and protective effects of small doses of barbiturates have not been demonstrated.

As yet, no one has been able to show any ameliorating effects of barbiturates given after a global ischemic or hypoxic cerebral insult. A preliminary communication reported improved neurologic outcome when large doses of thiopental were given 30 minutes after a global ischemic lesion in monkeys. As the control animals and the experimental animals had not been treated in the same manner, however, this study is not conclusive.[7,8]

There is today no clinical indication for treatment of cerebral insults with massive doses of barbiturates. "Thiopental loading" has been suggested for amelioration of brain damage after cardiac standstill. Since no protective effect has been demonstrated when barbiturates have been given after a global cerebral lesion, there is no evidence that such a treatment is even potentially beneficial. Theoretically, it would be possible to treat stroke patients with barbiturates. The doses required for protection in humans are not known. In all experimental studies, the doses required to achieve protection have been high, and there is no indication that the effective dose in humans would be lower.

Barbiturates have been used clinically to treat an increased intracranial pressure. The effect of barbiturates on the intracranial pressure, however, is probably mediated via their effect on the cerebral blood flow and not related to cerebral protection in hypoxia and ischemia.

MECHANISMS FOR CEREBRAL PROTECTION WITH BARBITURATES

Hypothermia, as well as barbiturates, has been shown to protect the brain in various hypoxic-ischemic models. Both hypothermia and barbiturates decrease cerebral metabolic rate, and the decrease in metabolism has generally been considered to be the main protective mechanism. Halothane also decreases cerebral metabolic rate; however, in a study on regional ischemia, halothane was not found to protect the brain. Unlike hypothermia and barbiturates, halothane is a vasodilator and increases cerebral blood flow. The increase in flow can contribute to edema formation. This in turn might explain why dogs under deep halothane anesthesia had a worse outcome than the awake, control animals.

Michenfelder and co-workers, based on their studies in dogs, postulated that anesthetics, including thiopental, alter $CMRO_2$ by altering neuronal electrical function only and not all of the energy-requiring processes in the cell. With a cessation of neuronal function (an isoelectric EEG), therefore, anesthetics would not have any further effect on cell metabolism, and no protective effect could be expected.[37]

Yatsu, however, injected methohexital in rabbits subjected to hypoxia and hypotension just as the EEG became flat.[66] He found that barbiturate-treated animals recovered without sequelae, while the control animals had severe brain damage. Hoff and co-workers found in their studies on a stroke model in monkeys that pentobarbital 60 mg/kg, which produced a flat EEG, was not protective, while animals that received pentobarbital, 90 mg/kg, were protected.[25] These results are in conflict with Michenfelder's postulation.

In another study, Michenfelder determined the quantitative relationship between the dose of thiopental and $CMRO_2$. He found that $CMRO_2$ decreases as the dose of barbiturate increases. The maximum decrease in $CMRO_2$ was 42%. Thereafter, despite continued infusion of thiopental, $CMRO_2$ did not decrease further. The point at which the curve leveled off was the same point at which a flat EEG was noted. In other words, in the presence of a flat EEG, no further decrease in $CMRO_2$ can be expected. If a decrease in $CMRO_2$ is the underlying mechanism in cerebral protection, then pentobarbital, 60 mg/kg, would have been expected to have the same protective effect as pentobarbital, 90 mg/kg, in the study of Hoff and co-workers.

In our study in rats, it was found that a 25% decrease in $CMRO_2$ produced by pentobarbital was not protective, while depression of $CMRO_2$ to the same degree by hypothermia gave good protection as judged by metabolic criteria in cerebral hypoxia.[22] Nordstrom and Rehncrona found that phenobarbital, given before the lesion, improved the recovery in rats after a severe ischemic lesion where the brain had been almost completely depleted of ATP for 25 minutes. Their conclusion is that, if barbiturates can protect the brain in a situation where there are no energy metabolites, thus no available energy, and very low blood flow to the brain, the main protective mechanism cannot be a decrease in $CMRO_2$ or cerebral blood flow. Other factors must be of major importance in cerebral protection.

One of the more recent proposed mechanisms for cerebral protection is that of free radical scavenging.[14] It has been suggested that the cell damage in hypoxia and ischemia is caused by free radicals. A free radical is any substance that has an unpaired electron in an outer orbit. Such highly reactive particles would presumably be formed in the respiratory chain in the mitochondria during hypoxia or ischemia. Oxygen is necessary for further free radical reactions. During the re-oxygenation after an hypoxic-ischemic insult, the free radicals would peroxidize the unsaturated fatty acids in the cell membrane and cause damage to the membrane. Several drugs have also been shown to scavenge free radicals in vitro; among them are barbiturates, vitamin C, and vitamin E.

It is important to stress that free radical reactions are very complicated, and since they are very rapid, they are too difficult to demonstrate. More research is, therefore, needed to find mechanisms of cell damage in cerebral ischemia and hypoxia. With more knowledge of these mechanisms, we hope it will be possible to find ways in which to ameliorate the effects of hypoxic-ischemic brain damage.

REFERENCES

1. Alexander, S. C., Smith, T. C., Strobel, G., and others: Cerebral carbohydrate metabolism of man during respiratory and metabolic alkalosis, J. Appl. Physiol. **24:**66, 1968.
2. Alexander, S. C., Colton, E. T., Smith, A. L., and others: The effects of cyclopropane on cerebral and systemic carbohydrate metabolism, Anesthesiology **32:**236, 1970.
3. Alexander, S. C., Smith, T. C., Strobel, G., and others: Cerebral carbohydrate metabolism of man during respiratory and metabolic alkalosis, J. Appl. Physiol. **24:**66, 1968.
4. Ames, A., III, Wright, R. L., Kowada, M., Thurston, J. M., and Majno, G.: Cerebral ischemia. II. The no-reflow phenomenon, Am. J. Pathol. **52:** 437, 1968.
5. Arnfred, I., and Secher, O.: Anoxia and barbiturates: tolerance to anoxia in mice influenced by barbiturates, Arch. Int. Pharmacodyn. Ther. **139:**67, 1962.
6. Atkinson, D. E.: The energy charge of the adenylate pool as a regulatory parameter, Bio-chemestry **7:** 4034, 1968.
7. Bleyaert, A. L., Nemoto, E. M., Stezpski, S. W., Alexander, H., and Safar, P.: Thiopental therapy after 16 minutes of global brain ischemia in monkeys, Crit. Care Med. **4:**130, 1976.
8. Bleyaert, A. L., Safar, P., Stezpski, S. W., Nemoto, E. M., and Moossy, J.: Amelioration of post-ischemic brain damage in the monkey by immobilization and controlled ventilation, Crit. Care Med. **6:**112, 1978.
9. Brunner, E. A., Passonneau, J. V., and Molstad, C.: The effect of volatile anesthetics on levels of metabolites and on metabolic rate in brain, J. Neurochem. **18:**2301, 1971.
10. Christiansen, M. S., Rasmussen, K., and Lassen, N. A.: Cerebral vasodilation by halothane anesthesia in man and its potentiation by hypotentiation by hypotension and hypocapnea, Br. J. Anaesthesiol. **39:**927, 1967.
11. Cohen, P. J.: The metabolic function of oxygen and biochemical lesions of hypoxia, Anesthesiology **148:**37, 1972.
12. Cohen, P. J., Wollman, H., Alexander, S. C., and others: Cerebral carbohydrate metabolism in man during halothane anesthesia, Anesthesiology **25:** 185, 1964.
13. Dawson, B., Michenfelder, J. D., and Theye, R. A.: Effects of ketamine on cerebral blood flow and metabolism: modification by prior administration of thiopental, Anesthesiology **50:**443, 1971.
14. Demopoulos, H. B., Milvy, P., Kakari, S., and Ransohoff, J.: Molecular aspects of membrane structure in cerebral edema. In Reulen, H. J., and Shurmann, K., editors: Steroids and brain edema, New York, 1972, Springer-Verlag, p. 29.
15. Ferrendelli, J. A., Gay, M. N., Sedgwick, W. G., and others: Quick freezing of the murine CNS: com-

parison of regional cooling rates and metabolite levels when using liquid nitrogen or freon-12, J. Neurochem. **19**:979, 1972.

16. Fink, B. R., and Haschke, R. H.: Anesthetic effects on cerebral metabolism, Anesthesiology **39**:199, 1973.

17. Folbergrova, J., Penten, U., Siesjo, B. K.: Patterns of changes in brain carbohydrate metabolites, amino acids and organic phosphates at increased carbon dioxide tension, J. Neurochem. **22**:1115-1125, 1974.

18. Gatfield, P. D., Lowry, O. H., Schulz, D. W., and others: Regional energy reserves in mouse brain and changes with ischaemia and anaesthesia, J. Neurochem. **13**:185, 1966.

19. Goldberg, N. D., Passonneau, J. V., and Lawry, U. H.: Effect of changes in brain metabolism on the levels of citric acid cycle intermediates, J. Biol. Chem. **241**:3997, 1966.

20. Goldstein, A., Jr., Wells, B. A., and Keats, A. S.: Increased tolerance to cerebral anoxia by pentobarbital, Arch. Int. Pharmacodyn. Ther. **161**:138, 1966.

21. Hagerdal, M., Harp, J. R., Nilsson, L., and others: The effect of hypothermia upon cerebral cortical blood flow and metabolism in the rat, J. Neurochem. in press.

22. Hagerdal, M., Welsh, F. A., Kegkhah, M. M., and others: Protective effects of ambitions of hypothermia and barbiturates in cerebral hypoxia, Anesthesiology in press.

23. Harp, J. R., and Siesjo, B. K.: Effects of anesthesia on cerebral metabolism, In Gordon, E., editor: A basis and practice of neuroanesthesia, New York, 1975, Exerpta Medica, pp. 83-116.

24. Heyman, A., Patterson, J. L., and Jones, R. W.: Cerebral circulation and metabolism in uremia circulation, **3**:588, 1951.

25. Hoff, J. T., Smith, A. L., Handinson, H. L., and Nielsen, S. L.: Barbiturate protection from cerebral infarction in primates, Stroke **6**:28, 1975.

26. Hossman, D.-A., and Kleihues, P.: Reversibility of ischemic brain damage, Arch. Neurol. **29**:375, 1973.

27. Jobes, D. R., Kennel, E., Bitner, R., and others: Effects of morphine nitrous oxide anesthesia on cerebral autoregulation, Anesthesiology **42**:30, 1975.

28. Keany, N. P., McDowall, D. G., Turner, J. M., and others: The time course of cerebral circulatory and metabolic changes with Althesin, Br. J. Anaesthesiol. **45**:117, 1973.

29. Kerr, S. E.: Studies on the phosphorus compounds of brain. I. Phosphorcreatine, J. Biol. Chem. **110**:625, 1935.

30. Kety, S. S., Polis, B. D., Nadler, C. S., and Schmidt, C. F.: The blood flow and oxygen consumption of the human brain in diabetic acidosis and coma, J. Clin. Invest. **27**:500, 1948.

31. Kety, S. S., Woodford, R. B., Harmel, M. H., and others: Cerebral blood flow and metabolism in schizophrenia, Am. J. Psychiatr. **104**:765, 1947-48.

32. MacMillan, B., and Seisjo, B. K.: The influence of hypocapnia upon intercellular pH and upon some

carbohydrate substrates and organic phosphates in the brain, J. Neurochem. **21**:1283, 1973.

33. Mangold, R., Sokoloff, L., Conner, E. L., Therman, P., and Kety, S. S.: The effects of sleep and lack of sleep in the cerebral circulation and metabolism in normal, young men, J. Clin. Invest. **34**:1092, 1955.

34. Mayman, C. J., Gatfield, P. D., and Breckenridge, B. M.: The glucose content of brain in anesthesia, J. Neurochem. **11**:483, 1964.

35. McHenry, L. W., Slocum, H. C., Owens, H. E., and others: Hyperventilation in awake and anesthetized man, Arch. Neurol. (Chic.) **12**:270, 1965.

36. Messick, J. M., and Theye, R. A.: Effects of pentobarbital meperidine on canine cerebral and total oxygen consumption rates, Can. Anaesthesiol. Soc. J. **16**:321, 1969.

37. Michenfelder, J. D.: The interdependency of cerebral functional and metabolic effects following massive doses of thiopental in the dog, Anesthesiology **41**:231, 1974.

38. Michenfelder, J. D.: Personal communication, 1978.

39. Michenfelder, J. D., Milde, J. H., and Sundt, T. M., Jr.: Cerebral protection by barbiturate anesthesia, Arch. Neurol. **33**:345, 1976.

40. Moyer, J. H., Pontius, R., Morris, G., and others: Effects of morphine and n-allynor-morphine on cerebral hemodynamics and oxygen metabolism, Circulation **15**:379, 1957.

41. Nemoto, E. M., Hoff, J. T., and Severinghouse, J. W.: Lactate uptake and metabolism by brain during hyperlactatemia and hypoglycemia, Stroke **5**:48, 1974.

42. Nilsson, L., and Seisjo, B. K.: Influence of anaesthetics on the balance between production and utilization of energy in the brain, J. Neurochem. **23**:29, 1974.

43. Owen, O. E., Reichard, G. A., Jr., Boden, G., and others: In Katzen, H. M., and Mahler, R. J., editors: Diabetes obesity and vascular diseases: metabolic and molecular interrelationships, vol. 2, New York, 1978, John Wiley & Sons, Inc., pp. 517-550.

44. Pierce, E. C., Lambertson, C. J., Deutsch, S., and others: Cerebral circulation and metabolism during thiopental anesthesia and hyperventilation in man, J. Clin. Invest. **41**:1664, 1962.

45. Ponten, U., Ratcheson, R. A., Salford, L. A., and others: Optimal freezing conditions for cerebral metabolites in rats, J. Neurochem. **21**:1127, 1973.

46. Ponten, U., Ratcheson, R. A., and Siesjo, B. K.: Metabolic changes in brains of mice frozen in liquid nitrogen, J. Neurochem. **21**:1121, 1973.

47. Sakabe, T., Kuramoto, T., Inove, S., and others: Cerebral effects of nitrous oxide in the dog, Anesthesiology **48**:195, 1978.

48. Schmidt, C. F., Kety, S. S., and Pennes, H. H.: The gaseous metabolism of the brain of the monkey, Am. J. Physiol. **143**:33, 1945.

49. Siesjo, B. K.: Metabolic control of intracellular pH, Scand, J. Clin. Lab. Invest. **32**:97-104, 1973.

50. Siesjo, B. K., Carlsson, C., Hagerdal, M., and others: Brain metabolism in the critically ill, Crit. Care Med. **4:**283, 1976.
51. Smith, A. L.: The mechanism of cerebral rasodilation by halothane, Anesthesiology **39:**581, 1973.
52. Smith, A. L., Neigh, J. L., Hoffman, J. C., and others: Effects of general anesthesia on autoregulation of cerebral blood flow in man, J. Appl. Physiol. **29:**665, 1970.
53. Smith, A. L., and Wollman, H.: Cerebral blood flow and metabolism: effects of anesthetic drugs and techniques, Anesthesiology **36:**378, 1972.
54. Sokoloff, L.: Circulation and energy metabolism of the brain. In Albers, R. W., Siegel, G. J., Katzman, R., and Agranoff, B. W., editors: Basic neurochemistry, ed. 1, Boston, 1972, Little, Brown and Co., pp. 299-325.
55. Sokoloff, L., Mangold, R., Wechsler, P. L., Kennedy, C., and Kety, S. S.: The effect of mental arithmetic on cerebral circulation and metabolism, J. Clin. Invest. **34:**1101, 1955.
56. Stone, W. E.: The effects of anaesthetics and of convulsants on the lactic acid content of the brain, Biochem. J. **32**(2):1908, 1938.
57. Stullken, E. H., Melde, J. H., Michenfelder, J. D., and others: The nonlinear responses of cerebral metabolism to low concentrations of halothane, enflurane, isoflurane, and thiopental, Anesthesiology **46:**28, 1977.
58. Takeshita, H., Michenfelder, J. D., and Theye, R. A.: The effects of morphine and n-allylnormorphine on canine cerebral circulation, Anesthesiology **37:**605, 1972.
59. Takeshita, H., Okuda, Y., and Atuo, D.: The effects of ketamine on cerebral circulatory and metabolic changes with althesin, Br. J. Anaesthesiol. **45:**117, 1972.
60. Theye, R. A., and Michenfelder, J. D.: The effect of nitrous oxide on canine metabolism, Anesthesiology **29:**119, 1968.
61. Veech, R. L., Harris, R. L., Veloso, D., and others: Freezeblowing: a new technique for the study of brain in vivo, J. Neurochem. **20:**183, 1973.
62. Wichsler, R. L., Dripps, R. D., and Kety, S. S.: Blood flow and oxygen consumption of the human brain during anesthesia produced by thiopental, Anesthesiology **12:**308, 1956.
63. Wollman, H., Alexander, S. C., Cohen, P. H., and others: Cerebral circulation during general anesthesia and hyperventilation in man, Anesthesiology **26:**329, 1965.
64. Wollman, H., Smith, A. L., and Hoffman, J. C.: Cerebral blood flow and oxygen consumption in man during electroencephalographic seizure patterns induced by anesthesia with Ethrane, Fed. Proc. **28:**356, 1969.
65. Wollman, H., Smith, A. L., and Punder, J. W.: Cerebral circulation and metabolism in man during general anesthesia with diethyl ether. Presented at The American Society of Anesthesiologists' Meeting, Washington, D.C., 1968.
66. Yatsu, F. M., Diamond, I., Graziano, C., and others: Experimental brain ischemia; protection from irreversible damage with a rapid acting barbiturate (Methohexital), Stroke **3:**726, 1972.

3

Cerebrospinal fluid mechanisms

GERALD HOCHWALD

The intracranial space is surrounded by the thick bones of the skull. The contents of this space can be divided into three fluid compartments: brain tissue water, cerebrospinal fluid (CSF), and intravascular blood. These compartments are contiguous and their volume changeable, but the contents are essentially incompressible. Within the framework of the Munro-Kellie doctrine the intracranial pressure does not rise if an increase or decrease in the size of one or more spaces is compensated for by equal and opposite changes in the size of the other space(s).[71] The intracranial space contains readily displaceable fluid in the form of blood and CSF. The intracranial blood volume is approximately 4%, and the CSF volume is 10% of the total intracranial volume.

Intracranial pressure may rise rapidly with increases in intravascular volume. The cerebral vasodilating effects of halothane and other volatile agents result in increases in cerebral blood flow and cerebral blood volume and may account for the increased intracranial pressure seen with anesthetic agents.[97,131] This response can increase intracranial pressure in the postinduction period. The elevated intracranial pressure is, however, of only limited duration. Compensatory adjustments that result in the return of intracranial pressure to normal values include a decrease in CSF volume and a fall in cerebral blood flow.[112] The degree to which compensatory mechanisms respond to changes in intracranial dynamics has been the subject of several symposia on intracranial pressure[14] and cerebral circulation and metabolism.[72]

By virtue of its larger volume, the capacity of the CSF to buffer increases if intracranial pressure is greater than that of cerebral intravascular blood. A net decrease in cerebrospinal fluid volume can be achieved by either an increase in CSF absorption rate, a decrease in CSF formation rate, or both. This chapter is intended to review some of the physiologic mechanisms of cerebrospinal fluid turnover. Other recent reviews* may be consulted for a more detailed account of specific aspects of related subjects, such as composition of CSF, regulation of CSF pH, physiologic functions regulated by CSF, and the pathophysiology of CSF in hydrocephalus.

CEREBROSPINAL FLUID SECRETION

Cerebrospinal fluid is continuously formed within the cerebral ventricles and is returned to the blood by way of the arachnoid villi. Although there is some argument concerning the exact sites of formation, the choroid plexus (Fig. 3-1) and the ependymal lining of the ventricle are considered the most likely sites. The secretory function of the choroid plexus can scarcely be doubted. In the plexus is an

---

*References 10, 20, 29, 74, 93, 124.

37

abundance of capillaries in close proximity to lining of epithelial cells containing microvilli on its apical CSF side, complex infoldings on the basal side, and tight junctions that encircle the apical ends of the epithelial cells and separate the CSF from the lateral intercellular spaces.[29,83] Despite the common embryologic origin of the epithelial cells lining the choroid plexus and the ventricles, it is doubtful whether these cells contain, at both of these sites, the same potential for secreting CSF. Except for tight junctions, the morphologic characteristics associated with the secretory function of the choroid plexus epi-

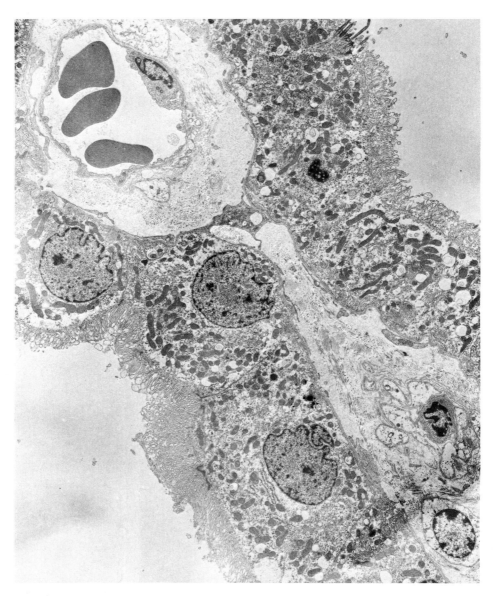

Fig. 3-1. Villus process from the choroid plexus of the lateral ventricle of a cat. The ependymal lining cells are located close to choroidal blood vessels and show a brush border at the ventricle surface. These cells contain numerous mitochondria and are separated from adjoining cells by extensions of the basal infoldings. (×6800.) (Courtesy Dr. H. Cravioto.)

thelium are wanting in the ventricular epithelium. If the brain is a source of CSF, then the fluid could be derived from the extracellular space. To prove this possibility it would be necessary to demonstrate in brain a source, a turnover, and a net flow of this fluid into the CSF compartment.

The composition of the fluid in the brain extracellular space is similar to that of CSF.[12,46] The mechanisms responsible for maintaining differences in composition between extracellular fluid and plasma at the blood-brain barrier and between CSF and plasma at the blood-CSF barriers seem to be similar. Therefore, both extracellular space fluid and choroid plexus fluid are products of secretion. Extrachoroidal sources of CSF include cerebral capillary endothelium,[87] which constitutes the blood-brain barrier to macromolecules, and the capillary-glia junction. Neither the sources nor the enzymic requirements for extrachoroidal CSF formation have been identified. It is also possible that the extracellular fluid is metabolic water derived from oxidative metabolism in the brain. It should be noted that any new statements on brain extracellular fluid as a source of CSF must take into consideration the fact that CSF formation has not been detected in the spinal subarachnoid space.[17,55,64]

Brain extracellular space fluid as a source of cerebrospinal fluid

A study of the turnover of brain extracellular fluid is very difficult. The extracellular space is small in diameter (180 Å), and the flow rate is probably too slow to allow direct physical measurement with present techniques. Cserr and her colleagues[19] made qualitative studies of the turnover of fluid in the brain by injecting dextran blue (MW 2 × 10⁶) intracerebrally as a visual marker for the bulk flow of extracellular fluid. This large-molecular-weight molecule has a low diffusion coefficient and a low permeability into cells. In 24 hours the injection site was characterized by a region of diffuse blue staining, some areas clearly continuous with larger blood vessels. They concluded that the movement of dye can be explained

neither by diffusion, as the distribution pattern is highly asymmetrical, nor by intracellular transport, as the pattern does not follow established fiber tracts. The most likely mechanism of dye movement, therefore, is bulk flow of extracellular fluid. Cserr and co-workers[22] also traced the movement of horseradish peroxidase after injection into the caudate nucleus. Results from electron microscopic analysis of the distribution of this protein suggested that extracellular fluid flowed from narrow intercellular clefts of the neuropil along a system of extracellular pathways, including perivascular and periventricular areas, and between fiber tracts (Fig. 3-2). It appeared that extracellular fluid drained into cerebrospinal fluid and possibly into fenestrated vessels within the brain.

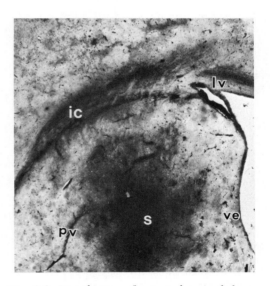

Fig. 3-2. Distribution of anionic horseradish peroxidase four hours after injection into the caudate nucleus demonstrating horseradish peroxidase near the injection site *(s)*, in the subependymal layer of the ventricular ependyma *(ve)*, at the dorsolateral angle of the lateral ventricle *(lv)*, surrounding the circumference of the caudate nucleus *(ic)*, and in a perivascular space *(pv)*. (30 μm section counterstained with hematoxylin and eosin, ×22.) (With permission from Cserr, H. F., Cooper, D. N., and Milhorat, T. H.: Exp. Eye Res. **25**(suppl.): 461, 1977. Copyright by Academic Press Inc. (London) Ltd.)

Quantitative measurements of fluid drainage from brain were also done to determine the brain efflux rate and route of injected radiolabeled extracellular markers, polyethylene glycol (MW 4,000) and dextran (MW 70,000). Cserr and co-workers[22] observed similar rates of removal of these markers from brain despite large differences in molecular weight. The results were consistent with removal from brain by bulk flow of extracellular fluid. A maximum of only 20% of the isotope cleared from brain could be recovered from CSF. This was thought to be in agreement with anatomic evidence that CSF may not be the sole route of extracellular fluid removal from brain.

Stern and colleagues[113] demonstrated a pathway in brain for the flow of extracellular fluid. In their experiments, they enhanced the volume flow of fluid by decreasing serum osmolality. Under these conditions, an increase in volume flow of CSF was also measured. Dextran blue was injected intracerebrally and the animals infused intravenously with anisotonic sucrose solutions. From observations made on dye patterns when serum osmolality was decreased, there is a movement of brain extracellular fluid, which contributes to the increase in CSF volume flow. Their conclusions were strengthened by the results of other experiments[119] in which quantitative estimations were made of the appearance in ventricular perfusion fluid of intracerebrally injected radiolabeled material.

Lymphaticlike function of cerebrospinal fluid

More than 50 years ago, Cushing[26] observed that the brain lacked a lymphatic system. It has been postulated that in its place CSF acts as "brain lymph" for removing lipid-insoluble substances and products of metabolism and transporting them back to the blood. It is important to demonstrate that a flow of brain extracellular fluid exists that drains the brain and is also part of the CSF circulation.[84]

There are some features of CSF such as composition and circulation that make a direct analogy between the function of the CSF and lymph somewhat difficult. As CSF composition is similar (Table 3-1) to that of brain extracellular fluid and both fluids are different from that of plasma, CSF formation from both choroidal and extrachoroidal sources are products of secretion. In organs other than those of the central nervous system the extracellular fluid is thought to be a filtrate of blood. The chemical composition of lymph is, therefore, similar to a filtrate of plasma. There are some unexplained inconsistencies concerning CNS extracellular fluid circulation. As indicated above, formation of CSF in the spinal subarachnoid space is undetectable. This suggests that a bulk flow of extracellular space fluid does not exist in this part of the central nervous system. With regard to the brain, however, circulation of this fluid in the spinal cord is more likely, but it becomes unclear how this fluid is returned to the blood.

Cerebrospinal fluid circulation

The circulation of CSF is not equal in the different CSF compartments. The rate and direction of CSF flow is dependent in part on the complex structure of the subarachnoid space, pressure gradients secondary to arterial and respiratory pulsations, and sudden changes in posture. CSF flows (Fig. 3-3) from its sources within the ventricles to the cisterna magna, where the cranial and spinal subarachnoid spaces are joined. Dandy and Blackfan[28] showed that dye injected into the lateral ventricles will appear within minutes in cisterna magna fluid. The fluid in the cisterna magna is continuous with that of the cranial and subarachnoid spaces. CSF is absorbed through the arachnoid villi of the dural sinuses. To reach those sinuses, fluid flows of necessity through the cranial subarachnoid space. Dye injection studies[65] show that cisterna magna fluid flows cephalad and basal around the brain stem and then toward the convexities of the cerebral and cerebellar cortex.

Some serious questions have been raised about the circulation of CSF in the spinal

Table 3-1. Composition of human cerebrospinal fluid, thoracic duct lymph, and serum*

	CSF	Lymph	Serum
Sodium (mEq/liter)	138.0	136.0	140.0
Potassium (mEq/liter)	2.8	3.5	4.0
Calcium (mEq/liter)	2.4	3.9	4.6
Magnesium (mEq/liter)	2.7	1.7	1.8
Chloride (mEq/liter)	124.0	100.0	99.0
Glucose (mg/dl)	60.0	95.0	90.0
Protein (g/dl)	0.015-0.050	4.89	7.08

*Average values derived from Fishman, R. A.: In Baker, A. B., and Baker, L. H., editors: Clinical neurology, vol. 1, 1973, Harper & Row, Publishers, and Yoffey, J. M., and Courtice, F. C.: Lymphatics, lymph and the lymphomyeloid complex, New York, London, 1970, Academic Press.

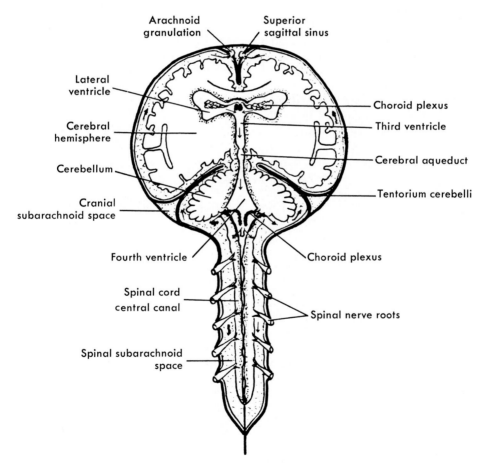

Fig. 3-3. Diagram of the pathways of the cerebrospinal fluid circulation. (Adapted from Millen and Woollam: The anatomy of the cerebrospinal fluid, London, New York, Toronto, 1962, Oxford University Press.)

subarachnoid space. Anatomic studies have shown the existence of spinal arachnoid villi in spinal nerve roots of humans,[56] dogs,[45] and monkeys.[129] It has been estimated on the basis of ventricular-to-lumbar subarachnoid space perfusion studies[17,55] and from brain compliance measurements[78] that only 10% to 15% of the total CSF absorption occurs in the spinal subarachnoid space. A small caudally directed flow in the spinal cord central canal was described in rabbits[12] but not in other species. In the immobile and intact animal, flow of CSF along the spinal cord is minimal.[54] It is likely that the forces involved in propagating CSF in cranial subarachnoid space are relatively ineffective in the spinal subarachnoid space. In experimental studies with immobilized, anesthetized cats, Grundy[54] saw, at laminectomy sites, very little movement of intrathecally injected dyes. Only when cats were shaken or tilted above the horizontal was there significant movement. (In the experimentally obstructed hydrocephalic cat,[44] however, the absorption of CSF occurs entirely in the spinal subarachnoid space.) In human studies with the aid of isotope scanning, Di Chiro[39] demonstrated that labeled protein passed up the lumbar subarachnoid space slowly but more rapidly than could be accounted for by diffusion.

The sluggish spinal CSF circulation was thought by Hochwald and co-workers[64] to be responsible for the protein concentration difference between cisterna magna and spinal subarachnoid space fluid in the cat. They concluded from determinations of albumin permeability coefficients of the two compartments that the higher protein concentration measured in the spinal subarachnoid space was due to a decreased rate of removal rather than an increased permeability to protein.

Cerebrospinal fluid absorption

As CSF is being continuously formed in the cerebral ventricles and as CSF pressure is relatively constant, it follows that there must be an absorption process that equals CSF formation. In 1875, Key and Retzius[70] suggested that Pacchionian bodies (arachnoid villi that are visible) protruding into venous sinuses were probably the site where CSF was returned to the blood. Weed's observations[123] on the localization of dye infused into the subarachnoid space provided evidence that the arachnoid villi are involved in CSF absorption. Although these sites are generally accepted, the mechanism by which CSF passes through these bodies is still controversial. In 1914, Cushing[25] thought the arachnoid villi had valves that permitted unidirectional movement of fluid into the blood of the sinuses. Subsequently, Weed[123] found no histologic evidence for this valvelike action and concluded that CSF passed into the venous sinuses by filtration. From experiments with monkeys, Welch and Friedman[127] proposed that the arachnoid villi consisted of a number of tubes varying in diameter from 4 to 12 μm. This structure provided a direct communication between the subarachnoid space and venous sinus and permitted a bulk flow of CSF back into the blood. When CSF pressure was lower than that of the venous sinuses, the channels in the arachnoid villi collapsed, and the back flow of blood into CSF was prevented. Welch and Pollay[128] also perfused particles of various sizes through arachnoid villi of excised dura mater and determined a limit to the size of the channels through which particulate matter could pass.

Results of electron microscopic analysis[2,3,105] suggested, however, that the arachnoid villi were covered by a membrane that was continuous with the endothelium of the venous sinus. These cells were joined by tight junctions, which made Welch's and Friedman's[127] and Welch's and Pollay's[128] findings of open channels connecting the subarachnoid space with the sinus doubtful. Therefore, a means other than a passive movement through potent channels was sought to explain how CSF, its content, and cells (under pathologic conditions) were transported back to the blood. This explanation had to include the findings of Heisey and co-workers[57] and of others[27,63] that CSF absorption increases linearly with increases in ventricular pressure. CSF absorption has been established as the means by which some poorly soluble substances not having access to a transport system exited the CSF compartment. (Conversely, the rates of disappearance of these test substances were used as evidence for bulk CSF absorption.) CSF absorption is driven by a hydrostatic force; under normal conditions CSF pressure exceeds that of the sagittal sinus.[108] Davson and co-workers[30] found that a difference in colloidal osmotic pressure between CSF and plasma had very little influence on CSF absorption rate. There appears to be no restriction to the movement of macromolecules such as dextran blue from CSF to blood.

The presence on arachnoid villi of an intact membrane separating CSF from the sagittal sinus seems to provide a formidable barrier to bulk absorption of CSF and passage of cells. Additional transport mechanisms such as pinocytosis[66] and energy-consuming processes[3] such as phagocytosis and degradation have been proposed. When Simmonds[110] injected isotope-labeled erythrocytes into the cisterna magna of dogs, intact erythrocytes appeared in the systemic circulation at a rate of 1% of the injected dose per hour. Similar results were obtained by Adams and Prawirohardjo.[1] When the arachnoid villi of these animals were examined, Alksne and Lovings[2] observed an accumulation of erythrocytes that were being degraded, but no fenestrations of the endothelial membrane were seen. Shabo and co-workers[105] showed that phagocytic activity developed in the core of arachnoid villi when homogenized brain tissue or horseradish peroxidase was injected into the subarachnoid space. With the aid of the electron microscope, Gomez and co-workers[51] observed that when the CSF-to-blood pressure gradient of monkeys and sheep was increased, the endothelial lining

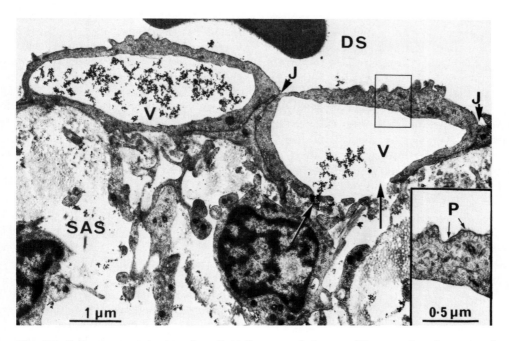

Fig. 3-4. Following an injection of a colloidally suspended tracer (Thorotrast) in the cisternal magna, the giant vacuoles *(V)* in the mesothelial lining of the arachnoid villus are readily filled with the tracer material. At this level of section, basal openings *(arrows)*, are seen in the vacuole on the right but not in the vacuole on the left. In contrast, the micropinocytotic vesicles *(P)* are essentially devoid of the tracer element, and no leakage is seen through the cell junction *(J)*. SAS, subarachnoid space; DS, dural sinus. (Transmission electron micrograph ×12,000; inset ×26,400.) (With permission from Tripathi, R. C.: Exp. Eye Res. **25**(suppl.):65, 1977. Copyright by Academic Press Inc. (London) Ltd.)

cells flattened and overlapping between them decreased. Gaps eventually developed between cells as the gradient increased further. The increased numbers of pinocytotic vesicles that appeared in the distended endothelial-lined tubules has also been advanced as the morphologic substrate of the pressure dependence of bulk flow drainage of CSF.[2,42,51,105]

Tripathi[115] has recently developed a theory of CSF drainage based on extensive light microscopic scanning and transmission electron microscopic examinations of the outflow pathway of the aqueous humor of the eye and CSF of the brain of mammals. There is a close similarity in formation and absorption of the fluid of the eye and brain. A search was made for pores in the membranes lining the canal of Schlemm and arachnoid villi through which fluid would drain the eye and brain. Tripathi[115] described giant vacuoles of several micrometers in size in the lining cells of both arachnoid villi and the Schlemm canal. These vacuoles (Fig. 3-4) were not considered to be artifacts but were thought to develop from invaginations of the basal cell surface. After gradual enlarging, the vacuoles open on the apical cell surface. This process (1) cleaves the cell, forming vacuolar transcellular channels that result in a dynamic system of pores, (2) is cyclical, (3) is hydrostatic pressure sensitive, and (4) controls the outflow of fluid and normal pressure by providing the requisite number of pores. Thus, in the absence of any other direct openings to explain the drainage of fluid, the vacuolar transcellular channels, and not micropinocytosis, phagocytosis, or passage through intercellular clefts, are thought to have the major role in the bulk flow of fluid across the arachnoid villi.

Methods to measure cerebrospinal fluid secretion

CSF formation has been studied by a variety of techniques. Most methods used were designed to study fluid formation from either choroidal or extrachoroidal sources. Ventriculocisternal perfusion is used most frequently because it is relatively easy to carry out and has been adapted for use in a variety of animals.[9,63,75,89,94] This method, however, measures total CSF production and cannot be used to determine fluid derived from either the choroid plexus or from the brain extracellular space. Perfusion of the cerebral ventricles was adapted by Pappenheimer and co-workers[89] for quantitative studies on CSF turnover. The ventricles of animals and humans[27] are perfused with an artificial spinal fluid containing a nondiffusible indicator substance, such as inulin, radiolabeled albumin, or dextran blue of known concentration. Perfusion is usually from the lateral ventricle to the cisterna magna of animals and at a known rate. From measurements of volume and of concentration of nondiffusible indicator substance in the fluid recovered from the cisterna magna, both CSF formation and absorption can be calculated. The rate of CSF formation, determined for a variety of species,[124] ranges from 350 $\mu l/min$ in humans[27,98] to 1.5 $\mu l/min$ in chickens.[7]

The technique of ventriculocisternal perfusion has also been used to measure the extrachoroidal formation of CSF. Curl and Pollay[23] perfused the isolated sylvian aqueduct of rabbits and found that in contrast to the results of others[4,86,102,125] the extrachoroidal contribution of fluid to the total CSF formation rate was greater than that of the choroid plexus. This result agreed primarily with that obtained during perfusion of previously plexecotomized animals.[82]

Rate of choroidal fluid secretion

Various techniques have been devised to measure CSF formation by the choroid plexus. These techniques have not been as popular because they require both extensive surgical manipulation and the development of microanalytical procedures.

With these methods, access to the choroid plexus is gained by removing the roof of either lateral ventricle. This preparation was used by Ames and co-workers[4-6] to collect and analyze nascent CSF from the cat's exposed choroid plexus. These investigators used a glass pipet to collect drops of newly formed fluid from the surface of the oil-covered choroid plexus. This method did not provide any quantitative data concerning

CSF formation rate by the choroid plexus. It did, however, demonstrate for the first time the role of the plexus in elaborating fluid and regulating CSF composition.

A more sophisticated technique was developed by Welch[125] for measuring CSF formation by the rabbit choroid plexus. Welch measured the secretion of fluid by determining the increase in hemoglobin concentration caused by the loss of fluid from blood flowing through the choroidal vessels. Hematocrit of plexus venous blood was compared with that of aortic blood. The choroidal vein was penetrated by micropuncture, and blood flow through these vessels was measured by timing the passage of spherules of 1-octanol over a measured length of vein. Thus, fluid formation by the choroid plexus was calculated as a product of choroidal blood flow and changes in hematocrit of choroidal venous blood. A mean blood flow of 2.86 cm^3/g was given, which was the first reported value of choroidal blood flow.

Several chambers were designed to encapsulate and isolate a part of the choroid plexus. These chambers fit around a portion of the plexus without interrupting the blood supply. Miner and Reed[86] used a chamber to encapsulate a portion of the exposed choroid plexus. They collected and analyzed the total fluid formed by that segment of plexus that was covered with oil and eliminated the possibility of exchange between newly formed fluid and the surrounding brain. Sahar[102] modified his capsule in order to perfuse its contents and measured CSF formation according to the same techniques and calculations used in ventriculocisternal perfusion.

In vitro preparations of the choroid plexus have been used to study movement of ions and nonelectrolytes across this organ. In the mounted tissue system the choroid plexus of the fourth ventricle is teased free from the surrounding brain and vascular supply and placed between two halves of a flux chamber. The ventricular surface of the plexus that is covered by ependymal cells is bathed by the fluid of one half of the chamber. The blood side of the plexus, which consists of blood vessels resting on connective tissue, is bathed by the fluid in the other half of the chamber. This technique has been used mainly by Wright and co-workers[134] to measure the rate of water flow and composition of nascent CSF by the frog choroid plexus. They developed procedures that allow nanoliter changes in volume of one chamber to be measured and a 0.1 to 0.5 nl sample of fluid to be analyzed for Na^+, K^+, and Cl^-. Welch and co-workers[126] used the roof membrane of the cat fourth ventricle (analogous to the frog's posterior choroid plexus) in a flux chamber to study potential difference across the membrane, conductance, ionic, and nonelectrolyte selectivity of the membranes. Criticisms aimed at in vitro preparations include edge damage of tissue mounted in the chamber, lack of response of CSF formation to acetazolamide (Diamox), unperfused blood vessels, and large unstirred layers.[104]

In the isolated choroid plexus preparation, the vessels are perfused with blood. This preparation removes some of the criticisms of the mounted choroid plexus method, inasmuch as blood vessels are perfused, unstirred layer effects are decreased, and so on. The choroid plexus of the sheep was used by Pollay and co-workers[95] to measure CSF secretion. Immediately after a sheep is killed, the brain is rapidly removed, and the internal carotid artery perfused with blood. The perfusion is limited to the anterior choroidal artery by ligating all vessels from the circle of Willis. The venous drainage is collected from the great vein of Galen. After the roof of the ventricle is reflected, the exposed choroid plexus is bathed with an artificial CSF. The preparation is technically difficult, and as nascent fluid is difficult to collect, CSF secretion is measured by the change in hematocrit of the blood perfusing the plexus.

Certain conclusions regarding the mechanism of CSF secretion by the choroid plexus have been reached from both in vivo and in vitro studies. A continuous volume of isotonic fluid is produced by the choroid plexus, which is coupled to the metabolic activity of its ependymal lining. The secretory activity of the choroid plexus has been established from the results of experiments in which it has been shown that flow continues against an osmotic gradient[16,57,120,130] and that metabolic inhibitors such as acetazolamide, ouabain, dinitrophenol[20,29,33,63,68] inhibit up to 70% of the total CSF formation. Welch,[125] Ames and co-workers[4] and Pollay and co-workers[95] showed that production of fluid by the plexus itself was virtually halted by acetazolamide. The remaining 30% is thought to be formed passively, flowing from brain extracellular space across the ventricular ependyma. If the extrachoroidal source of CSF is not affected by enzyme inhibitors (in contrast to the results of Curl and Pollay[23]), this fluid may be formed by hydrostatic forces in the cerebral capillaries. Hydrostatic forces may also play a role in CSF secretion by the choroid plexus. Davson[29] has proposed that the fluid made available for secretion by this organ arises as an ultrafiltrate from plasma.

The fraction of the total CSF formation rate attributed to either choroidal or extrachoroidal sources is still unresolved. From the descriptions of the methods used to examine this problem, it is easy to see how errors can be introduced by techniques that isolate this organ from its normal environment. Moreover, as pointed out by Welch,[124] calculations in these studies were often made from measurements of small differences between large quantities, and errors in measurement are subject to magnification. These reasons may explain why Welch,[125] Sahar,[102] and Miner and Reed[85] attribute to the choroid plexus virtually all of the CSF formation, while Curl and Pollay[23] and Milhorat[82] attribute only a relatively small fraction to it.

Mechanisms of fluid secretion by choroid plexus

The actual mechanism of CSF secretion by the choroid plexus is not completely understood. The forces involved in the movement of fluid from one body compartment to another belong to the more general problem of fluid transport across epithelial membranes. The secretory activity of the choroid plexus is linked to the metabolism of the epithelial lining. According to the epitheliologist (one who studies cell membranes by studying epithelial sheets rather than single cells), virtually all epithelia generate active transepithelial movement of solute.[35] This solute movement is accomplished by an osmotically coupled passive water flow.[36,38] In epithelia such as the choroid plexus the rate of water flow and movement of solute are such that the transported fluid is isotonic to the animal's plasma.[37] (An exception to this may be the recent results of Wright and co-workers,[134] who found that the frog choroid plexus mounted in a flux chamber secretes a hypertonic fluid.)

Most epithelial membranes are involved with secretion or absorption of fluid. The adjacent cells lining the membranes are joined to each other in a complex manner with the basal surfaces of the cells infolded.[92] The lateral and intercellular spaces are presently considered as important pathways for the coupling between salt and water and fluid flow. It has been proposed that an osmotic mechanism is responsible for the transport of water in transporting epithelium. As the fluid transported is isotonic, Diamond and Bossert[38] concluded that within the epithelium there is osmotic equilibrium between the transported solute and water. Curran and Mackintosh[24] and Patlak and co-workers[91] have described a double membrane model to account for isotonic water transport. The first of these in series membranes is relatively impermeable, and the second is very permeable to transported solute. An effective osmotic gradient is established by the active transport of solute across the first membrane. This gradient causes a flow of water, and the resultant hydrostatic pressure leads to a flow of isotonic fluid across the highly permeable membrane.

A more biologically acceptable model that takes the lateral spaces of adjacent epithelial cells into consideration was developed by Diamond and Bossert.[38] In epithelia such as the choroid plexus, morphologic tight junctions connecting adjacent ependymal cells were more leaky than thought. A paracellular shunt was therefore proposed to account for most of transepithelial ion conductance. Thus, these intercellular clefts can be penetrated by solute and are leaky because they are probably involved in coupling of water flow to actively transported solute. The standing gradient flow system is dependent on a long narrow channel, such as the basal infoldings of the cell or the lateral intercellular spaces, which are closed at one end. Lining the channels are pumps that determine the direction of the transported solute. In the "forward" operation system, which characterizes fluid-absorbing epithelia of the small intestine, solute is transported from the cell into the intercellular channel, making the channel fluid hypertonic. The solute diffuses down its concentration gradient toward the open end of the channel. Because the solute exerts an osmotic gradient, water enters the channel across its wall. A fluid of fixed osmolarity emerges from the open end and eventually passes into the blood. In the "backward" operation system, which characterizes secreting epithelia of the choroid plexus, solute is transported out of the intercellular channel, making the channel fluid hypotonic. The solute diffuses down its concentration gradient toward the closed end of the channel. Because of the osmotic pressure gradient, water leaves the channel across its wall. A fluid of fixed osmolarity will be secreted across its walls and into the CSF compartment.

The application of the standing osmotic gradient model to an understanding of the processes involved in CSF secretion by the choroid plexus presents some problems. The solute pumps are Na^+/K^+ dependent ATPase salt pumps that are responsible for the transport of sodium out of the intercellular clefts. Segal and Pollay[104] summarized some of the objections to the location of the sodium pumps. The salt-transporting regions are not limited but are spread throughout the intercellular clefts and into the basal infoldings of the ependymal cell. The tight junctions between the ependymal cells are probably leaky and may allow backflow of fluid. Other problems associated with this model include the means by which minor ion components and proteins are transported to CSF. Alternate, nonselective pathways for ions and vesicular pathways for proteins have been proposed.[104] Therefore, modifications to the standing gradient flow model have also been described.[100]

Segal and Pollay[104] have also made a summary of the processes that are thought to occur during CSF secretion by the choroid plexus cells and try to account for the movement of both ions and water. A filtrate of serum consisting of water, salts, and protein enters intercellular clefts and basal infoldings of the ependymal cells by capillary hydrostatic pressure. The composition of this fluid is altered as it passes through both cells and "leaky" tight junctions to become CSF. Sodium is pumped into the cell by pumps located in the walls of the clefts. A local osmotic gradient is created in this manner and draws water into the cell. Chloride can enter the cell coupled to sodium or can pass through the tight junction as a shunt pathway. Bicarbonate is formed within the cell by carbonic anhydrase, and both hydrogen and potassium ions are pumped back out of the cell as counter ions for the sodium pump. Ions present in CSF in lesser concentrations can pass through the tight junctions or have individual transport mechanisms. Protein is transported by the vesicle system of the cell.

On the apical surface of the ependyma cells[96] sodium pumps transport this ion out of the cell. A local osmotic gradient develops that draws water from the cell. It is not completely clear, however, how salt and water can couple on this side of the cell. Channels such as the intercellular clefts do not exist, and localized hypertonicity can therefore not be sufficiently maintained to draw water out of the cell. The microvilli present on this cell surface may, however, serve in this capacity and allow coupling between salt and water across the cell membrane.

Composition of cerebrospinal fluid

The concentrations and distribution ratios of ions between CSF and plasma[5,6,29] (Table 3-1) are significantly different from a dialysate of plasma. The difference in electrical potential between CSF and blood, measured in both mammalian[58] and nonmammalian species,[90] was thought to have an influence on the distribution of ions. The potential is, however, independent of pH of CSF or brain and only slightly dependent on CSF K^+ content.[58] This information lends strong support to the idea that CSF is secreted and not a product of passive ultrafiltration. In their studies on the sampling and analysis of newly formed choroid plexus fluid from the cat, Ames and co-workers[6] and Miner and Reed[85] found Na^+ at a slightly higher concentration in both nascent and mixed fluid than in a plasma dialysate. In mixed CSF the elevated concentration of Cl^- and lowered concentrations of HCO_3^- and K^+ may be imposed upon the fluid after it is secreted. Ca^{++} and Mg^{++} are subject to active homeostatic regulation by the choroid plexus.[13] The removal of Ca^{++} is thought to be independent of its CSF concentration[52] and occurs with a transport mechanism. The response of potassium in new choroidal fluid to changes in plasma concentration is not proportional.[4] The concentration of glucose in newly formed choroid plexus fluid of rabbits is similar to that of mixed fluid and is approximately 60% of that in blood.[101] This ratio remains constant until blood glucose is elevated to more than 15 to 20 mM. The transport mechanism[94] responsible for the movement of glucose from the cerebral ventricles to the surrounding brain and blood is thought by Brøndsted[15] to be Na^+-dependent and ouabain-sensitive. This transport mechanism may be located in the choroid plexus.[18]

CSF proteins are derived from serum; their concentration increases from 15 to 45 mg/100 ml in CSF samples taken from sites along the neuraxis from the cerebral ventricles to the spinal subarachnoid space.[81] Two proteins are present in higher concentration in human CSF than in blood.[61] They seem to be synthesized outside the central nervous system, but their function is unknown.[60]

FACTORS AFFECTING CEREBROSPINAL FLUID SECRETION

The effects of chemicals and physical factors on CSF formation were studied to learn something of the nature of the secretory process. Notably ouabain and acetazolamide were rather extensively investigated in this regard. The effects of acetazolamide on the

H^+-Na^+ exchange in the renal tubule and of cardiac glycosides on Na^+/K^+ activated ATPase are known. Acetazolamide effects on CSF dynamics were initially investigated by Tschirgi and co-workers,[116] who showed a decrease in both CSF pressure and CSF flow in experimental animals. After intravenous injection of 100 mg/kg of this drug reduction of CSF formation by 40% to 60% was found in a variety of animals[32,63,88] and in humans.[27,98] Acetazolamide was equally effective when it was alternately included in the mock CSF during ventriculocisternal perfusion[32] at a concentration of 0.2 to 1 mg/ml. Ames and co-workers[4] and Welch and co-workers[130] noted particularly that CSF secretion by the choroid plexus was markedly reduced. In their preparation of the exposed choroid plexus, fluid formation by this organ was inhibited when acetazolamide was either injected parenterally or applied topically. The Na^+ turnover rate in CSF, which is based largely on CSF turnover,[31,48] is also reduced. Wright,[132] however, was not able to show that acetazolamide inhibited the movement of Na^+ across the mounted, isolated choroid plexus of the frog.

Carbonic anhydrase inhibitors

The means by which acetazolamide reduces CSF formation is not yet clear. Insufficient information is available on how carbonic anhydrase is directly involved with the transfer of fluid and electrolytes. Macri and co-workers[76] argued that acetazolamide constricted choroidal blood vessels, implying that CSF production may be limited by the blood flow to this organ. However, Pollay and co-workers[95] observed that acetazolamide did not cause any increase in resistance to blood flowing through an in vitro preparation of the sheep choroid plexus, and yet CSF secretion was inhibited. In a series of studies on the transport rates of Na^+, Cl^-, and HCO_3^- from plasma to CSF, Maren[77] concluded that HCO_3^- formation from CO_2 is an essential feature of CSF secretion. This process is linked to 40% of the sodium transport. The inhibition of carbonic anhydrase by acetazolamide points to HCO_3^- formation rather than transport at the choroid plexus. The effect of acetazolamide on Na^+ and fluid production is therefore secondary to the drug's effect on HCO_3^- formation.

Cardiac glycosides

The choroid plexus contains large amounts of Na^+/K^+-activated ATPase,[11] and significant reductions in both CSF formation and enzyme activity were found when cardiac glycosides were applied topically to the plexus.[118] By inhibiting this enzyme activity and sodium transport, cardiac glycosides decrease fluid secretion. Both Ames and co-workers[4] and Welch[125] were able to show decreases in CSF formation with their exposed in situ choroid plexus preparation, as were Cserr[21] and Graziani and co-workers[53] when ouabain was added to the perfusion fluid during ventriculocisternal perfusion. Wright and co-workers[134] virtually inhibited CSF volume flow when ouabain was added to the ventricular compartment of their mounted frog choroid plexus preparation. When injected intravenously, ouabain produces toxic effects to the cardiovascular system before the necessary blood level is reached to effect secretion.

Effect of steroids

The inhibitory effects of steroids on CSF secretion have been demonstrated in cats[50] and dogs.[79,103] A reduction of CSF formation by approximately 50% is thought to be related to steroid inhibition of Na^+/K^+-activated ATPase activity in the choroid plexus and brain.[79]

Effects of other drugs

The effects of a number of other drugs on CSF formation have been examined—some because of effects on sodium transport; others because of effects on protein synthesis. Amiloride,[33,43] spironolactone (Aldactone),[33,43] furosemide (Lasix),[33,107] ethacrynic acid,[33,85] and vasopressin[33,43] reportedly decreased CSF formation rate. Not all of these results, however, have been confirmed; Wright[133] could not show an effect of furosemide, amiloride, or vasopressin on the frog choroid plexus, while Segal (quoted in Segal

and Pollay[104]) found ethacrynic acid ineffective on CSF formation and sodium transport in the rabbit. Actinomycin D, puromycin, or cyclohexamide were shown by Davson and Segal[33] to have no effect. Dinitrophenol was found to inhibit CSF production[20,29] and ependymal secretion[23] in the rabbit. However, Welch[125] could not show any consistent effect of this drug on the exposed choroid plexus.

Influence of temperature

The influence of changing body temperature on CSF formation rate was studied in several animal species. Most authors found that CSF formation declined with decreasing temperature.[34] Large reductions in body temperature (5° to 8° C) lowered formation rate by as much as 60%.[117] Fenstermacher and co-workers[47] virtually inhibited CSF production at a body temperature of 15° C. In cats undergoing ventriculocisternal perfusion, Snodgrass and Lorenzo[111] showed that between 41° C and 31° C, an 11% decrease in CSF formation was measured for every 1° change. They postulated that hypothermia decreases CSF secretion by the effects of temperature on either chemical reactions or cerebral blood flow. It is not clear, however, which mechanism has a greater influence on secretion.

Effect of hydrostatic pressure

The question of whether CSF formation rate is sensitive to changes in intraventricular hydrostatic pressure is still largely unresolved. Earlier studies on the effects of increased pressure were inconclusive inasmuch as techniques were not available to measure CSF formation independently of CSF absorption. Heisey and co-workers[57] subsequently adapted the method of ventriculocisternal perfusion to study CSF turnover. They demonstrated in goats that an intraventricular pressure of between -10 and 30 cm H_2O pressure had no influence on CSF production. Similar findings were reported by others using a variety of animals and humans. However, Calhoun and co-workers[16] and Frier and co-workers,[49] with calves, and Hochwald and Sahar,[59] with cats and rabbits, found a decrease in CSF formation with pressure under comparable conditions. When intraventricular pressure of cats was raised from -10 to $+25$ cm H_2O, Hochwald and Sahar[59] found that CSF formation rate decreased approximately 50%. Using an in situ preparation of the choroid plexus, Sahar[102] also demonstrated that CSF secretion rate in an isolation chamber is sensitive to pressure. Hochwald and Sahar[59] argued that in those experiments[9,57] in which the effects of ventricular pressure on CSF formation rate was examined the results were not statistically significant, because of the relatively small increments of pressure used to influence CSF secretion. The effect of pressure on formation was more apparent when the influence of larger pressure changes was measured in the same animal. Welch[124] has proposed that ventricular pressure may decrease CSF formation rate by reducing filtration from choroidal capillaries.

Effect of serum osmolality

Changes in osmolality of either ventricular fluid or serum are very effective means of altering CSF formation rate. DiMattio and co-workers[41] examined the effect of serum osmolality alteration on CSF bulk flow and brain water content. They infused glucose solutions of various osmolalities intravenously and measured CSF bulk flow with ventriculocisternal perfusion. Infusions of glucose in concentrations greater than 6 g/dl decreased fluid bulk flow rate. Glucose in concentrations less than 6 g/dl increased fluid bulk flow rate. At the extremes of induced serum osmolarities (290 and 360 mosmol/l), bulk flow rate was either increased more than double or was completely inhibited. Under the conditions of their experiments, brain cortical gray and white matter water content of cats increased when the infused glucose solution was 2.5 g/dl or less. Water content decreased when the infused solution was 10 g/dl or more. It was also observed that the infusion of either a 10 g/dl or 2.5 g/dl glucose solution alters serum osmolarity by 10%

or approximately 32 mosmol/l. Stern and Coxon[114] similarly found that guinea pig brain water content was affected only when plasma osmolarity was changed by 45 mosmol/kg H_2O. DiMattio and co-workers[41] concluded from these experiments that the increased bulk flow into the ventricles comes from the brain rather than directly from the blood. Evidence to support this conclusion was obtained from experiments[62] in which the effects of changes in serum osmolarity on bulk flow of fluid were studied under conditions in which CSF formation by the choroid plexus was partially or completely inhibited. Inhibition was accomplished either metabolically with acetazolamide or osmotically by perfusion with a hyposmolar (10 mosmol/l) solution. The results of those studies indicated that the increased bulk flow caused by a decrease in serum osmolarity is the same when the choroid plexus is or is not functioning. Thus Hochwald and co-workers[62] postulated that the apparent ease by which water passes from brain to CSF may explain the relative "resistance" of the brain to swelling during water intoxication.[40,99,122] Brain edema fluid caused by water intoxication may be vented to the CSF compartment, from where it is returned to the blood via bulk absorption. Thus, in water intoxication the sink action of CSF circulation may limit the degree to which water can accumulate in the structurally intact brain.

Influence of ventricular fluid osmolality

On the CSF side of the blood-CSF barrier, an osmotic gradient is also effective in altering CSF volume flow rate. However, the coefficient of osmotic flow obtained by altering perfusion fluid osmolality was 25% of that obtained by changing serum osmolality. The larger coefficient was probably the result of the differences of the relative brain-CSF and blood-CSF interface areas. Both Heisey and co-workers[57] and Welch and co-workers[130] were able to demonstrate a volume accretion into ventricular hypotonic perfusion or bathing fluid. The ability of the secretory process to move water uphill (against an osmotic gradient) was thus demonstrated. Curl and Pollay[23] also measured a volume flow of fluid into a hypotonic perfusion fluid and provided presumptive evidence for an extrachoroidal source of fluid, the underlying mechanism of which may be secretory. An increase in CSF volume flow into a hypertonic fluid was also shown. It is not clear to what extent choroidal or extrachoroidal sources of fluid are affected by increased ventricular fluid osmolality. Heisey and coworkers[57] attributed the increased flow rates, measured during perfusion of the ventricular system with hypertonic fluids, to osmotic flow through the ependymal walls of the ventricles. However, Welch and co-workers[130] have demonstrated that a 2.2-fold increase in bulk flow across the choroidal ependyma was possible when mannitol was substituted for NaCl in the fluid that bathed the choroid plexus. In a more extensive study of the influence of ventricular fluid osmolality on CSF turnover, Wald and co-workers[120] examined the effects of ventricular fluid osmolality on the bulk flow of nascent fluid into the cerebral ventricles of cats during ventriculocisternal perfusion. In their experiments, the newly formed fluid consisted of both CSF and fluid that resulted from an osmotic gradient between ventricular fluid and the blood and/or brain. Perfusions were carried out with solutions containing either sucrose, urea, or NaCl with osmolalities ranging from 6 to 780 mosmol. Differences between the normal bulk flow rate of nascent CSF and bulk flow rate measured during perfusion with anisotonic solutions were linearly related to corresponding differences in osmolality of the effluent fluid from the ventricles. The coefficients of osmotic flow were similar when sucrose and NaCl were used and were greater than when urea was used. During ventricular perfusion with sucrose, when effluent osmolality increased by 200 mosmol, bulk flow rate of nascent fluid increased by 200% of normal. Flow was undetectable when the effluent osmolality was 190 mosmol. Intravenous injection of acetazolamide reduced these coefficients to similar values for NaCl and for urea. In all experimental conditions no changes were found in cerebral water content. The authors concluded from their results that the increased bulk flow that occurs during perfusion with hypertonic solutions originates from the choroid plexus.

CLINICAL IMPLICATIONS

The results of recent experiments on the physiology of the cerebrospinal fluid make it increasingly apparent that despite the origin of the fluid from blood, CSF circulation and composition are independently regulated. This regulatory mechanism is probably indispensable in providing neurons with a fluid whose contents are essential for the normal function of these cells. The newly formed choroid plexus fluid contains electrolytes and nonelectrolytes in concentrations that are different from mixed CSF sampled at the cisterna magna. These substances enter the CSF compartment together with nascent CSF, and their concentrations in this fluid are further altered after its secretion. As noted above, this mechanism was used to explain the elevated concentration of Cl^- and lowered concentrations of HCO_3^- and K^+.

CSF is formed continuously and probably has a dual source. It is easy to reconcile the secretory process of the choroid plexus with its morphology; however, the mechanism responsible for the extrachoroidal flow of fluid is still unclear. CSF is in close communication with the fluid of the brain extracellular space. As flow is continuous and unidirectional, the fluid is probably important in the removal of metabolic waste produced by cells. CSF can function both in its "sink action" to limit the concentration in brain of various substances, including water, introduced into the blood and as a medium for the transport of humoral messages. For these and other reasons, a lymphatic role of the CSF was perceived. Similar to lymph, CSF is absorbed at a site distant from its origin. An obstruction to the flow of CSF results in the excessive accumulation of fluid—hydrocephalus. The pathophysiology of hydrocephalus has been recently reviewed by Welch.[124]

Osmotic disequilibrium states

An osmotic disequilibrium between blood and brain is not an uncommon clinical occurrence. Thus, clinical states associated with serum hypo-osmolarity can occur with pharmacologic agents (diuretics), excessive amounts of water, hypoglycemic agents, inappropriate secretion of large amounts of antidiuretic hormone, and so on. Hyperosmolarity is often the result of renal failure, hyperglycemia, or other conditions where more water than solute is lost from the body. Induced hyperosmolarity can be employed therapeutically to reduce intracranial pressure in patients with brain swelling. Commonly used agents include urea, mannitol, or glycerol. These substances are effective because they withdraw water from normal brain and thereby provide more room for the swollen brain. An osmotic pressure gradient between blood and brain can be readily established because of the presence of a rate-limiting barrier in the brain.[67] The barrier impedes the net movement into brain of electrolytes and other hydrophilic, osmotically active substances injected into the blood. The effectiveness of this osmotic pressure gradient is dependent mainly upon the rate in which the osmotically active material is injected and the ability of the substances to be excluded from the brain.

Hypo-osmolarity or hyponatremic states have been analyzed in greater detail in humans and animals[8] because of the association of these states with neurologic symptoms and with death. Reports on changes in both brain water and electrolyte content of experimental animals are conflicting, but this may be due to the species used or to the techniques employed to lower serum osmolarity. The most common method employed to induce and maintain a lowered serum osmolarity[99,122] is a subcutaneous injection of vasopressin followed by water injected either intraperitoneally or through a nasogastric tube. If the decrease in serum osmolarity is greater than 10%, an increase in brain water content will result.[62,114] When the induced serum-to-brain osmotic pressure gradient is large, death may ensue. If the animal survives this treatment and the water intoxication is continued, there is an adaptation to the osmotic disequilibrium. Under these conditions and in one to three days, brain edema increases, and there is some loss of brain potassium. Over a longer period of time, there is a greater loss of brain K^+, Na^+, and Cl^- and a decrease in brain osmolar content.[8] Neurologic symptoms are thought to occur when there is imbalance between brain water gain and brain electrolyte loss.

Effects of cerebrospinal fluid acid-base changes

In a review of CSF physiology, Plum and Siesjö[93] and Siesjö[109] summarized recent information on both the regulation of CSF pH and on the effects of CSF pH changes on cerebral blood flow and pulmonary ventilation. The mechanisms that regulate the pH of CSF include active transport of HCO_3^-, pH-dependent changes on both pulmonary ventilation and cerebral blood flow, and changes in CSF-to-plasma HCO_3^- ratio. Much of the recent work on factors determining CSF pH stemmed from experiments of Leusen,[73] who showed an increase in pulmonary ventilation when the cerebral ventricles were perfused with fluid high in P_{CO_2} or low in HCO_3^-. In a search for a neurogenic center regulating respiration, central nervous system chemoreceptors were localized on the ventrolateral surface of the medulla.[46] These receptors were shown to respond to changes in the pH of the brain extracellular space fluid.

Increased intracranial pressure

The measurement of CSF pressure in patients with intracranial pathology provides relatively little information about intracranial pressure dynamics. Marmarou and co-workers[78] have emphasized that the major parameters that control the resting level and rate of change of intracranial pressure are compliance of the CSF space (ratio of change in volume to the corresponding change in pressure) and resistance to absorption of CSF. A pressure-volume curve can be obtained by injecting or withdrawing known volumes into or out of the CSF space and measuring the corresponding rise or fall in pressure. For purposes of analysis, Marmarou and co-workers[78] have defined resistance as the difference in CSF and venous exit pressures divided by the rate of outflow. It should be noted that the determination of the outflow resistance is the basis of the intrathecal infusion test devised by Katzman and Hussey[69] to identify those patients with normal pressure hydrocephalus who will respond to CSF shunting.

Within limits, changes in either intracranial blood volume or CSF volume will be compensated for by an equal and opposite change in the volume of the other. Thus, a small increase in volume can be tolerated with only a small increase in intracranial pressure. In the presence of space-occupying lesions (cerebral edema, tumors, hematomas), the capacity of the intracranial space to compensate for an increase in volume declines. At high CSF pressure, the decrease in compliance is responsible for the marked increase in pressure that occurs with a net increase in volume, while at low CSF pressure the same increase in volume is followed by only a small rise in pressure. In patients with space-occupying lesions, increases in either the volume of intracranial blood or of the lesion produce increases in intracranial pressure that can compromise brain blood flow. Cerebral vasodilatation resulting from the use of certain volatile anesthetics or from increases in the partial pressure of CO_2 in blood can therefore have a deleterious effect on these patients.

The management of increased intracranial pressure in patients with a variety of conditions ranging from head trauma to Reye syndrome has become increasingly significant. Different modes of therapy have incorporated a variety of physiologic principles derived from neurology, anesthesiology, and neurosurgery. Some of the medical therapies involving the anesthetist in the treatment of increased intracranial pressure include hyperventilation, muscle paralysis, hypothermia, and barbiturate coma. The therapeutic goals of these approaches are to reduce intracranial pressure by (1) reducing arterial P_{CO_2} and maintaining adequate arterial P_{O_2} by controlled respiration and (2) reducing brain metabolic rate by hypothermia and barbiturate coma.[106]

REFERENCES

1. Adams, J. E., and Prawirohardjo, S.: Fate of red blood cells injected into cerebrospinal fluid pathways, Neurology **9**:561, 1959.
2. Alksne, J. F., and Lovings, E. T.: Functional ultrastructure of the arachnoid villus, Arch. Neurol. **27**:371, 1972.
3. Alksne, J. F., and White, L. E., Jr.: Electron-microscope study of the effect of increased intracranial pressure on the arachnoid villus, J. Neurosurg. **22**:481, 1965.
4. Ames, A., III, Higashi, K., and Nesbett, F. B.: Effects of P_{CO_2}, acetazolamide and ouabain on volume and composition of choroid-plexus fluid, J. Physiol. (Lond) **181**:516, 1965.
5. Ames, A., III, Higashi, K., and Nesbett, F. B.: Relation of potassium concentration in choroid-plexus fluid to that in plasma, J. Physiol. (Lond) **181**:506, 1965.
6. Ames, A., Sakanoue, M., and Endo, S.: Na^+, K^+, Ca^{2+} Mg^{2+} and Cl^- concentrations in choroid plexus fluid and cisternal fluid compared with plasma ultrafiltrate, J. Neurophysiol. **27**:672, 1964.
7. Anderson, D. K., and Heisey, S. R.: Clearance of molecules from cerebrospinal fluid in chickens, Am. J. Physiol. **222**:645, 1972.
8. Arieff, A. I., Llach, F., Massry, S. G.: Neurological manifestations and morbidity of hyponatremia: correlation with brain water and electrolytes, Medicine **55**:121, 1976.
9. Bering, E. A., Jr., and Sato, O.: Hydrocephalus: changes in formation and absorption of cerebrospinal fluid within the cerebral ventricles, J. Neurosurg. **20**:1050, 1963.
10. Bito, L. Z., Davson, H., and Fenstermacher, J. D., editors: Exp. Eye Res. **25**(suppl), 1977.
11. Bonting, S. L., Simon, K. A., and Hawkins, N. M.: Studies on sodium-potassium-activated adenosine triphosphatase. I. Quantitative distribution in several tissues of the cat, Arch. Biochem. Biophys. **95**:416, 1961.
12. Bradbury, M. W. B., and Lathem, W.: A flow of cerebrospinal fluid along the central canal of the spinal cord of the rabbit and communications between this canal and the sacral subarachnoid space, J. Physiol. **181**:785, 1965.
13. Bradbury, M. W. B., and Sarna, G. S.: Homeostasis of the ionic composition of the cerebrospinal fluid, Exp. Eye Res. **25**(suppl):249, 1977.

14. Brock, M., and Dietz, H., editors: Intracranial pressure, experimental and clinical aspects, Berlin, Heidelberg, New York, 1972, Springer-Verlag.
15. Brønsted, H. E.: Transport of glucose, sodium, chloride and potassium between the cerebral ventricles and surrounding tissues in cats, Acta Physiol. Scand. 79:523, 1970.
16. Calhoun, M. C., Hurt, H. D., Eaton, H. D., Rousseau, J. E., Jr., and Hall, R. C., Jr.: Rates of formation and absorption of cerebrospinal fluid in Holstein male calves, Storrs Agricultural Experiment Station, The University of Connecticut, Storrs, 1967, Bull. 401.
17. Coben, L. A., and Smith, K. R.: Iodide transfer at four cerebrospinal fluid sites in the dog: evidence for spinal iodide carrier transport, Exp. Neurol. 23:76, 1969.
18. Csaky, T. Z., and Rigor, B. M.: The choroid plexus as a glucose barrier, Prog. Brain Res. 29:147, 1967.
19. Cserr, H. F.: Bulk flow of cerebral extracellular fluid as a possible mechanism of CSF-brain exchange. In Cserr, H. F., Fenstermacher, J. D., and Fencl, V., editors: Fluid movement of the brain, New York, San Francisco, London, 1975, Academic Press, Inc.
20. Cserr, H. F.: Physiology of the choroid plexus, Physiol. Rev. 51:273, 1971.
21. Cserr, H.: Potassium exchange between cerebrospinal fluid, plasma and brain, Am. J. Physiol. 209:1219, 1965.
22. Cserr, H. F., Cooper, D. N., and Milhorat, T. H.: Flow of cerebral interstitial fluid as indicated by the removal of extracellular markers from rat caudate nucleus, Exp. Eye Res. 25(suppl):461, 1977.
23. Curl, F. D., and Pollay, M.: Transport of water and electrolytes between brain and ventricular fluid in the rabbit, Exp. Neurol. 20:558, 1968.
24. Curran, P. F., and Mackintosh, J. R.: A model system for biological water transport, Nature (Lond) 193:347, 1962.
25. Cushing, H.: Studies on the cerebrospinal fluid. I. Introduction, J. Med. Res. 31:1, 1914.
26. Cushing, H.: The third circulation, London, 1926, Oxford University Press.
27. Cutler, R. W. P., Page, L., Galicich, J., and Watters, G. V.: Formation and absorption of cerebrospinal fluid in man, Brain 91:707, 1968.
28. Dandy, W. E., and Blackfan, K. D.: Internal hydrocephalus, an experimental clinical and pathological study, Am. J. Dis. Child 8:406, 1914.
29. Davson, H.: Physiology of the cerebrospinal fluid, London, 1967, Churchill-Livingstone.
30. Davson, H., Hollingworth, J., and Segal, M. D.: The mechanism of drainage of the cerebrospinal fluid, Brain 93:665, 1970.
31. Davson, H., and Luck, C. P.: The effect of acetazolamide on the chemical composition of the aqueous humour and cerebrospinal fluid of some mammalian species and on the rate of turnover of ^{24}Na in these fluids, J. Physiol (Lond) 137:279, 1957.
32. Davson, H., and Pollay, M.: Influence of various drugs on the transport of ^{131}I and PAH across the cerebrospinal-fluid-blood barrier, J. Physiol. (Lond) 167:239, 1963.
33. Davson, H., and Segal, M. B.: The effects of some inhibitors and accelerators of sodium transport on the turnover of ^{22}Na in the cerebrospinal fluid and the brain, J. Physiol. (Lond) 209:131, 1970.
34. Davson, H., and Spaziani, E.: Effect of hypothermia on certain aspects of the cerebrospinal fluid, Exp. Neurol. 6:118, 1962.
35. Diamond, J. M.: The epithelial junction: bridge, gate and fence, Physiologist 20:10, 1977.
36. Diamond, J. M.: The mechanism of isotonic water transport, Symp. Soc. Exp. Biol. 19:329, 1965.
37. Diamond, J. M., and Bossert, W. H.: Functional consequences of ultrastructural geometry in "backwards" fluid-transporting epithelia, J. Cell Biol. 37:694, 1968.
38. Diamond, J. M., and Bossert, W. H.: Standing-gradient osmotic flow: a mechanism for coupling of water and solute transport in epithelia, J. Gen. Physiol. 50:2061, 1967.
39. Di Chiro, G.: Movement of the cerebrospinal fluid in human beings, Nature (Lond) 204:290, 1964.
40. Dila, C. J., and Pappius, H. M.: Cerebral water and electrolytes, an experimental model of inappropriate secretion of antidiuretic hormone, Arch. Neurol. (Chic) 26:85, 1972.
41. DiMattio, J., Hochwald, G. M., Malhan, C., and Wald, A.: Effects of changes in serum osmolarity on bulk flow of fluid into cerebral ventricles and on brain water content, Pflügers Arch. 359:253, 1975.
42. Domer, F. R.: Basic physiology of cerebrospinal fluid outflow, Exp. Eye Res. 25(suppl):323, 1977.
43. Domer, F. R.: Effects of diuretics on cerebrospinal fluid formation and potassium movement, Exp. Neurol. 24:54, 1969.
44. Eisenberg, H. M., McLennan, J. E., Welch, K., and Treves, S.: Radioisotope ventriculography in cats with kaolin-induced hydrocephalus, Radiology 110:399, 1973.
45. Elman, R.: Spinal arachnoid granulations with special reference to the cerebrospinal fluid, Bull. Johns Hopkins Hosp. 34:99, 1923.
46. Fencl, V., Miller, T. B., Pappenheimer, J. R.: Studies on the respiratory response to disturbances of acid-base balance, with deductions concerning the ionic composition of cerebral interstitial fluid, Am. J. Physiol. 210:459, 1966.
47. Fenstermacher, J. D., Li, C. L., and Levin, V. A.: Extracellular space of the cerebral cortex of normo-

thermic and hypothermic cats, Exp. Neurol. **27:** 101, 1970.

48. Fishman, R. A.: Factors influencing the exchange of sodium between plasma and cerebrospinal fluid, J. Clin. Invest. **38:**1698, 1959.

49. Frier, H. I., Gallina, A. M., Rousseau, J. E., Jr., and Eaton, H. D.: Rates of formation and absorption of cerebrospinal fluid in the very young calf, J. Dairy Sci. **55:**339, 1972.

50. Garcia-Bengochea, F.: Cortisone and the cerebrospinal fluid of noncastrated cats, Am. Surg. **31:** 123, 1965.

51. Gomez, D. G., Potts, G., Deonarine, V., and Reilly, K. F.: Effects of pressure gradient changes on the morphology of arachnoid villi and granulations of the monkey, Lab. Invest. **28:**648, 1973.

52. Graziani, L., Escriva, A., and Katzman, R.: Exchange of calcium between blood, brain, and cerebrospinal fluid, Am. J. Physiol. **208:**1058, 1965.

53. Graziani, L. J., Kaplan, R. K., Escriva, A., and Katzman, R.: Calcium flux into CSF during ventricular and ventriculocisternal perfusion, Am. J. Physiol. **213:**629, 1967.

54. Grundy, H. F.: Circulation of cerebrospinal fluid in the spinal region of the cat, J. Physiol. **163:**457, 1962.

55. Hammerstad, J. P., Lorenzo, A. V., and Cutler, R. W. P.: Iodide transport from the spinal subarachnoid fluid in the cat, Am. J. Physiol. **216:** 353, 1969.

56. Hassin, G. B.: Villi (Pacchionian bodies) of the spinal arachnoid, A.M.A. Arch. Neurol. Psychiatr. **23:**65, 1930.

57. Heisey, S. R., Held, D., and Pappenheimer, J. R.: Bulk flow and diffusion in cerebrospinal fluid system of the goat, Am. J. Physiol. **203:**775, 1962.

58. Held, D., Fencl, V., and Pappenheimer, J. R.: Electrical potential of cerebrospinal fluid, J. Neurophysiol. **27:**942, 1964.

59. Hochwald, G. M., and Sahar, A.: Effect of spinal fluid pressure on cerebrospinal fluid formation, Exp. Neurol. **32:**30, 1971.

60. Hochwald, G. M., and Thorbecke, G. J.: Autoradiography of immunoelectrophoresis in the study of the sites of formation of trace proteins in biological fluids. In Peeters, H. U. B., editor: Protides of the biological fluids, New York, 1962, Elsevier.

61. Hochwald, G. M., and Thorbecke, G. J.: Use of an antiserum against cerebrospinal fluid in demonstration of trace proteins in biological fluids, Proc. Soc. Exp. Biol. Med. **109:**91, 1962.

62. Hochwald, G. M., Wald, A., and Malhan, C.: The sink action of cerebrospinal fluid volume flow, Arch. Neurol. **33:**339, 1976.

63. Hochwald, G. M., and Wallenstein, M.: Exchange of albumin between blood, cerebrospinal fluid, and brain in the cat, Am. J. Physiol. **212:**1199, 1967.

64. Hochwald, G. M., Wallenstein, M. C., and Mathews, E. S.: Exchange of proteins between blood and spinal subarachnoid fluid, Am. J. Physiol. **217:**348, 1969.

65. Ingraham, F. D., Matson, D. D., Alexander, E., and Woods, P. P.: Studies in the treatment of experimental hydrocephalus, J. Neuropathol. **7:** 123, 1948.

66. Karnovsky, M. J., and Shea, S. M.: Transcapillary transport by pinocytosis, Microvasc. Res. **2:**353, 1970.

67. Katzman, R., Graziani, L., Ginsberg, S.: Cation exchange in blood, brain and CSF. In Lajtha, A., and Ford, D. H., editors: Progress in brain research, vol. 29, Amsterdam, 1968, Elsevier.

68. Katzman, R., Graziani, L., Kaplan, R., and Escriva, A.: Exchange of cerebrospinal fluid potassium with blood and brain; Study in normal and ouabain perfused cats, Arch. Neurol. **13:**513, 1965.

69. Katzman, R., and Hussey, F.: A simple constant-infusion manometric test for measurement of CSF absorption. I. Rationale and method, Neurology **20:**534, 1970.

70. Key, G., and Retzius, A.: Anatomie des nerven-systems und des bindegewebes, Stockholm, 1875.

71. Langfitt, T. W.: Pathophysiology of increased ICP. In Brock, M., and Dietz, H., editors: Intracranial pressure, experimental and clinical aspects, Berlin, Heidelberg, New York, 1972, Springer-Verlag.

72. Langfitt, T. W., McHenry, L. C., Jr., Reivich, M., and Wollman, H., editors: Cerebral circulation and metabolism, New York, Heidelberg, Berlin, 1975, Springer-Verlag.

73. Leusen, I. R.: Chemosensitivity of the respiratory center, Influence of CO_2 in the cerebral ventricles on respiration, Am. J. Physiol. **176:**39, 1954.

74. Leusen, I.: Regulation of cerebrospinal fluid composition with reference to breathing, Physiol. Rev. **52:**1, 1972.

75. Levin, V. A., Milhorat, T. H., Fenstermacher, J. D., Hammock, M. K., and Rall, D. P.: Physiological studies on the development of obstructive hydrocephalus in the monkey, Neurology (Minneap) **21:**238, 1971.

76. Macri, F. J., Politoff, A., Rubin, R., Dixon, R., and Rall, D.: Preferential vasoconstriction properties of acetazolamide on the arteries of the choroid plexus, Int. J. Neuropharmacol. **5:**109, 1966.

77. Maren, T. H.: Ion secretion into cerebrospinal fluid, Exp. Eye Res. **25**(suppl):157, 1977.

78. Marmarou, A., Shulman, K., and LaMorgese, J.: Compartmental analysis of compliance and outflow resistance of the cerebrospinal fluid system, J. Neurosurg. **43:**523, 1975.

79. Mayman, C. I.: Inhibitory effect of dexamethasone on sodium-potassium activated adenosine triphosphatase of choroid plexus in cat and rabbit, Fed. Proc. **31:**591, 1972 (abstract).

80. McDowall, D. G., Barker, J., and Jennett, W. B.: Cerebrospinal fluid pressure measurements during anaesthesia, Anaesthesia **21**:189, 1966.

81. Merritt, H. H., and Fremont-Smith, F.: The cerebrospinal fluid, Philadelphia, 1937, W. B. Saunders Co.

82. Milhorat, T. H.: Choroid plexus and cerebrospinal fluid production, Science **166**:1514, 1969.

83. Milhorat, T. H.: Structure and function of the choroid plexus and other sites of cerebrospinal fluid formation, Int. Rev. Cytol. **47**:225, 1976.

84. Milhorat, T. H.: The third circulation revisited, J. Neurosurg. **42**:628, 1975.

85. Miner, L. C., and Reed, D. J.: Composition of fluid obtained from choroid plexus tissue isolated in a chamber in situ, J. Physiol. (Lond) **227**:127, 1972.

86. Miner, L. C., and Reed, D. J.: The effect of ethacrynic acid on Na$^+$ uptake into the cerebrospinal fluid of the rat, Arch. Int. Pharmacodyn. Ther. **190**:316, 1971.

87. Oldendorf, W. H.: The blood-brain barrier, Exp. Eye Res. **25**(suppl):177, 1977.

88. Oppelt, W. W., Patlak, C. S., Zubrod, C. G., and Rall, D. P.: Ventricular fluid production rates and turnover in elasmobranchii, Comp. Biochem. Physiol. **12**:171, 1964.

89. Pappenheimer, J. R., Heisey, S. R., Jordan, E. F., and Downer, J. de C.: Perfusion of the cerebral ventricular system in unanesthetized goats, Am. J. Physiol. **203**:763, 1962.

90. Patlak, C. S., Adamson, R. H., Oppelt, W. W., and Rall, D.: Potential difference of the ventricular fluid in vivo and in vitro in the dogfish, Life Sci. **5**:2011, 1966

91. Patlak, C. S., Goldstein, D. A., and Hoffman, J. F.: Flow of solute and solvent across a two membrane system, J. Theor. Biol. **5**:426, 1963.

92. Pease, D. C.: Infolded basal plasma membranes found in epithelia noted for their water transport, J. Biophys. Biochem. Cytol. vol. 2, suppl 203, 1956.

93. Plum, F., and Siesjö, B. K.: Recent advances in CSF physiology, Anesthesiology **42**:708, 1975.

94. Pollay, M., and Davson, H.: The passage of certain substances out of the cerebrospinal fluid, Brain **86**:137, 1963.

95. Pollay, M., Stevens, A., Estrada, E., and Kaplan, R.: Extracorporeal perfusion of choroid plexus, J. Appl. Physiol. **32**:612, 1972.

96. Quinton, P. M., Wright, E. M., and Tormey, J. M.: Localization of sodium pumps in the choroid plexus epithelium, J. Cell Biol. **58**:724, 1973.

97. Rich, M., Scheinberg, P., and Belle, M. S.: Relationship between cerebrospinal fluid pressure changes and cerebral blood flow, Circ. Res. **1**:389, 1953.

98. Rubin, R. C., Henderson, E. S., Ommaya, A. K., Walker, M. D., and Rall, D. P.: The production of cerebrospinal fluid in man and its modification by acetazolamide, J. Neurosurg. **25**:430, 1966.

99. Rymer, M. M., and Fishman, R. A.: Protective adaptation of brain to water intoxication, Arch. Neurol. (Chic) **28**:49, 1973.

100. Sackin, H., and Boulpaep, E. L.: Models for coupling of salt and water transport, proximal tubular resorption in Necturus kidneys, J. Gen. Physiol. **66**:671, 1975.

101. Sadler, K., and Welch, K.: Concentration of glucose in new choroidal cerebrospinal fluid of the rabbit, Nature **215**:884, 1967.

102. Sahar, A.: The effect of pressure on the production of cerebrospinal fluid by the choroid plexus, J. Neurol. Sci. **16**:49, 1972.

103. Sato, O.: The effect of dexamethasone on cerebrospinal fluid production rate in the dog, Brain Nerve (Tokyo) **19**:485, 1967.

104. Segal, M. B., and Pollay, M.: The secretion of cerebrospinal fluid, Exp. Eye Res. **25**(suppl):127, 1977.

105. Shabo, A. L., Abbott, M. M., and Maxwell, D. S.: The response of the arachnoid villus to an intracisternal injection of autogenous brain tissue, an electron microscopic study in the macaque monkey, Neurology **19**:724, 1969.

106. Shapiro, H. M., Whyte, S. R., and Loeser, J.: Barbiturate-augmented hypothermia for reduction of persistent intracranial hypertension, J. Neurosurg. **40**:90, 1974.

107. Shaywitz, B. A., Katzman, R., and Escriva, A.: CSF formation and ^{24}Na clearance in normal and hydrocephalic kittens during ventriculocisternal perfusion, Neurology **19**:1159, 1969.

108. Shulman, K., Yarnell, P., and Ransohoff, J.: Dural sinus pressure in normal and hydrocephalic dogs, Arch. Neurol. **10**:575, 1964.

109. Siesjö, B. K.: The regulation of cerebrospinal fluid pH, Kidney Int. **1**:360, 1968.

110. Simmonds, W. J.: The absorption of labelled erythrocytes from the subarachnoid space in rabbits, Aust. J. Exp. Biol. Med. Sci. **31**:77, 1953.

111. Snodgrass, S. R., and Lorenzo, A. V.: Temperature and cerebrospinal fluid production rate, Am. J. Physiol. **222**:1524, 1972.

112. Sorensen, S. C., and Gjerris, F.: Adaptation of intraventricular pressure to acute changes in brain volume, Exp. Eye Res. **25**(suppl):387, 1977.

113. Stern, J., Hochwald, G. M., Wald, A., and Gandhi, M.: Visualization of brain interstitial fluid movement during osmotic disequilibrium, Fogarty Center Symposium on Ocular and Cerebrospinal Fluids, Washington, D.C., Exp. Eye Res. **25**(suppl):475, 1977.

114. Stern, W. W., and Coxon, R. V.: Osmolarity of brain tissue and its relation to brain bulk, Am. J. Physiol. **206**:1, 1964.

115. Tripathi, R. C.: The functional morphology of the outflow systems of ocular and cerebrospinal fluids, Exp. Eye Res. **25**(suppl):65, 1977.

116. Tschirgi, R. D., Frost, R. W., and Taylor, J. L.: Inhibition of cerebrospinal fluid formation by a carbonic anhydrase inhibitor, 2-acetylamino-1, 3, 4-thidiazole-5-sulfonamide (Diamox), Proc. Soc. Exp. Biol. Med. **87**:373, 1954.

117. Tsugane, R.: The production rate of cerebrospinal fluid under hypothermia, Brain Nerve (Tokyo) **20**:901, 1968.

118. Vates, T. S., Bonting, S. L., and Appelt, W. W.: Na-K activated adenosine triphosphatase and formation of cerebrospinal fluid in the cat, Am. J. Physiol. **206**:1165, 1964.

119. Wald, A., Hochwald, G. M., and Gandhi, M.: Evidence for the movement of fluid, macromolecules, and ions from the brain extracellular space to the CSF, Brain Res. **151**:283, 1978.

120. Wald, A., Hochwald, G. M., and Malhan, C.: The effects of ventricular fluid osmolality on bulk flow of nascent fluid into the cerebral ventricles of cats, Exp. Brain Res. **25**:157, 1976.

121. Wallace, G. B., and Brodie, B. B.: The distribution of iodide, thiocyanate, bromide and chloride in the central nervous system and spinal fluid, J. Pharmacol. Exp. Ther. **65**:220, 1939.

122. Wasterlain, C. G., Posner, J. B.: Cerebral edema in water intoxication, Arch. Neurol. (Chic) **19**:71, 1968.

123. Weed, L. H.: Studies on cerebro-spinal fluid. III. The pathways of escape from the subarachnoid spaces with particular reference to the arachnoid villi, J. Med. Res. **31**:51, 1914.

124. Welch, K.: The principles of physiology of the cerebrospinal fluid in relation to hydrocephalus including normal pressure hydrocephalus. In Friedlander, J., editor: Advances in neurology, vol. 13, New York, 1975, Raven Press.

125. Welch, K.: Secretion of cerebrospinal fluid by choroid plexus of the rabbit, Am. J. Physiol. **205**:617, 1963.

126. Welch, K., Araki, H., and Arkins, T.: Electrical potentials of the lamina epithelialis choroidea of the fourth ventricle of the cat in vitro: relationship to the CSF blood potential, Dev. Med. Child Neurol. **14** suppl 27:146, 1972.

127. Welch, K., and Friedman, V.: The cerebrospinal fluid valves, Brain **83**:454, 1960.

128. Welch, K., and Pollay, M.: Perfusion of particles through arachnoid villi of the monkey, Am. J. Physiol. **201**:651, 1961.

129. Welch, K., and Pollay, M.: The spinal arachnoid villi of the monkeys cercopithecus aethiops sabaeus and macaca irus, Anat. Rec. **145**:43, 1963.

130. Welch, K., Sadler, K., and Gold, G.: Volume flow across choroidal ependyma of the rabbit, Am. J. Physiol. **210**:232, 1966.

131. Wollman, H., Alexander, S. C., Cohen, P. J., Chase, P. E., Melman, E., and Behar, M. G.: Cerebral circulation of man during halothane anesthesia, Anesthesiology **25**:180, 1964.

132. Wright, E. M.: Ion transport across the frog posterior choroid plexus, Brain Res. **23**:302, 1970.

133. Wright, E. M.: Mechanisms of ion transport across the choroid plexus, J. Physiol. (Lond) **266**:545, 1972.

134. Wright, E. M., Wiedner, G., Rumrich, G.: Fluid secretion by the frog choroid plexus, Exp. Eye Res. **25**(suppl):149, 1977.

4

Intracranial pressure monitoring and interpretation

HUMBERT G. SULLIVAN
DONALD P. BECKER

On the basis of nearly ten years of experience with ICP monitoring in patients, it is our opinion that continuous monitoring of ICP has improved the management of patients with a broad spectrum of neurologic disease—brain tumor, head injury, intracranial aneurysm, Reye syndrome, stroke, and hydrocephalus. In some circumstances monitoring of ICP allows diagnosis of intracranial mass lesion (edema, recurrent hematoma) before the patient develops clinical symptoms. In these cases one is able to perform appropriate studies to define the etiology of increased ICP and then to treat the underlying cause of ICP elevation before the patient suffers adverse consequences. When elevated ICP is associated with clinical symptoms, therapy may be directed against the intracranial hypertension to reverse the adverse symtomatology. The reduction in ICP brought about by therapy may be weighed against changes in the patient's clinical condition. ICP monitoring is not foolproof and in this chapter we point out some of the pitfalls and shortcomings of ICP monitoring.

The term intracranial pressure (ICP) has become quite ingrained in common usage. Currently, the term intracranial pressure is employed to indicate supratentorial CSF pressure—either surface subarachnoid pressure or CSF pressure in the anterior horn of one lateral ventricle. The term intracranial pressure is, however, quite misleading in that it implies that supratentorial intracranial CSF pressure is the only pressure inside of the cranium. The term intracranial pressure leads, therefore, to a simple view of ICP dynamics in which ICP is regarded as the pressure inside of a closed fluid filled container. In actual fact, the level of ICP reflects complex physical interactions between the CSF space and its surroundings. In this chapter we will, for convenience, retain the term ICP but will take care, in each circumstance, to define how ICP was actually measured.

To fully understand current usage of ICP monitoring and current thinking regarding the mechanisms of ICP change, we believe that it is best to take a historical approach, integrating both laboratory and clinical studies. We believe that such an approach places ICP monitoring and interpretation into proper perspective and allows us to make some speculation regarding what the future holds in this area. We will not emphasize ICP monitoring technique, other types of physiologic monitoring currently available to complement ICP monitoring, or the therapy of intracranial hypertension. These subjects have been discussed thoroughly in other recent publications.[17,51,58]

BACKGROUND AND HISTORICAL PERSPECTIVE

The suggestion that ICP could reach levels as high as arterial blood pressure in patients with intracranial mass lesions probably stems from the work of Cushing[10] around the beginning of this century. Cushing induced ICP elevation by infusing normal salt solution into the lumbar CSF space and the cisterna magna of animals. In these experiments ICP was measured by a mercury manometer connected to the saline infusion line. The animals also had cranial windows so that the cortical surface could be observed at different levels of ICP. Cushing found that when ICP reached the level of arterial blood pressure, the cortex would blanch and a systemic vasomotor response would ensue so that arterial blood pressure was increased over ICP. There were concomitant increases in systemic arterial pulse pressure, bradycardia, and respiratory irregularities. If ICP were progressively elevated by saline infusion,

there was an associated progressive elevation of arterial blood pressure beginning at the time when ICP was nearly equal to systemic arterial blood pressure (Fig. 4-1). Cushing was impressed with the similarity of the above experimental observations to the blood pressure, pulse, and respiratory changes observed in patients with intracranial mass lesions. Cushing's work suggested that when systemic vasomotor responses were observed in patients with intracranial mass lesions, ICP was approaching the level of systemic blood pressure. This conclusion was hampered by the fact that Cushing did not evaluate the association between intracranial hypertension and the vasomotor response in patients by measuring ICP in humans demonstrating systemic vasomotor responses in association with intracranial mass lesions.

During the two or three decades following Cushing's observations, conflicting opinion developed regarding the importance of the systemic vasomotor response so often

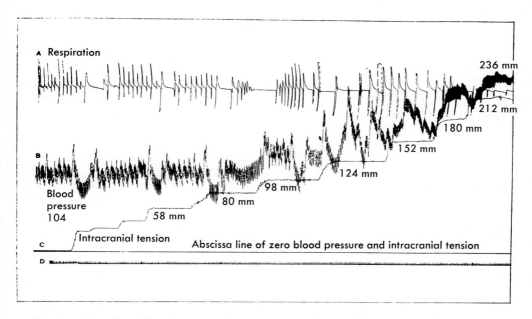

Fig. 4-1. The relationship between elevated intracranial pressure and blood pressure as observed by Cushing during normal saline infusion into the CSF space of animals. Notice that arterial blood pressure is unchanged until intracranial pressure approaches the level of diastolic blood pressure and that with further increases in intracranial pressure blood pressure increases as if to maintain perfusion pressure. (From Cushing, H.: Am. J. Med. Sci. **124:**383, 1902; courtesy Lea Brothers & Co., Philadelphia.)

seen in patients with intracranial mass lesions. The suggestion from Cushing's work that intracranial pressure could reach levels as high as systemic blood pressure did not appear valid in the clinical setting in view of conflicting data from pressure measurements by spinal fluid manometry in patients with intracranial mass lesions. In 1922 Jackson,[22] who advocated repeated lumbar puncture in the treatment of patients with severe traumatic brain injury, reported CSF pressure measurements by lumbar puncture in 33 cases with severe brain injury. The highest pressure measured by Jackson was 40 mm Hg. Most CSF pressures were less than 20 mm Hg, and many were near 10 mm Hg. In the eight fatal cases reported by Jackson, there was one lumbar CSF pressure as high as 50 mm Hg. The next highest was 40 mm Hg, and the other six fatal cases had lumbar CSF pressures of less than or equal to 22 mm Hg. McCreery and Berry[40] reported lumbar CSF pressures recorded in 400 of 520 patients with skull fracture. In this series a CSF pressure of 50 mm Hg was recorded in one patient, in 202 patients the pressures were between 20 and 30 mm Hg, and in 197 patients the pressure was less than 20 mm Hg. In 1928, McClure and Crawford[41] reported that of 382 lumbar CSF pressures in 148 cases of severe head trauma only 2% were greater than 30 mm Hg while 47% were less than 10 mm Hg. Furthermore, during the first three decades of this century, lumbar CSF pressure measured in patients with brain tumor was rarely higher than 30 mm Hg—certainly nowhere near systemic arterial blood pressure.[5,16,20]

In 1936, Browder and Meyers[6] reported the first systematic correlations of blood pressure, pulse, respirations, and temperature with sequentially measured lumbar CSF pressures in patients with severe head trauma. This report contained 23 cases of severe head injury. All cases received a lumbar CSF pressure measurement and vital sign check on admission. The pressure measurements and vital sign checks were repeated at intervals of approximately three hours. The purpose was to examine Cushing's tenet that

when systemic vasopressor responses occurred, the ICP was near the level of arterial blood pressure. The highest CSF pressure recorded by Browder and Meyers was 46 mm Hg—nowhere near the level of arterial blood pressure. Even of more interest, it was frequently noted that lumbar CSF pressure would decline at a time when systemic arterial blood pressure was increasing. Many of the patients with low lumbar CSF pressures had large intracranial hematomas or brain contusions. Fig. 4-2 demonstrates the changes in ICP and vital signs noted in three of the patients reported by Browder and Meyers. The case illustrated in Fig. 4-2, *A*, is especially interesting because there was an initial increasing lumbar CSF pressure that began to fall just as arterial pulse pressure widened and as blood pressure increased. Browder and Meyers concluded "Death, when it occurred, was not foreshadowed by a steadily mounting CSF pressure. . . . We are convinced that death in our cases was due to some as yet undetermined cerebral factor other than increased intracranial pressure."

The report of Browder and Meyers illustrates the tendency for physicians, during the first three decades of the twentieth century, to overlook the possibility that the intracranial space might be compartmentalized by tentorial and foramen magnum herniations so that pressure does not communicate freely within the CSF space. It is now clear that the declining lumbar CSF pressures observed by Browder and Meyers were probably associated with high intracranial pressure in the presence of transtentorial herniation. Appreciation of the need for monitoring of pressure from the supratentorial compartment is linked historically to the development of the concept that lumbar CSF pressure might be falsely low in the presence of transtentorial or foramen magnum brain herniations.

The first clear description of transtentorial herniation was published by Meyer[48] in 1920. Meyer presented photographs of autopsy specimens demonstrating brain herniations under the falx, through the tentorial

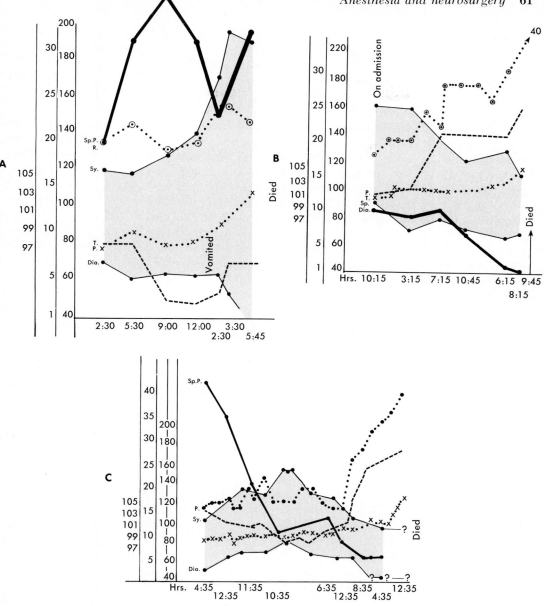

Fig. 4-2. Concomitant changes in lumbar CSF pressure and vital signs in three patients with severe head injury as reported by Browder and Meyers in 1936. Heavy line, CSF pressure; gray, systemic pulse pressure; dots and crosses, temperature; dots and open circles, respirations; heavy dotted line, pulse. Scale 1, temperature degrees F; scale 2, CSF pressure (mm H₂O) and respirations/min; scale 3, blood pressure (mm Hg) and pulse (beats/min). Note that all three patients show declining CSF pressure immediately prior to death associated with an intracranial mass lesion. Also note that when blood pressure was noted to increase (**A** and **C**); the level of lumbar CSF pressure was nowhere near the level of diastolic blood pressure. Subsequent studies have shown that these low, declining lumbar CSF pressures in patients with traumatic mass lesions were probably associated with compartmentalization of the CSF space by transtentorial herniation and that had ICP been measured in these patients, it would have been quite high. (From Browder, J., and Meyers, R.: Am. J. Surg. **31:**408, 1936.)

incisura, and into the foramen magnum. The photographs of Meyer clearly demonstrate grooving of the uncus by the free edge of the tentorium. Meyer also noted in one case with transtentorial herniation that lumbar puncture seemed to have accelerated the patient's demise. In 1929 Kernohan and Woltman[28] reported grooving of the midbrain by the free edge of the tentorium as a cause of upper motor neuron signs homolateral to a supratentorial lesion. In their first case there was a large left temporal lobe herniation into the tentorial hiatus. From the 1920s to the 1930s there were other sporadic reports of transtentorial herniation, but these reports as well as the descriptions of transtentorial herniation by Meyer and Kernohan were largely ignored and the possibility that different pressures might exist above and below the tentorium was not widely recognized until the late 1930s.

The first suggestion that pressure might be higher above than below the tentorium in patients with supratentorial mass lesions is probably contained in the important work of Moore and Stern in 1938.[59] This work defined the major pathologic lesions associated with transtentorial herniation: brain stem hemorrhage, hemorrhagic occipital infarction, and migration of the medial temporal lobe into the tentorial hiatus with grooving of the undersurface of the uncus by the free edge of the tentorium. Quoting from Moore and Stern, "It is suggested that sudden changes in the pressure relationship between the supra and infratentorial spaces leads to disturbance of circulation in the basilar artery."

In 1938, following closely on the report of Moore and Stern, Smyth and Henderson[82] reported simultaneous measurements of lumbar CSF pressure (LFP) and ventricular fluid pressure (VFP) in patients with brain tumors. The simultaneous response of LFP and VFP to jugular compression was also evaluated. All patients were in the lateral position and the two manometers were carefully brought to the same zero position. Of 39 patients evaluated, 8 patients were found

to have abnormal pressure dynamics. In two of these eight patients VFP was equal to LFP, but the rise in LFP following jugular compression was slow compared to the rise in VFP. VFP exceeded LFP in the remaining six of eight abnormal patients. These patients also had slow rise of LFP on jugular compression. Five of the six patients with VFP > LFP had supratentorial tumors, and all five had pathologic demonstration of transtentorial herniation. In the above six patients the difference between VFP and LFP ranged from 20 to 100 mm H_2O. The mortality in the group with obstruction was quite high compared to the other groups. Smyth and Henderson speculated that the aqueduct of Sylvius had become obstructed during the process of transtentorial herniation. The observations by Smyth and Henderson suggested that the falling or low LFP frequently observed by Browder and Meyers (Fig. 4-2) in patients with head injury may not have accurately reflected the true level of supratentorial pressure. As previously noted, unrecognized tentorial block may have been present in the patients reported by Browder and Meyers. The suggested link between ICP elevation and brain shift begins a story that we shall continue to trace throughout this chapter.

In 1938, shortly after the report by Smyth and Henderson, there followed the important paper by Jefferson[24] entitled the "Tentorial Pressure Cone." A similar term had been used two years previously by the French authors Vincent and Thiebaut.[93] Jefferson reported four cases: three cases of supratentorial tumor with autopsy-proven herniation of one or both temporal lobes through the incisura as well as one patient with progressive signs suggesting a tentorial pressure cone who was successfully treated by surgery. In two of the above cases, deterioration could be directly linked to lumbar puncture. Both the title of Jefferson's paper "Tentorial Pressure Cone" and his comment "lumbar puncture should be withheld in cases of high pressure even if the lesion is known to be hemispheral" emphasize the possibility of a pressure gradient across the tentorial hiatus in patients with supratentorial tumor. With the recognition by the late 1940s of transtentorial herniation as a common occurrence with intracranial mass lesions, it became clear that lumbar CSF pressure could no longer be trusted as an accurate index of intracranial pressure in patients with supratentorial mass lesions. Furthermore, lumbar puncture might be dangerous in these patients. During the next 10 years, it also became clear that there were other serious inadequacies in attempting to assess intracranial pressure by spinal puncture and manometry.

Dandy, in 1937, when reviewing his experiences with subtemporal decompression in 22 cases of pseudotumor cerebri, made note of the fact that there were extremely rapid fluctuations in the tension of the decompression site.[12] Dandy felt that these changes in intracranial tension were so rapid that they could only be explained by changes within the cerebral vascular bed. Two years later Cairns[7] reviewed the subject of raised intracranial pressure and presented a number of observations and hypotheses that would be the subject of much future study. Cairns hypothesized that intracranial herniations, even within the same compartment, were the result of local pressure gradients. He reported two surgical cases of sudden severe cerebellar swelling occasioned by an increase in the concentration of inspired CO_2. These cases stimulated him to study the effect of breathing 1%, 2.5% and 5% CO_2 on the level of lumbar CSF pressure in humans. The measurements were made by sequential observations of CSF pressure by spinal manometry. CO_2 tended to increase ICP, and the effect was proportional to the CO_2 concentration. Cairns also commented that cases of sudden severe brain swelling were analogous to the CO_2 response in that they probably represented a sudden dilatation of the brain vascular bed. The changes in ICP noted by Cairns confirmed similar changes noted in animals by Wolff and Lennox[98] and in humans by Cobb and Fremont-

Smith.[9] These reports made it clear that there could be rapid swings of intracranial pressure that could be totally missed by single measurements of CSF pressure using spinal manometry.

In 1943, O'Connell[60] demonstrated spinal manometry to be a highly inaccurate method of recording rapid changes in intracranial pressure. The intracranial system was modeled by a length of large bore rubber tubing attached to a fluid reservoir (Fig. 4-3). The pressure in this system was measured by a spinal needle and manometer. Pressure could be varied at any desired frequency by systematically changing the height of the fluid reservoir. When a 100 mm H_2O pressure shift was applied at a frequency of 20/min, the spinal needle recorded only a 2 to 3 mm Hg shift. O'Connell emphasized that the magnitude of cardiac and respiratory ICP fluctuations were probably much underestimated by spinal manometry. This hypothesis is in line with the common experience that at spinal manometry, cardiac fluctuations are hardly noticeable while with modern techniques we know that these fluctuations are on the order of 40 to 70 mm H_2O. Of course, the magnitude of rapid pathologic swings of ICP would also be obscured by spinal manometry. Furthermore, fluid displacement into the manometer might also lead to falsely low values of pressure.

Spinal manometry seemed to have the following poor qualities:

1. In the presence of transtentorial herniation spinal manometry does not measure a true ICP.
2. In patients with supratentorial mass lesions, lumbar puncture might accelerate the process of transtentorial herniation.
3. Single measurements might miss sporadically occurring short duration waves of elevated ICP.
4. Even if manometric observations are made over longer time periods, they seriously underestimate the magnitude of any rapid fluctuations of ICP, and chronic measurements with an open

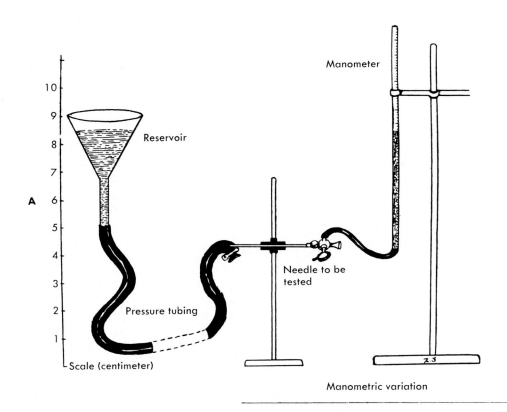

Shift or reservoir	Rate of shift	Wide bore tubing	Ventricular cannula	Lumbar puncture needle
10 mm	20 per minute	10 mm	1 mm	1 mm
	80 per minute	10 mm	4 mm	1 mm
100 mm	20 per minute	100 mm	100 mm	2-3 mm
	80 per minute	80 mm	50 mm	1 mm

Fig. 4-3. Apparatus (**A**) employed and results (**B**) reported by O'Connell in evaluating responsiveness of lumbar puncture needle and attached manometer to rapid fluctuations of CSF pressure. Using this apparatus pressure could be varied over a particular range at a chosen frequency simply by manipulating the reservoir. The spinal needle and manometer system failed to accurately record pressure shifts within the physiologic range for frequency and amplitude. (From O'Connell, J. E. A.: Brain **66:**211, 1943.)

manometer run a serious risk of infection.

5. Fluid displacement into the manometer has the potential to reduce the pressure.

The stage was clearly set for a departure from single measurements of ICP by spinal manometry. The strain gauge pressure transducer was the technical advance that made such a departure possible. The strain gauge pressure transducer allowed ICP to be monitored utilizing a closed system in which there was essentially no fluid displacement into the measuring device. Furthermore, the strain gauge pressure transducer allowed accurate measurement of the most rapid of physiologic variations.

The first continuous recordings of CSF pressure in humans via a strain gauge pressure transducer and ink writing polygraph reported in the English literature were probably those of Henry Ryder and his group in the early 1950s. Ryder and his colleagues recorded CSF pressure, arterial blood pressure, and jugular venous pressure continuously in patients during studies of CSF pressure dynamics.[64-70] The patients represented a broad spectrum of neurologic disease. The studies were usually of one to two hours' duration, and CSF pressure was monitored from either the lumbar sac or from the lateral ventricle. After two years over 200 patients had been studied. During these two years the Ryder group evaluated the effect of systemic vasodilators and vasoconstrictors, the Valsalva maneuver, normal saline infusion and CSF withdrawal, p.o. water load, and intravenous osmotic load upon ICP. One important observation made during these studies was that breathing CO_2 caused blood pressure and ICP to increase, while intravenous amyl nitrate lowered blood pressure and simultaneously increased ICP[64] (Fig. 4-4, *B*). It was concluded that increased cerebral blood volume was the factor leading to elevation of ICP at the time when blood pressure was falling. We have observed a similar phenomenon of increasing ICP and simultaneously decreasing blood pressure occurring spontaneously (Fig. 4-4, *C*). In the

same study, Ryder noted that hyperventilation decreased both ICP and BP while levarterenol (Levophed) decreased ICP but increased BP. Here ICP was postulated to fall, even in the face of increasing blood pressure, as a result of diminished cerebral blood volume. When fluid was infused or withdrawn from the CSF space, CSF pulse pressure was a linear function of mean ICP.[65] After fluid addition or withdrawal from the CSF space, ICP always returned to the same baseline value.[67] It was therefore appreciated that a condition of dynamic equilibrium existed with respect to ICP, and Ryder postulated that equilibrium pressure was maintained by increasing or decreasing CSF absorption as ICP deviated above or below equilibrium CSF pressure. Above venous pressure the change in CSF pressure with respect to volume (dP/dV) increased as mean ICP increases.[67] Ryder also observed that all observed variations of ICP tended to be larger when they started from a higher baseline ICP. Thus, Ryder and his colleagues speculated about the effect on ICP of cerebral blood flow, cerebral arterial blood volume, cerebral venous blood volume, and CSF absorption. Ryder[68] postulated the CSF pressure CSF volume curve to be hyperbolic. Many of the points touched on by Ryder and his group have been the subject of intense investigation during more recent years. We shall return to many of these points in more detail later in this chapter.

The final study reported by the Ryder group[70] involved the effects of artificially elevated CSF pressures in over 200 patients. CSF pressures were routinely raised by fluid infusion to values in the range of 45 to 60 mm Hg (600 to 800 mm H_2O). In a few patients pressure was elevated as high as 110 mm Hg (1500 mm H_2O). Ryder was impressed with the virtual absence of either cerebral or systemic symptoms associated with these high pressures and concluded, "There is no valid basis for two clinical inferences: first, fluid pressures within the range of normal indicate either the absence of or the correction of a grave disorder of the central nervous system; second, the proper treatment of condi-

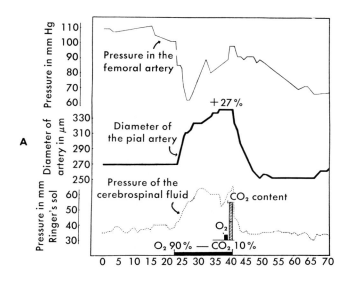

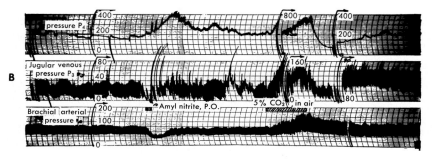

Fig. 4-4. Observations demonstrating that under certain circumstances ICP and blood pressure may vary in opposite directions. In these circumstances, it seems that changes in cerebral blood volume cause the increase in ICP. **A,** The work of Wolff and Lennox shows that when 10% CO_2 is added to the breathing mixture of an experimental animal, the increase in ICP parallels the dilatation of pial arteries as observed under a cranial window. As in this figure blood pressure may fall while ICP and arterial diameter are increasing. **B,** The work of Ryder and his associates shows that amyl nitrate will cause a simultaneous drop in systemic blood pressure and increase in ICP, while 5% CO_2 administration causes a parallel rise in both blood pressure and in ICP. **C,** Intracranial pressure recording from a patient with severe closed head injury showing spontaneous marked elevation of ICP and simultaneous fall in systemic blood pressure. Such a change probably represents the simultaneous occurrence of cerebral and systemic vasodilation. (**A** from Wolff, H. G., and Lennox, W. G.: Arch. Neurol. Psychiatr. **23:**1105, 1930, copyright 1930 American Medical Association; **B** from Ryder, H. W., Espey, F. F., Kimbell, F. D., and others: Arch. Neurol. Psychiatr. **68:**166, 1952, copyright 1952 American Medical Association; **C** from Thompson, R. A., and Green, J. B., editors: Advances in neurology, vol. 22, New York, 1979, Raven Press.)

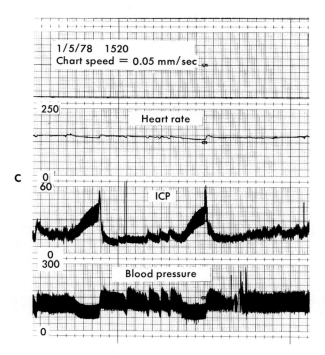

1/5/78   1520
Chart speed = 0.05 mm/sec

250

Heart rate

C   0
60

ICP

0
300

Blood pressure

0

Fig. 4-4, cont'd. For legend see opposite page.

tions associated with an abnormal fluid pressure consists in returning the pressure to normal." We speculate that these seemingly negative results caused the Ryder group not to pursue further CSF pressure studies in humans. It is unfortunate that Ryder and his colleagues did not appreciate that there might be considerable difference between raised ICP from CSF infusion and raised ICP associated with intracranial pathology. Furthermore, it seems that the concept of employing continuous recording of ICP as a monitoring tool was never appreciated by Ryder and his colleagues.

CONTINUOUS MONITORING OF INTRACRANIAL PRESSURE

The first report of continuous monitoring of ICP was probably by the French workers, Guillaume and Janny in 1951.[18] This work was largely unrecognized in English centers. Guillaume and Janny recorded human ventricular fluid pressure for long periods of time and observed large sporadic oscillations in the level of intracranial pres-

sure. Two types of ICP waves were observed —rapid waves with a frequency of 0.5 to 1.5/min and large sustained ICP elevations lasting eight minutes or longer. Guillaume and Janny ascribed the observed pressure waves to autonomous cerebral vasomotor activity.

In 1960, Lundberg[36] reported a safe method, developed in 143 neurosurgical cases, for continuous monitoring of ventricular fluid pressure. Among these patients was a wide variety of intracranial pathology excluding cerebral trauma. The patients were monitored for long periods of time—58 patients for more than one week, 17 patients for more than two weeks, and 4 patients for more than four weeks. In these initial cases, there was not a single instance in which intracranial hematoma or infection could be linked to the monitoring of ICP. VFP was recorded graphically on a continuous basis in 48 of Lundberg's initial 143 patients. These recordings demonstrated VFP to be a very unstable parameter that tended to exhibit three distinct spontaneous fluctuations: A waves (plateau

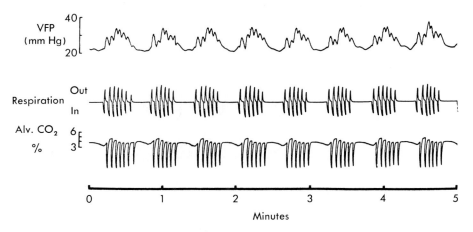

Fig. 4-5. Recordings made by Lundberg and his colleagues demonstrating the association between periodic respirations (Cheyne-Stokes) and B waves in the ICP record. This association was not thought to be cause and effect, but both the B waves and the periodic respirations were postulated to be the result of a common brain stem rhythm altering both respiratory pattern and cerebral vasomotor tone. (From Kjallgvist, A., Lundberg, N., and Pontén, U.: Acta Neurol. Scand. **40:**296, 1964, copyright © Munksgaard International Publishers Ltd., Copenhagen, Denmark.)

waves), B waves (one per minute waves), and C waves (six per minute waves). B and C waves were of small amplitude and were generally of limited usefulness in managing patients. B waves (Fig. 4-5) were found in association with Cheyne-Stokes respiration, and C waves (Fig. 4-6) were associated with Traube, Hering, Mayer blood pressure waves.[30] Both B and C waves were noted in association with depression in the level of consciousness—both natural and pathologic. A waves (Fig. 4-7), on the other hand, were of considerable importance both prognostically and in patient management.[36-39,62]

A waves (plateau waves) varied in magnitude from 50 to over 100 mm Hg, and the duration of these varied from 5 to 20 minutes. Plateau waves could occur at irregular intervals or they could occur in groups at a quite regular frequency (Fig. 4-7). Plateau waves did not have a characteristic frequency, and they were not uniformly associated with any abnormality of blood pressure or respiration. Plateau waves occurred only in the presence of an elevation of baseline ICP (>20 mm Hg) and were frequently associated with "pressure symptoms" and worsening of neurologic deficit. When the plateau waves were infrequent, the neurologic status would usually return to baseline between waves, but when these waves were frequent, an associated lasting deterioration in neurologic status was not uncommon. The most severe symptoms during plateau waves were apnea, respiratory arrest, decerebration, and marked depression in level of consciousness. Other symptoms frequently associated with plateau waves were headache, restlessness, incontinence, and purposeless movements. These attacks occurring with plateau waves could bear a striking resemblance to seizure activity, but subsequent studies revealed that the EEG did not show cortical seizure activity during plateau waves.[38] In general, A waves of less than 60 mm Hg were associated with mild symptomatology (headache and restlessness), while A waves of 80 to 100 mm Hg were associated with marked disorders of consciousness. However, some A waves in the 80 to 100 mm Hg range were not associated with any symptoms. Changes in blood pressure and pulse rate with A waves were inconsistent. Frequently, there was no change in systemic blood pressure

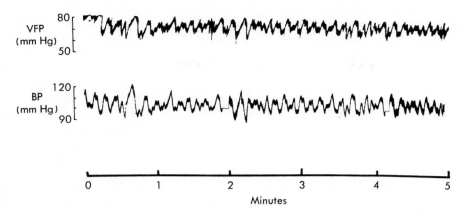

Fig. 4-6. Recordings made by Lundberg and his colleagues demonstrating the association between Traube, Hering, Mayer blood pressure waves and C wave (6 per minute waves) in the ICP. This association was not thought to be cause and effect, but both changes were postulated to be the result of a common brain stem rhythm altering both blood pressure and cerebral vasomotor tone. (From Kjallgvist, A., Lundberg, N., and Pontén, U.: Acta Neurol. Scand. **40**:299, 1964, copyright © Munksgaard International Publishers Ltd., Copenhagen Denmark.)

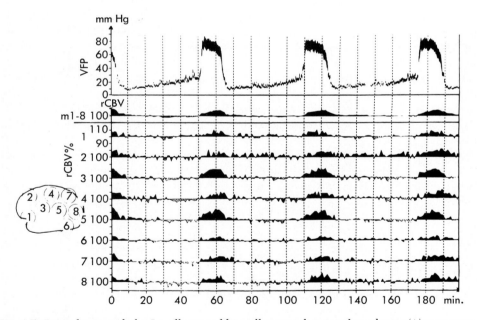

Fig. 4-7. Recordings made by Lundberg and his colleagues showing that plateau (A) waves are associated with a simultaneous increase in cerebral blood volume (CBV). The increase in CBV is thought to be the etiology of the plateau wave. (From Risberg, J., Lundberg, N., and Ingrav, D. H.: J. Neurosurg. **31**:303, 1969.)

even when ICP approached the level of systemic diastolic pressure, confirming what clinicians had long suspected: that elevation of systemic blood pressure had a poor correlation with raised ICP. Tachycardia was frequently noted at the peak of large plateau waves, refuting the notion that bradycardia was invariably associated with intracranial hypertension.[30]

Lundberg noted that the occurrence of A waves could be prevented by lowering the baseline ICP by drainage of CSF or by administration of osmotic diuretics. A waves were thought to represent a stage of decompensation of the intracranial system, and the major function of ICP monitoring was seen as the detection and prevention of plateau waves. On the basis of his experience with the initial 143 cases, Lundberg concluded that ICP monitoring was a significant adjunct to the management of patients with intracranial hypertension. A subsequent study allowed the same conclusion for patients with cerebral trauma.[39] The initial report also pointed out the usefulness of intraoperative ICP monitoring and the usefulness of ICP monitoring during pneumography, ventriculography, and angiography. Several of Lundberg's cases illustrate the fact that induction of anesthesia and anesthetic drugs may have an adverse effect on ICP. In a later report based on 848 cases Lundberg confirmed the conclusions of his initial study.[37] In that report he classified ICP levels as follows:

Normal	≤mm Hg
Slightly increased	11 to 20 mm Hg
Moderately increased	21 to 40 mm Hg
Severely increased	>40 mm Hg

We have found this classification useful in clinical work, and we actively investigate any patient with sustained elevation of ICP over 20 mm Hg.

Lundberg's work raised many questions that could only be approached experimentally. The high ICP values recorded by Lundberg were in conflict with previous recordings of spinal fluid pressure. This conflict demanded simultaneous recording of both

pressures during the inflation of a supratentorial mass. The seemingly capricious reaction of blood pressure to intracranial hypertension needed investigation. Did plateau waves produce symptomatology by ischemia, by increasing a tentorial pressure gradient, or by both mechanisms? Probably the most important question raised by Lundberg's work was just how did the occurrence of plateau waves and the baseline level of ICP relate to the volume of an intracranial mass lesion.

Beginning in the early 1960s Langfitt and his colleagues at the University of Pennsylvania performed a series of experiments in rhesus monkeys designed to answer the above questions. It was found that as supratentorial CSF pressure increased secondary to inflation of a supratentorial epidural balloon, there was a progressive divergence between the supratentorial CSF pressure and the CSF pressure recorded either in the cisterna magna or in the lumbar spinal sac.[34,35] Falling infratentorial pressures were observed at a time when supratentorial pressure was increasing. These results are reminiscent of the previously quoted observations by Browder and Meyers in which lumbar CSF pressure was noted to be decreasing in patients with traumatic intracranial mass lesions.[6] In Langfitt's experiments, lumbar and cisterna magna CSF pressure could be normal at a time when supratentorial pressure levels were as high as 200 mm Hg. The reason for the divergence of supratentorial pressures and infratentorial pressures was the occurrence of transtentorial herniation. Langfitt and co-workers[97] observed that the cause of the vasopressor response to increased ICP was multifactorial and did not necessarily depend on medullary ischemia as postulated by Cushing. The level of the vasopressor threshold could vary considerably depending upon experimental conditions. These experimental observations fit with the variability of blood pressure response observed by Lundberg in patients during plateau waves.[36,37]

A contribution that was to shape subsequent theoretical treatment of ICP change

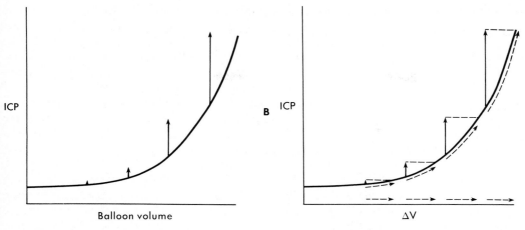

Fig. 4-8. Diagrams illustrating experiments done by Langfitt and his colleagues[34] that led to the hypothesis of a single pressure-volume curve for the intracranial system. **A,** Heavy line, plot of ICP versus volume of an extradural balloon; arrows, ICP changes noted at different baseline balloon volumes in response to hypercarbia, induced systemic hypertension, and rapid saline addition to the supratentorial CSF space. Notice that CO_2 blood pressure and saline challenges produce a larger rise in ICP as baseline balloon volume increases. **B,** The intracranial pressure-volume curve hypothesized by Langfitt to explain the results diagrammed in **A.** Notice that the abscissa has been changed to ΔV—the volume change of any intracranial compartment away from its equilibrium volume, which implies that volume changes in any number of different compartments are additive with respect to pressure. Dotted arrows indicate that CO_2, blood pressure, or saline challenge is seen as a volume addition along the abscissa, which is additive with baseline volume of the balloon explaining the observed results (**A**). The volume-pressure response (VPR) developed by Miller and his colleagues[53] was initially thought of as the pressure change produced by adding 1 ml volume to the CSF space along the abscissa of this curve. For proof that the concept of a single P-V curve is not valid, see Fig. 4-14 and text.

was the pressure-volume curve obtained by Langfitt[34] when supratentorial CSF pressure was plotted as a function of the volume of an expanding epidural balloon. This curve had an initial flat portion and a final steep portion where there were large increases in ICP associated with small volume additions to the epidural balloon (Fig. 4-8, *A*). During the steep portion of this curve, incremental but cumulative balloon loading would set off waves of ICP and blood pressure. In these experiments three spontaneous plateaulike waves were observed during the steep portion of the curve. Hypercarbia, pharmacologic elevation of blood pressure, and small saline injections into the CSF space produced little CSF pressure change at balloon volumes corresponding to the flat portion of the ICP versus balloon volume

curve, but these same maneuvers produced increasingly larger ICP changes at balloon volumes corresponding to the flat portion of the ICP versus balloon volume curve. These results are shown diagrammatically in Fig. 4-8, *A*. The CSF pressure responses to CO_2, blood pressure, and saline injection challenge suggested that volume additions to the intracranial space were additive, and it was proposed that the plot of ICP versus balloon volume was valid for volume additions anywhere within the supratentorial space. Fig. 4-8, *B* shows how this postulate would explain the experimental observations. The curve was referred to as the "intracranial volume pressure relationship" and was frequently denoted simply as the pressure-volume curve. Langfitt summarized the importance of the proposed pressure-volume curve as follows: "It is important to note that this relationship (the P-V curve), irrespective of the source of extraneous volume and transition from the horizontal to the vertical portion of the curve, explains many of the observations to follow." The flat part of the intracranial P-V curve was taken to represent the situation in which CSF and blood were available to compensate for mass volume added to the intracranial system; the steep part of this curve was taken to represent the situation where compensation by loss of CSF and blood was limited or no longer available. The dynamics of CSF bulk flow, which were defined simultaneous to Langfitt's experiments by Pappenheimer and his colleagues[19] in the goat and subsequently by Cutler[11] in humans, seemed to support the concept of CSF as an intracranial safety valve. According to the dynamics of CSF bulk flow, whenever ICP exceeds CSF equilibrium pressure, CSF absorption increases to exceed CSF formation so that CSF volume decreases to bring ICP back toward the equilibrium CSF pressure level. One can easily envision this process of diminishing CSF volume taking place along the flat portion of the intracranial pressure volume curve. Presumably blood volume would decrease by collapse of parenchymal vessels (veins) contiguous to the developing mass. It should be noted that the hypothesis of a single P-V curve for the intracranial space was never validated experimentally by observing the same pressure change as a result of equivalent volume loading of two different intracranial compartments.

Lundberg and his associates[38] employed Langfitt's intracranial pressure-volume curve to explain the occurrence of plateau waves. This explanation was advanced as follows: "plateau waves occur when the interrelations between pressure and volume are represented on the steep part of the intracranial pressure-volume curve where small increases in volume . . . give rise to a relative great increase of intracranial pressure." To further investigate the etiology of plateau waves Lundberg and his colleagues made measurements of cerebral blood flow (CBF) and regional cerebral blood volume (rCBV) during and between plateau waves[62]. Plateau waves were found to coincide with an increase in rCBV (Fig. 4-7) and paradoxically with a decrease in CBF. The peak of regional CBV did not coincide with the peak of the plateau wave. The peak of rCBV occurred at a time when CSF pressure was falling. In one patient there was a clear tendency for the plateau wave to begin at a threshold level of VFP (Fig. 4-7). It was hypothesized that plateau waves were set off by a stimulus to cerebral vasodilation such as reaching a threshold level of ICP or more nonspecific stimuli such as pain, arousal, mental activity, or hypoventilation. Because pressure volume relationships were seen as operating on the steep part of the pressure volume curve, it was proposed that vasodilatation caused a rapid rise in ICP with concomitant obstruction of cerebral venous drainage resulting in the paradoxical combination of increased rCBV and decreased CBF. It was proposed that ICP could fall before rCBV reached a peak because of rapid CSF absorption caused by the high pressure associated with the wave.

Around this time McDowell, Jennett, and their colleagues[15,25,26,42] were studying the effects of the volatile anesthetic agents halothane, trichlorethylene, and methoxyflurathane on intracranial pressure, contrasting patients with normal ICP dynamics and those with intracranial mass lesions. They found that in patients with brain tumors, any of the above volatile anesthetic agents produced a severe increase in intracranial pressure whether or not ICP had been elevated at the start of the study. In contrast, in patients without mass lesion the administration of these agents produced only a small increase in ICP. These results are shown in Fig. 4-9. Other studies[43,99] demonstrated that these anesthetic agents produced cerebral vasodilatation. Therefore, the large induced pressure rises were similar to plateau waves. The observations on volatile anesthetic agents fit well with the concept of a single intracranial pressure-volume curve as proposed by Langfitt—flat initially and then becoming quite steep at higher volumes.

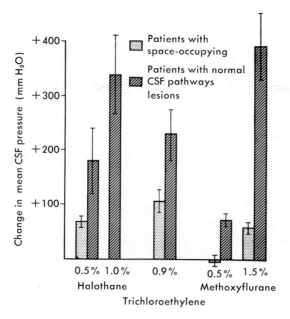

Fig. 4-9. Effect of volatile anesthetics on intracranial pressure in patients with normal CSF pathways and in patients with space-occupying lesions. Much larger increases of ICP occur in patients with intracranial mass lesions than in patients with normal pathways. These results are similar to those observed in animals by Langfitt (see Fig. 4-8, **A**). (From McDowall, D. G., and Fitch, W.: Inter. Anesth. Clin., vol. 7, no. 3, Boston, 1969, Little, Brown and Co.)

With the widespread adoption of ICP monitoring there can no longer be any doubt that intracranial hypertension with CSF pressures ranging up to 100 mm Hg is a common occurrence in cases of head injury, brain tumor, encephalitis, metabolic cerebral disturbances, stroke, and intracranial hemorrhage.* It remains to be decided whether the adverse neurologic sequelae of the above disorders are a consequence of increased ICP by itself, the effect of ICP on cerebral blood flow, or the consequence of brain shift and distortion so often associated with elevated ICP. Patients with benign intracranial hypertension tolerate surprisingly large elevations of ICP without impressive symptomatology. As noted previously, large elevations of ICP may be produced by saline infusion into the CSF space without alarming symptoms. In patients with brain shift, minor fluctuations in ICP can produce considerable change in neurologic function. It appears, therefore,

that there is an interaction between ICP and brain shift in causing neurologic dysfunction. Whatever the interrelationship between elevated ICP and brain shift, substantial evidence has accumulated linking these two parameters with death and disability in many neurologic disorders. For example, Finne and Walker[14] report 88% of patients who die from glial tumors show transtentorial herniation. Adams and Graham[1] show a similar high incidence of brain herniations in patients dying from head injury. In our clinical study[51] of 160 patients with severe head injury in whom intracranial pressure was monitored continuously, we believe that we have established beyond doubt the importance of intracranial hypertension as a significant factor in determining both morbidity and mortality from head injury.

A major difficulty with ICP monitoring is that ICP may be normal or only slightly elevated at a time when the patient harbors a sizeable intracranial mass lesion. This difficulty is to be anticipated on the basis of the

---

*References 1, 21, 27, 29, 33, 36, 39, 61, 63, 91, 92.

intracranial pressure-volume curve postulated by Langfitt (Fig. 4-8). Sullivan[83] reported ICP versus balloon volume plots for cats in which an occipital epidural balloon was inflated at a rate such that pupillary dilatation occurred in 88 ± 7 (SD) minutes. In these animals the phase of rapidly increasing ICP was not reached until 57 ± 8 (SD) minutes had elapsed. ICP elevation therefore preceded the clinical sign of pupillary dilation, but ICP remained low until mass volume was greater than one-half of that required to dilate the pupil. In our experience the above laboratory study is representative of what is seen in patients in that elevated ICP may precede clinical signs, but a normal level of ICP does not exclude a sizeable mass lesion. Under these circumstances, it is only reasonable that methods should be sought to make ICP monitoring a more sensitive tool.

CONTROLLED PERTURBATIONS OF THE CSF SPACE

In view of the fact that ICP could be normal in the presence of a sizeable intracranial mass lesion, Miller and his colleagues* set about to improve the sensitivity of continuous ICP monitoring by evaluating the ICP

*References 49, 50, 52, 53, 55, 56.

change resulting from the injection of a small volume of fluid into the patient's ventricular catheter. This method seemed quite natural since small fluid volumes were already employed to flush the ventricular catheter. The volume pressure response (VPR) was defined as the pressure change resulting from a bolus injection of 1 ml of fluid (0.07% of intracranial volume, 0.7% of total CSF volume) into the ventricular catheter. A VPR of greater than 4 mm Hg/ml was almost always associated with an intracranial mass lesion.[49,50,54,57] Specifically, in the situation of low ICP and high VPR, the elevated VPR almost always indicated the presence of a previously unexpected intracranial mass lesion. It was postulated that the VPR could be related to the intracranial pressure volume curve as defined by Langfitt.[49,50] The level of VPR was taken as a reflection of the steepness of a small segment of the intracranial pressure volume curve. This relationship is seen in Fig. 4-8, *B*.

The finding of low ICP and high VPR suggested that VPR might change independent of the baseline ICP. Proof that VPR could change independent of changes in ICP came from measurements of VPR and ICP in patients in whom intracranial hypertension was treated either by steroids or by mannitol.

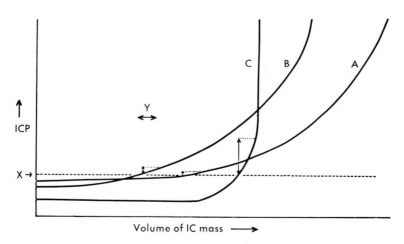

Fig. 4-10. Diagram drawn by Miller showing how a pressure volume curve of variable inflection would explain how VPR could change independent of CSF pressure. Arrows, pressure change due to addition of fixed volume. (From Wilkins, R. A., editor: Clin. Neurosurg., vol. 22, 1975.)

Steroids lowered VPR before changes were noted in mean ICP, and mannitol lowered VPR out of proportion to the change in mean ICP.[54] The fact that VPR could change independent of ICP was seen as indicating that the intracranial pressure volume curve was not of fixed configuration but that the shape of this curve could change depending on the intracranial mileau (Fig. 4-10).

In our recent series of 160 consecutive severe head injuries an elevated value of VPR identified all patients who were harboring missed intracranial hematomas.[51] In this same series of patients the VPR was not helpful in identifying and treating those patients without surgical mass lesion who went on to die from malignant intracranial hypertension. Such patients represented nearly one-sixth of the patients in our series. Clearly, the situation of low ICP and high VPR should be considered unsafe, but the condition of low ICP and low VPR cannot be considered safe. There is a need for a method that will identify those patients with low ICP and low VPR who will go on to develop malignant intracranial hypertension and brain shift.

VPR data also provided insight into the mathematical relationship between CSF pressure and CSF volume. VPR from a large number of patients plotted against the mean CSF pressure in these same patients seemed to follow a linear relationship.[49] This data is shown in Fig. 4-11. Since VPR may be taken as an estimate of the slope (dP/dV) of the tangent to the CSF pressure–CSF volume curve at a particular point on that curve, the linear relationship between VPR and CSF pressure suggested an exponential relationship between CSF pressure and CSF volume. Thus, one would expect the following equations to express the relationship between CSF pressure (P) and CSF volume (V) or between CSF pressure and any deviation of CSF volume (ΔV) away from baseline CSF volume.

$$dP/dV = bP \qquad VPR \simeq dP/dV \qquad (1)$$
$$\ln P = b\Delta V + C$$
$$P = Ke^{bV} \qquad P = P_oe^{b\Delta V}$$

where K, b, and C are constants

$$P_o = P \text{ when } \Delta V = 0$$

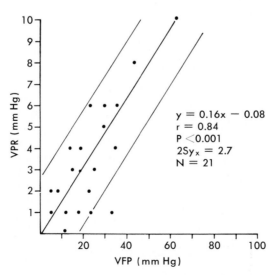

$$y = 0.16x - 0.08$$
$$r = 0.84$$
$$P < 0.001$$
$$2Sy_x = 2.7$$
$$N = 21$$

Fig. 4-11. Data from Miller and associates showing that VPR (an estimate of dP/dV) tends to increase linearly with ventricular fluid pressure (VFP). Scatter of data is probably due to the fact that each point represents a different patient. The linear relationship between VPR and ICP suggests that the CSF pressure–CSF volume curve is exponential. (From Leech and Miller, J. Neurol. Neurosurg. Psychiatr. **37:**1094, 1974.)

According to Langfitt's hypothesis of a single pressure volume curve for the intracranial system, we should be able to let ΔV represent the volume change of any intracranial compartment. The resulting curve is not like the hyperbolic relationship described by Langfitt. This discrepancy suggests that the plot of CSF pressure versus CSF volume and the plot of CSF pressure versus the volume of an epidural balloon should be considered as two separate relationships. Because of the scatter of data among the patients reported by Miller, a more direct confirmation of the relationship between dp/dV (VPR) and ICP was required.

Marmarou[44] made such a direct evaluation of equation 1 in six cats by plotting lnP as a function of ΔV. In these animals a relatively greater volume could be evaluated than in humans. The plot of lnP versus ΔV was found to be linear over a volume range of up to 3% of intracranial volume (≈ 40 cc in man) and over a CSF pressure range of from 0 to 40 mm Hg. Sullivan[86] has confirmed this finding in 15 cats for the same volume range and over a CSF pressure range of from 0 to 50 mm Hg. Sklar and Elashvili[78] have confirmed the linearity of the plot of lnP versus ΔV in dogs for a pressure range of from 0 to 40 mm Hg. Data for the experimental plots of lnP versus ΔV is shown in Fig. 4-12. For the convenience of utilizing log base 10, Marmarou and Shulman[44-47,79,80] have defined the pressure volume index (PVI) as follows:

$$\text{PVI} = \ln 10/_b \qquad (2)$$
$$\text{PVI} = \Delta V/[\log P_p/P_o]$$

where

b = as defined in equation 1
P_p = peak CSF pressure after a bolus volume addition of ΔV to the CSF space
P_o = as defined in equation 1

Thus, PVI was defined so that it represented the volume addition to the CSF space required to change ICP by ten-fold.

Marmarou[44] combined equation 1 with the well-known linear equations for CSF bulk flow to derive equations allowing calculation of CSF outflow resistance (R_{csf}), CSF elastance (E_{csf}; VPR is an estimate of E_{csf}), and rate of CSF formation (F_{csf}) on the basis of simple volume perturbations of the CSF space. PVI, R_{csf}, and E_{csf} could be defined from a single intraventricular bolus injection. Calculation of F_{csf} required both bolus injection and withdrawal of fluid. Marmarou and his colleagues[79] proposed that the PVI would provide a sensitive indicator of impending intracranial volumetric decompensation and that knowledge of PVI, R_{csf}, and F_{csf} would allow "tailored" treatment of intracranial hypertension in patients.

Marmarou and his group[79] evaluated the clinical usefulness of PVI in 52 patients undergoing continuous monitoring of intracranial pressure. In this study the following observations were reported:

1. Plateau waves did not occur if the PVI exceeded 15 ml ($n = 36$).
2. About one half of patients (7/16) with PVI less than 15 ml experienced plateau waves.
3. PVIs of less than 10 ml (n = 4) were "uniformly" associated with unsatisfactory clinical outcomes eventuating either in chronic vegetative states or death.
4. Patients ($n = 4$) demonstrating a reduction of PVI during the period of study had "new intracerebral pathology."
5. "Ten patients treated with mannitol experienced a rise in PVI (9.8 ml to 14.4 ml)," which "was independent of ICP change"—an observation in line with Miller's notion of a pressure volume curve of variable infection.

In this same study, it was reported that when CSF outflow resistance (calculated by the bolus method) exceeded 12 mm Hg/ml/min, ICP could be effectively lowered by CSF diversion. No comment was made regarding the usefulness of knowledge of CSF formation rate in management of these patients. It should be noted that defining the PVI, F_{csf}, and R_{csf} requires large bolus injections (5 to 10 ml) into the CSF space.

Sullivan studied the methods of Marmarou and his colleagues in both animals and in patients. As previously noted, Marmarou's initial experiment was repeated in 15 cats, reconfirming the exponential nature of the CSF pressure–CSF volume relationship over a pressure range of from 0 to 50 mm Hg and a volume range of up to 3% of intracranial volume.[85] PVI, CSF elastance, and CSF outflow resistance by the bolus technique were evaluated sequentially in seven cats during the constant rate inflation of an epidural bal-

loon.[83] In these studies the PVI during balloon inflation was no better an indicator of the presence of a mass lesion than was the ICP by itself. The PVI remained very stable until the phase of rapidly increasing ICP and then the PVI *increased* with increasing balloon volume. According to Marmarou, a large value of PVI should indicate the ability of the system to absorb a large volume increase with very little CSF pressure

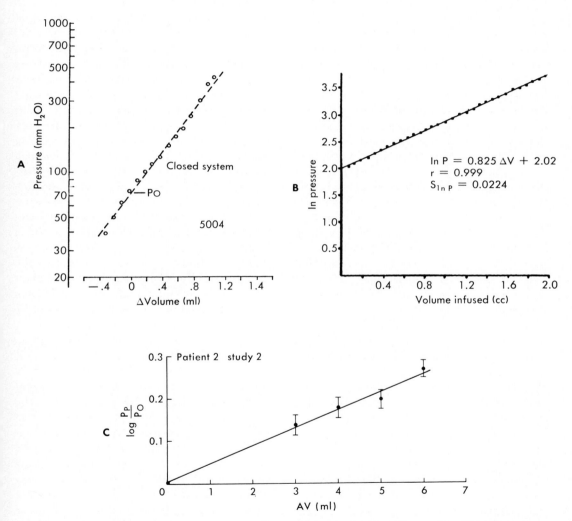

Fig. 4-12. Data from different authors demonstrating that the plot of lnP versus ΔV is linear, where P = ICP and ΔV = CSF volume change (see equation 1 in text). **A,** Plot of lnP versus ΔV for the cat. **B,** Plot of lnP versus ΔV for the dog. **C,** Plot of lnP versus ΔV for a patient with a severe head injury. (**A** courtesy Anthony Marmarou, M.D.; **B** from Sklar, F. H.: J. Neurosurg. **47:**672, 1977; **C** from Sullivan, H. G.: Surg. Neurol. **9:**50, 1977, Paul C. Bucy and Associates.)

change—a situation that does not seem compatible with increasing mass volume and increasing ICP. These observations cast doubt on the validity of the mathematical relationships defining PVI in the situation of a slowly accumulating epidural mass lesion and lead one to pose the question of whether the equation defining PVI would be valid in all patients undergoing continuous monitoring of ICP.

Sullivan[84] reported a pilot study to evaluate the validity of the "PVI relationship" in patients undergoing ICP monitoring. Of the six patients studied, five clearly followed the relationship defining PVI while one patient probably did not follow this relationship. This last patient was of particular interest in that at the time of the study he had an undiagnosed extraaxial hematoma. Had PVI been calculated in this patient, solely on the basis of single volume injections into the CSF space, the value of this index would have been normal—an interesting parallel with the PVI changes noted during balloon inflation in cats. The VPR in the above patient with an undiagnosed extraaxial hematoma was clearly elevated (8 mm Hg) and correctly indicated the presence of the missed hematoma. In all but the above-noted patient the VPR allowed an accurate calculation of the PVI (equation 1).

In the above study, Sullivan reported a major practical difficulty in making PVI and related determinations. At least one hour is required to make an accurate assessment of PVI. Even more time is required if one wishes to determine CSF outflow resistance by the bolus technique. In practical terms we have found that a patient's response to a trial of CSF drainage is as useful as knowledge of the magnitude of the patient's CSF outflow resistance. The mechanism that Marmarou described for determining CSF formation rate involves ventricular drainage to relatively low CSF pressures. The authors have been unable to accomplish drainage to such low pressures without a high incidence of catheter blockage.

With the bolus technique Marmarou[79] reported a normal CSF outflow resistance

(R_{csf}) of 2.54 ± 0.45 (SE) mm Hg/ml/min^{-1}. Based on isotope clearance data in 11 patients, Cutler and co-workers[11] reported a normal R_{csf} value of 9.7 ± 1.0 (SE) mm Hg/ml/min^{-1}. Ekstedt,[13] on the basis of 470 steady state perfusions in patients, reported a normal R_{csf} value of 10.4 mm Hg/ml/min^{-1}, which is in good agreement with the results of the isotope technique. Sullivan[86] compared R_{csf} by the bolus technique against R_{csf} by the steady state perfusion method in 18 cats. In these animals the bolus technique underestimated the value of R_{csf} given by the steady state method. The underestimate increased as the value of R_{csf} increased. In these experiments the magnitude of the error in determining R_{csf} by the bolus technique was as high as 50%. It appears that the bolus technique does not provide an accurate assessment of R_{csf}. Sullivan[86] postulated that the failure of the bolus technique to yield an accurate assessment of CSF outflow resistance is most likely due to a "relaxation" occurring within brain tissue as CSF pressure decays toward equilibrium after a bolus intraventricular fluid load. The phenomenon of "brain tissue relaxation" in circumstances where the brain is deformed illustrates the importance of mechanical properties of brain tissue in determining what particular level of CSF pressure will result after specific changes within the craniospinal system.

In a well-equipped intensive care unit an accurate determination of VPR requires about 15 minutes. Furthermore, a check of the VPR involves small volumes that are generally well tolerated by patients. On the other hand, an accurate determination of PVI will require at least one hour; the patient is subjected to relatively large loading volumes, uncertainty may remain as to the validity of underlying assumptions, and in the presence of extraaxial lesions the PVI may be no more sensitive than ICP alone. Reliable values of R_{csf} cannot be calculated by the bolus method, and more often than not attempts to determine F_{csf} result in catheter blockage. Presently the PVI and related measurements do not seem practical for clinical use. The proof that Marmarou provided of the exponential nature of the CSF pressure volume relationship remains an important contribution to our understanding of CSF pressure volume dynamics and stands as a proven contradiction to the so-called intracranial pressure volume curve proposed by Langfitt.

For practical purposes the VPR is the only perturbation of the CSF space that functions well as an adjunct to continuous monitoring of ICP. With the present state of knowledge, an elevated value of VPR (>4 mm Hg/ml) must raise the suspicion of an undiagnosed intracranial mass lesion. As previously noted, patients with low values of VPR cannot be considered safe from a future, possibly devastating episode of intracranial hypertension. We have observed patients with normal values of VPR progress on to death as a consequence of intracranial hypertension. It is important, therefore, to employ methods other than the VPR to identify all patients who are at risk from intracranial hypertension.

SPONTANEOUS FLUCTUATIONS IN INTRACRANIAL PRESSURE

At the First International Symposium on ICP, Janny[23] remarked that "an increase in ICP is paralleled by an increase in the amplitude of its fluctuations." This observation immediately raises the question of whether analysis of these spontaneous fluctuations of ICP would provide information of use in the management of intracranial hypertension. Many such spontaneous fluctuations are available for analysis—the ICP pulse wave, the ICP respiratory wave, fluctuations associated with coughing, position changes, or straining, as well as the large ICP changes recorded as plateau wave phenomena. Analysis of these spontaneously occurring ICP fluctuations generally demands some application of computer technology to ICP monitoring.

Initial studies by Janny[23] and Kullberg[32] employed computer averaging techniques to evaluate random fluctuations in ICP. In these studies ICP pulse and respiratory variations were eliminated by averaging over long-time intervals or simply by the small size of pulse and respiratory fluctuations in comparison with other spontaneous ICP fluc-

tuations. Both Janny and Kullberg employed a 24- to 48-hour frequency histogram technique for analyses of ICP data. Both authors found that the ICP frequency histogram does not follow a normal distribution. In most patients there was a skew toward higher pressures or there was a bimodal distribution with a second smaller ICP peak occurring at higher values of mean ICP. The authors have employed frequency histograms in the analysis of clinical ICP data, and it has been our feeling that a simple ICU alarm system set to warn whenever ICP crosses a low maximum will quickly inform the personnel that there is a tendency for ICP to increase. The changes seen on a frequency histogram cannot precede actual changes in the ICP; therefore ICP frequency histograms cannot provide advance warning of intracranial decompensation.

Szewczykowski[87,88] has developed an online computer method for detecting intracranial decompensation. This method plots the mean standard deviation ($\overline{SD}$) in ICP against the mean ICP ($\overline{ICP}$), where the mean values of ICP are grouped at 2 mm Hg intervals. On the basis of these plots Szewczykowski distinguished two ICP zones. The initial zone (zone A) of the plot of $\overline{SD}$ versus $\overline{ICP}$ showed little change in $\overline{SD}$ as $\overline{ICP}$ increased while the final zone (zone B) of this plot demonstrated increasing $\overline{SD}$ with increasing $\overline{ICP}$. The critical ICP level at which SD began to increase with $\overline{ICP}$ varied widely. The above method suffers from the same fault as the previous methods in that it depends on ICP fluctuations that can be detected with an adequate alarm system. Three years have passed since Szewczykowski first published the method, and there have been no further published data supporting the method as a valuable adjunct to clinical ICP monitoring.

Cardiac systole provides a recurring perturbation of the intracranial system. It is well established that the magnitude of ICP pulse pressure (PP) increases with the level of mean ICP. The normal waveform of the ICP pulse has also been described. It remains to be determined whether in the presence of a

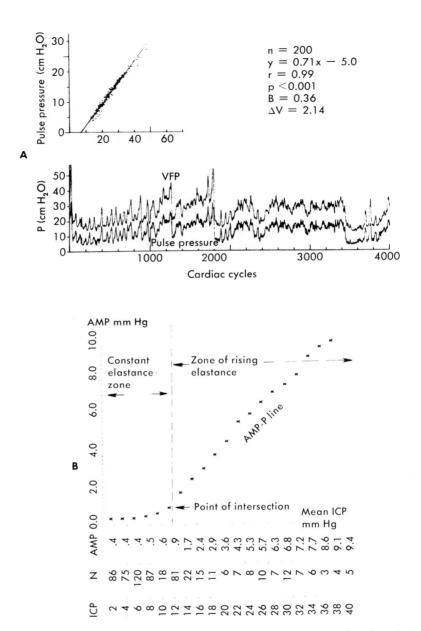

Fig. 4-13. Data demonstrating that beyond the baseline CSF pressure the plot of ICP pulse pressure versus ICP is linear. **A,** Pulse pressure versus ICP plot and ICP versus cardiac cycles plot in a patient with a glioma. Note that the X intercept of the pulse pressure versus ICP plot is based only on extrapolation of data at higher pressures (see equation 3). **B,** Computer printout of ICP pulse pressure (AMP) versus mean ICP for a normal patient. The relationship is linear above baseline mean ICP. Below baseline mean ICP there is no change in pulse pressure with decreasing ICP. (**A** from Avezaat, C. J. J., and others. In Beks, J. W. F., Bosch, D. A., and Brock, M., editors: Intracranial pressure III, Berlin, Heidelberg, New York, 1976, Springer-Verlag; **B** from Szewczykowski, J. Neurosurg. **47**:22, 1977.)

pathologic process, changes in the waveform or magnitude of PP will precede changes in $\overline{ICP}$. If such were the case, monitoring of PP or wave form characteristics might provide a valuable addition to our armamentarium. Analysis of ICP-PP magnitude or waveform generally requires computer averaging techniques.

Avezaat[2] has employed a computer system to monitor PP in 31 patients who were undergoing continuous recording of ICP. In all patients there was a linear relationship between PP and $\overline{ICP}$. The X intercept of this line was in most cases significantly different from zero. This intercept was based on an extrapolation of the regression line for PP versus $\overline{ICP}$ to the $\overline{ICP}$ axis. There was no data demonstrating that the PP versus $\overline{ICP}$ plot actually followed this extrapolation. These data are shown in Fig. 4-13, *A*. As we shall point out later, there is good evidence to support the conclusion that the linear plot of PP versus $\overline{ICP}$ fails near the equilibrium ICP. On the basis of the observed linear relationship between PP and $\overline{ICP}$ and on the basis of an assumed exponential relationship between CSF pressure and intracranial volume, Avezaat derived an equation for PP as a function of $\overline{ICP}$.

$$PP = (\overline{ICP} - ICP_0)(e^{B\Delta V} - 1) \qquad (3)$$

where

ICP_0 = the "x" intercept of the plot of PP versus $\overline{ICP}$

B = a fundamental constant expressing the ease with which the system will accept a given volume load

ΔV = any change of volume within the system

Avezaat proposed that a change in the slope of the computer plot of PP versus $\overline{ICP}$ could alert the physician to possibly deleterious events within the intracranial system. Such a change in slope could be due to either a change in the volume of blood (ΔV, equation 3) entering the head with each systole or the change in slope could be due to a change in how readily the system will accept a recurring fixed volume load (B, equation 3). Avezaat concluded that when there is a

change in the slope of the plot of PP versus $\overline{ICP}$ the only method of determining which parameter (B or ΔV) is involved is to make a measurement of the volume pressure response (VPR = $\Delta P/\Delta V$ for 1 ml bolus fluid injection into the CSF space). Thus, the elaborate method of Avezaat is really no better than the simple approach of making sequential measurements of the VPR. Furthermore, as with previous methods, the success of this method depends upon the actual spontaneous occurrence of pathologically high values of $\overline{ICP}$.

In addition to evaluating the plot of $\overline{SD}$ versus $\overline{ICP}$, Szewczykowski[89,90] has developed a computer method for analysis of PP amplitude as a function of $\overline{ICP}$. This method may find more practical application than previous computer-based methods. Szewczykowski utilizes infusion or drainage of CSF to provide, over a reasonably short time period, a suitable range of $\overline{ICP}$ over which one may evaluate the magnitude of PP. Two zones of PP change in response to increasing ICP were described. Above the baseline CSF pressure the plot of PP versus $\overline{ICP}$ was linear, PP increasing as $\overline{ICP}$ increased. However, below baseline $\overline{ICP}$ there was very little change in PP with decreasing values of $\overline{ICP}$. Szewczykowski's method evaluates intracranial compensatory reserves according to the slope of the linear regression of PP versus $\overline{ICP}$ above baseline $\overline{ICP}$ (Fig. 13, *B*). In 10 normal patients this slope factor was 0.329 ± 0.084 (SD) over an $\overline{ICP}$ range from 0 to 30 mm Hg and over a PP range of from 0 to 10 mm Hg. An abnormally high slope factor (0.551) was measured in one patient with normal $\overline{ICP}$ and an unsuspected epidural hematoma. The above method offers the opportunity to evaluate PP at $\overline{ICP}$ values that do not occur spontaneously and for this reason it might be anticipated that changes in the slope factor would precede changes in ICP. This study has not resolved the problem of a change in loading volume (cerebral blood volume change with systole) altering the slope factor. Another problem with the study as done by Szewczykowski is that addition and withdrawal of CSF was made via the lumbar route. In patients undergoing continuous monitoring of ICP such fluid additions and withdrawals must be made through the ventricular catheter. On the basis of the data relating ICP and PP Szewczykowski developed an equation for CSF pressure as a function of blood volume change. This relationship is different from the relationship determined independently by Marmarou, Sullivan, Miller, and Sklar for CSF pressure as a function of CSF volume—another bit of experimental evidence indicating that the single pressure volume curve for the intracranial space is an invalid concept.

ICP pulse pressure waveform has been investigated as a possible adjunct to ICP monitoring. The ICP pulse pressure waveform is composed of a main initial peak (P_1) followed by three smaller peaks (P_2, P_3, P_4) decreasing in amplitude. P_1 is thought to be directly related to arterial input, while P_2 to P_4 are thought to be venous in origin.[8] Castel and Cohadon[8] utilized Fourier's harmonic analysis to study ICP PP waveform in 44 patients.

When ICP was changed artificially by CSF infusion or withdrawal, Castel and Cohadon noted that P_2 became the largest of the four peaks. With hydrocephalus, the four peaks become less distinct while with mass lesions the peaks become even more distinct. It was suggested that the ICP PP waveform could be employed as a diagnostic tool in defining the etiology of intracranial hypertension. Castel and Cohadon were, however, not able to provide an explanation for their observations. The question of whether analysis of ICP pulse pressure waveform will eventually be of value in patient monitoring remains unanswered. Since the waveform of ICP pulse pressure reflects rather poorly understood, complex physical interactions, we doubt that observation of the ICP waveform alone will contribute substantially to progress in the management of intracranial hypertension.

PARADOXICAL OBSERVATIONS

In order to appreciate the discussion that follows, the reader should recall that the VPR is the CSF pressure change resulting from a bolus injection of 1 ml of fluid into the CSF space, and when the VPR is low, it is implied that the CSF space will accept large volumes of fluid with only a small change in CSF pressure. If one accepts the concept, as proposed by Langfitt, modified by Miller, and assumed by many authors, of a single intracranial pressure volume curve expressing CSF pressure as a function of volume change in any intracranial compartment, then a low VPR would imply that changes in cerebral blood volume such as those caused by spontaneous vasodilation of the cerebrovascular bed, by head turning or by neck compression should result in small elevations of intracranial pressure. During the past several years of ICP monitoring in patients, we have been impressed by a number of paradoxical phenomena that simply cannot be explained on the basis of a single intracranial pressure volume curve. Some patients with relatively low values of ICP and VPR develop alarmingly large increases in ICP with light neck compression or head turning. Other patients (on controlled ventilation with stable blood gases) with low ICP and low VPR have unexpectedly developed large plateau waves. Patients in the terminal phases of intracranial hypertension have demonstrated a seemingly paradoxical drop in VPR as ICP continues to increase to levels near arterial blood pressure.

The above observations suggest that volume changes within the cerebrovascular bed or within a mass lesion may have a quite different effect on CSF pressure than volume changes within the CSF space. Sullivan[85] tested the hypothesis that equal volume change in two different intracranial compartments will cause different effects on CSF pressure. This study was conducted by comparing the peak CSF pressure produced by bolus loading of the CSF space with the peak CSF pressure produced by equivalent bolus loading of an epidural balloon. Both spaces were loaded at the same rate. The rate of loading was such that CSF absorption was insignificant. Loading of both spaces always began at the same baseline pressure. When baseline balloon volume was low, equivalent loading of both compartments produced the

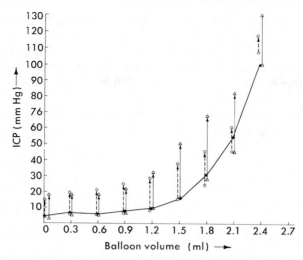

Fig. 4-14. Direct test of the hypothesis of a single pressure volume curve demonstrating this hypothesis to be invalid. Heavy curve, plot of ICP versus epidural balloon volume; open circles and dotted arrows, CSF pressure change with rapid loading of the CSF space; triangles and solid arrows, CSF pressure change after equivalent loading of epidural balloon. Loading is so rapid that essentially no CSF absorption takes place during either balloon or CSF space loading. Beginning at a baseline balloon volume of 1.5 ml, balloon loading causes a much larger CSF pressure change than does equivalent loading of the CSF space. Notice also that the absolute magnitude of the CSF pressure change decreases as balloon volume increases. (From Sullivan, H. G., and others: Am. J. Physiol. **234:**R167-171, 1978.)

same CSF pressure change. On the other hand, when baseline balloon volume was slightly higher, equivalent loading of the balloon produced a much larger increase in CSF pressure compared with the increase in CSF pressure following loading of the CSF space. These results are illustrated in Fig. 4-14 and provide proof for the concept that CSF pressure volume plots are different, depending on which intracranial volume compartments are being considered.

We believe that in defining intracranial pressure volume curves one should take great care to state precisely just which curves are being considered. To help standardize terminology we suggest the following names for two commonly discussed pressure volume curves:

1. CSF pressure volume curve for the plot of CSF pressure versus CSF volume. This curve is exponential (for rapid volume changes) under normal circumstances.

2. Mass lesion pressure volume curve for the plot of CSF pressure versus mass volume. For epidural balloon inflation this curve is hyperbolic.

The curve has not been defined for other types of mass lesions. We suggest that one should also state the type of mass under consideration. Since elastance is the slope of a pressure volume curve at a given point and compliance is the slope of a volume pressure curve at a given point, it is clear that when using the term elastance in relation to the intracranial system one should state clearly just which pressure volume curve is being considered. Such ambiguous terms as brain elastance or intracranial elastance should be avoided. In these terms, the VPR is an estimate of the elastance of the CSF pressure volume curve and we term this elastance the CSF space elastance (Ecsf).

The discrepancies (low VPR and large change in ICP with head turning, low VPR associated with spontaneous plateau waves) noted above between the CSF P-V curve and the plot of CSF pressure versus cerebral blood volume indicate that a critical situation may be present in the cerebral parenchyma where small volume changes within brain tissue may induce decompensation at a time when manipulations within the CSF space would suggest that the patient is not in danger. These observations suggest that effort should be directed at evaluating the mechanical properties of cerebral parenchyma more directly.

As the reader will recall, another seemingly paradoxical observation was that when the steady state equations for CSF bulk flow were combined with the known exponential relationship (for rapid changes in CSF volume) between CSF pressure and CSF volume, a relationship emerged that significantly underestimated the true value of CSF outflow resistance.[86] The brain seemed to undergo a type of "tissue relaxation" when deformed by ventricular enlargement secondary to a bolus fluid injection into the CSF space. These observations also point to the importance of the mechanical properties of brain tissue in determining just how CSF pressure will change in response to any particular alteration within the intracranial system.

Schettini[71-77,94-96] has employed a method for evaluation of in vivo brain tissue mechanical properties in dogs and has demonstrated that brain tissue mechanical response properties (viscoelastic response parameters—mechanically the brain is a viscoelastic material[30,73]) were severely altered by hypoosmotic brain edema, drug-induced hypotension, hypercarbia, drug-induced hypertension, hypercarbic anoxia, and cerebral vasodilation at a time when ICP was normal. Schettini's studies also demonstrate the significance of the phenomenon of brain tissue relaxation.[74] These studies are promising, but further work remains to be done before clinical application is possible. Other methods of evaluating the internal milieu of brain tissue include measurement of CBF and CBV, monitoring cerebral edema accumulation and resolution with serial CAT scans, continuous monitoring of EEG and evoked potentials, and repeated determinations of cerebral metabolic rate for O_2 and glucose. A host of other parameters could also be listed. Many of the above parameters can only be sampled intermittently and *not* monitored continuously. Furthermore, many of these techniques are cumbersome and time consuming and are not suited to the odd hours and the rapidity with which decompensation can occur in neurologically ill patients. These features considerably diminish the usefulness of many potentially available tools.

SUMMARY

We believe that in future studies aimed at preventing volumetric decompensation within the intracranial system, attention must be directed away from the CSF space toward the brain tissue itself. Techniques must be developed that will detect and identify accumulating edema, changes in cerebral blood volume, and changes in cerebral blood flow as well as other potentially adverse changes within the internal environment of brain tissue long before changes in intracranial pressure occur. These techniques must allow continuous monitoring of the internal environment of brain tissue and the techniques must be simple and easily repeatable in the working environment of a neurologic intensive care unit. For the present, it must be stated that ICP monitoring, in spite of its flaws, remains a useful tool in managing neurologically ill patients, being an aid in clinical management, in cases of brain tumor, stroke, hydrocephalus, metabolic encephalopathy, intracranial aneurysm, and hydrocephalus. We also believe that for the technique of continuous monitoring of ICP to be employed most beneficially physicians responsible for ICP monitoring in patients must be aware of both the limitations and advantages of the method.

REFERENCES

1. Adams, H., and Graham, D. I.: The relationship between ventricular fluid pressure and the neuropathology of raised intracranial pressure. In Brock, M., and Deitz, H., editors: Intracranial pressure, Berlin, Heidelberg, New York, 1972, Springer-Verlag, pp. 250-253.

2. Avezaat, C. J. J., van Eijndhoven, J. H. M., de Jong, D. A., and Moolenaar, W. C. J.: A new method of monitoring intracranial volume pressure relationship. In Beks, J. W. F., Bosch, D. A., and Brock, M., editors: Intracranial pressure III, Berlin, Heidelberg, New York, 1976, Springer-Verlag, pp. 308-313.

3. Aoki, Y., and Lombroso, C. T.: Prognostic value of electroencephalography in Reye's syndrome, Neurology 23:333, 1973.

4. Becker, D. P., Vries, J. K., Young, H. F., and Ward, J. D.: Controlled cerebral perfusion pressure and ventilation in human mechanical brain injury: prevention of progressive brain swelling. In Lundberg, N., Ponten, U., and Brock, M., editors: Intracranial pressure II, Berlin, Heidelberg, New York, 1975, Springer-Verlag, pp. 480-484.

5. Brain, W. R.: A clinical study of increased intracranial pressure in sixty cases of cerebral tumor, Brain 48:105, 1925.

6. Browder, J., and Meyers, R.: Observations on behavior of the systemic blood pressure, pulse and spinal fluid pressure following craniocerebral injury, Am. J. Surg. 31:403-427, 1936.

7. Cairns, H.: Raised intracranial pressure: hydrocephalic and vascular factors, Br. J. Surg. 27:275-294, 1939.

8. Castel, J. P., and Cohadon, F.: The pattern of cerebral pulse: automatic analysis. In Beks, J. W. F., Bosch, D. A., Brock, M., editors: Intracranial pressure III, Berlin, 1976, Springer-Verlag, pp. 303-305.

9. Cobb, S., and Fremont-Smith, F.: Cerebral circulation: changes in human circulation and in the pressure of cerebrospinal fluid during inhalation of mixture of carbon dioxide and oxygen, Arch. Neurol. Psychiatr. 26:731-736, 1931.

10. Cushing, H.: Some experimental and clinical observations concerning states of increased intracranial tension, Am. J. Med. Sci. 124:375-400, 1902.

11. Cutler, R. W. P., Page, L., Galicich, J., and Watters, G. V.: Formation and absorption of cerebrospinal fluid in man, Brain 91:707-720, 1968.

12. Dandy, W. E.: Intracranial pressure without brain tumor, Brain 106:492-513, 1937.

13. Ekstedt, J.: CSF hydrodynamics studied by means of constant pressure infusion technique. In Lundberg, N., Ponten, U., and Brock, M., editors: Intracranial pressure II, Berlin, Heidelberg, New York, 1975, Springer-Verlag, pp. 35-41.

14. Finney, L. A., and Walker, E. A.: Transtentorial herniation, Springfield, Ill., 1962, Charles C Thomas, Publisher.

15. Fitch, W., and McDowall, D. G.: Hazards of anesthesia in patients with intracranial space occupying lesions. In McDowall, D. G., editor: International anesthesia clinics, vol. 7, no. 3, Boston, 1969, Little Brown & Co., pp. 639-662.

16. Fremont-Smith, F., and Hodgson, J. S.: Combined ventricular and lumbar puncture in the diagnosis of brain tumor, Assoc. Res. Nerv. Dis. Proc. 4:172-184, 1924.

17. Griffith, R. L., and Becker, D. P.: Physiological monitoring of the head injury patient. In Thompson, R. A., and Green, J. B., editors: Advances in neurology, vol. 17, Raven Press, New York (in press).

18. Guillaume, J., and Janny, P.: Manométrie Intracranienne Continue Intérêt de la Méthode et Premiers Résultats, Rev. Neurol. 84:131-142, 1951.

19. Heisey, S. R., Held, D., and Pappenheimer, J. R.: Bulk flow and diffusion in the cerebrospinal fluid system of the goat, Am. J. Physiol. 203:775-781, 1962.

20. Hodgson, J. S.: The relationship between increased intracranial pressure and increased intraspinal pressure; changes in cerebrospinal fluid in increased intracranial pressure, Assoc. Res. Nerv. Dis. Proc. 8:182-188, 1927.

21. Horta, M. P., and Mello, P. A.: Intracranial pressure in Reye's syndrome. In Beks, J. W. F., Bosch, D. A., and Brock, M., editors: Intracranial pressure III, Berlin, Heidelberg, New York, 1976, Springer-Verlag, pp. 327-329.

22. Jackson, H.: The management of acute cranial injuries by the early exact determination of intracranial pressure and its relief of lumbar drainage. Surg. Gynecol. Obstet. 34:494-508, 1922.

23. Janny, P., Jouan, J. P., Janny, L., Gourgand, M., and Gueit, A. M.: A statistical approach to longterm monitoring of intracranial pressure. In Brock, M., and Dietz, H., editors: Intracranial pressure, Berlin, 1972, Springer-Verlag, pp. 50-64.

24. Jefferson, G.: The tentorial pressure cone, Arch. Neurol. Psychiatr. 40:857-875, 1938.

25. Jennett, W. B., Barker, J., Fitch, W., and McDowall, D. G.: Effect of anesthesia on intracranial pressure in patients with space-occupying lesions, Lancet 1:61-64, 1969.

26. Jennett, W. B., McDowall, D. G., and Barker, J.: The effects of halothane on intracranial pressure in cerebral tumors; report of two cases, J. Neurosurg. 26:270-274, 1967.

27. Johnston, I. H., Johnston, J. A., and Jennett, W. B.: Intracranial pressure following head injury, Lancet 2:433-436, 1970.

28. Kernohan, J. W., and Woltman, H. W.: Incisure of the crus due to contralateral brain tumor, Arch. Neurol. Psychiatr. 21:274-287, 1921.

29. Kindt, G. W., Waldman, J., Kohl, S., Baublis, J., and Tucker, R. P.: Intracranial pressure in Reye's syndrome, J.A.M.A. 231:822, 1975.

30. Kjallgvist, A., Lundberg, N., and Pontén, U.: Respiratory and cardiovascular changes during spontaneous variations of ventricular fluid pressure in patients with intracranial hypertension, Acta Neurol. Scand. 40:291-317, 1964.

31. Koeneman, J. B.: Viscoelastic properties of brain tissue (master's thesis), 1966, Case Institute of Technology.

32. Kullberg, G.: A method for statistical analysis of

intracranial pressure recordings. In Brock, M., and Dietz, H., editors: Intracranial pressure, Berlin, 1972, Springer-Verlag, pp. 59-64.

33. Langfitt, T. W., Kumar, V. S., James H. E., and Miller, J. D.: Continuous recording of intracranial pressure in patients with hypoxic brain damage. In Brierley, J. B., and Mildrum, B. S., editors: Brain hypoxia, London, 1971, Heinemann, pp. 118-135.

34. Langfitt, T. W., Weinstein, J. D., and Kassell, N. F.: Cerebral vasomotor paralysis produced by intracranial hypertension, Neurology (Minneap) **15:**622-641, 1965.

35. Langfitt, T. W., Weinstein, J. D., Kassell, N. F., and Simeone, A.: Transmission of increased intracranial pressure. I. Within the craniospinal axis, J. Neurosurg. **21:**989-997, 1964.

36. Lundberg, N.: Continuous recording and control of ventricular fluid pressure in neurosurgical practice, Acta Psychiatr. Neurol. Scand. (Suppl.), pp. 146-149, 1960.

37. Lundberg, N.: Monitoring of the intracranial pressure. In Critchley, M., O'Leary, J. L., and Jennett, B., editors: Scientific foundations of neurology, Philadelphia, 1972, F. A. Davis, pp. 356-371.

38. Lundberg, N., Crongvist, K., and Jallquist, A.: Clinical investigations on interrelations between intracranial pressure and intracranial hemodynamics. In Luyendijk, W., editor: Progress in brain research, vol. 30, Amsterdam, 1968, Elsevier, pp. 69-75.

39. Lundberg, N., Troupp, H., and Lorin, H.: Continuous recording of ventricular-fluid pressure in patients with severe acute traumatic brain injury; a preliminary report, J. Neurosurg. **22:**581-590, 1965.

40. McCreery, J. A., and Berry, F. B.: A study of 520 cases of fracture of the skull, Ann. Surg. **88:**890-901, 1928.

41. McClure, R. D., and Crawford, A. S.: The management of craniocerebral injuries, Arch. Surg. **16:**451-468, 1928.

42. McDowall, D. G., Barker, J., and Jennett, W. B.: Cerebrospinal fluid pressure measurements during anesthesia, Anesthesia **21:**189-201, 1966.

43. McDowall, D. G., and Harper, A. M.: Blood flow and oxygen uptake of the cerebral cortex of the dog during anesthesia with different volatile agents, Acta Neurol. Scand. (Suppl.)**14:**146, 1965.

44. Marmarou, A.: A theoretical and experimental evaluation of the cerebrospinal fluid system, Philadelphia, 1973, Ph.D. thesis.

45. Marmarou, A., Shapiro, K., and Shulman, K.: Isolating factors leading to sustained elevations of the ICP. In Beks, J. W. F., Bosch, D. A., and Brock, M., editors: Intrancranial Pressure III, Berlin, Heidelberg, New York, 1976, Springer-Verlag, pp. 33-35.

46. Marmarou, A., Shulman, K., and LaMorgese, J.: A compartmental analysis of compliance and outflow resistance and the effects of elevated blood pressure. In Lundberg, N., Ponten, U., and Brock, M.,

editors: Intracranial Pressure II, Berlin, Heidelberg, New York, 1975, Springer-Verlag, pp. 86-88.

47. Marmarou, A., Shulman, K., and LaMorgese, J.: Compartmental analysis of compliance and outflow resistance of the cerebrospinal fluid system, J. Neurosurg. **43:**523-534, 1976.

48. Meyer, A.: Herniation of the brain, Arch. Neurol. Psychiatr. **4:**387-400, 1920.

49. Miller J. D.: Volume and pressure in the craniospinal axis. In Wilkins, R. H., editor: Clinical Neurosurgery, vol. 22, Baltimore, 1975, The Williams & Wilkins Co., pp. 76-105.

50. Miller, J. D.: Intracranial pressure-volume relationships in pathological conditions, J. Neurosurg. Sci. **20:**203-209, 1976.

51. Miller, J. D., Becker, D. P., Ward, J. D., Sullivan, H. G., Adams, W. E., and Rosner, M. J.: Significance of intracranial hypertension in severe head injury, J. Neurosurg. **47:**503-516, 1977.

52. Miller, J. D., and Garibi, J.: Intracranial volume-pressure relationships during continuous monitoring of ventricular fluid pressure. In Brock, M., and Deitz, H., editors: Intracranial pressure, Berlin, Heidelberg, New York, 1972, Springer-Verlag, pp. 270-274.

53. Miller, J. D., Garibi, J., and Pickard, J. D.: The effects of induced changes of cerebrospinal fluid volume during continuous monitoring of ventricular pressure, Arch. Neurol. **28:**265-269, 1973.

54. Miller, J. D., and Leech, P. J.: Assessing the effects of mannitol and steroid therapy on intracranial volume-pressure relationships, J. Neurosurg. **42:**274-281, 1975.

55. Miller, J. D., Leech, P. J., and Pickard, J. D.: Volume-pressure response in various experiments and clinical conditions. In Lundberg, N., Ponten, U., and Brock, M., editors: Intracranial pressure II, Berlin, Heidelberg, New York, 1975, Springer-Verlag, pp. 97-100.

56. Miller, J. D., and Pickard, J. D.: Intracranial volume-pressure studies in patients with head injury, Injury **5:**265-269, 1974.

57. Miller, J. D., Sakalas, R., Ward, J. D., Young, H. F., Adams, W. E., Vries, J. K., and Becker, D. P.: Methylprednisolone treatment in patients with brain tumors, Neurosurgery **1:**114-117, 1977.

58. Miller, J. D., and Sullivan, H. G.: Severe intracranial hypertension. In Trubuhovich, R. V., editor: Management of acute intracranial disasters, Boston, 1979, Little, Brown & Co., pp. 19-75.

59. Moore, M. T., and Stern, K.: Vascular lesions in brain stem and occipital lobe occurring in association with brain tumors, Brain **61:**70-98, 1938.

60. O'Connell, J. E. A.: The vascular factor in intracranial pressure and the maintenance of the cerebral spinal fluid circulation, Brain **66:**204-228, 1943.

61. Richardson, A., Hide, T. A. H., and Eversden, I. D.: Long-term continuous intracranial pressure monitoring by means of a modified subdural pressure transducer, Lancet **2:**687-690, 1970.

62. Risberg, J., Lundberg, N., and Ingrav, D. H.: Re-

gional cerebral blood volume during acute transient rises of the intracranial pressure (plateau waves), J. Neurosurg. **31**:303-310, 1969.

63. Rossanda, M., Collice, M., Porta, M., AND Boselli, L.: Intracranial hypertension in head injury, clinical significance and relation to respiration. In Lundberg, N., Ponten, U., and Brock, M., editors: Intracranial pressure II, Berlin, Heidelberg, New York, 1975, Springer-Verlag.

64. Ryder, H. W., Espey, F. F., Kimbell, F. D., Penka, E. J., Rosenauer, A., Podolsky, B., and Evans, J. P.: Influence of changes in cerebral blood flow on the cerebrospinal fluid pressure, Arch. Neurol. Psychiatr. **68**:165-169, 1952.

65. Ryder, H. W., Espey, F. F., Kimbell, F. P., Penka, E. J., Rosenauer, A., Podolsky, B., and Evans, J. P.: Modification of the effect of cerebral blood flow on cerebral spinal fluid pressure by variations in craniospinal blood volume, Arch. Neurol. Psychiatr. **68**:170-174, 1952.

66. Ryder, H. W., Espey, F. F., Kimbell, F. D., Penka, E. J., Rosenauer, A., Podolsky, B., and Evans, J. P.: Effect of changes in systemic venous pressure on cerebrospinal fluid pressure, Arch. Neurol. Psychiatr. **68**:175-179, 1952.

67. Ryder, H. W., Espey, F. F., Kimbell, F. D., Penka, E. J., Rosenauer, A., Podolsky, B., and Evans, J. P.: The mechanism of the change in cerebrospinal fluid pressure following an induced change in the volume of the fluid space, J. Lab. Clin. Med. **41**:428-435, 1953.

68. Ryder, H. W., Espey, F. F., Kimbell, F. D., Renka, E. J., Rosenauer, A., Podolsky, B., Hirget, P., and Evans, J. P.: The elasticity of the craniospinal venous bed, J. Lab. Clin. Med. **42**:944, 1953.

69. Ryder, H. W., Espey, F. F., Kimbell, F. D., Penka, E. J., Rosenauer, A., Podolsky, B., and Evans, J. P.: The mechanism of the effect of changes in blood osmotic pressure on the cerebrospinal fluid pressure, J. Lab. Clin. Med. **41**:543-549, 1953.

70. Ryder, H. W., Rosenauer, A., Penka, E. J., Espey, F. F., and Evans, J. P.: Failure of abnormal cerebrospinal fluid pressure to influence cerebral function, Arch. Neurol. Psychiatr. **70**:563-586, 1953.

71. Schettini, A., and Furniss, W. W.: Dynamic response of the intracranial system in the conscious dog to papaverine hydrochloride, Stroke **7**:618-625, 1976.

72. Schettini, A., MacKay, L., Majors, R., Mahig, J., and Nevis, A.: Experimental approach for monitoring surface brain pressure, J. Neurosurg. **34**:38-47, 1971.

73. Schettini, A., Mahig, J., and Moreshead, G.: Influence of cerebral vascular factors on brain-relative stiffness. In Brock, M., and Dietz, H., editors: Intracranial pressure, Berlin, 1972, Springer-Verlag, pp. 27-32.

74. Schettini, A., and Walsh, E. K.: Pressure relaxation of the intracranial system in vivo, Am. J. Physiol. **225**:513-517, 1973.

75. Schettini, A., and Walsh, E. K.: Experimental identification of the subarachnoid and subpial compartments by intracranial pressure measurements, J. Neurosurg. **40**:609-616, 1974.

76. Schettini, A., and Walsh, E. K.: Simultaneous pressure-depth measurements of the intracranial system made epidurally. In Lundberg, N., Ponten, U., and Brock, M., editors: Intracranial pressure II, Berlin, 1975, Springer-Verlag, pp. 409-413.

77. Schettini, A., Walsh, E. K., and Furniss, W. W.: The influence of methylmethacrylate on brain elastic response *in vivo*, Ann. Biomed. Engl. **5**: 111-121, 1977.

78. Sklar, F. H., and Elashvili, I.: The pressure-volume function of brain elasticity; physiological considerations and clinical applications, J. Neurosurg. **47**: 670-679, 1977.

79. Shapiro, K., Marmarou, A., and Shulman, K.: Clinical applications of the pressure volume index, paper no. 75, The American Association of Neurological Surgeons' Meeting, San Francisco, 1976.

80. Shulman, K., and Marmarou, A.: Pressure-volume considerations in infantile hydrocephalus, Dev. Child. Neurol. **13**(suppl. 25):90-95, 1971.

81. Smyth, C. N.: The guard-ring tocodynamometer; absolute measurement of intraamniotic pressure by a new instrument, J. Obstet. Gynecol. Br. Emp. **64**:59-66, 1957.

82. Smyth, G. E., and Henderson, W. R.: Observations on the cerbrospinal fluid pressure and on simultaneous ventricular and lumbar punctures, J. Neurol. Psychiatr. **1**:226-237, 1938.

83. Sullivan, H. G., Miller, J. D., Becker, D. P., Flora, R. E., and Allen, R. A.: The physiological basis of ICP change with progressive epidural brain compression; an experimental evaluation in cats, J. Neurosurg. **47**:532-550, 1977.

84. Sullivan, H. G., Miller, J. D., Griffith, R. L., and Becker, D. P.: CSF pressure-volume dynamics in neurosurgical patients; a preliminary evaluation in six patients, Surg. Neurol. **9**:47-54, 1977.

85. Sullivan, H. G., Miller, J. D., Griffith, R. L., and Becker, D. P.: CSF pressure transients in response to epidural and ventricular volume loading, Am. J. Physiol. **234**:R167-171, 1978.

86. Sullivan, H. G., Miller, J. D., Griffith, R. L., Carter, W., and Rucker, S.: Bolus versus steady-state infusion for determination of CSF outflow resistance, Ann. Neurol. **5**:228-238, 1979.

87. Szewczykowski, J., Dytho, P., Dunicki, A., Korsak-Sliwka, J., Sliwka, S., Dziduszko, J., and Bozena, A.: Determination of critical ICP levels in neurosurgical patients: a statistical approach. In Lundberg, N., Ponten, U., and Borck, M., editors: Intracranial pressure II, 1975, Berlin, Springer-Verlag, pp. 391-393.

88. Szewczykowski, J., Dytko, P., Kunicki, A., and others: A method of estimating intracranial decompensation in man, J: Neurosurg. **45**:155-158, 1976.

89. Szewczykowski, J., Korsak-Sliwka, J., Kunicki, A.,

Dytho, P. W., Sliwka, A., and Dziduszho, J.: Computer-assisted determination of optimum ICP levels. In Beks, J. W. F., Bosch, D. A., Brock, M., editors: Intracranial pressure III, Berlin, 1976, Springer-Verlag, pp. 295-299.

90. Szewczykowski, J., Sliwka, S., Kunicki, A., Dytko, P., and Lorsak-Sliwka, J.: A fast method of estimating the elastance of the intracranial system; a practical application in neurosurgery, J. Neurosurg. **47:** 19-26, 1977.

91. Troupp, H.: Intraventricular pressure in patients with severe brain injuries, J. Trauma **5:**373-378, 1965.

92. Vapalahti, M., and Troupp, H.: Prognosis for patients with severe brain injuries, Br. Med. J. **3:** 404-407, 1971.

93. Vincent, C., David, M., and Thiebaut, F.: Le cone de pression temporal dans les tumeurs des hemispheres cérébraux, Rev. Neurol., 1936.

94. Walsh, E. K., Furniss, W. W., and Schettini, A.: On the measurement of brain elastic response in vivo, Am. J. Physiol. **232:**R27-R30, 1977.

95. Walsh, E. K., and Schettini, A.: A pressure-displacement transducer for measuring brain tissue properties in vivo, J. Appl. Physiol. **38:**187-189, 1975.

96. Walsh, E. K., and Schettini, A.: Elastic behavior of brain tissue in vivo, Am. J. Physiol. **230:**1058-1061, 1976.

97. Weinstein, J. D., Langfitt, T. W., and Kassell, N. F.: Vasopressor response to increased intracranial pressure, Neurology **14:**1118-1131, 1964.

98. Wolff, H. G., and Lennox, W. G.: Cerebral circulation. XII. The effect on pial vessels of variations in the oxygen and carbon dioxide content of the blood, Arch. Neurol. Psychiatr. **23:**1097-1120, 1930.

99. Wollman, H., Alexander, S. C., Cohen, P. J., Chase, P. E., Melman, E., and Behar, M. G.: Cerebral circulation of man during halothane anesthesia, Anesthesiology **25:**180, 1964.

5

Intracranial pressure control

DAVID A. ROTTENBERG
JEROME B. POSNER

Although disorders of the third circulation have been recognized and treated by physicians and surgeons since the dawn of recorded medical history, until recently our understanding of the cerebrospinal fluid (CSF) system was based almost entirely upon empirical observations, and there was no uniformly successful treatment for intracranial hypertension or hypotension. The last 30 years have witnessed a virtual explosion of scientific interest in CSF formation, bulk flow and absorption, and intracranial pressure, as a result of which it is now possible to describe (model) the CSF system in mathematical terms and to accurately predict its responses to a variety of pathologic perturbations. Furthermore, a number of surgical techniques and pharmacologic agents for the treatment of patients with raised intracranial pressure have recently become available. Although we cannot yet account for the efficacy of some of these treatment modalities, the effectiveness of many others can be explained in precise physiologic terms. Unfortunately, advances in our understanding of CSF physiology and in the treatment of disease states associated with increased/decreased intracranial pressure have not always found their way into neurologic and neurosurgical practice, and much of the treatment currently offered patients with intracranial hypertension or hypotension remains essentially empirical.

This review attempts to survey—within the context of our present understanding of CSF statics and dynamics—the clinical problems associated with altered intracranial pressure relationships and to describe in pathophysiologic terms various therapeutic approaches to the patient with increased or decreased intracranial pressure.

A recent monograph[11] updates the anatomy and physiology of the cerebrospinal fluid system. Since any discussion of intracranial pressure relationships assumes a basic knowledge of neuroanatomy and CSF physiology, the essential anatomic and physiologic features of the cerebrospinal fluid system will be described before proceeding further.

In the normal adult the ventriculosubarachnoid space contains approximately 125 to 150 ml of CSF. CSF is formed at a constant rate of about 0.35 ml/min and derives, in large part, from the choroid plexuses of the cerebral ventricles; although cerebral endothelial cells and the ependyma may also contribute to total CSF bulk flow, the contribution of these extrachoroidal sources remains in dispute. Cerebrospinal fluid produced within the ventricular system passes through the outflow foramina of the fourth ventricle and circulates throughout the cerebrospinal subarachnoid space, ultimately being absorbed into the venous system through the arachnoid villi associated with dural venous sinuses and spinal nerve roots.

The skull and spinal canal, which contain the substance of the brain and spinal cord and the cerebrospinal vasculature as well as the CSF, constitute a semirigid compartment vented to the atmosphere indirectly by means of the cardiovascular system. Although the intracranial and intraspinal contents are not entirely rigid, an increase or decrease in the volume of any one of the three "compartments" mentioned above (brain/spinal cord, blood, CSF) implies a concomitant decrease or increase in the volume of one or another compartment. In general, because the brain and spinal cord volumes are relatively insensitive to rapid compression or decompression, an increase or decrease in the volume of CSF usually implies a reciprocal decrease or increase in the volume of the craniospinal venous bed. Similarly, fluctuations in cerebral blood volume (CBV) may be compensated by reciprocal fluctuations in CSF volume.

Under normal resting conditions, CSF pressure (CSFP) measured by lumbar puncture in the lateral recumbent position is equal to 100-160 mm H_2O. Sudden changes in lumbar CSFP are produced in normal individuals by coughing, straining, changes in position, and hyperventilation or hypoventilation. Thus, both static and dynamic factors contribute to the production of CSFP, and *both* static and dynamic considerations must be invoked to explain the pathogenesis of intracranial hypertension or hypotension and the appearance of clinical symptoms in disease states associated with abnormal increases or decreases in CSFP.

HISTORICAL PRECEDENTS

The history of neurologic and neurosurgical interest in the ventricular system, cerebrospinal fluid, and intracranial pressure (ICP) may be conveniently divided into three phases: (1) a *descriptive* phase beginning in antiquity, possibly with ritual trepanation, and ending in the eighteenth century with the recognition of CSF as a normal constituent of the central nervous system (CNS) circulating within anatomically defined pathways; (2) a *clinical* phase beginning in 1768 with the publication of Robert Whytt's *Observations on the Dropsy in the Brain* and culminating in the work of Harvey Cushing; and (3) an *experimental* phase beginning in 1842 with the publication of François Magendie's famous monograph, *Recherches physiologiques et cliniques sur le liquide céphalo-rachidien ou cérébrospinal,* and continuing to the present day. During the past 25 years, the distinctions between phases 2 and 3 have become increasingly blurred as a succession of technological advances has, in effect, brought the laboratory to the bedside.

Although CSF was probably mentioned in a gloss on the Edwin Smith Surgical Papyrus (c. 3000 BC), Galen's account of the ventricular system is the first detailed one we possess. Galen conceived of the "anterior ventricles" as elaborating the psychic pneuma (animal spirit) and, at the same time, as constituting "an olfactory organ and a channel for the outflow of superfluities." The Galenic theory that CSF was in some way associated with animal spirits and cerebral waste products persisted for more than a millennium and was echoed in the writings of Massa (1536), who provided the first modern description of the cerebrospinal fluid, and by Willis (1664), who naively (but correctly) suggested that the choroid plexuses secrete ventricular CSF. One hundred years after the publication of Willis' *Cerebri anatome*, Domenico Cotugno (1764) described the spinal subarachnoid space and concluded that "those waters which the cerebellar ventricle receives, whether from the larger ventricles of the cerebrum through the lacuna and the aqueduct of Sylvius, whether from special exhaling arteries, are . . . mixed with the waters of the spine."

Magendie's anatomic, physiologic, and clinical researches during the second quarter of the nineteenth century ushered in the modern era of CSF physiology and set the stage for Luschka (1855), who confirmed that CSF was secreted by the choroid plexuses, and for Key and Retzius (1875-1876), who established by means of gelatin dye injections that CSF is absorbed into the venous system by way of the Pacchionian villi. The introduction of percutaneous lumber puncture by Quincke in 1891[124] provoked widespread interest in the clinical concomitants of increased ICP, which were catalogued by Kocher[72] 10 years later. Kocher subdivided the symptoms and signs of cerebral compression into three clinical stages that he related to progressive medullary anemia, but it remained for Cushing[25-27] to quantify Kocher's observations and introduce them into neurosurgical practice. The classic Kocher-Cushing signs of cerebral compression were enumerated by Cushing in a sequel to the Mutter Lecture for 1901[25]: ". . . headache, vertigo, restlessness, roaring in the ears, a disturbed sensorium with excitement or delirium, an unnatural sleep . . . distention and tortuosity of the veins radiating from the optic papilla" and "slowing of the pulse with or without a certain rise in blood pressure" (stage I); a rise in systemic blood pressure, "vagus symptoms" (bradycardia), "respiratory disturbances", intermittent stupor, and "rhythmic alterations in size of the pupils" (stage II); and "falling blood pressure, irregular cardiac and respiratory efforts, deep coma . . . complete muscular relaxation, wide pupils" and, ultimately, cardiorespiratory failure (stage III).

Cushing's conception of the physiologic response to increased ICP was all but universally accepted until Browder and Meyers[12] published the results of their experiments on postoperative neurosurgical patients with bulging decompression sites. These authors concluded that "increases in intracranial pressure below the level of mean systemic pressure have no effect on the pulse rate, respiratory rate or systemic blood pressure." Evans and co-workers[40] were likewise unable to induce hypertension, bradycardia, or apnea (the Cushing phenomenon) in human subjects by artificially elevating ICP to the level of mean systemic blood pressure. On several occasions they "elevated the intracranial pressure to 2,000 mm of saline (147 mm Hg) without the subject's awareness of any sensation." They concluded, therefore, that "signs and symptoms other than the Cushing phenomenon must be depended on for the proper handling of the emergency patient with high intracranial pressure." Subsequently, Weinstein and co-workers[168] studied the vasomotor response to induced intracranial hypertension in rhesus monkeys and discovered that the threshold for this response varied with (1) the depth of anesthesia, (2) the experimental method whereby intracranial hypertension was produced (extra-axial versus intra-axial balloon, subarachnoid saline injection), and (3) the presence or absence of transtentorial herniation. These authors argued that "local compression or ischemia of many parts of the central nervous system may cause arterial hypertension which shows little relationship to the level of intracranial pressure." They thought it unlikely that either medullary ischemia (Cushing) or brain stem distortion (Thompson and Molina[161]) was primarily responsible for the observed vasopressor response to increased ICP.

A careful reading of his early publications on the vasopressor response reveals that Cushing clearly recognized that "the brain does not transmit the pressure from . . . a localized foreign body equally in all directions"; "the dislocation downward of the brain, and consequent blocking of the foramen magnum, plays a certain part in shutting off the spinal fluid from the effects of tension existent within the cranial chambers"; "in the clinical states representing conditions of general compression, such as meningitis, acute cerebral edema, (subarachnoid) hemorrhage, etc., the tension of the fluid in the lumbar meninges more nearly corresponds with the intracranial tension"; and "the ophthalmoscope offers a method of determining in clinical cases the presence or absence of intracranial venous stasis inasmuch as the congestion is transmitted to and is easily observable in the veins of the fundus."

Adolph Meyer[104] recognized that obstructive hydrocephalus, cerebral edema, and hemispheral tumors may produce "subtentorial herniation of the uncus." He also suggested that "impingement on the calcarine branch of the posterior cerebral artery" by an uncal hernia might give rise to "secondary hemianopsia," and hinted at the danger of lumbar puncture in the presence of increased ICP. But it remained for Jefferson[64] to define the clinical syndrome of the "tentorial pressure cone" and stress the urgency of its early recognition with a view toward neurosurgical intervention. Jefferson concluded that "lumbar puncture should be withheld in cases of high pressure, even if the lesion is known to be hemispheral, unless it is believed to be essential to the diagnosis"—a caveat that still bears repeating. He also recognized that the absence of papilledema did not exclude the presence of "high intracranial pressure." McNealy and Plum[101] described two distinct clinical syndromes (the so-called uncal and central syndromes) of progressive brain stem dysfunction in patients with supratentorial mass lesions. They minimized the role of raised ICP in the pathogenesis of these syndromes and argued that the inexorably progressive rostral-caudal deterioration of brain stem function that they observed resulted from "a spreading disturbance from an initial source rather than any sudden displacement- or distortion-producing disturbances at sites remote from those already impaired."

Although Magendie was well aware of the "pression que supporte et que transmet le liquide céphalorachidien" (cerebrospinal fluid pressure) and discussed the effects of pathologically increased CSF pressure on brain and spinal cord function, it remained for subsequent generations of physiologists and clinical investigators to quantify his astute observations and to fully appreciate their diagnostic and therapeutic significance. With the advent of electromanometry and ICP monitoring (Guillaume and Janny[53]), it became apparent that ventricular fluid pressure (VFP) varies from moment to moment; that periodic elevations of VFP ("par-

oxysmes hypertensifs") occur in patients with chronically elevated ICP and are occasionally, but not necessarily, associated with a wide range of clinical symptoms and signs; and that sustained elevations of ICP are frequently observed during sleep. The pioneering work of Guillaume and Janny was extended by Lundberg,[86] who standardized the techniques of ICP recording and studied the relationship between variations in VFP and "general pressure symptoms." Lundberg described spontaneous fluctuations of VFP in patients with space-occupying intracranial lesions and intracranial hypertension of other etiologies. Two predominant wave forms were identified: plateau waves (A waves) of irregular occurrence and without premonitory symptoms or obvious precipitating factors, ranging in amplitude from 50 to 100 mm Hg and lasting for 5 to 20 minutes, and one-per-minute waves (B waves, occurring mainly in association with Cheyne-Stokes respirations and varying in amplitude from "discernibility" to 50 mm Hg). Lundberg concluded that the continuous monitoring of VFP in neurosurgical patients may provide valuable clinical information and allow for the rational control of intracranial hypertension by intermittent ventricular drainage.

Although Masserman's[100] clinically oriented studies of "cerebrospinal hydrodynamics" provided the impetus for a reevaluation of the prevailing anatomically oriented concepts of CSF formation and absorption, it was Ryder[140] who first proposed that CSFP was "an equilibrium pressure, in the sense that any fluid exchange into or out of the craniospinal space (is) balanced." Ryder[139] also recognized that pressure and volume within the craniospinal compartment are not linearly related and that the shape of the pressure-volume curve is largely determined by the elasticity of the craniospinal venous bed ("not . . . the skull or . . . limiting membranes"). The introduction of ventriculocisternal perfusion in 1962[58,118] provoked renewed interest in CSF formation and absorption and led, ultimately, to a

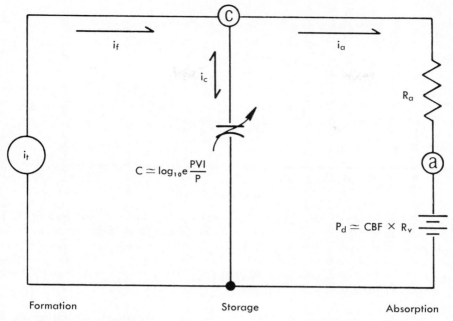

Fig. 5-1. Cerebrospinal fluid system. $I_{(total)}$ represents the mechanism of CSF formation, which is essentially pressure independent. CSF "storage" depends upon the variable (nonlinear) capacitance, C, and CSF absorption occurs across the pressure-independent outflow resistance, R_a. P_d represents the sagittal sinus pressure, which varies with cerebral blood flow (CBF) and extracerebral venous resistance (R_v). (Adapted from Marmarou, A., and others: J. Neurosurg. 48:332-344, 1978.)

mathematical analysis of CSF statics and CSF dynamics.*

DEFINITIONS

intracranial pressure (P_{CSF}) The pressure (relative to atmospheric pressure) within the ventriculosubarachnoid space (mm H_2O).

I_a, I_c, **and** I_f The rates of CSF absorption, CSF accumulation (storage), and CSF formation (ml/min). (See Fig. 5-1).

P_d The sagittal sinus venous pressure (or arachnoid villus opening pressure, whichever is greater) (mm H_2O); P_d varies with cerebral blood flow (CBF) and extracerebral venous resistance (R_v). (See Fig. 5-1.)

R_a CSF absorption resistance (mm H_2O-min/ml), defined functionally as $P_{CSF} - P_d)/I_f$. (See Fig. 5-1.)

PVI Pressure-volume index—the volume increment or decrement required to produce a

ten-fold change in CSF pressure (ml). (See Fig. 5-2.)

CSF statics Considerations that apply to the cerebrospinal fluid system in the steady state (when $I_c = O$ and $I_a = I_f$); under these conditions, $P_{CSF} = P_d + I_f R_a$.

CSF dynamics Considerations that apply to the cerebrospinal fluid system during the course of volume additions or volume withdrawals (i.e., when $I_c \neq O$); under these conditions, $P_2 = P_1 10^{\Delta V/PVI}$.

PATHOPHYSIOLOGY OF INTRACRANIAL HYPERTENSION AND INTRACRANIAL HYPOTENSION

The CSF system can be described in both static and dynamic terms (see above definitions), and both static and dynamic considerations must be invoked to explain the pathogenesis of intracranial hypertension or hypotension and the appearance of clinical symptoms in various disease states associ-

*References 7-9, 29, 54, 93, 94.

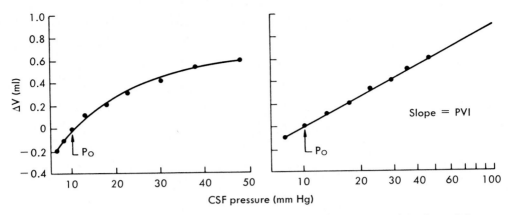

Fig. 5-2. Pressure-volume index. Linear *(left)* and semilogarithmic *(right)* plots of the relationship between pressure and volume within the craniospinal compartment. Note that the pressure-volume index (PVI) is equal to the volume increment or decrement required to produce a ten-fold change in CSF pressure. The first derivative of the pressure-volume curve (dV/dP) is termed compliance. (Adapted from Marmarou, A., and others: J. Neurosurg. **48**:332-344, 1978.)

ated with abnormal increases or decreases in CSFP. The following is a summary account of the CSF system, emphasizing both its "static" and "dynamic" properties. The CSF system is schematized in Fig. 5-1.

CSF statics

In the steady state, when $I_c = 0$, that is, when the rate of CSF absorption equals the rate of CSF formation, the following relationship is obtained[93,94]: $P_{CSF} = P_d + I_f R_a$, which implies that resting CSFP is equal to the dural venous sinus pressure (P_d) plus the product of the CSF formation rate (I_f) and the CSF absorption resistance (R_a). Thus, sustained elevations of ICP can only result from an increase in the dural sinus pressure (sagittal sinus occlusion), an increased rate of CSF formation (choroid plexus papilloma), or an increase in the resistance to CSF absorption (subarachnoid hemorrhage, meningeal carcinomatosis). CSF hypotension, on the other hand, may result from a decrease in sagittal sinus venous pressure (dehydration with low central venous pressure), a decrease in the rate of CSF bulk flow (following the administration of drugs such as acetazolamide or digoxin), or a decrease in the resistance to CSF absorption (CSF fistula). Two clinical examples illustrate how pathologic alterations in P_d and R_a affect ICP:

1. If mastoiditis is complicated by an isolated (dominant) sigmoid sinus thrombosis, P_d may rise transiently from 70 mm H_2O to 270 mm H_2O; if I_f and R_a are normal (e.g., 0.35 ml/min and 100 mm H_2O-min/ml, respectively), then P_{CSF} will rise from 105 mm H_2O (70 + 0.35 × 100) to 305 mm H_2O (270 + 0.35 × 100).

2. A head injury associated with a basal skull fracture may be complicated by a dural tear, which allows CSF to escape through the nose. P_d and I_f remain normal (70 mm H_2O and 0.35 ml/min, respectively), but R_a falls. If, for example, R_a decreases from 100 to 25 mm H_2O-min/ml, P_{CSF} will fall from 105 mm H_2O (70 + 0.35 × 100) to 79 mm H_2O (70 + 0.35 × 25).

CSF dynamics

Although CSF statics adequately describe intracranial pressure relationships when the rate of CSF formation is equal to the rate of CSF absorption, additional (dynamic) considerations must be invoked when $I_c \neq 0$, that is, when the rate of CSF formation exceeds the rate of CSF absorption or vice versa. Dynamic states are associated with rapid changes in cerebral blood and/or brain volume and can be mimicked experimentally by rapid volume additions to or withdrawals from the craniospinal compartment. Changes in the volume of the intracranial contents lead to predictable changes in CSFP, which depend not only on the magnitude of the volume increment or decrement (ΔV) but also on the craniospinal compliance. Compliance refers to the first derivative of the pressure-volume curve (dV/dP), which varies inversely with pressure according to the relationship $C = \log_{10}e$ PVI/P_{CSF}, where PVI is the pressure-volume index (see below) and P_{CSF} is the resting CSFP.[93,94] Compliance may also be understood as a measure of the stiffness or rigidity of the craniospinal compartment, which derives in large part from the elasticity of the craniospinal venous bed.[84,85,93,139,140] Meningeal elasticity and the viscoelastic properties of the brain and spinal cord may also contribute to craniospinal compliance.[54,82,83,154] The craniospinal compartment becomes noncompliant ("tight") when an increase in cerebral (venous) blood volume is not accompanied by a proportional reduction in cerebral blood flow (CBF) (jugular compression, superior vena cava syndrome) or, alternately, when the total volume of the cerebral venous reservoir is permanently reduced (chronic hydrocephalus, cerebral atrophy).* In contrast, compliant ("slack") brains are associated with a reduction in CBF (profound hypotension) or a significant increase in meningeal elasticity (e.g., following craniectomy). Because of its pressure dependence, compliance is not as useful a quantity as the pressure-volume index (PVI) for routine computational purposes.

The PVI[93] is defined as the volume increment or decrement (ΔV) required to produce a ten-fold change in CSF pressure (Fig. 5-2); in mathematical terms, $PVI = \dfrac{\Delta V}{\log P_2/P_1}$. Thus, a sudden volume increment, ΔV, produces a rise in CSFP so that $P_2 = P_1 10^{\Delta V/PVI}$ (Table 5-1); the magnitude

---

*Cerebral edema also reduces craniospinal compliance, but the mechanism is poorly understood.

Table 5-1. Peak pressure responses to graded volume injections as a function of PVI

$P_1 = 150$ mm H_2O	Pressure-volume index (ml)		
ΔV, ml	15	20	25
1	175	168	164
5	323	267	238
10	696	474	377
15	1500	844	597
20	3232	1500	946

P_2, mm H_2O

of the pressure change depends upon the initial resting pressure (P_1), the magnitude of the volume increment (ΔV), and a measure of the craniospinal compliance (PVI).

Table 5-1 illustrates the effect of compliance (PVI) on intracranial pressure-volume relationships. With reference to Table 5-1, suppose that a patient suffers an acute 15 ml subarachnoid or intracerebral hemorrhage. If the preictal CSFP is 150 mm H_2O (P_1) and the PVI is normal (25 ml), CSFP rises acutely to 597 mm H_2O (P_2). If, on the other hand, the brain is tight (PVI = 15 ml), then CSFP peaks at 1500 mm H_2O.

Dynamic considerations apply in physiologic as well as in pathologic states. Inhalation of 5% CO_2 rapidly increases cerebral blood volume and thereby leads to an increase in CSFP; as indicated in Table 5-1, this increase in pressure will be much smaller in a normal than in a tight brain. Hyperventilation, on the other hand, rapidly lowers CSFP by reducing CBV. Not surprisingly, when controlled hyperventilation is employed in the treatment of intracranial hypertension, the observed fall in CSFP is most marked in patients with noncompliant brains.

In most clinical situations, both static and dynamic considerations apply; changes in P_d, I_f, and R_a are frequently accompanied by changes in PVI. For example, an acute subarachnoid hemorrhage has two immediate effects on the cerebrospinal fluid system: (1) R_a increases because blood constituents and plasma proteins increase CSF viscosity[29] and plug arachnoid villi[32,45] and

(2) the rapid addition of subarachnoid blood (ΔV) to the intracranial contents leads to a rise in CSFP that depends primarily upon the magnitude of craniospinal compliance (PVI).

An appreciation of the static and dynamic factors that modify P_{CSF} allows one to resolve a number of clinical paradoxes, such as the measurement of normal CSFP in a patient with multiple intracranial mass lesions. A slowly enlarging intracranial mass will increase CSFP only if it (1) increases P_d by compromising or occluding the sagittal sinus or dominant lateral sinus or (2) increases R_a by compressing the Sylvian aqueduct or by obliterating the convexity subarachnoid space. Any diminution in craniospinal compliance (PVI) that might result from local and/or distant effects on the cerebral vasculature would be manifest only transiently during volume additions to or withdrawals from the craniospinal compartment (e.g., during Valsalva maneuvers, postural changes).

To summarize the clinical situation, each patient has a resting CSFP principally determined by P_d, I_f, and R_a, that is, CSF statics. Superimposed upon that equilibrium pressure are transient fluctuations in CSFP (lasting seconds to minutes) produced by physiologic or pathologic changes in the volume of the intracranial contents and predicted by the formulas for CSF dynamics. Dynamic considerations apply in *physiologic states* when blood volume is altered as a result of changes in arterial P_{CO_2} (hyperventilation or hypoventilation), changes in cerebral venous pressure (spontaneous respirations, coughs, Valsalva maneuvers), or changes in posture (assumption of the upright or recumbent position). Dynamic considerations account for the oscillations of the fluid meniscus that one observes in a small-bore manometer at the time of lumbar puncture as well as the pressure drop (opening pressure [OP]–closing pressure [CP]) that ensues after the removal of spinal fluid. The amplitude of the manometric oscillations as well as the magnitude of the OP-CP difference are determined by the cranio-

spinal compliance. Thus, large fluctuations in CSFP coincident with the heartbeat or with spontaneous respirations suggest a diseased or tight brain. Assuming that the lumbar subarachnoid space is in open communication with the ventricular system and supratentorial subarachnoid space, a large drop in CSFP following the removal of spinal fluid at lumbar puncture also suggests diminished craniospinal compliance; however, a large post-lumbar-puncture drop in CSFP does not, as Ayala argued, reflect a decrease in total CSF volume. Conversely, small changes in CSFP following the removal of large volumes of CSF suggest an increase in craniospinal compliance and not an increase in total CSF volume.

In *pathologic states*, acute changes in CSFP probably reflect the intermittent failure of CBF autoregulation and are associated with sudden changes in CBV. When the PVI is low, small changes in CBV may be associated with large oscillations in CSFP. Transient vasomotor paralysis in the setting of diminished craniospinal compliance provides an adequate explanation for the plateau waves that Lundberg[86] observed in patients with bilateral papilledema and pathologically elevated mean VFP. These plateau or A waves (1) typically occur "during a fairly advanced state of intracranial hypertension . . . and only if the mean intracranial pressure is substantially elevated (>20 mm Hg)"*; (2) may be induced in susceptible patients by the rapid injection of gas or fluid into the ventriculosubarachnoid space; and (3) frequently coincide with "an arousal reaction in the behavior of the patient, as well as in the EEG"[60]; (4) are terminated by CSF drainage and are often aborted by spontaneous or induced hyperventilation; (5) tend to diminish or disappear after subtemporal decompression "in spite of the mean

---

*The various pressure waves observed in patients with normal pressure hydrocephalus[18,56,159] probably reflect the effects of transient vasomotor instability in diseased brains, whereas the secondary pressure waves described by Magnaes[92] (in patients without known CNS disease) following sudden postural changes reflect the physiologic latency of cerebral vasomotor regulation.

pressure remaining at about the same level as before the operation"[87]; (6) may be observed in the absence of an appreciable change in systemic arterial blood pressure; and (7) are accompanied by a significant reduction in CBF.[87] Lundberg, Cronqvist, and Kjallquist[87] performed serial angiograms on patients with spontaneous plateau waves and observed arterial dilatation but no increase in the diameter of large parasagittal veins. Based on their studies of regional CBF and VFP during spontaneous plateau waves, Risberg, Lundberg, and Ingvar[133] concluded that pressure peaks are associated with paroxysmal increases in CBV occasioned by intermittent vasomotor paralysis. They

suggested that "an initial vasodilatation" (in the setting of increased CSFP provoked by hypercapnia, emotion, pain, physical or mental activity, arousal, seizures, or REM sleep) may transiently destabilize cerebral vasomotor regulation.

CAUSES OF ALTERED INTRACRANIAL PRESSURE

With reference to the above mentioned physiologic considerations, one can describe the major causes of altered intracranial pressure in pathophysiologic terms (Table 5-2). Thus, chronic elevations of CSFP imply an increase in dural venous sinus pressure, an increase in CSF absorption resistance,

Table 5-2. Some causes of altered intracranial pressure

Perturbation	Proximate cause	Clinical examples
Increased dural sinus venous pressure ($\uparrow P_d$)	Sinus compression/occlusion	Sagittal sinus thrombosis Otitic hydrocephalus Brain tumors
	Increased sinus blood flow	CO_2 retention Arteriovenous malformations[76]
	Increased peripheral venous pressure	Internal jugular vein occlusion Superior vena cava syndrome Congestive heart failure
Decreased dural sinus venous pressure ($\downarrow P_d$)	Decreased sinus blood flow	Dehydration Shock Hyperventilation
	Decreased peripheral venous pressure	Dehydration
Increased CSF absorption resistance ($\uparrow R_a$)	Ventricular outflow obstruction	Brain tumor Aqueductal stenosis
	Obliteration of the cisternal and/or convexity subarachnoid space	Meningitis Extradural/subdural masses Cerebral edema
	Plugging of the arachnoid villi	Subarachnoid hemorrhage Infectious polyneuritis Spinal cord tumors
Decreased CSF absorption resistance ($\downarrow R_a$)	Diversion of CSF from the ventriculosubarachnoid space	External ventricular drainage Ventriculosystemic shunts Lumbar puncture headache Dural tears and CSF fistulas
Increased rate of CSF formation ($\uparrow I_f$)	Increased choroidal CSF formation	Choroid plexus papilloma
	Increased extrachoroidal CSF formation	Hypo-osmolality Cerebral edema
Decreased rate of CSF formation ($\downarrow I_f$)	Choroidal "atrophy"	? Chronic hydrocephalus[106]
	Decreased extrachoroidal CSF formation	Hyperosmolality ? Dehydration

or an increase in the rate of CSF formation. Dural sinus pressure rises when the sagittal sinus or another major venous sinus is compressed or occluded. Dural sinus occlusions complicate head trauma,[6,98] local or generalized sepsis[44,160] (e.g., lateral sinus thrombosis following otitis media), or physiologic or pathologic states associated with blood hypercoagulability[16,49,98a,150,151] (e.g., the puerperium, oral contraceptive use, inflammatory bowel disease, and systemic cancer). Hematomas, neoplasms,[71,112,142] and hydrocephalic ventricles[116,149] may compress the sagittal or lateral sinuses and thereby increase CSFP. Extracranial disease processes may also increase pressure in the dural venous sinuses. Head and neck tumors or their cervical metastases may compress and/or invade the internal jugular veins, leading to increased jugular venous and dural sinus pressure; unilateral or bilateral resection of the internal jugular vein in the treatment of head and neck cancer may also lead to intracranial hypertension.[95,153] Moreover, elevations in extracranial venous pressure associated with superior vena cava obstruction and chronic congestive heart failure may be reflected in an increase in sagittal sinus venous pressure and in CSFP.

Increased CSF absorption resistance results from ventricular outflow obstruction (e.g., aqueductal stenosis/compression, posterior fossa tumors, and transtentorial herniation) and/or from obliteration of the subarachnoid CSF pathways at the base or over the cerebral convexities (e.g., following subarachnoid hemorrhage, meningitis or meningeal carcinomatosis, and in patients with subdural tumor, hematoma, or empyema). Primary brain tumors and parenchymal cerebral metastases with their attendant edema may increase brain volume and obliterate the cisternal and/or convexity subarachnoid space, increasing R_a and, in consequence, raising ICP. This is the mechanism whereby most mass lesions (and, perhaps, pseudotumor cerebri) raise ICP. The plugging up of arachnoid villi by large (protein) molecules might also be expected to increase R_a and CSFP,[32,45,114] since in-

creased ICP and papilledema occasionally develop in patients with infectious polyneuritis[68] and in patients with a variety of spinal cord tumors,[3,48,90,126] the common denominator being an increase in CSF protein concentration.*

Increased CSF formation is an uncommon cause of increased ICP. Papillomas of the choroid plexus, which frequently hemorrhage into the ventricular system, may also raise ICP by increasing I_f.[4,39,47,107,164] Hochwald, Wald, and Malhan[59] demonstrated that serum hypo-osmolality significantly increases CSF bulk flow and argued that the CSF functions as a sink, limiting intracellular water accumulation during water intoxication. Thus, the increase in CSFP occasionally observed in patients with severe hyponatremia[158] may derive in part from an increase in I_f.

Intracranial hypotension is less important clinically than intracranial hypertension, and its causes are fewer. Intracranial pressure is reduced when dural venous sinus pressure falls in consequence of a drop in central venous pressure (dehydration) or of a diminution in CBF (shock). A decrease in CSF absorption resistance will also lead to subnormal CSFP, and this is the mechanism of intracranial hypotension following lumbar puncture or the development of traumatic CSF fistulas. Finally, CSFP will fall if the rate of CSF formation is reduced, and this may be one mechanism whereby intracranial pressure is lowered by systemic diuretics, hyperosmolar agents, glucocorticoids, acetazolamide, and cardiac glycosides (see below).

Lumbar CSFP may not accurately reflect ICP, and in patients with mass lesions who have begun to herniate, lumbar CSFP may be normal or low despite grossly elevated supratentorial CSFP; impaction of the temporal lobes into the tentorial incisura and/or of the cerebellar tonsils into the foramen magnum prevents the transmission of ICP

---

*Sullivan and Reeves[155] recently reported a patient with normal CSF protein, increased ICP, and the Guillain-Barré syndrome.

into the lumbar subarachnoid space.[78] Of the patients described by Duffy[37] fully half herniated after lumbar puncture and had normal opening pressures "despite raised intracranial pressure later being proved."

SYMPTOMS AND SIGNS OF INTRACRANIAL HYPERTENSION/ HYPOTENSION

Strictly speaking, there are no pathognomonic symptoms or signs of increased or decreased CSFP. Nevertheless, the observation of such frequently associated symptoms and signs as headache, papilledema, unilateral pupillary dilatation, oculomotor or abducens paresis, irregular respirations, and so on should give rise to a clinical suspicion of abnormally elevated or reduced CSFP, which can be confirmed only by direct measurement. Most of the signs and symptoms traditionally associated with intracranial hypertension are related to traction on cerebral blood vessels, distortion of pain-sensitive dura mater, impending herniation and intermittent vascular compression, or midline shifts or axial distortion of the brain stem, and are not due to increased ICP per se.

Papilledema, when present, is the most reliable sign of increased ICP. However, many patients with raised ICP fail to develop papilledema,[19,37,80]* and in some patients with pseudotumor cerebri, papilledema develops and then subsides spontaneously, although CSFP remains elevated.[42] Why papilledema fails to develop in every patient with persistently elevated CSFP remains unclear, although several potential explanations, including increased intraocular pressure,[19,38] anomalous ocular venous drainage, and anatomic abnormalities of the optic nerve sheath that interfere with the transmission of CSFP into the orbit,[165] have been advanced. It should also be noted that papilledema is not synonymous with raised intracranial pressure.

*In our experience, patients over the age of 50 and patients with chronically elevated cerebral venous pressure infrequently develop papilledema, even when CSFP is markedly and persistently elevated.

Ocular hypotony,[20,31] orbital venous stasis,[20,57] retrobulbar tumors,[20,157,165] and granulomatous inflammation within or cystic lesions of the optic nerve sheath[152] may produce papilledema in the absence of intracranial hypertension. Retinal venous pulsations, when present, imply that CSFP is normal or not significantly elevated.[70,81,166] Unfortunately, the sign is insufficiently reliable[113,163,173] to obviate the need for direct pressure measurements. The absence of spontaneous venous pulsations is not helpful diagnostically.

The most common symptom associated with increased ICP, namely headache that is worse in the early morning and subsides as the day wears on, is likewise not a sign of raised intracranial pressure per se. Kunkle and co-workers[74,75] studied the relationship between increased ICP and headache and concluded that "when headache is associated with increased intracranial pressure, the headache is not caused by the increase in pressure." These authors examined 72 patients with brain tumors and found that (1) headache occurred almost as frequently in patients with normal CSFP as in patients with increased CSFP; (2) some patients had increased ICP but did not complain of headache; and (3) artificially raising ICP by injecting normal saline into the lumbar subarachnoid space failed to produce headache in four normal erect subjects or in one patient with a left parietal oligodendroglioma and a resting CSFP of 175 mm H_2O. From these observations, they concluded that brain tumor headache results from traction on or displacement of pain-sensitive intracranial structures and is independent of CSFP per se.

Patients with intracranial hypotension also complain of headache, although this headache is not caused by a decrease in CSFP. The low-pressure headache associated with lumbar puncture or CSF fistulas results, as does the headache associated with intracranial hypertension, from traction on pain-sensitive structures. Patients suffering from lumbar-puncture headache do not complain of pain in the recumbent position; their headache develops only upon arising, when leakage of CSF through a dural tear allows the brain to settle within the skull, with the result that pain-sensitive structures at the base and vertex are put on stretch. The abducens palsies occasionally observed in patients with intracranial hypertension and in patients with intracranial hypotension[15] are almost certainly the result of traction on the sixth cranial nerve at some point along its course from pons to orbit.

Ryder and co-workers[141] investigated the relationship between ICP and symptoms of CNS dysfunction in patients "with and without abnormal pressures and disorders of the central nervous system." Only 15 (9%) of their patients complained of headache when lumbar CSFP was increased, and in 9 of these 15 the pain was localized to the region of a skull fracture or other skull defect; such headaches were exacerbated by increasing and relieved by lowering CSFP. Restlessness, anxiety, and back pain ("the jitters") occurred in 18% of patients regardless of their underlying neurologic condition. This reaction was not associated with persistently elevated lumbar CSFP, and withdrawal of CSF did not abort it. Shock, apnea, nausea, and vomiting were not observed. The authors concluded that (1) acute elevations of ICP per se do not interfere with cerebral function; (2) there is no specific neurologic syndrome associated with raised ICP; (3) pressure-sensitive afferents do not exist in the human CNS; and (4) "stretching, distortion or translation of craniospinal structures"—not intracranial hypertension—gives rise to those symptoms and signs traditionally associated with "abnormal fluid pressures."

A number of transient symptoms and rapidly evolving signs of neurologic dysfunction (other than headache and papilledema) traditionally associated with increased ICP result, instead, from volume additions to the intracranial contents that precipitate or accelerate midline shifts, brain herniations, and vascular compression. Adams and Graham[1] studied the relationship between VFP and the pathologic sequelae of trans-

tentorial herniation and found a high correlation between the level of VFP during life and postmortem evidence of pressure necrosis in the parahippocampal and cingulate gyri and of infarction of medial occipital cortex (secondary to compression of the posterior cerebral artery). The appropriate conclusion to be drawn from this study is that increased VFP exacerbates preexisting transcompartmental pressure gradients and predisposes to brain herniation—*not* that increased VFP per se produces pressure necrosis and cerebral infarction.

Adson and Lillie[2] attempted to correlate clinical symptoms and signs with intraventricular pressure in a patient with a large right parietal glioma. They observed that "simultaneously with an increase in intracranial pressure, the patient would become restless, confused, and more or less irrational, and muscular twitchings with convulsions would occur." Since drainage of ventricular CSF through their manometer "failed to alter the neurologic phenomena," they were unable to relate their clinical observations to changes in VFP. Subsequently, Browder and Meyers[12] challenged the generally accepted view that elevations of ICP to the level of the diastolic or mean systolic arterial blood pressure produce hypertension, bradycardia, slow deep respirations, vomiting, headache, and "mental torpor, stupor and, later, coma." They demonstrated that experimental elevations of ICP far in excess of those usually encountered in clinical practice failed to produce striking alterations of either the systemic blood pressure or pulse rate. A cardiovascular response was observed only when CSFP was raised to the level of mean systemic arterial pressure; moreover, this response "was not necessarily in accord with the classic pattern." Browder and Meyers concluded that variations in systemic blood pressure, pulse, respiratory rate, and level of consciousness —either alone or in combination—do not allow one to reliably infer that ICP is rising or falling.

Ethelberg and Jensen[41] described nonepileptic paroxysmal phenomena (crescendo headache, visual obscurations, photopsia, chalastic/hypertonic fits, impairment of consciousness, sensory hallucinations, and "brainstem phenomena") in 140 patients with verified intracranial neoplasms. These phenomena were commonly associated with parieto-occipital and subtentorial tumors and were often precipitated by sudden postural changes (especially the rapid assumption of an upright position), head movement, straining, or lumbar puncture. In general, the prevalence of obscurations increased with increasing CSFP and with the severity of papilledema (diopters disc elevation); however, in middle-aged and elderly patients with visual obscurations, supratentorial CSFP was frequently normal or only slightly elevated. The authors reasoned that visual obscurations and other nonepileptic paroxysmal phenomena are associated with transient circulatory disturbances consequent upon transtentorial herniation and/or brain stem displacement and distortion. The development of transtentorial CSF pressure gradients after rapid postural changes or lumbar puncture—not intracranial hypertension per se—was thought to explain the pathogenesis of these phenomena.*

Lundberg[86] described a variety of transient symptoms that appeared or were exacerbated by spontaneous plateau waves (see box, p. 102); he also noted the occurrence of residual depression of consciousness and persistent alterations in muscle tone. Subsequently, Ingvar and Lundberg[60] continuously monitored VFP and the electroencephalogram in six patients with CNS neoplasms and increased ICP and established that the above mentioned paroxysmal phenomena are not associated with cortical

epileptiform discharges. These authors concluded that "the primary disturbance might put an imprint upon the syndrome developing during a paroxysmal increase in the ventricular fluid pressure" and that the paroxysmal cerebral symptoms accompanying plateau waves "would . . . seem to originate in subcortical (probably brainstem) structures which do not have, or are transiently disconnected from, an immediate influence upon the cortical electrical activity."

Lundberg[86] observed that plateau waves occurred during natural sleep and under general anesthesia. To explain why symptoms of intracranial hypertension are commonly accentuated during sleep and why nighttime deterioration and early morning headache occur in patients with raised ICP, Cooper and Hulme[22] continuously monitored VFP and the electroencephalogram in 15 patients with intracranial mass lesions and pseudotumor cerebri during nighttime sleep and noted the occurrence of spontaneous plateau waves during REM and, in patients with mean CSF pressures in excess of 500 mm H_2O, stage II sleep. They related the increased incidence of spontaneous plateau waves during sleep to intermittent cerebral vasodilatation induced by sleep-related increases in cerebral metabolic activity.

The frequent concurrence of plateau waves and paroxysmal symptoms of CNS dysfunction such as those described by Ethelberg and Jensen[41] and Lundberg[86] may be explained as follows: When mass lesions or brain hernias begin to obstruct the tentorial incisura or foramen magnum, CSFP is no longer equally transmitted throughout the ventriculosubarachnoid space, and pressure gradients develop between the supratentorial and infratentorial compartments and/or between the posterior fossa and spinal subarachnoid space.[78] This compartmentalization leads, in turn, to a significant loss of craniospinal compliance[85,94] with the result that small intracompartmental volume increments (such as might result from transient cerebral vasodilatation) lead to marked increases in intracompartmental pressure,

---

* Magnaes[92] studied the effects of rapid postural changes on lumbar and ventricular CSFP in patients with cervical spondylosis, subarachnoid hemorrhage, and hydrocephalus and discovered that plateau waves and craniospinal block could be induced by rapid tilting from the supine to the sitting position and vice versa. In some of his patients with elevated ICP, rapid postural changes were associated with clinical symptoms that coincided with large transient or stationary CSF pressure waves; such symptoms were aggravated by the development of craniospinal block.

PAROXYSMAL SYMPTOMS IN PATIENTS WITH INTRACRANIAL SPACE-OCCUPYING LESIONS*

Impairment of consciousness
Trancelike state
Feeling of unreality/warmth
Confusion, disorientation
Restlessness, agitation
Disorganized motor activity, crocidismus
Sense of suffocation, air hunger
Cardiovascular/respiratory disturbances
Headache
Pain in the neck and shoulders
Nasal itch
Blurring of vision, amaurosis
Mydriasis, pupillary areflexia
Nystagmus
Oculomotor/abducens paresis
Conjugate deviation of the eyes
External ophthalmoplegia
Dysphagia, dysarthria
Nuchal rigidity
Retroflexion of the neck

Opisthotonus, trismus
Rigidity and tonic extension/flexion of the arms and legs
Bilateral extensor plantar responses
Sluggish/absent deep tendon reflexes
Generalized muscular weakness
Facial twitching
Clonic movements of the arms and legs
Facial/limb paresthesias
Rise in temperature
Nausea, vomiting
Facial flushing
Pallor, cyanosis
Sweating
Shivering and "goose flesh"
Thirst
Salivation
Yawning, hiccoughing
Urinary and fecal urgency/incontinence

*Modified from Lundberg, N.: Continuous recording and control of ventricular fluid pressure in neurosurgical practice, Acta Psychiatr. Neurol. Scand. (Suppl.) **149:**1-193, 1960.

the enhancement of preexisting intercompartmental pressure gradients, and brain herniations, vascular compression, axial distortion of the brain stem, and so on. For example, in a patient with supratentorial metastases and signs of impending transtentorial herniation, resting VFP and lumbar CSFP are both 300 mm H_2O ($P_d = 90$, $I_f = 0.30$, $R_a = 700$) and PVI = 20. Cerebral vasodilatation leads to a sudden 10 ml increase in supratentorial blood volume, transient herniation occurs, and VFP peaks at 950 mm H_2O (plateau wave). Later, when incisural obstruction is virtually complete, R_a rises to 1000 mm H_2O-min/ml, and resting VFP and lumbar CSFP rise to 390 mm H_2O; now, however, as the parahippocampal gyri impact into the tentorial incisura, the PVI falls to 15 ml, and an increase of 10 ml in supratentorial blood volume leads to a pressure peak of 1810 mm H_2O; the peak transtentorial pressure gradient, previously 650 (950 − 300) mm H_2O is now 1420 (1810 − 390) mm H_2O.

MANAGEMENT OF PATIENTS WITH INCREASED INTRACRANIAL PRESSURE

Since, in the presence of an intracranial mass lesion, the symptoms and signs traditionally associated with increased ICP are produced by secondary distortions, displacements, and herniations, the treatment of increased ICP should be primarily directed at reducing the bulk of the offending mass lesion or, alternately, of adjacent normal tissues. The initial treatment of any patient with increased ICP whose neurologic status is deteriorating rapidly is aimed at reducing the volume of the intracranial contents acutely (within minutes) in order to prevent irreversible brain damage. Once the patient's condition has stabilized, additional treatment modalities are employed in an

Table 5-3. Effects of various antihypertensive treatment modalities on P_d, I_f, R_a, and PVI*

	P_d	I_f	R_a	PVI
Systemic diuretics	0	↓	0	0
Hypertonic solutions	?↑	↓	0	↑
Corticosteroids	0	↓	?↑	↑
Acetazolamide	0	↓↓	0	0
Barbiturates	?↓	0	0	0
Controlled hyperventilation	?↓	↓	0	0
Hypothermia	↓	↓	0	0
CSF diversion	?↓[121]	0	↓↓	?↑
Surgical decompression	↓	0	↓	↑

*Symbols: Major effect, ↑↑ or ↓↓; minor or secondary effect, ↑ or ↓; questionable effect, ?↑ or ?↓; no information, 0.

effort to consolidate the gains of emergency treatment and to allow the physician ample opportunity (hours to days) to deal with the underlying pathologic process. Although a variety of medical and surgical treatments have been advocated for the relief of symptoms and signs associated with increased ICP, the rational use of specific treatment modalities depends upon an understanding of their effects on the previously defined physiologic parameters P_d, I_f, R_a, and PVI (Table 5-3). Whatever treatment modalities he or she employs, the physician must recognize that increased ICP per se is not the cause of the patient's distress but rather the consequence of a preexisting pathologic process.

Systemic diuretics

Several recent reports[23,103,111,172] have advocated the use of furosemide and ethacrynic acid in the management of patients with intracranial hypertension. These systemic diuretics may reduce ICP in one of several ways. Firstly, diuresis per se will reduce the volume of the intracranial contents in proportion as the percentage amount of total body water decreases: in a 70 kg patient in whom $P_{CSF} = 350$ mm H_2O and PVI = 15 ml, a furosemide-induced diuresis of 500 ml will reduce the volume of the intracranial

contents by approximately 15 ml and lower CSFP from 350 to 35 mm H_2O.* Secondly, both furosemide and ethacrynic acid have been reported to decrease I_f (by 45% and 60%, respectively)[35,119,127]; extrachoroidal as well as choroidal CSF formation may be affected, although the mode of action of these drugs on I_f is unknown. Finally, both furosemide and ethacrynic acid have been shown to reduce cerebral edema, and a direct effect on edema resolution has been postulated.[131] Meinig and co-workers[103] followed the resolution of peritumoral edema on serial computed tomographic (CT) scans during chronic treatment with dexamethasone and furosemide and concluded that combined therapy was more effective than either steroid or diuretic therapy alone. In another study,[132] dexamethasone and ethacrynic acid were administered to patients with brain tumors, and the former was found to be more effective in the resolution of perifocal (white-matter) edema and the alleviation of neurologic symptoms. Cottrell and co-workers[23] compared the effect of furosemide and mannitol on ICP in anesthetized neurosurgical patients and concluded that furosemide consistently reduced CSFP without producing marked elevations of serum osmolality or serious electrolyte disturbances. Significant reductions in ICP were observed at the peak of diuresis (5.4 ± 1.4 torr) and at the completion of diuresis (4.7 ± 1.7 torr).

It would appear that IV furosemide and ethacrynic acid are highly effective in acutely reducing ICP (e.g., in the operating room prior to or during neurosurgery). Their ability to reduce ICP without increasing blood osmolality or cerebral blood flow (CBF) may constitute a theoretical advantage over hyperosmolar agents in some clinical settings (see p. 104). The role of systemic diuretics in the chronic management of

---

*A similar reduction in ICP could be achieved with IV mannitol by acutely increasing blood osmolality from 285 to 289 mOsm/l; assuming that the "rapid equilibrium volume" of mannitol is 20% of total body weight, such a 4 mOsm/l increase would be anticipated following the administration of 10 g of mannitol.

raised ICP has not been fully established and awaits further study.

Hyperosmolar agents

The serendipitous discovery by Weed and McKibben[167] that the intravenous administration of hypertonic salt and glucose solutions to etherized cats precipitated a marked drop in cisternal CSFP led to the introduction of hyperosmolar agents into neurosurgical practice. These agents lower CSFP by reducing the volume of the intracranial contents and the rate of CSF formation. Moreover, hyperosmolar agents may also increase craniospinal compliance.

The rapid oral or parenteral administration of an osmotic load of any crystalloid substance will induce transient plasma hyperosmolality and—to the extent that the substance in question does not cross the blood-brain barrier (BBB)—lead to the establishment of an osmotic gradient between blood on the one hand and CSF/brain on the other.[137] The volume of water "withdrawn" from the intracranial compartment along this osmotic gradient (ΔV) depends upon (1) the numerical value of the integral $\int_0^T g(t)dt$, where g(t) is the magnitude of the osmotic gradient as a function of time and T is the total time during which the gradient exists and (2) the proportional integrity of the BBB. To the extent that the BBB is disrupted (i.e., by tumor, infarction, or brain injury), plasma crystalloids will not be excluded from CSF/brain, and an osmotic gradient will not be established in spite of persisting plasma hyperosmolality.

Osmotic dehydrating agents such as mannitol and glycerol also lower CSFP by reducing the rate of CSF formation. DiMattio and co-workers[34] studied the effects of changes in serum osmolarity on CSF bulk flow in cats during ventriculocisternal perfusion and found that CSF bulk flow varied inversely with serum osmolarity. At high induced serum osmolarities bulk flow was almost completely inhibited. A similar, if transient, effect might be anticipated in human subjects following the administration of large osmolar loads of IV mannitol or oral glycerol.

Miller and Leech[109] found that 0.5 g/kg doses of intravenous mannitol reduced the "volume-pressure response" (VPR, the increment in VFP produced by a rapid 1 ml increase in ventricular CSF volume), which they considered as a measure of periventricular elastance, in eight patients with brain tumors, head injuries, hydrocephalus, and benign intracranial hypertension. The percentage reduction in VPR was significantly greater than the percentage reduction in VFP following mannitol administration, implying a mannitol-induced increase in the PVI.[154]

Three potential "side effects" in addition to a rebound increase in CSFP[137] may be observed following the administration of hyperosmolar agents. Osmotically induced cerebral vasodilatation[67,171] together with an increase in plasma volume may transiently increase CBV and CSFP.[23] A diminution in cerebrovascular resistance (consequent upon cerebral vasodilatation and/or diminished blood viscosity) may increase CBF[14,50] and CSFP.[23,172] (Because hyperosmolar agents increase CBF, their use would seem to be *relatively* contraindicated in patients with vascular lesions such as aneurysms and epidural or subdural hematomas.) Finally, a rapid reduction in the volume of normal brain and CSF without a concomitant reduction in the volume of a coexisting intracranial mass lesion (such as an epidural or subdural hematoma) may allow for expansion of the mass lesion, which had previously been tamponaded by underlying brain.

Because of their demonstrated efficacy, relative safety and ease of administration, intravenous mannitol and oral glycerol have been used more frequently than other hypertonic agents in the management of patients with increased ICP. James and co-workers[62] reported the results of 73 administrations of hypertonic mannitol (0.18 to 2.5 g/kg over 2 to 10 min) to 44 patients: ICP was reduced an average of 52% on 67 occasions, and the time to maximum reduction varied from 20 to 360 minutes. A rebound increase in ICP to 10% or more above the control value occurred in only three patients. No other complications of therapy were reported. Oral glycerol is a safe and effective cerebral dehydrating agent, and a single 1 g/kg dose is adequate to lower raised ICP acutely, although its effect is short-lived. Continuous administration of oral glycerol must be carefully monitored to avoid the establishment of a reverse osmotic gradient, secondarily increased ICP, and clinical deterioration.[137] Oral glycerol (just as intravenous hypertonic solutions) is most effective in patients with markedly increased ICP, and the duration of the pressure-lowering effect is related both to the gram per kilogram dose and to the pretreatment CSFP.

Corticosteroids

In spite of the fact that corticosteroids have been used to treat patients with cerebral edema and increased ICP for almost 20 years, the effect of their administration on CSFP per se and the mechanism by which they reduce cerebral edema have yet to be defined. Weinstein and co-workers[169] measured the lumbar CSFP in eight patients with metastatic brain tumors before and at one and two weeks after the institution of daily dexamethasone therapy (16 to 24 mg qd). Six of these patients had initial pressures greater than 180 mm H_2O. Although clinical improvement was associated with a fall in lumbar CSFP, the latter phenomenon probably related to a steroid-mediated reduction in total mass effect rather than to any specific effect of steroid therapy on the cerebrospinal fluid system. Kullberg and West[73] studied the effect of high-dose dexamethasone and betamethasone therapy on ventricular CSFP in seven patients with malignant brain tumors and "symptoms of intracranial hypertension." VFP was continuously monitored and the relationship between steroid dose and mean ventricular CSFP studied. The authors failed to observe any "discernible immediate changes of the VFP curve, even when large steroid doses

were injected intravenously." However, in five of their seven patients VFP decreased during steroid therapy after a variable latency (one to eight days); in four patients the reduction in VFP was associated with a reduction in the frequency and amplitude of spontaneously occurring plateau waves. Symptomatic improvement was usually observed pari passu with a reduction in mean VFP, although this relationship did not always obtain. The authors concluded that the most conspicuous effect of high-dose corticosteroids on VFP was "the reduction of the high-pressure episodes, the plateau waves, whereas the basic pressure level was less markedly affected." The delay between steroid administration and the observed lowering of VFP suggests that the latter phenomenon depends upon a reduction in peritumoral edema or, conceivably, upon an oncolytic effect of the steroids themselves.[146]

Garcia-Bengochea[43] studied the effect of chronic corticosteroid administration on the rate of CSF formation in adult cats by catheterizing the spinal subarachnoid space and collecting the effluent CSF for prolonged periods before and after a two-week course of parenteral cortisone acetate. He found that cortisone treatment produced a consistent and statistically significant reduction in the rate of CSF formation. Subsequently, Sato[143] utilized a ventriculocisternal perfusion technique to monitor the effect of IV dexamethasone on CSF bulk flow in dogs. Although he observed a 50% reduction in the rate of CSF formation within 30 minutes after dexamethasone administration, he failed to observe any diminution in cisternal CSFP in nonperfused animals given the same steroid dose. Weiss and Nulsen[170] demonstrated that CSF bulk flow was reduced in normal and in hydrocephalic dogs following intravenous corticosteroid administration; after a single intravenous dose of either dexamethasone or methylprednisolone, CSF bulk flow was reduced by approximately 50%, with a gradual return to baseline levels after six hours. That a similar reduction in CSF bulk flow was obtained by

Sato and co-workers,[144] who perfused the spinal subarachnoid space of anesthetized dogs, suggests an extrachroidal effect of steroids on CSF formation.*

After studying the fate of blue dextran and radioiodinated serum albumin (RISA) injected into the caudate nucleus of rats, Cserr and Tang[24] concluded that, in the presence of "local brain edema," bulk flow of cerebral interstitial fluid (ISF) significantly contributes to CSF formation. However, these authors were unable to observe any such contribution in rats pretreated with dexamethasone. It may be, therefore, that steroids indirectly lower CSFP in patients with brain lesions and intracranial hypertension through an effect on ISF bulk flow.

Johnston and co-workers[65] have suggested that chronic administration and acute withdrawal of corticosteroids may increase CSF absorption resistance (Table 5-2). Miller and Leech[109] demonstrated that intramuscular betamethasone reduced the volume-pressure response in patients with brain tumors, head injuries, and benign intracranial hypertension—without lowering mean VFP. A similar effect of methylprednisolone was observed by Miller and co-workers[110] in seven patients with glioblastoma multiforme and metastatic carcinoma. These data suggest that corticosteroids may alter CSF dynamics by increasing the PVI.

The optimal dosage of corticosteroids for patients with raised ICP has not been established. For the treatment of intracranial hypertension associated with brain tumors most physicians prescribe (the equivalent of) 10 to 20 mg of dexamethasone initially, followed by 16 mg a day in divided doses. Our experience and that of others[130] suggests that patients who fail to respond to 16 mg a day may respond to 32 or 64 mg a day— or to even higher doses. The low incidence of serious complications associated with the administration of high-dose corticosteroids to patients with increased ICP has been

recently documented by Marshall and co-workers.[97]

Since the mechanism of action of corticosteroids probably differs from that of systemic diuretics or hyperosmolar agents, corticosteroids should be combined with systemic diuretics or hyperosmolar agents in the emergency treatment of malignant intracranial hypertension. For less severely ill patients and for patients with chronically elevated ICP, steroids alone are usually sufficient.

Acetazolamide

Tschirgi and co-workers[162] observed a significant and sustained reduction in CSF bulk flow and in cisternal CSFP following the intravenous administration of acetazolamide to lightly anesthetized cats and rabbits. They demonstrated that the acetazolamide effect was independent of inspired CO_2 tension and hypothesized that acetazolamide inhibited the enzymatic hydration of CO_2 produced by cellular metabolism, leading to a diminished entry of isotonic sodium chloride into the interstitial compartment. Pollay and Davson[120] administered acetazolamide to anesthetized rabbits during ventriculocisternal perfusions with an isotonic salt solution and obtained unequivocal evidence of an acetazolamide effect; intravenous acetazolamide (100 mg/kg) reduced CSF bulk flow by 49%, whereas the rate of CSF formation fell 41% when acetazolamide (20 mg/100 ml) was added to the ventriculocisternal perfusion fluid.

Subsequently, Rubin and co-workers[138] assessed the effect of acetazolamide on the rate of CSF formation in three patients using an inulin dilution technique. They concluded that "the degree of response varied in individual test subjects" and that "the maximum response was always achieved within the first 90 minutes and the duration of the response was not longer than 30 minutes." Neblett and co-workers[115] observed a sustained reduction in the amount of daily ventricular drainage collected from two hydrocephalic children receiving unspecified doses of acetazolamide. Of interest, a more pro-

---

* Martins and co-workers[99] were unable to demonstrate an effect of single large intravenous doses of dexamethasone on the rate of CSF formation in rhesus monkeys.

nounced reduction in ventricular drainage occurred when digoxin or digitoxin was administered to these same children and to an adult with postoperative intracranial hypertension. When administered simultaneously, acetazolamide and digoxin were no more effective in reducing ventricular drainage than was digoxin alone. These observations await confirmation by other investigators.

Birzis and co-workers[10] reported that "high doses of acetazolamide were . . . very effective in lowering spinal fluid pressure of hydrocephalics." Unfortunately, the authors relied on CSFP data obtained at lumbar puncture (often performed "under mild pentobarbital sedation"), and no attempt was made to administer acetazolamide to the various control and treatment groups in a double-blind double-crossover fashion. A subsequent prospective double-blind study of acetazolamide in 32 newborn infants with myelomeningocele[102] failed to demonstrate an acetazolamide effect on the incidence of hydrocephalus, the rate of head enlargement, or the requirement for ventriculovenous shunting. In another study, Schain[145] administered acetazolamide (20 to 55 mg/kg/day for three months) to four hydrocephalic children with intracranial hypertension and concluded that it had no significant therapeutic value in the treatment of chronic hydrocephalus.

Thus, there is both experimental and clinical evidence to suggest that acetazolamide reduces the rate of CSF formation in humans, but there is, at best, contradictory evidence regarding its usefulness in the treatment of patients with intracranial hypertension.

Barbiturates

Although Shenkin and Bouzarth[148] stated that "properly administered thiopental sodium has no effect on CSF pressure," recent evidence suggests that barbiturates may provide a rapid "pharmacological decompression" in patients with acute elevations of ICP.[13,96] Single bolus doses of barbiturates (e.g., 1.5 mg/kg of thiopental or pentobar-

bital) may be effective when intracranial hypertension cannot be controlled by diuretics, osmotherapy, corticosteroids, and hyperventilation.[13,147] Moreover, barbiturate-induced lowering of ICP usually occurs without a simultaneous reduction in cerebral perfusion pressure. Barbiturates may potentiate the vasoconstrictor effects of norepinephrine on the cerebral vasculature,[123] and Shapiro and co-workers[147] hypothesized that barbiturates reduce ICP by reducing intracranial blood volume.

When barbiturates are employed to lower ICP, both CSFP and systemic arterial pressure (SAP) must be continuously monitored to ensure that cerebral perfusion pressure (SAP − CSFP) is not reduced. Since, in the doses required to lower ICP, barbiturates interfere with synaptic transmission and may mask signs of neurologic deterioration, Bruce and co-workers[13] recommend that their use be reserved for patients in coma "such that the neurologic exam is not beneficial in the selection of therapy."

Controlled hyperventilation

Lowering arterial P_{CO_2} by passive hyperventilation produces cerebral vasoconstriction, increasing cerebral vascular resistance and leading to a marked reduction in CBF and in CBV.*[128,135] Hyperventilation tends to increase arterial P_{O_2} and, thus, potentially improves cerebral oxygenation. Unfortunately, however, controlled hyperventilation is frequently ineffective in lowering ICP, and when effective is often only transiently so. There are several reasons for this lack of efficacy. The cerebral vasculature of severely brain-injured patients does not respond normally to hypocapnia (vasoparalysis).[88,132] James and co-workers[62] found that hyperventilation was ineffective in lowering ICP in four of seven patients with cerebral vascular disease (aneurysms and arteriovenous malformations) and in 4 of 13 head-injured patients. Moreover, excessive hyper-

---

*A failure of the blood supply to the choroid plexus may explain the reduction in I_f observed by Oppelt and co-workers[117] in rabbits during experimental respiratory alkalosis (P_{CO_2} = 10 mm Hg).

ventilation may result in reduced cerebral oxygenation. Gotoh and co-workers[51] studied the effects of hyperventilation on the electroencephalogram in 13 patients with a variety of neurologic disorders and concluded that EEG slowing, which appeared when internal jugular venous PO_2 fell below 21 mm Hg, reflected cerebral hypoxia rather than cerebral alkalosis. Despite the high arterial oxygen tensions achieved during hyperventilation with 100% O_2, EEG slowing appeared whenever internal jugular venous PO_2 fell below this threshold value. In another study, EEG slowing failed to occur in eight normal young volunteers who hyperventilated while breathing 100% oxygen at 3 atmospheres absolute pressure, whereas EEG slowing was observed in six of these same eight volunteers during hyperventilation at an ambient pressure of 3 atmospheres absolute but with an inspired oxygen concentration of 7% (PO_2 160 mm Hg).[129] These data suggest that the EEG changes that occur during hyperventilation represent mild and reversible cerebral hypoxia.

It should be recalled that most severely brain-injured patients are already hyperventilating and "optimally" hypocarbic; additional, passive hyperventilation will not further reduce ICP and may, as noted above, reduce cerebral oxygenation and exacerbate preexisting brain damage. The pressure-lowering effect of controlled hyperventilation is frequently evanescent[61,88] because (1) the cerebral vasculature adapts rapidly to hypocapnia, CBF reverts toward normal,[125] and P_d (which varies with CBF) increases and (2) an hyperventilation-induced decrement in CBV is rapidly replaced by nascent CSF.

Despite its limitations, many patients do respond to hyperventilation, and some physicians believe that the combination of dexamethasone and moderate hypocapnia may promote the restoration of cerebral autoregulation and lower ICP. We recommend that controlled hyperventilation (after endotracheal intubation) be reserved for comatose patients who are receiving hyperosmolar agents and corticosteroids and who are not hyperventilating sufficiently to maintain

their arterial PCO_2 in the range of 25 to 30 mm Hg (see below).

Hypothermia

Rosomoff and Gilbert[134] demonstrated that hypothermia reduces brain volume in dogs and that cisternal CSFP falls pari passu with body temperature. However, they were unable to relate the hypothermia-induced reduction in brain volume to the observed fall in CSFP, inasmuch as systemic blood pressure and external jugular venous pressure also fell progressively as body temperature was lowered. Lundberg and co-workers[89] described two patients with severe closed head injuries in whom VFP was continuously monitored for a period of nine to ten days. In each case, a rapid reduction in VFP and a cessation of spontaneously occurring plateau waves were associated with the induction and maintenance of hypothermia. In one patient, VFP fell from 60 to 90 mm Hg to near-normal levels, and plateau waves ceased entirely when the rectal temperature fell below 29° C. Lemmen and Davis[79] monitored lumbar CSFP in 22 patients during the induction of anesthesia and hypothermia preparatory to intracranial surgery. Although they concluded that induced hypothermia was not a practical means of reducing the increased ICP associated with space-occupying lesions, no firm conclusions can be drawn from their published data because of the multiplicity of uncontrolled variables. James and co-workers[62] found that hypothermia was effective in reducing ICP by 10% or more in 17 of 40 trials and that among responders the percentage reduction in ICP was comparable to the results obtained with hypertonic mannitol and controlled hyperventilation. The observed decrease in ICP "paralleled the decrease in body temperature in nearly all cases." Mild hypothermia (32° to 36° C) was nearly as effective as moderate hypothermia (27° to 31° C), but the time to maximum reduction of ICP was shorter with moderate as compared to mild hypothermia (150 versus 516 min), because body temperature was reduced as rapidly as possible in moderate-hypothermia patients.

Induced hypothermia may lower ICP acutely by reducing CBF and CBV. A more sustained lowering of ICP may result from a temperature-related fall in dural sinus venous pressure and/or in the rate of CSF formation.[30] At the present time, hypothermia is seldom used to lower ICP, and its value in the management of neurosurgical patients is far from established. Certainly, febrile patients with increased ICP should be treated with a cooling blanket, and because of its potentially salutary effect on CSFP, moderate hypothermia may have a place in the chronic management of severely brain-injured patients.

CSF diversion

In patients with raised ICP, the rapid removal of ventricular CSF invariably reduces CSFP.[61,62,86] External ventricular drainage and ventriculosystemic shunts reduce ICP by providing a low-resistance pathway for CSF absorption. Chronic CSF diversion is most effective and, therefore, specifically indicated when CSF absorption resistance is greatly increased. On theoretical grounds, ventriculoatrial shunts are preferable to ventriculoperitoneal shunts, since right atrial pressure probably varies less with position and activity than does intra-abdominal pressure.

Given the equivalent circuit diagrammed in Fig. 5-1, ventriculosystemic shunting is best understood in terms of the resistance network illustrated in Fig. 5-3.[136] Assuming that the internal resistance of "battery" P_d can be neglected, CSF bulk flow through the shunt apparatus is inversely proportional to the flow resistance designated R_s and is directly proportional to the preexisting absorption resistance R_A, where R_A is equal to $\dfrac{R_a R_e}{R_a + R_e}$. Moreover, an increased proportion of total CSF bulk flow traverses a ventriculovenous shunt when P_d rises in consequence of an increase in R_v (see Fig. 5-1).

It should be noted that shunt patency is *not* synonymous with shunt function and that even "low-pressure" shunt systems will

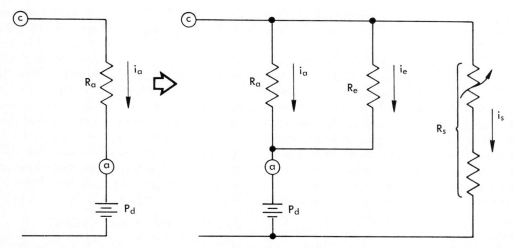

Fig. 5-3. Hypothetical equivalent circuit in a patient with communicating hydrocephalus following the placement of a ventriculovenous shunt. R_a, resistance to CSF absorption across the arachnoid villi; R_e, resistance to CSF absorption across the ventricular/choroidal ependyma; R_s, resistance to CSF efflux through the ventriculovenous shunt. Note that R_s is composed of a fixed resistance representing the shunt tubing and reservoir and a variable (nonlinear) resistance representing the shunt valve. CSF bulk flow through the arachnoid villi, ventricular/choroidal ependyma, and ventriculovenous shunt is represented by i_a, i_e, and i_s, respectively.

Table 5-4. The effect of ventriculovenous shunting on CSF pressure in hypothetical patients with pseudotumor cerebri and normal-pressure hydrocephalus*

	CSF pressure when			
	$R_s = \infty$	$R_s = 1000$	$R_s = 100$	$R_s = 10$
Pseudotumor cerebri				
Case I: $P_d = 70$, $I_f = 0.35$, $R_A = 1000$	420 (0)	245 (0.18)	102 (0.32)	73.5 (0.35)
Case II: $P_d = 385$, $I_f = 0.35$, $R_A = 100$	420 (0)	417 (0.03)	403 (0.18)	388 (0.32)
Normal-pressure hydrocephalus				
Case I: $P_d = 70$, $I_f = 0.25$, $R_A = 100$	95 (0)	92.7 (0.02)	82.5 (0.13)	72.3 (0.23)
Case II: $P_d = 35$, $I_f = 0.25$, $R_A = 240$	95 (0)	83.4 (0.05)	52.7 (0.18)	37.4 (0.24)

*R_s is the resistance to CSF efflux through the ventriculovenous shunt (see Fig. 5-3). P_d, I_f, and R_A are defined in the text. CSF pressure and P_d are expressed as mm H_2O; R_s and R_A as mm H_2O − min/ml; and I_f as ml/min. The figures in parentheses represent CSF bulk flow through the ventriculovenous shunt (ml/min). Note that an increasing proportion of I_f is shunted as R_s/R_A becomes smaller.

not significantly lower VFP (regardless of the absolute value of R_s) unless R_s is $<<$ than R_A. The effect of shunt resistance on CSFP depends upon the relative magnitudes of R_A and R_s as well as the absolute magnitude of P_d (Table 5-4). The relationship between flow and pressure in two standard ventriculosystemic shunt systems is illustrated in Fig. 5-4.

Failure to appreciate that all patent shunts are not necessarily functioning shunts has led to confusion in the literature regarding the indications for shunting patients with normal-pressure hydrocephalus. When a patient with the preoperative diagnosis of normal-pressure hydrocephalus fails to improve after shunting, one should not jump immediately to the conclusion that (1) the diagnosis was incorrect (i.e., the patient had cerebral atrophy and not normal-pressure hydrocephalus) or (2) shunting was not indicated. The neurosurgeon must know not only that a shunt is patent but that its flow resistance, R_s, is low enough to divert a significant portion of the total CSF bulk flow at normal or "subnormal" CSF pressures. In practice, one can estimate R_s by measuring the resistance to CSF absorption before and after reversible occlusion of the shunt system.[122,136]

Surgical decompression

Removal of part of the skull (external decompression) or part of the brain (internal decompression) has been advocated for uncontrollable brain swelling, especially in patients with severe craniocerebral trauma. Although decompressive surgery is often performed with an eye to reducing ICP, the major effect of such surgery—and the reason for its occasional success—is the reduction of midline shift, brain herniation, and/or brain stem displacement. Although subtemporal decompression was advocated by Dandy in 1937[28] for the treatment of pseudotumor cerebri, the efficacy of this procedure remains to be demonstrated.[63] Indeed, Dandy himself was surprised "that the increased pressure usually sets its limit within the bounds afforded by subtemporal decompression"; in one of his cases "this was certainly not true, for the vision was lost when the decompression became . . . tense." Recent evidence[42] would suggest that CSFP may remain elevated for years following subtemporal decompression in the absence of headache or papilledema.

TREATMENT OF IMPENDING HERNIATION IN ACUTELY DECOMPENSATING PATIENTS

The physician faced with an acutely decompensating neurologic patient must act quickly and decisively to reduce the volume of the intracranial contents and reverse the signs and symptoms of herniation. Our recommendations are listed in the boxed

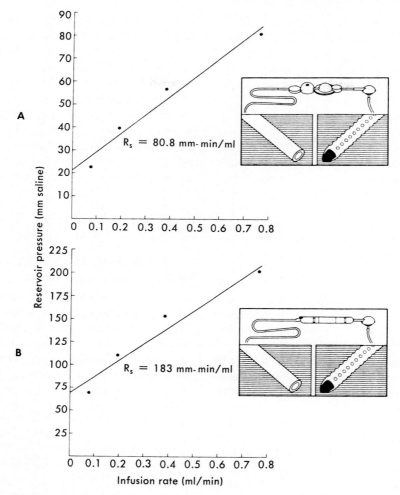

Fig. 5-4. Relationship between pressure and flow in two standard ventriculoatrial shunt systems. **A,** Pudenz ventricular catheter, Rickham reservoir, "medium-pressure" Heyer-Schulte multipurpose valve, Holter type A atrial catheter. **B,** Pudenz ventricular catheter, Rickham reservoir, "medium-pressure" Holter valve, and Holter type A atrial catheter. Each shunt system was perfused with normal saline through its ventricular catheter. Pressure measurements were made in the Heyer-Schulte (**A**) or Rickham (**B**) reservoir. Steady-state pressures were recorded at various infusion rates; each data point represents the mean of three experiments. Least-squares regression lines were drawn in order to define an approximate shunt flow resistance (R_s) within the range 0.0764 to 0.764 ml/min. In fact, all of the pressure-flow curves are nonlinear.

material on p. 112. Hyperosmolar agents appear to be more effective than systemic diuretics in reducing the volume of the intracranial contents, and they represent the first line of treatment. The choice of an hyperosmolar agent is less important than the rapidity with which the chosen agent is employed; however, mannitol would seem to be the best choice at present, since it crosses the blood-brain barrier more slowly than either urea or glycerol, and rebound increases in ICP are therefore less likely to occur.[62,137] An initial dose of 0.5 to 2.0 g/kg should be administered IV as rapidly as possible (preferably within 15 minutes), and the patient's clinical response or—if one is fortunate enough to

have an indwelling ventricular cannula—
VFP closely monitored. Additional 25 g
doses may be given as necessary to control
clinical symptoms and/or to abort symptomatic plateau waves. Central venous pressure should also be monitored, especially in
older patients and in patients with a history
of cardiac disease.

Intravenous glucocorticoids should be administered together with mannitol, but here
again the dose is not well established. There
is increasing evidence that higher doses
than those usually employed may be more
effective than conventional doses in the treatment of primary and metastatic brain tumors,[130] and we would recommend 100 mg
of dexamethasone (or its equivalent) as a
loading dose, to be followed by 100 mg qd
in divided doses, depending upon the patient's clinical response. As the patient's
condition stabilizes or improves, this daily
dose may be rapidly tapered.

The volume of the intracranial contents
may be rapidly reduced by hyperventilation,
and in comatose patients, reducing the
PCO_2 to 25 to 30 mg Hg seems desirable;
in such patients effective hyperventilation
requires endotracheal intubation. Although
the pressure-lowering effect of hyperventilation is frequently transient, its institution
may allow time for corticosteroids to begin
reducing cerebral edema. However, many
herniating patients are already hyperventilating and sufficiently hypocarbic so as not
to benefit from passive hyperventilation.
The role of barbiturates and hypothermia in
the acute treatment of herniation associated

with cerebral mass lesions has not yet been
established, and carefully controlled studies
will be required before these modalities can
be recommended for routine clinical use.

The definitive treatment of increased ICP
is ultimately determined by the nature of
the underlying pathologic process. Whenever feasible, surgical extirpation of a mass
lesion and/or CSF diversion are the treatments of choice. Corticosteroids—in the
lowest possible doses—are also useful. The
chronic use of hyperosmolar agents or of
systemic diuretics is probably undesirable,
inasmuch as rebound effects and electrolyte
imbalance are not uncommon.

INTRACRANIAL PRESSURE MONITORING

Continuous recording of VFP for diagnostic and therapeutic purposes was introduced by Lundberg in 1960,[86] and the desirability and clinical utility of ICP monitoring has been debated ever since.[13,22,77,108]
The use of CSFP monitoring has been extended to preoperative and postoperative
neurosurgical patients and to patients with
craniocerebral trauma, pseudotumor cerebri,
hydrocephalus, occlusive cerebrovascular
disease, Reye syndrome, meningitis, encephalitis, diabetic ketoacidosis, and even
anorexia nervosa.* The major arguments in
favor of continuously monitoring ICP were
advanced by Langfitt in 1973[77]: "to provide
information that will permit better management of the individual patient" and to collect data "on the incidence and clinical significance of increased ICP in patients with
various types of intracranial pathology."

It should be recognized, however, that
even in the best of hands, intracranial pressure monitoring is not without significant
risks.[62,156] The limitations of intracranial
pressure monitoring have been recently re-
stated by Cooper and Ransohoff.[21] These
authors point out that intercompartmental
and intracompartmental pressure gradients
are common but are inadequately defined
by monitoring techniques and that neu-

**TREATMENT OF IMPENDING
HERNIATION IN ACUTELY
DECOMPENSATING PATIENTS**

Osmotherapy Mannitol, 0.5 to 2.0 g/kg IV
stat followed by 25 g prn
Corticosteroids Dexamethasone, 100 mg IV
push followed by 100 mg qd in divided
doses
Hyperventilation lower PCO_2 to 25 to 30
mm Hg

---

*References 5, 13, 56, 66, 89, 105.

rologic deterioration cannot always be related to elevations of ICP. Strategically situated lesions, such as medial temporal lobe tumors, may be life threatening by virtue of their location adjacent to the incisura and brain stem but may produce no measurable increase in intracranial pressure; conversely, patients with markedly elevated ICP (e.g., patients with pseudotumor cerebri) may remain alert and entirely asymptomatic. It remains to be demonstrated that intracranial hypertension per se is harmful in the absence of symptomatic reductions in cerebral perfusion pressure. Since CBF is probably not significantly reduced until ICP exceeds 70 torr,[52] clinically encountered elevations of CSFP seldom lead to a critical reduction in cerebral perfusion pressure.

MANAGEMENT OF PATIENTS WITH DECREASED INTRACRANIAL PRESSURE

Inasmuch as symptomatic decreases in ICP almost always result from the leakage of CSF, the management of low-pressure states is usually directed at repairing a CSF leak. In most instances (e.g., post-lumbar-puncture headache[91]) the leak will repair itself with time, and the patient is instructed to remain horizontal or semierect in bed, depending upon whether CSF is leaking from the lumbar sac or from the cranial cavity. Occasionally, however, spontaneous or traumatic leaks do not repair themselves, and symptoms persist. These leaks require definitive treatment. The leak must first be located, usually by the subarachnoid injection of radionuclides[33,46,69] or water-soluble contrast agents,[36] followed by serial scanning of the neuraxis. Once the leak is located, surgical repair should be carried out. Some authors[17,69] have advocated sealing post-lumbar-puncture CSF leaks with an "epidural blood patch," that is, an epidural injection of the patient's own blood. We have no experience with this therapeutic technique and are not enthusiastic about its use for theoretical reasons. Blood is a noxious substance, and the accidental injection of blood into the subarachnoid space may produce a severe inflammatory response. It is possible that a similar response may follow injection of blood into the subdural or epidural space.

REFERENCES

1. Adams, J. H., and Graham, D. I.: The relationship between ventricular fluid pressure and the neuropathology of raised intracranial pressure, Neuropathol. Appl. Neurobiol. **2:**323-332, 1976.
2. Adson, A. W., and Lillie, W. I.: The relationship of intracranial pressure, choked disc, and intraocular tension, Trans. Am. Acad. Ophthalmol. Otolaryngol. **30:**138-154, 1927.
3. Arseni, C., and Maretsis, M.: Tumors of the lower spinal cord associated with increased intracranial pressure and papilledema, J. Neurosurg. **27:**105-110, 1967.
4. Barge, M., Benabid, A. L., de Rougemont, J., and others: L'hyper-production de LCR dans les papillomes du plexus choroïde de l'enfant, Neuro-Chirurgie **6:**639-644, 1976.
5. Beks, J. W. F., Journée, H. L., Albarda, S., and others: The significance of ICP-monitoring in the post-operative period. In Beks, J. W. F., Bosch, D. A., and Brock, M., editors: Intracranial pressure III, New York, 1976, Springer-Verlag, pp. 251-258.
6. Beller, A. J.: Benign post-traumatic intracranial hypertension, J. Neurol. Neurosurg. Psychiatr. **27:**149-152, 1964.
7. Benabid, A. L., de Rougemont, J., and Barge, M.: La pression intracrânienne. I. Etude théorique, J. Physiol. (Paris) **68:**655-669, 1974.
8. Benabid, A. L., de Rougemont, J., and Barge, M.: La pression intracrânienne. II. Vérification expérimentale d'un modèle mathématique, J. Physiol. (Paris) **70:**41-59, 1975.
9. Benabid, A. L., de Rougemont, J., and Barge, M.: La pression intracrânienne. III. Essai d'une théorie généralisée, J. Physiol. (Paris) **70:**61-75, 1975.
10. Birzis, L., Carter, C. H., and Maren, T. H.: Effect of acetazolamide on CSF pressure and electrolytes in hydrocephalus, Neurology **8:**522-528, 1958.
11. Bito, L. Z., Davson, H., and Fenstermacher, J. D., editors: The ocular and cerebrospinal fluids, New York, 1977, Academic Press, Inc.
12. Browder, J., and Meyers, R.: Behavior of the systemic blood pressure, pulse rate and spinal fluid pressure associated with acute changes in intracranial pressure artifically produced, Arch. Surg. **36:**1-19, 1938.
13. Bruce, D. A., Berman, W. A., and Schut, L.: Cerebrospinal fluid pressure monitoring in children: physiology, pathology and clinical usefulness. In Barness, L. A., editor: Advances in pediatrics, vol. 24, Chicago, 1977, Year Book Medical Publishers, Inc., pp. 233-290.

14. Bruce, D. A., Langfitt, T. W., Miller, J. D., and others: Regional cerebral blood flow, intracranial pressure, and brain metabolism in comatose patients, J. Neurosurg. **38**:131-144, 1973.

15. Bryce-Smith, R., and Macintosh, R. R.: Sixth-nerve palsy after lumbar puncture and spinal analgesia, Br. Med. J. **1**:275-276, 1951.

16. Buchanan, D. S., and Brazinsky, J. H.: Dural sinus and cerebral venous thrombosis; incidence in young women receiving oral contraceptives, Arch. Neurol. **22**:440-444, 1970.

17. Cass, W., and Edelist, G.: Postspinal headache, successful use of epidural blood patch 11 weeks after onset, J. Am. Med. Assoc. **227**:786-787, 1974.

18. Chawla, J. C., Hulme, A., and Cooper, R.: Intracranial pressure in patients with dementia and communicating hydrocephalus, J. Neurosurg. **40**:376-380, 1974.

19. Cogan, D. G.: Neurology of the visual system, Springfield, Ill., 1976, Charles C Thomas, Publisher.

20. Cogan, D. G., and Kuwabara, T.: Papilledema. In Bito, L. Z., Davson, H., and Fenstermacher, J. D., editors: The ocular and cerebrospinal fluids, London, 1977, Academic Press, Inc., pp. 419-433.

21. Cooper, P. R., and Ransohoff, J.: Limitations of intracranial pressure monitoring. In Morley, T. P., editor: Current controversies in neurosurgery, Philadelphia, 1976, W. B. Saunders Co., pp. 658-666.

22. Cooper, R., and Hulme, A.: Intracranial pressure and related phenomena during sleep, J. Neurol. Neurosurg. Psychiatr. **29**:564-570, 1966.

23. Cottrell, J. E., Robustelli, A., Post, K., and others: Furosemide- and mannitol-induced changes in intracranial pressure and serum osmolality and electrolytes, Anesthesiology **47**:28-30, 1977.

24. Cserr, H. F., and Tang, D. T.: Evidence for bulk flow of cerebral interstitial fluid and its possible contribution to cerebrospinal fluid production. In Lundberg, N., Ponten, U., and Brock, M., editors: Intracranial pressure II, New York, 1975, Springer-Verlag, pp. 24-27.

25. Cushing, H.: The blood-pressure reaction of acute cerebral compression, illustrated by cases of intracranial hemorrhage, Am. J. Med. Sci. **125**:1017-1044, 1903.

26. Cushing, H.: Concerning a definite regulatory mechanism of the vaso-motor centre which controls blood pressure during cerebral compression, Johns Hopkins Hosp. Bull. **12**:290-292, 1901.

27. Cushing, H.: Some experimental and clinical observations concerning states of increased intracranial tension, Am. J. Med. Sci. **124**:375-400, 1902.

28. Dandy, W. E.: Intracranial pressure without brain tumor; diagnosis and treatment, Ann. Surg. **106**:492-513, 1937.

29. Davson, H., Hollingsworth, G., and Segal, M. B.: The mechanism of drainage of the cerebrospinal fluid, Brain **93**:665-678, 1970.

30. Davson, H., and Spaziani, E.: Effect of hypothermia on certain aspects of the cerebrospinal fluid, Exp. Neurol. **6**:118-128, 1962.

31. Dellaporta, A.: Fundus changes in postoperative hypotony, Am. J. Ophthalmol. **40**:781-785, 1955.

32. Denny-Brown, D. E.: The changing pattern of neurologic medicine, N. Engl. J. Med. **246**:839-846, 1952.

33. Di Chiro, G.: New radiographic and isotopic procedures in neurological diagnosis, J. Am. Med. Assoc. **188**:524-529, 1964.

34. DiMattio, J., Hochwald, G. M., Malhan, C., and others: Effects of changes in serum osmolarity on bulk flow of fluid into cerebral ventricles and on brain water content, Pflügers Arch. **359**:253-264, 1975.

35. Domer, F. R.: Effects of diuretics on cerebrospinal fluid formation and potassium movement, Exp. Neurol. **24**:54-64, 1969.

36. Drayer, B. P., Wilkins, R. H., Boehnke, M., and others: Cerebrospinal fluid rhinorrhea demonstrated by metrizamide CT cisternography, Am. J. Roentgenol. **129**:149-151, 1977.

37. Duffy, G. P.: Lumbar puncture in the presence of raised intracranial pressure, Br. Med. J. **1**:407-409, 1969.

38. Ectors, L., and Bégaux-Van Boven, C.: Glaucome et papille de stase, Ophthalmologica **108**:113-120, 1944.

39. Eisenberg, H. M., McComb, G., and Lorenzo, A. V.: Cerebrospinal fluid overproduction and hydrocephalus associated with choroid plexus papilloma, J. Neurosurg. **40**:381-385, 1974.

40. Evans, J. P., Espey, F. F., Kristoff, F. V., and others: Experimental and clinical observations on rising intracranial pressure, Arch. Surg. **63**:107-114, 1951.

41. Ethelberg, S., and Jensen, V. A.: Obscurations and further time-related paroxysmal disorders in intracranial tumors; syndrome of initial herniation of parts of the brain through the tentorial incisure, Arch. Neurol. Psychiatr. **68**:130-149, 1952.

42. Foley, K. M.: Is benign intracranial hypertension a chronic disease? Neurology **27**:388, 1977.

43. Garcia-Bengochea, F.: Cortisone and the cerebrospinal fluid of noncastrated cats, Am. Surg. **31**:123-125, 1965.

44. Garcin, R., and Pestel, M.: Thrombo-phlébites cérébrales, les thromboses artérielles, Paris, 1955, Masson et Cie Editeurs, pp. 503-533.

45. Gardner, W. J., Spitler, D. K., and Whitten, C.: Increased intracranial pressure caused by increased protein content in the cerebrospinal fluid; an explanation of papilledema in certain cases of small intracranial and intraspinal tumors, and in the Guillain-Barré syndrome, N. Engl. J. Med. **250**:932-936, 1954.

46. Gass, H., Goldstein, A. S., Ruskin, R., and others: Chronic postmyelogram headache; isotopic demonstration of dural leak and surgical cure, Arch. Neurol. **25:**168-170, 1971.
47. Ghatak, N. R., and McWhorter, J. M.: Ultrastructural evidence for CSF production by a choroid plexus papilloma, J. Neurosurg. **45:**409-415, 1976.
48. Gibberd, F. B., Ngan, H., and Swann, G. F.: Hydrocephalus, subarachnoid haemorrhage and ependymomas of the cauda equina, Clin. Radiol. **23:**422-426, 1972.
49. Goldman, J. A., and Eckerling, B.: Intracranial dural sinus thrombosis following intrauterine instillation of hypertonic saline, Am. J. Obstet. Gynecol. **112:**1132-1133, 1972.
50. Goluboff, B., Shenkin, H. A., and Haft, H.: The effects of mannitol and urea on cerebral hemodynamics and cerebrospinal fluid pressure, Neurology **14:**891-898, 1964.
51. Gotoh, F., Meyer, J. S., and Takagi, Y.: Cerebral effects of hyperventilation in man, Arch. Neurol. **12:**410-423, 1965.
52. Grubb, R. L., Raichle, M. E., Phelps, M. E., and others: Effects of increased intracranial pressure on cerebral blood volume, blood flow, and oxygen utilization in monkeys, J. Neurosurg. **43:**385-398, 1975.
53. Guillaume, J., and Janny, P.: Manométrie intracranienne continue; intérêt de la méthode et premiers résultats, Rev. Neurol. **84:**131-142, 1951.
54. Guinane, J. E.: An equivalent circuit analysis of cerebrospinal fluid hydrodynamics, Am. J. Physiol. **223:**425-430, 1972.
55. Guinane, J. E.: Cerebrospinal fluid pulse pressure and brain compliance in adult cats, Neurology **25:**559-564, 1975.
56. Hartmann, A., and Alberti, E.: Differentiation of communicating hydrocephalus and presenile dementia by continuous recording of cerebrospinal fluid pressure, J. Neurol. Neurosurg. Psychiatr. **40:**630-640, 1977.
57. Hayreh, S. S.: So-called 'central retinal vein occlusion'. II. Venous stasis retinopathy, Ophthalmologica **172:**14-37, 1976.
58. Heisey, S. R., Held, D., and Pappenheimer, J. R.: Bulk flow and diffusion in the cerebrospinal fluid system of the goat, Am. J. Physiol. **203:**775-781, 1962.
59. Hochwald, G. M., Wald, A., and Malhan, C.: The sink action of cerebrospinal fluid volume flow, Arch. Neurol. **33:**339-344, 1976.
60. Ingvar, D. H., and Lundberg, N.: Paroxysmal symptoms in intracranial hypertension, studied with ventricular fluid pressure recording and electroencephalography, Brain **84:**446-459, 1961.
61. James, H. E., Langfitt, T. W., and Kumar, V. S.: Analysis of the response to therapeutic measures to reduce intracranial pressure in head injured patients, J. Trauma **16:**437-441, 1976.

62. James, H. E., Langfitt, T. W., Kumar, V. S., and others: Treatment of intracranial hypertension; analysis of 105 consecutive continuous recordings of intracranial pressure, Acta Neurochir. **36:**189-200, 1977.
63. Janeway, R., and Kelly, D. L.: Papilledema and hydrocephalus asociated with recurrent polyneuritis, Arch. Neurol. **15:**507-514, 1966.
64. Jefferson, G.: The tentorial pressure cone, Arch. Neurol. Psychiatr. **40:**857-876, 1938.
65. Johnston, I., Gilday, D. L., and Hendrick, E. B.: Experimental effects of steroids and steroid withdrawal on cerebrospinal fluid absorption, J. Neurosurg. **42:**690-695, 1975.
66. Johnston, I., and Paterson, A.: Intracranial pressure monitoring in patients with benign intracranial hypertension. In Lundberg, N., Ponten, U., and Brock, M., editors: Intracranial pressure II. New York, 1975, Springer-Verlag, pp. 500-521.
67. Jonsson, O.: Extracellular osmolality and vascular smooth muscle activity, Acta Physiol. Scand. (suppl.) **359:**1-48, 1970.
68. Joynt, R. J.: Mechanism of production of papilledema in the Guillain-Barré syndrome, Neurology **8:**8-12, 1958.
69. Kadrie, H., Driedger, A. A., and McInnis, W.: Persistent dural cerebrospinal fluid leak shown by retrograde radionuclide myelography: case report, J. Nucl. Med. **17:**797-799, 1976.
70. Kahn, E. A., and Cherry, G. R.: The clinical importance of spontaneous retinal venous pulsation, Univ. Mich. Med. Bull. **16:**305-308, 1950.
71. Kinal, M. R.: Infratentorial tumors and the dural venous sinuses, J. Neurosurg. **25:**395-401, 1966.
72. Kocher, T.: Hirnerschutterung, hirndruck und chirurgische eingriffe bei hirnkrankheiten, Vienna, 1901, Alfred Holder.
73. Kullberg, G., and West, K. A.: Influence of corticosteroids on the ventricular fluid pressure, Acta Neurol. Scand. (suppl. 13, Part II) **41:**445-452, 1965.
74. Kunkle, E. C., Ray, B. S., and Wolff, H. G.: Experimental studies on headache: analysis of the headache associated with changes in intracranial pressure, Arch. Neurol. Psychiatr. **49:**323-358, 1943.
75. Kunkle, E. C., Ray, B. S., and Wolff, H. G.: Studies on headache: the mechanisms and significance of the headache associated with brain tumor, Bull. N.Y. Acad. Med. **18:**400-422, 1942.
76. Lamas, E., Lobato, R. D., Esparza, J., and others: Dural posterior fossa AVM producing raised sagittal sinus pressure; case report, J. Neurosurg. **46:**804-810, 1977.
77. Langfitt, T. W.: Summary of First International Symposium on Intracranial Pressure, Hanover, Germany, July 27-29, 1972, J. Neurosurg. **38:**541-544, 1973.
78. Langfitt, T. W., Weinstein, J. D., and Kassell, N. F.: Transmission of increased intracranial pres-

sure. I. Within the craniospinal axis, J. Neurosurg. **21**:989-997, 1964.

79. Lemmen, L. J., and Davis, J. S.: Studies of cerebrospinal fluid pressure during hypothermia in intracranial surgery, Surg. Gynecol. Obstet. **106**: 555-558, 1958.

80. Levatin, P.: Increased intracranial pressure without papilledema, Arch. Ophthalmol. **58**:683-688, 1957.

81. Levin, B. E.: The clinical significance of spontaneous pulsations of the retinal vein, Arch. Neurol. **35**:37-40, 1978.

82. Lim, S. T., Potts, D. G., Deonarine, V., and others: Ventricular compliance in dogs with and without aqueductal obstruction, J. Neurosurg. **39**:463-473, 1973.

83. Lofgren, J.: Mechanical basis of the CSF pressure-volume curve. In Lundberg, N., Ponten, U., and Brock, M., editors: Intracranial pressure II, New York, 1975, Springer-Verlag, pp. 79-81.

84. Lofgren, J., von Essen, C., and Zwetnow, N. N.: The pressure-volume curve of the cerebrospinal fluid space in dogs, Acta Neurol. Scand. **49**:557-574, 1973.

85. Lofgren, J., and Zwetnow, N. N.: Cranial and spinal components of the cerebrospinal fluid pressure-volume curve, Acta Neurol. Scand. **49**:575-585, 1973.

86. Lundberg, N.: Continuous recording and control of ventricular fluid pressure in neurosurgical practice, Acta Psychiatr. Neurol. Scand. (Suppl.) **149**:1-193, 1960.

87. Lundberg, N., Cronqvist, S., and Kjallquist, A.: Clinical investigations on interrelations between intracranial pressure and intracranial hemodynamics. Prog. Brain Res. **30**:69-75, 1968.

88. Lundberg, N., and Kjallquist, A.: Reduction of increased intracranial pressure by hyperventilation, a therapeutic aid in neurological surgery, Acta Psychiatr. Neurol. Scand. (Suppl.) **139**:1-64, 1959.

89. Lundberg, N., Troupp, H., and Lorin, H.: Continuous recording of the ventricular-fluid pressure in patients with severe acute traumatic brain injury, a preliminary report, J. Neurosurg. **22**:581-590, 1965.

90. Luzecky, M., Siegal, B. A., Coxe, W. S., and others: Papilledema and communicating hydrocephalus; association with a lumbar neurofibroma, Arch. Neurol. **30**:487-489, 1974.

91. MacRobert, R. G.: The cause of lumbar puncture headache, J. Am. Med. Assoc. **70**:1350-1353, 1918.

92. Magnaes, B.: Body position and cerebrospinal fluid pressure. I. Clinical studies on the effect of rapid postural changes, J. Neurosurg. **44**:687-697, 1976.

93. Marmarou, A., Shulman, K., and LaMorgese, J.: Compartmental analysis of compliance and outflow resistance of the cerebrospinal fluid system, J. Neurosurg. **43**:523-534, 1975.

94. Marmarou, A., Shulman, K., and Rosende, R. M.: A nonlinear analysis of the cerebrospinal fluid system and intracranial pressure dynamics, J. Neurosurg. **48**:332-344, 1978.

95. Marr, W. G., and Chamber, R. G.: Pseudotumor cerebri syndrome following unilateral radical neck dissection, Am. J. Ophthalmol. **51**:605-611, 1961.

96. Marshall, L. F., Bruce, D. A., Bruno, L., and others: Role of intracranial pressure monitoring and barbiturate therapy in malignant intracranial hypertension; case report, J. Neurosurg. **47**:481-484, 1977.

97. Marshall, L. F., King, J., and Langfitt, T. W.: The complications of high-dose corticosteroid therapy in neurosurgical patients; a prospective study, Ann. Neurol. **1**:201-203, 1977.

98. Martin, J. P.: Signs of obstruction of the superior longitudinal sinus following closed head injuries (traumatic hydrocephalus), Br. Med. J. **2**:467-470, 1955.

98a. Martin, J. P.: Thrombosis in the superior longitudinal sinus following childbirth, Br. Med. J. **4**:537-540, 1941.

99. Martins, A. N., Ramirez, A., Solomon, L. S., and others: The effect of dexamethasone on the rate of formation of cerebrospinal fluid in the monkey, J. Neurosurg. **41**:550-554, 1974.

100. Masserman, J. H.: Cerebrospinal hydrodynamics. IV. Clinical experimental studies, Arch. Neurol. Psychiatr. **32**:523-553, 1934.

101. McNealy, D. E., and Plum, F.: Brainstem dysfunction with supratentorial mass lesions, Arch. Neurol. **7**:10-32, 1962.

102. Mealey, J., Jr., and Barker, D. T.: Failure of oral acetazolamide to avert hydrocephalus in infants with myelomeningocele, J. Pediatr. **72**:257-259, 1968.

103. Meinig, G., Aulich, A., Wende, S., and others: The effect of dexamethasone and diuretics on peritumor brain edema: comparative study of tissue water content and CT. In Pappius, H. M., and Feindel, W., editors: Dynamics of brain edema, New York, 1976, Springer-Verlag, pp. 301-305.

104. Meyer, A.: Herniation of the brain, Arch. Neurol. Psychiatr. **4**:387-400, 1920.

105. Mickell, J. J., Reigel, D. H., Cook, D. R., and others: Intracranial pressure: monitoring and normalization therapy in children, Pediatrics **59**:606-613, 1977.

106. Milhorat, T. H.: Hydrocephalus and the cerebrospinal fluid, Baltimore, 1972, The Williams & Wilkins Co.

107. Milhorat, T. H.: Pediatric neurosurgery, Philadelphia, 1978, F. A. Davis Co.

108. Miller, J. D., Becker, D. P., Ward, J. D., and others: Significance of intracranial hypertension in severe head injury, J. Neurosurg. **47**:503-516, 1977.

109. Miller, J. D., and Leech, P.: Effects of mannitol and steroid therapy on intracranial volume-pres-

sure relationships in patients, J. Neurosurg. **42**: 274-281, 1975.

110. Miller, J. D., Sakalas, R., Ward, J. D., and others: Methylprednisolone treatment in patients with brain tumors, Neurosurgery **1**:114-117, 1977.

111. Miyazaki, Y., Suematsu, K., and Yamaura, J.: Effect of ethacrynic acid on lowering of intracranial pressure, Arzneimittelforschung **19**:1961-1965, 1969.

112. Mones, R. J.: Increased intracranial pressure due to metastatic disease of venous sinuses, a report of six cases, Neurology **15**:1000-1007, 1965.

113. Moreno Cadierno, M., and Crespí Cárcar, F.: Sobre la significación del pulso venoso en el síndrome hipertensivo intracraneal, Arch. Soc. Oftal. Hisp. Am. **19**:499-505, 1959.

114. Morley, J. B., and Reynolds, E. H.: Papilloedema and the Landry-Guillain-Barré syndrome, case reports and a review, Brain **89**:205-222, 1966.

115. Neblett, C. R., McNeel, D. P., Waltz, T. A., Jr., and others: Effect of cardiac glycosides on human cerebrospinal-fluid production, Lancet **4**:1008-1009, 1972.

116. Norrell, H., Wilson, C., Howieson, J., and others: Venous factors in infantile hydrocephalus, J. Neurosurg. **31**:561-569, 1969.

117. Oppelt, W. W., Maren, T. H., Owens, E. S., and others: Effects of acid-base alterations on cerebrospinal fluid production, Proc. Soc. Exp. Biol. Med. **114**:86-89, 1963.

118. Pappenheimer, J. R., Heisey, S. R., Jordon, E. F., and others: Perfusion of the cerebral ventricular system in unanesthetized goats, Am. J. Physiol. **203**:763-774, 1962.

119. Pollay, M.: Formation of cerebrospinal fluid; relation of studies of isolated choroid plexus to the standing gradient hypothesis, J. Neurosurg. **42**: 665-673, 1975.

120. Pollay, M., and Davson, H.: The passage of certain substances out of the cerebrospinal fluid, Brain **86**:137-150, 1963.

121. Portnoy, H. D., and Croissant, P. D.: Pre- and postoperative cerebrospinal fluid absorption studies in patients with myelomeningocele shunted for hydrocephalus, Child's Brain **4**:47-64, 1978.

122. Portnoy, H. D., Schulte, R. R., Fox, J. L., and others: Anti-siphon and reversible occlusion valves for shunting in hydrocephalus and preventing post-shunt subdural hematomas, J. Neurosurg. **38**:729-738, 1973.

123. Price, M. L., and Price, H. L.: Effects of general anesthetics on contractile responses of rabbit aortic strips, Anesthesiology **23**:16-20, 1962.

124. Quincke, H.: Die lumbalpunction des hydrocephalus, Berl. Klinische Wochenschrift **38**:929-968, 1891.

125. Raichle, M. E., Posner, J. B., and Plum, F.: Cerebral blood flow during and after hyperventilation, Arch. Neurol. **23**:394-403, 1970.

126. Raynor, R. B.: Papilledema associated with tumors of the spinal cord, Neurology **19**:700-704, 1969.

127. Reed, D. J.: The effect of fuorsemide on cerebrospinal fluid flow in rabbits, Arch. Int. Pharmacodyn. **178**:324-330, 1969.

128. Reivich, M.: Regulation of the cerebral circulation, Clin. Neurosurg. **16**:378-418, 1969.

129. Reivich, M., Cohen, P. J., and Greenbaum, L.: Alterations in the electroencephalogram of awake man produced by hyperventilation: effects of 100% oxygen at 3 atmospheres (absolute) pressure, Neurology **16**:304, 1966.

130. Renaudin, J., Fewer, D., Wilson, C. B., and others: Dose dependency of Decadron in patients with partially excised brain tumors, J. Neurosurg. **39**:302-305, 1973.

131. Reulen, H. J.: Vasogenic brain oedema, Br. J. Anaesth. **48**:741-752, 1976.

132. Reulen, H. J., Hadjidimos, A., and Schurmann, K.: The effect of dexamethasone on water and electrolyte content and on rCBF in perifocal brain edema in man, In Beks, J. W. F., Klatzo, I., Long, D. M., Pappius, H. M., and Ransohoff, J., editors: Steroids and brain edema, New York, 1972, Springer-Verlag, pp. 239-252.

133. Risberg, J., Lundberg, N., and Ingvar, D. H.: Regional cerebral blood volume during acute transient rises of the intracranial pressure (plateau waves), J. Neurosurg. **31**:303-310, 1969.

134. Rosomoff, H. L., and Gilbert, R.: Brain volume and cerebrospinal fluid pressure during hypothermia, Am. J. Physiol. **183**:19-22, 1955.

135. Rosomoff, H. L.: Distribution of intracranial contents with controlled hyperventilation: implications for neuroanesthesia, Anesthesiology **24**: 640-645, 1963.

136. Rottenberg, D. A.: A dynamic approach to ventricular shunting, Neurology **27**:360, 1977.

137. Rottenberg, D. A., Hurwitz, B. J., and Posner, J. B.: The effect of oral glycerol on intraventricular pressure in man, Neurology **27**:600-608, 1977.

138. Rubin, R. C., Henderson, E. S., Ommaya, A. K., and others: The production of cerebrospinal fluid in man and its modification by acetazolamide, J. Neurosurg. **25**:430-436, 1966.

139. Ryder, H. W., Espey, F. F., Kimbell, F. D., and others: The elasticity of the craniospinal venous bed, J. Lab. Clin. Med. **42**:944, 1953.

140. Ryder, H. W., Espey, F. F., Kimbell, F. D., and others: The mechanism of the change in cerebrospinal fluid pressure following an induced change in the volume of the fluid space, J. Lab. Clin. Med. **41**:428-435, 1953.

141. Ryder, H. W., Rosenauer, A., Penka, E. J., and others: Failure of abnormal cerebrospinal fluid pressure to influence cerebral function, Arch. Neurol. Psychiatr. **70**:563-586, 1953.

142. Sahs, A. L., and Joynt, R. J.: Brain swelling of unknown cause, Neurology **6**:791-803, 1956.

143. Sato, O.: The effect of dexamethasone on cerebrospinal fluid production rate in the dog, Brain and Nerve (Tokyo) **19**:485-492, 1967.

144. Sato, O., Hara, M., Asai, T., and others: The

effect of dexamethasone phosphate on the production rate of cerebrospinal fluid in the spinal subarachnoid space of dogs, J. Neurosurg. **39**:480-484, 1973.

145. Schain, R. J.: Carbonic anhydrase inhibitors in chronic infantile hydrocephalus, Am. J. Dis. Child **117**:621-625, 1969.

146. Shapiro, W. R., Posner, J. B.: Corticosteroid hormones, Arch. Neurol. **30**:217-221, 1974.

147. Shapiro, H. M., Whyte, S. R., and Loeser, J. D.: Barbiturates and hypothermia for persistently increased intracranial pressure. In Lundberg, N., Ponten, U., and Brock, M., editors: Intracranial-pressure II, New York, 1975, Springer-Verlag, pp. 365-367.

148. Shenkin, H. A., and Bouzarth, W. F.: Clinical methods of reducing intracranial pressure; role of the cerebral circulation, N. Engl. J. Med. **282**:1465-1471, 1970.

149. Shulman, K., and Ransohoff, J.: Sagittal sinus venous pressure in hydrocephalus, J. Neurosurg. **23**:169-173, 1965.

150. Sigsbee, B., and Rottenberg, D. A.: Sagittal sinus thrombosis as a complication of regional enteritis, Ann. Neurol. **3**:450-452, 1978.

151. Sigsbee, B., and Posner, J. B.: Nonmetastatic superior sagittal sinus thrombosis in patients with cancer, Neurology **29**:139-146, 1979.

152. Smith, J. L., Hoyt, W. F., and Newton, T. H.: Optic nerve sheath decompression for relief of chronic monocular choked disc, Am. J. Ophthalmol. **68**:633-639, 1969.

153. Sugarbaker, E. D., and Wiley, H. M.: Intracranial pressure studies incident to resection of the internal jugular veins, Cancer **4**:242-250, 1951.

154. Sullivan, H. G., Miller, J. D., Becker, D. P., and others: The physiological basis of intracranial pressure change with progressive epidural brain compression, an experimental evaluation in cats, J. Neurosurg. **47**:532-550, 1977.

155. Sullivan, R. L., Jr., and Reeves, A. G.: Normal cerebrospinal fluid protein, increased intracranial pressure, and the Guillain-Barré syndrome, Ann. Neurol. **1**:108-109, 1977.

156. Sundbarg, G., Kjallquist, A., Lundberg, N., and others: Complications due to prolonged ventricular fluid pressure recording in clinical practice. In Brock, M., and Dietz, H., editors: Intracranial pressure, experimental and clinical aspects, New York, 1972, Springer-Verlag, pp. 348-352.

157. Susac, J. O., Smith, J. L., and Walsh, F. B.: The impossible meningioma, Arch. Neurol. **34**:36-38, 1977.

158. Swanson, A. G., and Iseri, O. A.: Acute encephalopathy due to water intoxication, N. Engl. J. Med. **258**:831-834, 1958.

159. Symon, L., Dorsch, N. W. C., and Stephens, R. J.: Pressure waves in so-called low-pressure hydrocephalus, Lancet **4**:1291-1292, 1972.

160. Symonds, C. P.: Otitic hydrocephalus, Brain **54**:55-71, 1931.

161. Thompson, R. K., and Molina, S.: Dynamic axial brain-stem distortion as a mechanism explaining the cardiorespiratory changes in increased intracranial pressure, J. Neurosurg. **16**:664-675, 1959.

162. Tschirgi, R. D., Frost, R. W., and Taylor, J. L.: Inhibition of cerebrospinal fluid formation by a carbonic anhydrase inhibitor, 2-acetylamino-1,3, 4-thiadiazole-5-sulfonamide (Diamox), Proc. Soc. Exper. Biol. Med. **87**:373-376, 1954.

163. Van Uitert, R., and Eisenstadt, M. L.: Retinal venous pulsations in patients with increased intracranial pressure (letter to the editor), Arch. Neurol. **35**:550, 1978.

164. Vigouroux, A.: Écoulement de liquide céphalorachidien. Hydrocéphalie. Papillome des plexus choroides du IVe ventricule, Rev. Neurol. **16**:281-285, 1908.

165. Walsh, F. B., and Hoyt, W. F.: Clinical Neuro-ophthalmology, ed. 3, Baltimore, 1969, The Williams & Wilkins Co.

166. Walsh, T. J., Garden, J. W., and Gallagher, B.: Obliteration of retinal venous pulsations during elevation of cerebrospinal-fluid pressure, Am. J. Ophthalmol. **67**:954-956, 1969.

167. Weed, L. H., and McKibben, P. S.: Pressure changes in the cerebrospinal fluid following intravenous injection of solutions of various concentrations, Am. J. Physiol. **48**:512-530, 1919.

168. Weinstein, J. D., Langfitt, T. W., and Kassell, N. F.: Vasopressor response to increased intracranial pressure, Neurology **14**:1118-1131, 1964.

169. Weinstein, J. D., Toy, F. J., Jaffe, M. E., and others: The effects of dexamethasone on brain edema in patients with metastatic brain tumors, Neurology **23**:121-129, 1973.

170. Weiss, M. H., and Nulsen, F. E.: The effect of glucocorticoids on CSF flow in dogs, J. Neurosurg. **32**:452-458, 1970.

171. Willerson, J. T., Curry, G. C., Atkins, J. M., and others: Influence of hypertonic mannitol on ventricular performance and coronary blood flow in patients, Circulation **51**:1095-1100, 1975.

172. Wilkinson, H. A., Wepsic, J. G., and Austin, G.: Diuretic synergy in the treatment of acute experimental cerebral edema, J. Neurosurg. **34**:203-208, 1977.

173. Williamson-Noble, F. A.: Venous pulsation, Trans. Ophthalmol. Soc. U. K. **72**:317-326, 1952.

6

Central nervous system and spinal cord neuroradiologic diagnostic tools

JOSEPH P. LIN
IRVIN I. KRICHEFF

Since the discovery of x ray by Wilhelm Konrad von Röntgen in 1895[7], x ray has been used for the diagnosis of neurologic disorders. The first ventriculogram was performed by Dandy in 1918[8] by injecting air into the lateral ventricles. In 1919, Dandy[9] injected air into the spinal subarachnoid space through the lumbar region to study the spinal and cerebral subarachnoid spaces, procedures that became known as the air myelogram and the pneumoencephalogram. With these techniques, the intracranial and intraspinal cerebrospinal-fluid-containing spaces in living subjects could be visualized and investigated for the first time. In 1922, Sicard and Forestier[39] incidentally injected Lipiodol, a radiopaque iodinated substance, into the spinal subarachnoid space to obtain the first positive contrast myelogram. Moniz[44] in 1927 performed the first successful carotid angiogram by direct injection of 22% solution of sodium iodide after surgical exposure of the artery. Since then, the technique of cerebral angiography has been markedly improved and has become an important diagnostic procedure in neuroradiology. Houdart, Djindjian, and co-workers[24] and later Djindjian and co-workers[15,16] in early 1962 developed aortography and then superselec-tive techniques of spinal cord angiography in conjunction with subtraction techniques that enabled us to study the vascular supply to the spinal cord and its pathology in living human beings. Di Chiro and co-workers[11,12] developed the technique of selective spinal cord angiography in this country in 1964.

In 1973 Hounsfield[25] combined the technology of the computer and a well-collimated x-ray beam to produce a head scanner that could differentiate the attentuation coefficients of intracranial tissues of less than 2%. This new technical breakthrough enabled physicians for the first time to visualize the detailed anatomy of the intracranial structures in a living human being without introducing contrast material into the patient. This new diagnostic tool was called computed tomography (CT) of the head.

From the discovery of x ray to the introduction of computed tomography, one basic and most important requirement for obtaining a satisfactory and interpretable neuroradiologic study, whether it is a skull film, spine film, tomogram, ventriculogram, pneumoencephalogram, myelogram, cerebral angiogram, or computed tomogram of the head, is the immobilization of the patient to be examined. Any motion of the patient

119

during the examination not only interferes with the study but also increases the complication rate through repetition of the examination and subjects the patient to unnecessary radiation exposure. In pediatric cases and with apprehensive or uncooperative patients, general anesthesia is frequently employed for the purpose of obtaining an interpretable neuroradiologic study. General anesthesia is also used when the vasculature to be studied supplies areas, such as the face, that are rich in pain receptors. Anesthesiologists also play an important role in prevention and emergency management of patients who have anaphylactic reaction to the iodinated contrast material during a neuroradiologic examination. Occasionally, hyperventilation or apnea is required during a procedure for a special purpose such as to slow the cerebral circulation time[19], to relieve arterial spasm[17], to demonstrate the abnormal vascularity of a brain tumor[18,26,43], or to obtain perfect subtraction films in spinal cord angiogram[16], which can only be achieved by apnea under general anesthesia. Therefore, anesthesiologists should be familiar with neuroradiologic diagnostic tools, positions of patients in various neuroradiologic procedures, and anaphylactic reactions to iodinated contrast material in order to provide the best patient care and to obtain the best studies to help the neuroradiologist to reach the correct diagnosis.

In this chapter, no attempt is made to describe the radiologic features of different disease entities. Only the positions of the patients in various neuroradiologic procedures are described.

PNEUMOENCEPHALOGRAPHY

Since the introduction of computed tomography of the head in 1973, the number of pneumoencephalograms and ventriculograms performed in various institutions has markedly decreased. However, pneumoencephalography still plays an important role in detecting small suprasellar mass lesions and small mass lesions in the cerebellopontine angle cistern region.[40] In places where computed tomography of the head

is not available, complete pneumoencephalography may still be carried out. Therefore, anesthesiologists should be familiar with the positions of patients during this examination. The indications for pneumoencephalography are congenital intracranial anomalies, hydrocephalus, cerebral atrophy, low pressure hydrocephalus, acoustic neuromas, brain stem mass, sellar and suprasellar masses, intraventricular masses, parasagittal masses, and cerebral hemispheric masses. Masses causing obstructive hydrocephalus are usually studied by ventriculography.

Though the "routine" pneumoencephalogram does not actually exist as such, certain basic procedures generally apply. It should be kept in mind that numerous specialized techniques exist for studying specific areas, and these should be employed when specific problems are being studied. A few of the more common problems will be alluded to subsequently.

Following the securing of the patient in the pneumoencephalographic chair, which can perform 360-degree forward or backward somersault maneuvers, the examiner will perform a spinal tap at whatever lumbar level he or she considers to be the most convenient. Following the spinal tap, a minimum of CSF (less than 1 ml) should be obtained in the laboratory tube for the study of cells. It is necessary to do this at this time because the instillation of air rapidly causes pleocytosis. Excessive removal of fluid in the initial stages of the examination seems to increase the incidence of nonfilling of the ventricular system.

The patient's head is so positioned that the orbitomeatal baseline (a line connecting the midpoints of the orbit and external ear orifice) makes a 30-degree angle with the horizontal line, and 5 cc of air are slowly instilled. The relationship of the baseline to the floor is then altered by tilting the patient backward or tilting his or her head backward so that the baseline now makes a reverse 10-degree or greater angle with the floor. An additional 5 cc of air is instilled in this position and several seconds allowed for the air to rise into the basal subarachnoid space. Next the patient is returned to the original position, and the last 5 cc of air are slowly instilled. This procedure permits the air to demonstrate (1) the size of the lateral ventricles, (2) the basal subarachnoid space, (3) the fourth ventricle, aqueduct, and posterior third ventricle (all on the first study), and (4) the position of the cerebellar tonsils. At this time the technician obtains four films consisting of a lateral, a lateral tomogram, and two degrees of half-axial projections.

If the cerebellar tonsils appear normal in position, assessment of the size of the ventricular system is made, and an additional 15 cc of air is injected for normal-sized ventricles (more for larger ventricles) for the study of the anterior third ventricle and lateral ventricles. The patient is then placed in the brow-up position to equalize the air across the foramen of Monro, and the technician takes a hyperextended lateral view, a straight frontal view, and a half-axial film. The patient is next placed in the erect position, and the same three views are obtained. This is repeated in the brow-down position. A forward somersault is then accomplished to fill the temporal horns. The technician then obtains a minus 15 degrees (Caldwell), half-axial, and stereo lateral views demonstrating the temporal horns.

When the initial brow-up views demonstrate sufficient air in the ventricles, one can then remove the needle because the somersaulting chair permits repositioning of air at any time. The remainder of CSF removal for laboratory analysis may be done at any time beginning with the second instillation of air. Once the area of interest has been well demonstrated or sufficient air is in place in a general study, one should proceed promptly through the entire examination without stopping at each position. Films should be processed as soon as they are done and checked by the physician as they are developed. A very important rule to always keep in mind is that when a specific problem is being studied, one should go immediately to the evaluation of the specific area of interest and not proceed with the remainder of the study until that area is thoroughly evaluated.

The problem of ventricular filling

Should the ventricles not fill using the techniques initially described, one should assess where the air is going. If the air is located anterior to the brain stem, the problem is probably one of inadequate flexion and the patient should then be tilted so that the baseline makes a greater angle with the floor. A larger angle is not deleterious for this will direct the air into the cisterna magna; once this is filled it will overflow into the vallecula and hence into the fourth ventricle. Should one note that air is going only into the cisterna magna, then one is probably dealing with a large cisterna magna and the further instillation of air and complete filling of the cisterna magna will then allow air to overflow into the fourth ventricle. If the cisterna magna is completely full and some air has even escaped from it anteriorly but the ventricles remain unfilled, place the patient well forward, brow down, and slowly rotate the head as far as it will go to either side. If air is noted to be escaping from the cisterna magna into the superior cerebellar cistern or occipital cisterns, then one is dealing with the very difficult problem of an incompetent cisterna magna. Fortunately, this is rare for it leads to considerable difficulties in ventricular filling. The only solution here is to sit the patient completely erect so that the baseline is parallel to the floor and to very slowly instill relatively large quantities of air. The bulk of the air will go into the subarachnoid space, but generally 10 to 15 cc will enter the ventricle. To study the fourth ventricle in a situation such as this, one must obtain films as the air is being instilled or with a backward somersault. The lateral views of the first set of films should always be studied for the location of the cerebellar tonsils. If these are noted to be below the foramen magnum, the study is frequently aborted. The referring physician or attending neurosurgeon should be consulted immediately.

Specific diagnostic problems

Suprasellar mass. One should attempt initially to place air only in the ventricular system. Seven to 10 cc of air is injected with the patient in the 30-degree position. The air should be instilled very slowly. The technician obtains a half-axial, lateral, and lateral tomogram projections, and then the patient is immediately placed in the brow-up hanging head position where a lateral, lateral tomogram, and whatever frontal views can be obtained are exposed. Following the viewing of these films and visualization of the anterior recesses of the third ventricle, the patient is placed in the erect position and further air is instilled into the subarachnoid space. The brow-up sequence is now repeated. If this procedure is not followed, then the air in the chiasmatic cistern will obscure the anterior recesses of the third ventricle. However, tomographic cuts of the sella turcica and suprasellar region in frontal and lateral projections with a complex motion tomographic unit should be obtained at this time to better delineate the anterior third ventricle, the suprasellar cisterns, the pituitary fossa, and the stalk of the pituitary gland. Following these two procedures, sufficient air can then be placed into the ventricular system to permit adequate visualization of the anterior horns and temporal horns of the lateral ventricles.

Acoustic neuroma. Study of the acoustic neuroma requires excellent visualization of the fourth ventricle in the lateral projection and in several varying degrees of half-axial projections to enable the examiner to make use of parallax in analyzing air-filled structures. In addition, it is essential that the air be placed into the cerebellar pontine angle cisterns if this can possibly be done. Placing air in these cisterns is accomplished by having the patient's head in the extended position while instilling air and estimating the length of time—a few seconds—it will take the air to reach the interpeduncular cistern. At the examiner's estimate of this time, the patient is then placed in the 30- to 40-degree angle position so that this air will pass posteriorly into the cerebellopontine angle cisterns. If one cistern fails to fill, this procedure may be repeated with a slight tilting with the head to make that side superior. One should not proceed with the rest of the study until the angles are well studied. A negative study should be completed with tomography of the air-filled CP angles.

Small acoustic neuroma[40]. A small quantity (approximately 7 cc) of air is introduced via lumbar spinal tap with the patient lying prone and the patient's head in flexion with the canthomeatal line perpendicular to the table top of a tilting complex motion tomographic table. The table is tilted upward about 30 to 45 degrees. Then the head of the patient is rotated 15 to 20 degrees toward the side to be examined and resting on the table in order to elevate the corresponding cerebellopontine angle cistern slightly to let the air fill the intracanicular portion of the internal auditory canal and the cerebellopontine angle cistern. Tomographic cuts of the corresponding internal auditory canal and cerebellopontine cistern are taken. Small intracanicular acoustic neuroma or its extension in the cerebellopontine angle cistern can be well demonstrated.

Incisural block. Evaluation of patients for obstruction of the flow of CSF through the incisural notch cannot be accomplished on a casual basis. If this diagnosis is suspected, one must thoroughly flood the basal cisterns with a large amount of air (15 to 25 cc) and have the patient sitting in the erect position moving his or her head actively or passively for at least 15 to 20 minutes before films are obtained. Films should also be obtained following this maneuver in the brow-up and brow-down positions.

Inadequate instillation of air. When one is incapable of placing enough air in the ventricles, additional views and additional positions must be obtained, for one of the basic rules is that all portions of the ventricular system must be obtained. The anterior portion of the third ventricle can be filled by using the hanging head position and central portions of the ventricle can be filled by slight forward and backward tilts of the patient.

The examiner should not accept rotated or poorly exposed films from the technician, for he or she will be considered responsible for the technique. The most difficult views to obtain straight fashion are the brow-down. Procedures usually are more rapidly completed when the examining physician assists the technician through every stage of the procedure in the positioning of the patient and the transferring of cassettes. The physician should see to it that the first films obtained are rapidly processed and shown to the technician so that he or she can make any adjustment of exposure factors that may be required.

Films are numbered together in groupings. All views taken with the same amount of air and the head in the same position have the same number. Any change of either the amount of air or the head position should change the number.

Complications

Headache, nausea, and vomiting are the common complications experienced by patients during pneumoencephalography. Headaches can usually be relieved by bed rest and analgesics. Nausea and vomiting may be treated with trimethobenzamide (Tigan), 200 mg IM. If nausea and vomiting are due to postural hypotension, maintenance of a normal blood pressure and Trendelenburg's position will usually help. One must always be aware of the possibility of cerebellar tonsil herniation during pneumoencephalography. The scout films must be carefully viewed to ascertain the normal positions of the cerebellar tonsils before instillation of more air into the lumbar subarachnoid space. If the cerebellar tonsils are low, the procedure must be discontinued and the neurosurgeon must be notified immediately for the possibility of decompression to relieve the increased intracranial pressure. Very rarely, subarachnoid hemorrhage may occur during pneumoencephalogram. Local infection at the site of needle puncture and aseptic or bacterial meningitis have been reported.

VENTRICULOGRAPHY

Ventriculography is usually performed in those instances in which there is clinical evidence of a posterior fossa or posterior third ventricle mass obstructing the ventricular system. In the presence of enlarged ventricles and elevated pressure, it is frequently

dangerous and difficult to fill the ventricular system by the instillation of air from below. The burr holes and insertion of a soft ventricular needle (Scott needle) are accomplished by members of the neurosurgical service. Air (25 cc) is instilled into the ventricles with the patient secured in the pneumoencephalographic chair.

Following the instillation of air, the patient is placed in the brow-up position. Films are obtained in the lateral, straight frontal, and angled frontal view (Towne). The patient is then tilted backward into the "hanging head" position and a single lateral film centered over the anterior third ventricle is obtained. Next, a backward somersault is performed with the patient ending up in the brow-down position. The patient should now be in a position where the fastigium of the fourth ventricle is the highest point of the posterior fossa ventricular system. During the somersault, the physician assisting the technician should take the responsibility of seeing to it that the patient's head is maintained in a straight, nonrotated position and that it is guided through the somersault to avoid excess movement. When the somersault is completed and the patient is in a brow-down position, four films are obtained. There should be no delay between the sets of films taken in the brow-up and brow-down positions. It is not necessary to wait to observe the initial films for, in most cases, this merely delays the procedure. Should a block of the ventricular system and/or displacement of the fourth ventricle and aqueduct be well demonstrated, the examination is completed. Should the air pass through the fourth ventricle into the sacral subarachnoid space during the somersault, one can sit the patient up in such fashion that the baseline makes a 30-degree angle with the floor and air may now enter the fourth ventricle from below. If it is desired that the now subarachnoid air enter the anterior cisterns (cisterna pontis and interpeduncularis), the patient should be seated erect in the hyperextended, slightly backward tilted, position.

If the initial backward somersault followed by the sitting up "30 degree head position" does not fill the fourth ventricle (a fact that can be checked by using Polaroid or image intensification), the patient may be somersaulted again in an effort to orient the fastigium as the highest point at the end of the study. Should the ventricular catheter actually be in the third ventricle, the patient may be placed in the brow-down position and additional air instilled directly into the third ventricle. As the third ventricle fills, air will then move into the aqueduct and the fourth ventricle.

Another way of getting air from the lateral ventricles into the posterior third and fourth ventricles when no block exists is similar to the method just described and avoids somersaulting. After 20 to 30 cc of air is placed in the lateral ventricles and brow-up films are obtained, the patient is turned forward slowly into a downward hanging head position. The air will then pass through the foramen of Monro into the posterior third ventricle, aqueduct, and fourth ventricle. This is probably a better system for filling the posterior third and fourth ventricles and the aqueduct than the backward somersault in those instances in which no obstruction is present. This method may be tried if somersaulting fails.

Positive contrast material ventriculogram

Occasionally, water-soluble or oily iodinated contrast material is used instead of air for ventriculograms. In these instances, the patient can be studied on a stretcher, radiographic table, or pneumoencephalographic chair. However, if a true lateral tomogram is desired, the patient should be studied in the pneumoencephalographic chair. Three milliliters of the contrast material is introduced via the soft ventricular needle with the patient in the upright position, and the patient's head is flexed in order to collect the contrast material in the frontal horn of the lateral ventricle of the injected side. Then, by gradual tilting the head to the noninjected side and backward, the contrast material will flow along the medial portion of the frontal horn into the foramen of Monro to enter the third ventricle. This can be done under fluoroscopic control. After the third ventricle is filled, slowly hyperextend the patient's head and put the patient in the brow-up and semiupright position to let the contrast material flow toward the aqueduct and fourth ventricle. At this time, films are obtained for evaluation.

PANTOPAQUE MYELOGRAPHY[10,20,27,38]

The indications for Pantopaque myelography are congenital spinal anomalies, spinal cord and vertebral tumors, vascular lesions of the spinal cord, degenerative disc diseases, spinal trauma, and inflammatory lesions.

Surgical aspects

All the attendants in the myelographic room should wear surgical masks and lead aprons at all times. Before beginning the procedure it is the physician's responsibility to inquire about allergies to local anesthetics and iodinated compounds.

The proper needle placement into the lumbar subarachnoid space is more critical in myelography than in any other examination performed by spinal tap. This is so because the needle must be well positioned to stay in place during the examination and permit the removal of contrast material when the examination is completed if one uses a nonabsorbable material such as Pantopaque. No spinal tap should be performed without viewing of frontal and lateral films of the lumbosacral area by the individual performing the tap. This is necessary to permit evaluation of anomalies or degenerative changes that may make the tap difficult.

The spinal tap for lumbar myelography is most accurately performed under fluoroscopic control with the patient in the prone position at the L3-L4 interspace, unless the clinical history indicates pathology at that level, in which case the tap shall be performed at the L2-L3 level. For thoracic or cervical myelography the spinal tap should be accomplished at the most easily palpated level, this being either L4-L5 or L5-S1. A few milliliters of CSF should be collected for laboratory examination.

Following the instillation of contrast material (Pantopaque) (lumbar, 24 ml; thoracic, 36 ml; cervical, 24 ml), the stylus should be replaced and the hub of the needle covered with a sterile gauze pad. If a complete block is suspected on the basis of clinical information, only 3 ml should be instilled, for this is all that is necessary.

The patient is then placed prone on the table with head extended, and necessary securing devices are applied.

Removal of contrast material

After the adequacy of the films has been ascertained, the contrast material may be removed under fluroscopic control. The table may be tilted up or down to center the bulk of the contrast material below the tip of the needle except in those cases where the needle is in the lowest point of the lumbar lordotic curve.

It should be clearly understood that sterile surgical techniques should be maintained throughout the procedure. Any break in technique by the examining physician should require a change of gloves and, if necessary, a change of tray.

RADIOGRAPHIC AND FLUOROSCOPIC EXAMINATIONS
Lumbar myelogram

Lumbar myelogram fluoroscopic spot films should be obtained that demonstrate the contrast material filling the lumbar sac in the AP projection. Films should be obtained with the contrast material *centered* over the L5-S1 interspace and again *centered* over the L4-L5 interspace in the AP projection with the x-ray table and the patient in upright or semiupright position. Oblique films to the right and to the left should be obtained with the contrast material *centered* at the L5-S1 intervertebral disc space level and additional films with the contrast material *centered* at the L4-L5 intervertebral disc space level. It is important that the patient be truly oblique at approximately 45 degrees. The x-ray table is then lowered and frontal films with the contrast material covering the levels from L3-L4 up to about T8 or T10, depending on the curvature of the patient's back, will complete the examination. Should any abnormalities

be seen at these higher levels, appropriate spot films should be obtained. Simultaneous translateral films should be taken using the lateral spot film unit at the pathologic levels if a biplane fluoroscopic unit is available.

In rare instances decubitus translateral films may be of value in assessing the axillae and nerve roots. This may be necessary in patients with exceptionally wide lumbar subarachnoid space. Both decubitis films should be obtained for comparison.

Thoracic myelogram

A few lead markers should be placed along the paraspinal area to orient the level of the spot films. Large spot films of the entire thoracic area in frontal and cross table translateral projections should be obtained with the contrast material filling the subarachnoid space. It should be noted that films are only adequate if the contrast material truly distends the sac. Unfortunately, this is usually adequate only in the upper and lower thoracic areas with the midthoracic contrast material streaming through centrally due to the kyphotic thoracic curve. Therefore, in most cases, it is necessary that both right and left decubitus films be obtained. The patient should be placed in the decubitus position with the contrast material in the lumbar area and then be tilted slightly, head down, so that the material flows along the lowermost gutter into the thoracic area. During this procedure, the patient's head should be propped upward and supported on a pillow to prevent any possible contrast material from entering the skull. Usually the entire thoracic spine can be covered on one film. A vertical 14-by-14 and horizontal beam 14-by-14 film should then be obtained using the overhead tube. The contrast material is then run down into the lumbar area and the procedure repeated in the opposite decubitus position. It is generally unsatisfactory to merely turn the patient on the opposite side without fluoroscopic positioning of contrast material due to curvatures of the back. Occasionally, one can fill the entire thoracic subarachnoid space by introducing large amounts of contrast material in upright position.

Should any suspicious dorsal findings be

seen, or in instances where an arteriovenous malformation of the thoracic area is suspected, the needle should be removed from the back and the patient placed supine for fluoroscopic spot films of the dorsal surface of the thoracic subarachnoid space.

When a lesion is demonstrated in the thoracic area, it is necessary to mark this level for surgical localization. Locate the level of the lesion accurately fluoroscopically by placing the edge of the lead glove at the level or with the extended finger. Turn on the light, making sure the glove or finger does not move. Inject a drop of sky blue dye subperiosteally in the spinous process at the level of the block. Place a lead marker over the block level and take a 14-by-17 or a 7-by-17 film of the area for documentation.

Cervical myelogram

The patient's head should be hyperextended prior to downward tilting and the technician should be requested to see that the head position is maintained. All fixative devices should be checked before tilting the patient downward. It is also helpful to explain to the patient the definitions of flexion and extension and try to remember to use terms such as "bring your head up" or "move your head down." All patients should also be instructed to bring their heads down slowly and to bring their heads up rapidly. After the head is positioned, the patient is tilted downward enough for the contrast material to negotiate the kyphotic curve and run into the cervical area. Do not hesitate to tilt the patient way down, for it is more comfortable to do this somewhat promptly than to tilt very slowly so that the patient is in a head-down position for a prolonged period of time. Furthermore, prompt tilting allows flow of the entire bolus of contrast material into the cervical area without its breaking up into small bubbly masses. Once the contrast material has reached the cervical region the patient should be placed in the horizontal position and the head should be brought down until the mandible is superimposed on the lowermost point of the occiput. This will permit viewing of the greatest amount of the

cervical spine. Spot films in frontal and cross table translateral projections are then obtained to cover the cervical area from C2 to approximately T3 with swimmer's view. (Swimmer's view is a lateral view of the lower cervical and upper thoracic region with one arm of the patient at his or her side and one arm over the head to separate the shoulder shadows for the x-ray beam to penetrate.) The area can be well covered with no more than approximately 10- to 20-degree tilting in either direction. The fluoroscopic examiner must carefully assess the cord shadow for pulsations and comment on increased, absent, or decreased pulsation. These findings should be recorded in the fluoroscopist's preliminary report notes and included in the final report. Should nerve root sleeves seem to be unfilled, contrast material should be "juggled" up and down slightly to attempt to fill nerve root sleeves. Should an extradural block be encountered in the cervical area in patients with cervical spondylosis, one should first have the patient flex his or her head into neutral position and tilt the table slightly down. Next, obliqueing of the neck from side to side may permit the contrast material to move past along the lateral gutters. Should these maneuvers fail to clear the block, the patient is placed erect and the entire downward tilting maneuver repeated.

Cervical examinations to include the foramen magnum are probably the most difficult myelographic examinations to perform properly. To perform this examination properly and prevent the spillage of the contrast material into the middle fossa of the skull, it is necessary to align the clivus in such a manner as to make a continuous curve with the cervical spine under the control of a lateral fluoroscopic unit or bilateral filming. Polaroid films are helpful in speeding up this procedure when lateral fluoroscopy is not available. Both oblique views at the level of the foramen magnum should be taken while tilting the patient's head downward slowly and when the contrast material is flowing through the foramen magnum. After the spot film is taken, tilt the table up immediately to allow the contrast material to return to the midcervical region. The same maneuver is repeated for the other oblique view.

COMPLETE BLOCK

Should a complete block with a neurologic level be suspected clinically prior to examination, 3 ml of contrast material will usually suffice for the examination. After insertion of the material, the patient should be tilted with the head down until the block is encountered and then brought back as far to the horizontal as is possible while keeping the contrast material against the block. Frontal and lateral films taken with the patient still prone at the level of the block are sufficient. If the block is in the thoracic area, it should be marked as described in the section for thoracic myelography.

Sometimes neurosurgeons wish to see the upper extent of the lesion that causes the complete block. Then lateral cervical puncture at C1-C2 level[34] or cisternal puncture should be carried out to introduce the contrast medium from the high cervical region. Three milliliters of contrast material also should be adequate for this. The patient may be in the prone or supine position for lateral C1-C2 puncture but for cisternal puncture, the patient is in either prone or in the lateral decubitus position with the head flexed to open the occipitocervical junction for the puncture.

If the patient is under general anesthesia, close cooperation between the anesthesiologist and the fluoroscopist is important. Each time the x-ray table is tilted up or down or the patient's head is turned to either side, the anesthesiologist must be informed *before* the action is taken.

Complications. Local infections at the site of needle puncture, aseptic or bacterial meningitis, venous intravasation of Pantopaque, headache, adhesive arachnoiditis, and allergic reaction to the iodinated contrast material are the complications encountered in Pantopaque myelography.[27]

Water-soluble positive contrast material myelography. Water-soluble iodinated contrast materials and gas or air are the only contrast materials used for myelograms in Scan-dinavian and non-English-speaking European countries. However, in the early days, the water-soluble contrast material, Abrodil or methiodal sodium, could only be used for lumbar myelogram in conjunction with spinal anesthesia because of its severe local irritable properties and neurotoxicity.[3,38,41] In recent years (1960s and 1970s) Conray[1] and Dimer X (Dimeray)[2] have replaced methiodal sodium for lumbar myelography. No spinal anesthesia is needed, but special precaution must be taken to confine the contrast material below the level of conus medullaris to avoid the local irritation to the spinal cord.[1,2,41,42] Most recently (1972), Metrizamide or Amipaque, a water-soluble, nonionic iodinated contrast material, has been used in Europe.[41] Metrizamide can be used for complete myelography, posterior fossa studies, ventriculogram, and cisternogram with relatively few complications such as headache, nausea, vomiting, and hypotension.[3,41,42] It outlines the spinal cord and nerve roots very clearly, and withdrawal of the contrast material becomes unnecessary. However, the procedure must be completed within a relatively shorter period before the contrast material is diluted by the cerebrospinal fluid and absorbed into the bloodstream.

The technique for metrizamide myelography is similar to the Pantopaque technique except that the quality of cervical myelogram will be better if metrizamide is introduced via a C1-C2 puncture.

Complications of metrizamide (Amipaque) myelography. Adhesive arachnoiditis is less frequently noticed[41] in metrizamide myelography than in Pantopaque myelography or Dimer-X myelography.[3] Headache usually occurs three to six hours after the introduction of metrizamide into the spinal subarachnoid space.[3] Very rarely, seizures may develop following a metrizamide myelogram.[3] Metrizamide myelography should not be carried out in patients under the medication of Phenothiazine. The synergistic interaction between these two substances may precipitate epileptic seizure attacks. Nausea, vomiting, and hypotension may also occur after metrizamide myelography. Again the allergic reactions to the iodinated contrast material, local infection, and aseptic or bacterial meningitis may happen.

Metrizamide has been clinically investigated in several institutions in the United States since 1975. These data have been submitted to the Food and Drug Administration for evaluation. Hopefully, metrizamide will be commercially available for clinical use in the near future.

Posterior fossa Pantopaque study for small acoustic neuroma.[5,6,31] A small quantity (1 to 3 ml) of Pantopaque is instilled via lumbar puncture and under fluoroscopic control. Pantopaque is directed to the cervical region by tilting the x-ray table head down with the patient's chin hyperextended. Then the table is tilted back to the horizontal position to keep the Pantopaque in the midcervical region. Position the patient's head in either 45-degree obliquity or completely lateral decubitus with the side to be studied lying on the table. The x-ray table is slowly tilted head down. The Pantopaque column will flow toward the intracranial cavity and fill the internal auditory canal of the side on the x-ray table. Translateral films in transorbital, basal, or Stenver's views with the patient remaining in this position are taken and reviewed. If the other side is to be studied as well, the table should be tilted head up to let the Pantopaque flow back down to the cervical region. Then the same maneuver is carried out with the side of the patient's head to be studied lying on the table. While some investigators have suggested using larger quantities of Pantopaque, it is our belief that since the advent of CT this is no longer necessary.

Gas myelography

Gas myelography is used extensively in Scandinavian and other non-English-speaking countries. However, it is not as popular in this country because of significant patient discomfort, poor delineation of nerve root shadows, requirement of a sophisticated tomographic unit, and hesitance to perform cisternal or C1-C2 puncture.[21] Gas myelography is superior to the Pantopaque myelography in outlining the spinal cord shadow. In patients with a history of allergy to the iodinated contrast material, gas myelography is the method of choice.

There are two gas myelography techniques: single needle or double needle. Single needle technique requires instilling the gas through either lumbar spinal tap[35,36] or high cervical (C1-C2) tap.[21] Only one needle is used, and the cerebrospinal fluid is exchanged with approximately the same amount of gas (oxygen or air)[21] or the cerebrospinal fluid is completely removed before the instillation of a large quantity of air.[35,36] The intraspinal pressure should not exceed 300 mm H_2O[21] to 500 mm H_2O.[36] With the two needle technique one instills the gas through the lumbar needle and drains the cerebrospinal fluid from the cervical needle to achieve a better filling of the entire spinal subarachnoid space with gas. The patient is placed in a lateral decubitus position with the head flexed and rests on a sponge to prevent the escape of gas into the intracranial cavity. The x-ray table should be tilted head down about 15 degrees. The patient should be positioned with the help of sponges to make the spinal canal parallel to the table top of the x-ray table in order to allow a long segment of the spine in focus for tomographic cuts. The tomographic cuts are taken at 2 mm intervals through the entire spinal canal. Occasionally frontal tomographic cuts may be obtained. After the films are viewed and considered to be satisfactory, the needle(s) is removed and the patient is transferred to the stretcher in the prone position for a few hours to prevent gas or air from entering the ventricles and anterior intracranial subarachnoid spaces. It is our belief that consistently successful cervical gas myelography is best accomplished by C1-C2 puncture, for the single needle lumbar technique frequently fails to adequately fill the cervical theca.

Spinal cord angiography

Spinal cord angiography is used in investigating vascular lesions of the spinal cord such as arteriovenous malformations and hemangioblastomas, in demonstrating the artery of the lumbar enlargement (artery of Adam-kiewicz), in spinal trauma or scoliosis before the surgery, and in investigating ischemia of the spinal cord and vertebrospinal tumors.[16]

The success of a spinal cord angiogram depends heavily on obtaining good subtraction films. It is essential to eliminate the overlying shadows of the vertebrae and other spinal bony structures in order to be able to visualize the small intraspinal vessels. Therefore, during the filming, the patient must be kept apneic for a few seconds to allow perfect filming without any motion of the patient. The first film of the serial angiogram is taken before the injection of contrast material and is used as the base film. By reversing the image of this film and then superimposing it on the subsequent films of the serial spinal cord angiogram, the overlying spinal bony structures will be subtracted or eliminated from the films.[23,33] The small intraspinal vessels then will be clearly visualized. Therefore, spinal cord angiography is frequently carried out under general anesthesia to control the respiratory movement of the patient during the angiogram. Furthermore, intercostal injections of contrast material are quite painful and the physician must consider the patient's reaction to the pain, general condition, and how extensive an examination is to be done when deciding on the form of anesthesia or analgesics to be used. Local and general adverse reaction such as paroxysmal tetaniclike contractions of the abdomen and lower extremities after inadvertent injection of a large quantity of contrast material into the intercostal artery supplying the Adamkiewicz artery can be controlled by an in situ injection of 5 mg of diazepam (Valium) through the angiographic catheter.

Equipment. A fluoroscopic unit with spot film device, biplane serial film changers, angiographic catheters, and iodinated angiographic water-soluble contrast material (we use 60% meglumine iothalamate) is needed.

Technique. The patient is placed in supine position on the x-ray table. The angiographic catheter is introduced via femoral artery puncture into the aorta. Selective catheter-izations of ileolumbar, lateral sacral, intercostal, and vertebral arteries are carried out according to the underlying pathology and the suspected regions under fluoroscopic control. Two to three spot films of each vessel are taken (one film without contrast material, one in arterial phase, and one in later phase) utilizing the spot film device. Subtraction films of the arterial phases of each vessel are immediately obtained for viewing to determine which vessel if any should be studied by serial angiogram. During spot filming and serial angiogram, the anesthetist will be asked to stop the patient's respiratory movement for a short period for the reasons mentioned above. Spinal cord angiography is a long and tiring procedure. If all vessels cannot be catheterized at one time and an excessive quantity of contrast material is used, the procedure can be completed on another day.

Cerebral angiography

In recent years, selective catheterization of the individual carotid or vertebral artery via femoral or, rarely, axillary artery puncture has gradually replaced the direct percutaneous puncture of carotid, vertebral, subclavian, or brachial arteries.[29] The femoral catheter approach permits one to catheterize selectively the vertebral artery, the internal carotid artery, and individual branches of the external carotid artery and to inject several vessels at one setting with only one arterial puncture. The patient is also more comfortable and more easily positioned for filming without dislodging the catheter from the selected vessel. However, direct percutaneous puncture of the extracranial portions of cerebral vessels plays an important role in elderly patients and in cases when the catheter cerebral angiography fails.

Equipment for cerebral angiography includes serial film changers (single or biplane), x-ray tubes, generators, image intensifier with television monitor (for catheter work), floating angiographic table top for catheterization to position various anatomic areas over the film changer or image intensifier, automatic injector for injecting contrast medium during the serial angiogram, angiographic needles, angiographic catheters, (the catheters should be soft and small to lessen the complication rate), guide wires for introducing and threading the catheter, and water-soluble iodinated contrast medium (60% Conray, Renografin 60, Hypaque meglumine 60%).

Cerebral angiography is used to investigate cerebral vascular lesions, that is, aneurysm, arteriovenous malformation, artherosclerotic cerebral vascular disease, brain tumor, head trauma, congenital cerebral anomalies, and cerebral infection. Since the introduction of computed tomography of the head in 1972,[25] the use of cerebral angiography has decreased somewhat, but it is still an essential diagnostic tool for investigating intracranial aneurysms, cerebral arteriovenous malformations, cerebral vascular occlusive diseases and, to a lesser extent, intracranial space-occupying lesions.

Standard radiographic projections. For lateral views of the head in cerebral angiography the central ray of the x-ray tube is perpendicular to the sagittal plane of the skull with the patient's head in straight position. For the anteroposterior view of the head in carotid angiography, the central ray of the x-ray tube is angled 25 degrees caudad to the infraorbitomeatal line. For the anteroposterior view of the head in retrograde brachial or vertebral angiography, the central ray of the x-ray tube is 35 degrees caudad to the infraorbitomeatal line.[29]

Techniques. The patient is placed supine on the angiographic table. The area to be punctured is cleansed with antiseptic solution. For direct percutaneous carotid artery puncture, the patient's head is hyperextended with the aid of an inflatable rubber bag under the patient's shoulders. The degree of the hyperextension can be controlled by the quantity of air within the rubber bag. The skin at the site of puncture and the subcutaneous tissue behind and just on either side of the carotid artery are anesthetized with 1% xylocaine or procaine. This placement of anesthetic tends to elevate and immobilize the artery, and the artery is punctured. After the needle is threaded in

the carotid artery, the rubber bag is deflated. The patient's head is positioned according to the standard projections just described. The head of the patient should be flexed with his or her chin as close to the chest as possible for a good anteroposterior view. If the patient is under general anesthesia, there may be some difficulty in bringing the patient's chin down against the chest because of the presence of an endotracheal tube. In cases of intracranial aneurysms and head trauma, oblique and occasionally basal views may be obtained for additional information.[28]

Retrograde brachial angiogram is the safest procedure among all the cerebral angiograms.[28] However, it is not a selective angiogram. Right retrograde brachial angiogram fills the right subclavian, right vertebral, innominate, and right common carotid arteries. Although the left retrograde brachial angiogram only fills the left vertebral artery and the left subclavian artery, the filling of the posterior circulation is not adequate for detailed evaluation. It is, however, quite adequate for the investigation of cerebral vascular occlusive disease. The brachial artery is punctured in the midportion of the upper arm with a 16-gauge brachial needle. A Polaroid film is taken to ascertain the position of the needle.

Catheter cerebral angiography. The success of catheter cerebral angiography depends on the skill of the angiographers in placing the catheter in the selected vessel. The angiographers should be familiar with various curvatures of the catheter tip in order to catheterize individual cerebral arteries in different age groups. The catheter is introduced through a femoral artery puncture (rarely the axillary artery is used) using the Seldinger technique,[37] and with the aid of a guide wire is threaded into the ascending aortic arch under fluoroscopic control. Then the guide wire is withdrawn and the catheter is cleansed and flushed with heparinized normal saline. The desired vessel is identified by placing the catheter in the orifice of the vessel and injecting 1 to 2 ml of contrast medium. Some catheters can now be threaded up the vessel themselves; others require a guide wire. The guide wire is reintroduced through the catheter into the selected vessel. The catheter is threaded along the guide wire into the vessel up to the desired level. Serial angiography will then be carried out. Frequent flushing of the needle or catheter every one or two minutes with normal saline or heparinized normal saline must be strictly enforced to prevent the formation of blood clot within the lumen of the needle or catheter. The advantage of catheter cerebral angiography is the ability to study several vessels at one session and the patient is subjected to less discomfort as compared with other direct percutaneous puncture cerebral angiographies.

Occasionally, hyperventilation of the patient during the serial cerebral angiography has been employed to demonstrate the abnormal vascularity of the brain tumor or cerebral arteriovenous malformations,[18,26,43] to improve the quality of the cerebral angiogram,[19] or to relieve experimentally the vascular spasm in patients with ruptured intracranial aneurysm[17] by altering the arterial carbon dioxide tension. This can only be achieved by intermittent positive pressure ventilation under general anesthesia.

Complications. Local infection or hematoma formation at the site of needle puncture, arterial occlusion distal to the site of

needle puncture, septicemia, cerebral embolism, anaphylatic reactions to the iodinated contrast material and, rarely, seizures or death are the complications of cerebral angiography.

Computed tomography (CT) of the head

Since 1972, computed tomography of the head has been extremely useful in the diagnosis of neurologic diseases.[4,25,30] Recently, computed tomography of the body has been used to investigate paraspinal and intraspinal pathologies.[13,14,22,32] The innocuous nature of the technique and its ability to detect differences of the radiation absorption of various intracranial tissues with an order of sensitivity of about 100 times that of conventional x rays make CT an ideal tool to study intracranial disorders.

Computed tomography utilizes a well-collimated narrow x-ray beam that projects x rays through the object of interest from many angles of incidence. The x-ray beam passes through the part of the body to be examined in an axial plane, and the transmitted photons are detected by highly sensitive solid or gas detectors that are analogous to a fluoroscopic screen or radionuclide gamma camera in that they emit a light signal or ions proportional to the amount of x rays impinging upon them. These readings are

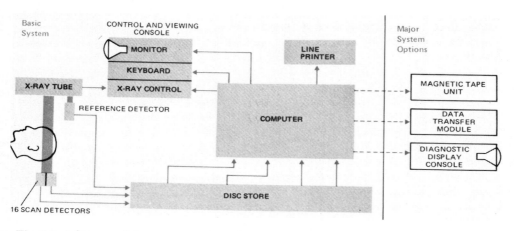

Fig. 6-1. A diagram of the operating principles of EMI Scanner CT 1010. (Courtesy EMI Medical, Inc.)

continuously fed to the system's computers, which rapidly calculate the absorption values of the material within each slice relative to its location, the location of the x-ray source and detectors and the radiation output (Fig. 6-1). These data are then used to build a picture that may be displayed on a TV monitor or a hard copy.[25] This image is actually made up of many small blocks or pixels, which represent the average absorption value of the tissues in the slice under examination in that block. The absorption coefficients of various tissues are converted to a number of ± 500 in the EMI CT head scanners and ± 1000 in most other scanners with water as zero reference. Using the ± 500 scale, CSF = 0 to +4, normal brain +18 to +28, extravasated blood +20 to +45, calcium +30 to +90, and fat −50.

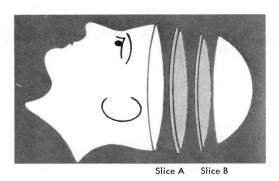

Slice A   Slice B

Fig. 6-2. A drawing of cross-section slices of the head during a single scan in EMI Scanner 1010. (Courtesy EMI Medical, Inc.)

The patient lies on an adjustable table or couch with his or her head in the round opening of the gantry. In the original Mark I EMI scanner, the head was in a latex cap surrounded by a plastic box containing water. The orbitomeatal line (a line drawn from the external auditory canal to the lower rim of the orbit) is used as a baseline to obtain a correct angulation. The head of the patient is flexed or the gantry is tilted to obtain an angulation of 25 degrees between the orbitomeatal line and the x-ray beam in most brain examinations (Figs. 6-2 to 6-4). Zero degree angulation is used for studies of orbits and sellar and suprasellar regions. Intravenous administration of water-soluble iodinated contrast material has been proven to be very helpful in enhancing intracranial vascular lesions, neoplasms, infarct, and abscesses[30] (Figs. 6-5 to 6-7). The enhancement test is carried out after rapid bolus (three to five minutes) or intravenous drip infusion (four to eight minutes) of water-soluble iodinated contrast material to deliver 28 to 44 g of iodine. Typically, 200 to 300 ml of 30% solution, or half the amount of 60% solution, is used. Some institutions deliver 28 g rapidly and infuse an additional 16 g slowly during the examination to maintain a constant blood iodine level. Ordinarily, only eight to ten slices are obtained. However, if both noncontrast and contrast studies are desired, the time of examination is doubled. Therefore, uncooperative patients and children under 8 to 10 years of age should be given heavy sedation or be under

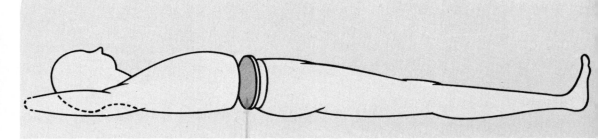

Fig. 6-3. A drawing of a single slice of the cross-section of the body during a single scan in EMI Scanner 5005. (Courtesy EMI Medical, Inc.)

general anesthesia to prevent any motion during the examination.

RADIATION HAZARDS

The anesthesiologist generally remains in the radiographic room throughout fluoroscopy and frequently during angiographic filming. Thus, radiation protection must be considered. The wearing of a lead apron is mandatory, for it results in a factor of 30 in radiation attenuation for the wearer. Just as important as the wearing of an apron is the distance from the radiation source. Radiation dose is related inversely to the square of the distance from the source. Thus, an individual standing immediately adjacent to a table during fluoroscopy would typically receive 30 mR per hour at eye level and 100 mR per hour at table top level, measured without a lead apron attenuation. Were this individual to move 2 feet from the side of the table, the eye dose would be reduced to 5 mR per hour and table top dose would be reduced to 15 mR per hour. At 6 feet from the table side, the dose would be less than 1 mR per hour. These measured doses are also decreased when measured at the

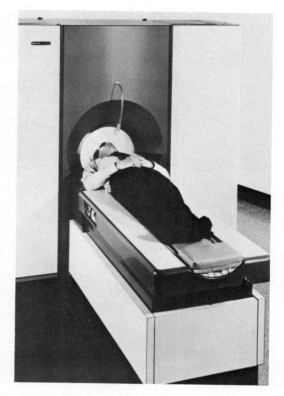

Fig. 6-4. Patient lying on the table of a EMI Scanner 5005. (Courtesy EMI Medical, Inc.)

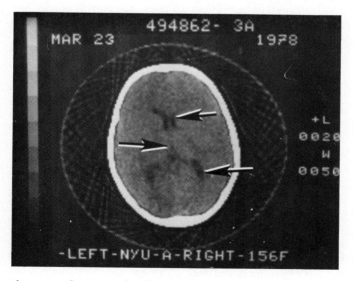

Fig. 6-5. Normal computed tomography of a transaxial section of the brain at the level showing frontal horns *(upper right arrow)* and occipital horns *(lower right arrow)* of the lateral ventricle and the third ventricle *(left arrow)*.

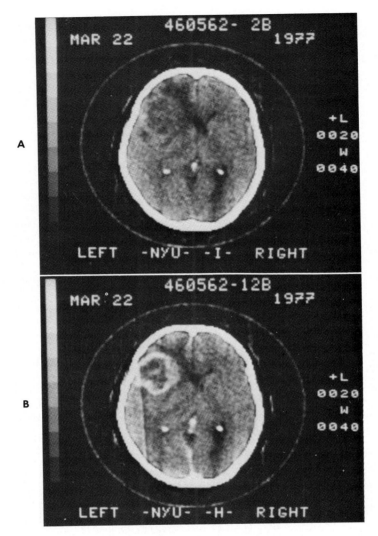

Fig. 6-6. Computed tomography of a glioma. **A,** Noncontrast CT shows frontal horn on the side of mass lesion to be compressed and shifted to the opposite side. An ill-defined area of low attenuation coefficient is seen in the frontal region (**B**). Contrast enhancement CT shows the peripheral zone of the tumor is markedly enhanced. Central lucency represents either central necrosis of the tumor or nonenhanced portion of a solid tumor.

head and/or foot of the table with the patient in place, for there is considerable attenuation of scattered radiation by the body of the patient. When one takes into account distance from fluoroscopy unit to the head of the table, the attenuation by the patient and the reduction factor by the apron, one calculates exceedingly low exposure levels.

Angiographic filming usually requires a minimum of 24 radiographic exposures. The radiation dose level for such a series of exposures is roughly equivalent to one hour of fluoroscopy at 2 mA. It should be kept in mind that the radiation dose levels indicated above may vary by ± 50% depending upon the equipment used and the size of the patient in the field. The radiation dose for computed tomography of the head is about

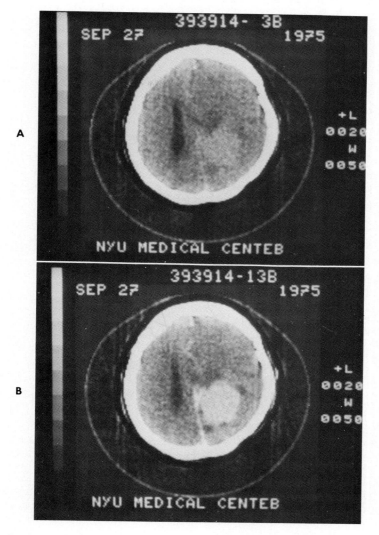

Fig. 6-7. Computed tomography of a falx meningioma (**A**). Noncontrast CT shows an area of slightly increased attenuation coefficient located in the right occipitoparietal region near the midline. Right lateral ventricle is obliterated, and there is lateral displacement of left lateral ventricle. **B,** Contrast enhancement CT shows this falx meningioma to be markedly enhanced.

2 to 10 rads for a complete study of the head. Because of the well-calibrated x-ray tubes used in CT, the radiation dose to the anesthesiologist wearing protective lead apron should be negligible. In summary, while radiation exposure should always be kept to a minimum, the anesthesiologist taking proper precautions of wearing an apron and standing 2 or more feet away from the table

top should not approach permissible dose levels.

CONCLUSION

Anesthesiologists are indispensible in assisting neuroradiologists to obtain a satisfactory and interpretable study on uncooperative patients and on patients under the age of about 12. Repeating the procedures not only increases the complication rates and the radiation to the patients but also prolongs the hospital stay, which in turn will increase the financial burden on the patients and will make hospital beds unavailable for other patients. Anesthesiologists also play an important role in prevention and treatment of untoward reactions to the iodinated contrast material or manipulations carried out during the neuroradiologic examination. Only close cooperation between the anesthesiologists and the neuroradiologists ensures the delivery of the best care possible to the patient.

REFERENCES

1. Ahlegren, P.: Lumbale Myelographie mit Conray Meglumin 282, Fortschr. Geb. Roentgenstr. Nuklearmed. **111**:270, 1969.
2. Ahlegren, P.: Dimer-X: a new contrast medium for lumbar myelography without spinal anesthesia, Acta Radiol. (Diag) **13**:753, 1972.
3. Ahlegren, P.: Amipaque myelography: the side effects compared with Dimer-X, Neuroradiology **9**:197, 1975.
4. Ambrose, J.: Computerized transverse axial scanning (tomography). II. Clinical application, Br. J. Radiol. **46**:1023, 1973.
5. Baker, H. L.: Cerebellopontine angle myelography, J. Neurosurg. **36**:614, 1972.
6. Britton, B. H., and Fluitisma, B.: Iophendylate examination of the posterior fossa, Radiol. Clin. North Am. **12**:431, 1974.
7. Christensen, E. E., Curry, T. S., and Nunnally, J.: An introduction to the physics of diagnostic radiology, Philadelphia, 1972, Lea & Febiger.
8. Dandy, W.: Ventriculography following the injection of air into the cerebral ventricles, Ann. Surg. **68**:4, 1918.
9. Dandy, W.: Roentgenography of the brain after the injection of air into the spinal canal, Ann. Surg. **70**:397, 1919.
10. Davis, D. O., and Rumbaugh, C. L.: Pantopaque myelography, Semin. Roentgenol. **7**:197, 1972.
11. Di Chiro, G., Doppman, J., and Ommaya, A. K.: Selective arteriography of arteriovenous aneurysms of spinal cord, Radiology **88**:1065, 1967.
12. Di Chiro, G., and Wener, L.: Angiography of the spinal cord, J. Neurosurg. **39**:1, 1973.
13. Di Chiro, G., and Schellinger, D.: Computed tomography of spinal cord after lumbar intrathecal introduction of metrizamide (computer assisted myelography), Radiology **120**:101, 1976.
14. Di Chiro, G., Doppman, J. L., and Wener, L.: Computed tomography of spinal cord arteriovenous malformations, Radiology **123**:351, 1977.
15. Djindjian, R., Hurth, M., and Julian, H.: Problèmes techniques posés par la mise en évidence des vaisseaux de la moelle épiniére, J. Neuro-radiol. Anvers **5**:6, 1965.
16. Djindjian, R.: Angiography of the spinal cord, Baltimore, 1970, University Park Press.
17. du Boulay, G., Edmonds-Seal, J., and Bostick, T.: The effect of intermittent positive pressure ventilation upon the calibre of cerebral arteries in spasm following subarachnoid hemorrhage—a preliminary communication, Br. J. Radiol. **41**:46, 1968.
18. du Boulay, G. H., and Symon, L.: The anesthetist's effect upon the cerebral arteries, Proc. Roy. Soc. Med. **64**:77, 1971.
19. Edmonds-Seal, J., du Boulay, G., and Bostick, T.: The effect of intermittent positive ventilation upon cerebral angiography with special reference to the quality of the films—a preliminary communication, Br. J. Radiol. **40**:957, 1967.
20. Epstein, B. S.: The spine, ed. 4, Philadelphia, 1976, Lea & Febiger.
21. Goldman, R. L., and Heinz, E. R.: Gas myelography, Semin. Roentgenol. **7**:216, 1972.
22. Hammerschlag, S. B., Wolpert, S. M., and Carter, B. L.: Computed tomography of the spinal canal, Radiology **121**:361, 1976.
23. Hehman, K. N.: Subtraction in cerebral angiography, Semin. Roentgenol. **6**:14, 1971.
24. Houdart, R., Djindjian, R., Julian, H., and Hurth, M.: Données nouvelles sur la vascularisation de la moelle dorso-lumbaire, Rev. Neurol. **112**:472, 1965.
25. Hounsfield, G. N.: Computerized transverse axial scanning (tomography). I. Description of system, Br. J. Radiol. **46**:1016, 1973.
26. Huber, P.: Functional tests in angiography of brain tumours, Neuroradiology **1**:132, 1970.
27. Lin, J. P., Ramos, M., and Guzman, E.: Radiography of the spine, Wilmington, Dela., 1966, E. I. du Pont de Nemours & Co., Inc.
28. Lin, J. P., and Kricheff, I. I.: Angiographic investigation of cerebral aneurysms (technical aspect), Radiology **105**:69, 1972.
29. Lin, J. P.: Techniques of cerebral angiography, Radiol. Clin. North Am. **12**:223, 1974.
30. Lin, J. P.: Computed tomography of the head in adults, Postgrad Med. **60**:113, 1976.
31. Long, J. M., Kier, E. L., and Hilding, D. A.: Pitfalls of posterior fossa cisternography using 2 cc of iophendylate (Pantopaque), Radiology **102**:71, 1972.
32. Nakagawa, H., Huang, Y. P., Malis, L. I., and Wolf, B. S.: Computed tomography of intraspinal and paraspinal neoplasms, J. Computer Assist. Tomo. **1**:377, 1977.
33. Principles of subtraction (in radiology), Wilmington, Dela., E.I. du Pont de Nemours & Co., Inc.
34. Rosomoff, H. L., Carroll, F., Brown, J., and Sheptak, P.: Percutaneous radiofrequency cervical cordotomy technique, J. Neurosurg. **23**:639, 1965.

35. Roth, M.: Gas myelography by the lumbar route, Acta Radiol. (Diag). **1:**53, 1963.

36. Roth, M.: Pneumomyelography. In Shapiro, R., editor: Myelography, ed. 3, Chicago, 1975, Year Book Medical Publishers, Inc.

37. Seldinger, S.: Catheter replacement of needle in percutaneous arteriography: new technique, Acta Radiol. **39:**368, 1953.

38. Shapiro, R.: Myelography, ed. 3, Chicago, 1975, Year Book Medical Publishers, Inc.

39. Sicard, J. A., Forestier, J., et Laplane, V.: Radioscopie du lipiodol rachidien, Rev. Neurol. **31:**244, 1924.

40. Siew, F. P., Kricheff, I. I., and Chase, N. E.: Demonstration of small acoustic neuromas using negative contrast medium with tomography, Radiology **91:**764, 1968.

41. Skalpe, I., and Amundsen, P.: Lumbar radiculography with metrizamide, Radiology **115:**91, 1975.

42. Skalpe, I., and Amundsen, P.: Thoracic and cervical myelography with metrizamide, Radiology **116:**101, 1975.

43. Wende, S., Nakayama, N., Palvölgyi, R., and Schindler, K.: Comparison of cerebral scintigraphy with magnification angiography under hyperventilation in cerebral tumors, Neuroradiology **6:**781, 1973.

44. Zulch, K. J.: Editorial, Neuroradiology **8:**245, 1975.

7

Anesthesia for neuroradiologic procedures

BERNARD WOLFSON
WILLIAM D. HETRICK

The bony skull and vertebral column protect the cerebrospinal axis not only from trauma but from diagnostic probing. Routine radiographic procedures have little value except to diagnose such relatively simple lesions as fractures or dislocations of the bony skeleton. Because of this, the many more sophisticated diagnostic procedures described in a previous chapter have been devised. Although most neurodiagnostic procedures are invasive to some degree, they are not traumatic or painful enough always to require general anesthesia. If a patient is unwilling or unable to remain still during any portion of the procedure or the subsequent x-ray exposures, general anesthesia may be required. Small children and some older children or adults will not cooperate because of fear or lack of comprehension of what the procedure involves. Lack of cooperation may also be due to disease-related impairment of cerebral function; the semicomatose patient who responds to pain but cannot be reached on a thinking level is an extreme and striking example.

Even in cooperative patients, it may at times be considered preferable to use general endotracheal anesthesia to ensure complete airway protection. In certain poor risk patients, a conventional general anesthesia may be less hazardous than intravenous sedatives or tranquilizers, which may have effects unpredictable in intensity or duration. Some comatose or semicomatose patients may be intubated without anesthesia. However, because this maneuver may increase intracranial pressure significantly, the use of anesthetics and muscle relaxants to mitigate this effect must be considered. Thiopental may be of particular value since it may protect the brain against the metabolic effects of cerebral ischemia[53] and can reduce intracranial pressure.[50] Because most radiologic suites have not been designed as anesthetizing locations, general anesthesia for neurodiagnostic procedures often presents extra problems: space is often limited, and bulky x-ray apparatus is always present; vacuum suction may not be available; and personnel are not adapted to existing facilities. The temptation to "make do" under these circumstances must be scrupulously avoided. Ventilation, monitoring, and resuscitation equipment must be equivalent to that used in the general operating room. Electrocardiographic monitoring is essential, especially if controlled ventilation is to be used, since arrhythmia may be the earliest sign of pressure on the brain stem. A defibrillator should be immediately available. If general anesthesia is not used, it is common to use sedation during

138

neurodiagnostic procedures. It is important to be certain that the airway is adequately protected and respiration remains optimum to avoid carbon dioxide–induced increases in intracranial pressure. Maintenance of adequate cardiovascular parameters is essential, and monitoring should be just as intense as when general anesthesia is used.

Evaluation of a patient who is to undergo any of the diagnostic procedures to be discussed should be along the same lines as that for any patient requiring general anesthesia, since it may be necessary to convert local analgesia plus sedation to a general anesthetic at some time during the procedure. As all these patients are being investigated because of the possibility of neurologic disease, additional factors must be considered. If an intracranial lesion is present, intracranial pressure should be evaluated. Papilledema and headache may be present and suggestive of increased intracranial pressure. Cerebrovascular disease may be inferred in patients with systemic vascular disease. Conversely, a history of transient ischemic attacks may suggest concurrent generalized arteriosclerotic disease. Where prolonged bed rest has been enforced, either due to trauma or neurologic disease, the possibility of general debility compounding the cardiovascular depressant effect of anesthesia and the hyperkalemic response to succinylcholine should be remembered. Many cases of acute trauma present for neuroradiologic investigation, especially CAT scanning, and are often complicated because the state of consciousness precludes adequate history taking. In the absence of specific information to the contrary, a full stomach must be assumed; in addition, multiple organ damage must be considered.

The decision to use general or local anesthesia should be made following discussion between neurosurgeon, radiologist and anesthesiologist. When possible, patient preference should be considered.

PNEUMOENCEPHALOGRAPHY

The indications and technique for pneumoencephalography have been described in Chapter 6. Although the number of pneumoencephalograms has been reduced by the CAT scanner, this diagnostic procedure is used from time to time. It is important to avoid marked increases in intracranial pressure whether due to anesthetic agents or techniques or side effects such as retching or coughing, since such increases exert pressure on the ventricles, decrease air entry, or actually empty air.

The investigation is not without hazard. In a personal series of 4000 cases, Davidoff and Dyke[11] reported nine deaths, a mortality rate of 0.22%. Coleman and co-workers[7] reported 31 fatalities associated with pneumoencephalography. Five occurred during the procedure—four due to air embolism. Whittier[56] reported 24 deaths in a series of 2490 pneumoencephalograms, of which only 6 were thought to be related directly to the pneumoencephalogram. Jacoby and co-workers[27] reported six deaths during 1196 pneumoencephalograms performed under general anesthesia. In four instances, air embolism was confirmed at autopsy. In a fifth case, air embolism was suspected, but no autopsy was obtained. The sixth patient died following herniation of the brain stem. A seventh patient suffered this complication but was resuscitated. The exact diagnosis may be difficult to make, since both these complications result in abrupt respiratory and cardiac embarrassment that may be followed almost immediately by cardiac arrest. These authors suggest that when such signs occur after lumbar puncture, but before injection of air, herniation of the brain stem should be diagnosed. If air has just been injected, embolism should be considered. The possibility of collapse due to anesthesia should be considered, but treatment for this should be concurrent with that for other diagnoses. This includes placing the patient with the left side down in the Trendelenburg position for air embolism or reinjection of CSF or saline for brain stem herniation. Herniation should not occur in the absence of increased intracranial pressure. Pneumoencephalography should not be performed when intracranial pressure is

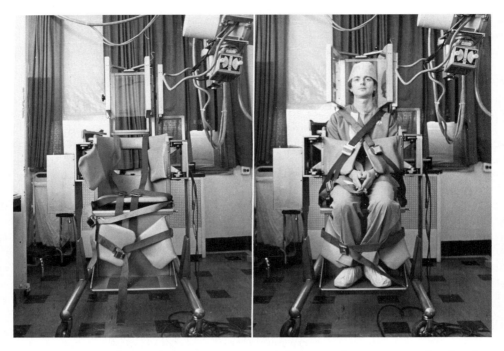

Fig. 7-1. Chair used in performing pneumoencephalograms. The patient may be placed in this special apparatus and be rotated into all positions necessary to obtain adequate films.

increased. Air embolism is due either to absorption through a dural sinus[30] or to intravascular placement of the lumbar needle.[27] The presence of a functioning ventriculoatrial shunt[64] may increase risk of air embolism. Cardiac arrest has followed rapid injection of a large bolus of air.[44] Slow air injection is commonly followed by hypertension, headache, nausea, and vomiting. Hypotension, bradycardia, and syncope have been reported in the unanesthetized patient.[61] Small children who are usually anesthetized for air studies may also be particularly prone to these latter complications.[54]

General anesthesia or local analgesia plus sedation may be used. Airway management during anesthesia may be difficult because of the proximity of x-ray apparatus. The patient may be placed in a special apparatus, which may be rotated into all positions necessary to obtain adequate films.[44,58] The chair used in our institution is shown in Fig. 7-1. If this or a similar apparatus is not available, the patient must be moved to an x-ray table to make prone and supine exposures.

Any anesthetic technique may interfere with normal cardiovascular responses to positional change.[6,44,58] Wilson and co-workers[58] reported decreases in blood pressure associated with the sitting position but felt this was not usually serious because of concurrent increases in cardiac output. Campkin and Turner[6] related the severity of pressure changes to the type of anesthesia and concluded that controlled ventilation using nitrous oxide, oxygen, and pancuronium was most supportive and therefore the preferred technique. Ramsay and co-workers,[44] using the Phillips isocentric chair and employing spontaneous respiration with oxygen and halothane, recorded statistically significant pressure change only following the move from prone to sitting position. The authors believed that this was related to the use of the Phillips chair and not to light anesthesia. It may be noted, however, that normal PCO_2 readings were recorded, while Campkin's and Turner's[6] spontaneously breathing group had elevated arterial PCO_2. This finding, plus the absence of nitrous oxide, suggests to the present authors that light anesthesia may indeed have been a factor. This is of more than theoretical interest because light anesthesia with the possibility of attendant coughing and straining could be hazardous.

The use of nitrous oxide during air encephalography was questioned by Saidman and Eger[47] because the markedly higher blood solubility of nitrous oxide than nitrogen (approximately 30:1) results in expansion of the injected air and possibly a pressure rise within the cranium. The extent of the volume change depends on the concentration of nitrous oxide inhaled. They reported a death in a child that might have been due to nitrous oxide–induced elevation in intracranial pressure. Increase in intracranial pressure associated with nitrous oxide has been reported by other investigators.[6,25] Campkin and Turner[6] showed that the magnitude of the pressure elevation was greater during spontaneous ventilation with nitrous oxide, oxygen, and halothane than with a muscle relaxant—controlled ventilation technique. Gordon and Greitz[25] demonstrated similar elevations during controlled ventilation with nitrous oxide, oxygen, and halothane and also during neuroleptic anesthesia. However, both groups considered that the effect of nitrous oxide was not significant in the absence of previously increased intracranial pressure.

Following experiments in dogs with a number of anesthetic gases, Aird[3] suggested that nitrous oxide might be a satisfactory contrast medium for encephalography. He demonstrated that injected nitrous oxide disappeared within an hour, whereas air remained for approximately seven days. However, Newman[40] obtained poor results with nitrous oxide because of its rapid ventricular absorption. He obtained better results with ethylene. General anesthesia was not administered for these examinations. Saidman and Eger[47] suggested that pressure changes dur-

ing nitrous oxide anesthesia would not occur if nitrous oxide was used as contrast medium. This contention was later shown to be accurate.[13] The clinical use of nitrous oxide as the contrast medium in two groups of children has been reported.[19,29] In both groups more than the usual amount of gas had to be injected because of absorption of nitrous oxide from the ventricles. However, as nitrous oxide was also used as part of the general anesthetic technique, this absorption was relatively slow and adequate films were obtained. Although it was difficult to assess,[6] morbidity was thought to be reduced,[29] as was duration of hospitalization.[19] These reports are in accord with the findings of Davidoff and Dyke,[11] who suggested that the duration of postpneumoencephalography morbidity was related to the duration of contact between the contrast medium and the ventricles. In a study of postpneumoencephalography headache, Wolfson and co-workers[60] concluded that this was related in part to the contrast medium but also to the spinal tap and subsequent CSF leakage. Headache occurs with frequency and may last for many days (Fig. 7-2). Nitrous oxide for encephalography has not gained widespread popularity, presumably because of technical difficulties.

Soon after its introduction into clinical practice, ketamine was suggested as a very useful agent for neurologic diagnostic studies, especially in children.[8,57] The advantages claimed were satisfactory blood pressure, pulse and respiration, maintenance by the patient of a clear airway without the need for intubation, and avoidance of nitrous oxide. However, well-documented increases in intracranial pressure following the use of ketamine,[24,33,51,20,62] including one with resultant apnea,[33] tempered this initial enthusiasm. The success of ketamine in so many of these investigations may be because it was not used in the presence of increased intracranial pressure. The ease with which ketamine may be used, however, should not be allowed to disguise the fact that monitoring by skilled and informed personnel is essential and administration by those carry-

	Pure spinal		Mixed		Nonspinal		Total	
	DOCA (%)	Placebo (%)	DOCA (%)	Placebo (%)	DOCA (%)	Placebo (%)	DOCA (%)	Placebo (%)
Day 1	30	23	38	54	8	7	76	84
Day 2	24	25	41	47	11	9	76	81
Day 3	14	16	24	30	3	7	41	53

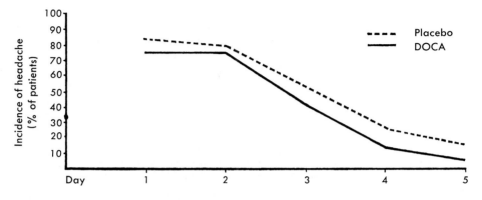

Fig. 7-2. Total incidence of headache after pneumoencephalography in patients receiving DOCA or a placebo. (From Wolfson, B., Siker, E. S., and Gray, G. H.: Anaesthesia **25**:328, 1970.)

ing out the pneumoencephalogram should be discouraged. If it is felt that ketamine is the indicated technique, it should be remembered that elevations in intracranial pressure may, at least temporarily, be controlled by thiopental.[62,51] A technique involving use of thiopental and lidocaine with spontaneous respiration has also been recommended.[45]

If general anesthesia is required for pneumoencephalography, the patient should be treated as would any other with a potential intracranial pathologic condition, except that nitrous oxide should be omitted. This involves a smooth induction in a flaccid, nonresponsive patient, with subsequent controlled ventilation, using a nondepolarizing muscle relaxant. Anesthesia can be maintained with either incremental thiopental, diazepam (Valium), or neuroleptic agents. The use of a short-acting narcotic such as fentanyl (Sublimaze), which may be antagonized at the end of the anesthetic, will reduce overall drug requirements and permit rapid recovery. Muscle relaxants permit light planes of anesthesia to be used without the attendant problems of coughing and vom-

iting. Controlled ventilation, by reducing arterial Pco_2, may counteract the increase in intracranial pressure due to the anesthetic or contrast medium. Halothane and oxygen with controlled ventilation may be used in children if the intravenous route is not considered technically feasible. Ketamine should not be considered when intracranial hypertension is present.

Because of problems already noted and because observation of state of consciousness is a valuable monitor in any patient with presumed neurologic disease, it is common in many centers to use local analgesia plus sedation for the performance of pneumoencephalography. This presumes a cooperative patient. Patients treated in this way are by no means immune to complications. Hypotension may still occur in the sitting position and be intensified by drugs used for sedation. Hypertension is common following the injection of air into the subarachnoid space,[61] and severe headache, nausea, and vomiting are common. Numerous drugs or combinations of drugs have been used in an attempt to reduce the incidence and severity of headache and nausea to acceptable proportions while maintaining consciousness, the ability to cooperate, and a patent airway. Wolfson and co-workers[61] reported on the use of droperidol (Inapsine) and fentanyl. This technique had a high incidence (21%) of hypotension requiring vasopressors or fluid treatment in 65% of patients. Seventeen percent of patients interviewed after receiving this drug combination said the examination was unbearable. Wolfson and co-workers[59] later described the use of subhypnotic doses of ketamine with diazepam and droperidol to reduce hallucinations and nausea. Patient acceptance was much better, but 37.5% of patients hallucinated. Thirty-three percent of the reported hallucinations were decidedly unpleasant. Fifty-one percent of patients lost consciousness at some time during the procedure, making this technique unacceptable. The authors concluded that the most satisfactory technique involved the use of diazepam as a tranquilizer and amnesic, combined with alphaprodine for headache, plus droperidol as an antinauseant. Hypotension occurring prior to the injection of air was treated with metaraminol. After the injection of air, hypotension was relatively uncommon; hypertension was more of a problem. This usually responded either to narcotic or to droperidol. Although the incidence of amnesia with this technique was less than with higher doses of diazepam alone, lack of cooperation because of drowsiness occurred less frequently, and patient acceptance was excellent.[18]

ANGIOGRAPHY

Angiography in neurodiagnostic practice may be used to delineate the cerebral or spinal cord vasculature. Complications of the arterial puncture or catheterization may occur: spasm, hematomas, or embolization of arteriosclerotic plaques or thrombosis or injection into the wall of the vessel with intimal stripping and compression of smaller branching vessels.[21] The contrast medium used may itself produce pain and burning in the vascular distribution site. With the almost universal use of meglumine iothalamate (Conray), the severity of these reactions has been much reduced. In cerebral angiography the incidence is further reduced by selective internal carotid artery catheterization. This eliminates facial discomfort in the distribution area of the external carotid artery, but burning behind the eye may still occur. More serious contrast-induced complications include arterial spasm and anaphylactic reactions. Spasm may be especially dangerous in the presence of a leaking intracerebral aneurysm where existing spasm may be markedly intensified. Anaphylaxis is less common following intra-arterial than intravenous injection, but hypotension, bradycardia, arrhythmia, and pulmonary edema may occur. In addition, convulsions, paralysis or paresis, and loss of speech or sight may develop either immediately or in the postexamination period.

Central nervous system damage following angiography is partially due to a direct necrotizing effect associated with hypoxic microvascular damage.[36] The concentration of the medium is the critical factor involved.[37] The least toxic agent in a series investigated was meglumine iothalamate.[38] In this study vasopressor administration prior to the injection of contrast markedly enhanced spinal cord damage with virtually all available media,[38] presumably by constricting other parts of the vascular bed and effectively increasing the concentration of the contrast agent in the brain and cord. Conversely, by increasing the total vascular bed, vasodepressor drugs have been shown to decrease spinal cord toxicity.[63] In a study in monkeys, Doppman[15] used vasopressors deliberately in an effort to produce better delineation of spinal cord vessels, and in some instances vessels that could not be seen with more common techniques were well visualized. There was no spinal toxicity observed in this study. This technique has not gained popularity in humans. Selective angiography combined with subtraction techniques described in the previous chapter are the commonly accepted methods of choice today. It is unlikely, therefore, that more data will become available on the effects of vasopressors in the clinical situation, and it may be prudent to avoid the use of vasoconstrictors during angiography. If one is necessary, a predominantly beta-acting drug such as ephedrine may be the agent of choice. Hypotension and bradycardia occurring during dye injection may be vagal in origin and respond to atropine.[34]

These complications have definite implications for the anesthesiologist. He may be called upon urgently to treat a life-threatening anaphylactic reaction or an equally threatening respiratory tract obstruction due to a large hematoma in the neck. In this litigious time he will almost certainly be involved in any legal action arising from neurologic sequelae. It is essential, therefore, in this regard, that hypoxia or other factors that may cause nervous system damage be rigorously avoided, and adequate documentation of meticulous technique (for example, FI_{O_2}) is to be encouraged. In addition, lines of communication must be kept open between anesthesiologist and operator. Each must be made immediately aware of any problems being encountered by the other so that he may plan accordingly.

Cerebral angiography may be carried out by percutaneous puncture of the common carotid or vertebral arteries or by retrograde catheterization of brachial, axillary, or most commonly the femoral artery. The femoral artery catheterization technique is less disturbing to the patient, permits selective angiography, and has fewer complications than direct puncture techniques.[41] Local or general anesthesia may be used.

Advantages of general anesthesia include increased patient comfort and immobility during x-ray exposures. Angiogram quality may be enhanced by hyperventilation.[10,17,46] Hypocarbia, by slowing cerebral circulation, allows greater concentration of the contrast medium[17] and by constricting cerebral vessels improves clarity.[10] Mechanical hyperventilation itself, by increasing venous pressure, may also slow cerebral circulation and improve angiographic quality even during normocarbia. Hyperventilation to less than

30 mm Hg P_{CO_2} does not produce a further decrease in cerebral vessel caliber but does prolong circulation time.[10] This was particularly well demonstrated in children with increased cerebral blood flow where good angiograms are often difficult to obtain. Hyperventilation may improve angiographic quality in patients with brain tumor by provoking an intracerebral steal.[10,46] Hypocarbia does not usually constrict tumor vessels, and hyperventilation shunts blood and contrast medium to the tumor, which becomes well delineated. A similar effect has been demonstrated with meningiomas supplied by extracerebral vessels.[46] Less well-defined angiograms have also been demonstrated in spontaneously breathing adults in whom arterial P_{CO_2} is greater than 45 mm Hg.[10] An effect similar to that of hypercarbia might be anticipated during the use of potent inhalation agents, all of which produce cerebral dilatation. Dallas[10] was unable to demonstrate statistically significant differences in radiographic quality between trichlorethylene- and nitrous oxide–anesthetized patients at comparable arterial P_{CO_2}. However, only small numbers were involved in the study, and the trend in the results seemed to favor the nitrous oxide group.

Hypotension induced by nitrous oxide, oxygen, and halothane during cerebral angiography may make carotid puncture difficult.[32] The hypotension was particularly troublesome in patients with cerebrovascular lesions, and it was concluded that the technique was not suitable for such patients. These factors point to the use of a controlled ventilation method using nitrous oxide and narcotics whenever possible. In fact, some investigators[10] advocate the use of hyperventilation in all cases. Others avoid it in the presence of a presumed ruptured intracranial aneurysm because they believe that the related spasm and impaired cerebral circulation may be further worsened by hypocarbia-induced cerebral vasoconstriction.[46] du Boulay and co-workers[16] have reported variable effects of changes in arterial P_{CO_2} on spastic intracerebral vessels.

Most often, a CO_2 increase dilates these vessels, but in some instances constriction or no response was seen. Normocarbic general anesthesia is probably appropriate in such a patient. This question may soon be academic, if it is not so already, since radiologists and neurosurgeons are reluctant to perform prolonged angiography during the early posthemorrhagic stage, preferring to rely on CAT scanning and limited angiography for initial diagnosis.

A major disadvantage of general anesthesia is that consciousness cannot be used to monitor neurologic state. A secondary disadvantage is that intracranial pressure may be acutely increased. These factors have made local anesthesia with or without sedation the method of choice in some centers in the United States. In Britain, on the other hand, general anesthesia is usually commonly preferred and is considered essential for vertebral or arch angiography.

Local anesthesia still requires close circulatory and respiratory monitoring. Supplemental sedation, frequently necessary for patient comfort or procedural necessity, can be done with a tranquilizer. Diazepam is widely used, even though it has hypnotic but no analgesic properties. Hypnosis without analgesia in a patient undergoing painful stimuli frequently produces restlessness. Narcotics may be added in small enough doses to maintain consciousness and voluntary cooperation. Respiratory depression must be considered to accompany any use of narcotic, and is therefore contraindicated in the presence of mass lesions.

Spinal cord angiography is almost always done using selective angiography, usually with subtraction techniques. Many patients have cord damage or are paraplegic prior to cord angiography. Contrast medium-induced spinal cord damage is a significant hazard. Djindjian,[13] a pioneer of this technique, believes that general anesthesia with total apnea during angiogram exposure is essential to obtain adequate results. Djindjian[13] reported 240 selective angiographies of the spinal cord with one death, which he attributed to an allergic reaction to the contrast medium. There were no permanent neurologic deficits, although some patients developed paroxysmal lower limb contractures during anterior spinal artery angiography. The paroxysms responded to injection of diazepam, 5 mg, directly to the angiography catheter. Diazepam produces no tissue toxicity when injected into the renal or mesenteric arteries in dogs.[14] Spinal cord damage must be accepted as a possible complication of spinal angiography. Local analgesia allows the patient to be assessed for neurologic damage or irritation after each vessel is injected.

MYELOGRAPHY

Myelography is accompanied by some discomfort during lumbar puncture and during final aspiration of the contrast medium. Cauda equina nerve roots may be manipulated. Usually, moderate sedation is all that is required.

Anesthesia is usually limited to children and an occasional adult who is unwilling or unable to cooperate. The primary problems involved are maintaining respiratory and cardiovascular stability during multiple positional changes. Ketamine can be useful in children.

COMPUTERIZED AXIAL TOMOGRAPHY

The introduction of computerized axial tomography (CAT scanning), also referred to as computer or computed tomography (CT), cerebral computer tomography (CTT), or EMI scanning (electric and musical industries limited), has greatly enhanced the diagnostic armamentarium of the neuroradiologist. The patient is placed on a couch with the head in a cap surrounded by a water-containing bag or cuff. These are in turn encircled by a rotating gantry that contains the detecting system of the scanner. A complete rotation of the gantry takes approximately four and one-half minutes (Fig. 7-3). Anesthesia personnel might receive a skin dose of 1 to 2 mrad per hour.[2] The use of a lead apron allows safe participation in a full daily schedule. Except for the intrave-

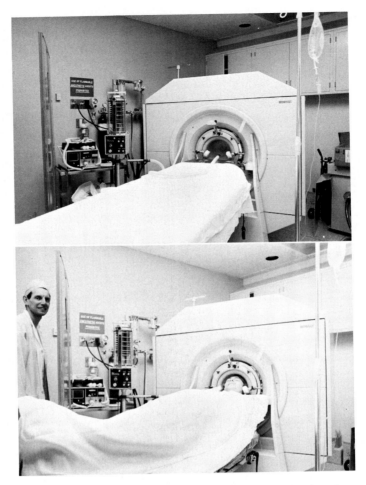

Fig. 7-3. CT scanner used for scanning of the head and neck.

nous injection, the procedure is noninvasive. Few adult patients need general anesthesia, and 17% of all patients receiving anesthesia have suffered acute head trauma.[2] A new generation of scanners now in production has eliminated the need for the water-containing bag and has reduced the time of each rotation to approximately one minute. The radiologist needs complete immobility during each "cut." General anesthesia is indicated where this cannot be guaranteed by other means. Unfortunately, this usually means the patient is either a small child or has some neurologic problem, either acute or chronic, which precludes cooperation.

Anesthesia considerations include factors already discussed, such as general medical and neurologic status, and, in trauma cases, the presumed presence of a full stomach and possible concomitant injuries. The problem of shortage of space already mentioned is often particularly applicable in the case of CAT scanning because the scanner has been a recent addition to the radiology department and often has had to utilize available space, without consideration for the requirements of anesthesia. The approach to this problem in our institution may be seen in Fig. 7-3. Anesthetic gases have been piped in, and a wall bracket has been used to mount flow meters and a halothane vaporizer. We have further conserved space by utilizing a single tube anesthesia system (Bain circuit). This has the added advantage of being very lightweight, making it easy to stabilize the endotracheal tube, and Pco$_2$ may be predetermined by correlating respiratory rate and minute volume as suggested by the manufacturers. The lead glass screen and the defibrillator-monitor are routinely present. In addition, most of the anesthesia staff wear a lead apron.

The choice of anesthetic techniques is a personal one. We favor a pentothal, nitrous oxide, oxygen relaxant sequence technique.[2] Controlled ventilation, usually with moderate hyperventilation, can facilitate intracranial pressure control. In children, an inhalation induction may be utilized with careful temperature monitoring, warm water in the head bag,[2] and heating lamps. It may be difficult to stabilize the infant's head, and in children with severe hydrocephalus visualization of the posterior fossa may be difficult.[4] Even in adults, examination of this region may require extreme head flexion.[42] This may cause discomfort in the conscious patient, kink the tube in the intubated patient, or produce brain stem compression in the presence of a large infratentorial tumor.[50] Many CAT scans are performed on an outpatient basis, and the same meticulous medical assessment and anesthetic considerations should be applied.

An anesthesiologist may be called upon to sedate or monitor the patient, especially where contrast medium is to be injected and a reaction is feared. The problems with sedation have been described.

ADVERSE REACTIONS TO CONTRAST MEDIA

Reactions to contrast material vary from mild skin rashes to anaphylactoid reactions that include wheezing, syncope, and vasomotor collapse. Nausea, tingling, and giddiness as well as transient hypotension may be seen. In a prospective study reported by the Committee on Contrast Media of the International Society of Radiology,[52] of 27,628 vascular studies, nonfatal reactions occurred in 2.33%. Four fatal reactions occurred, one during venography, two during angiocardiography, and one during cerebral angiography. Repeat studies in patients with a previous history of untoward response were associated with three times as many reactions as in the general population. The exact mechanism of these reactions is unknown, although they have not been shown to be IgE mediated. There are no predictive tests available.

Intradermal testing for prediction of these reactions is unreliable and has been virtually abandoned. Intravenous test doses immediately prior to the procedure is not a sure method of detection.[23] Steroids (150 mg prednisone or its equivalent per day), starting 18 hours before and continuing 12 hours after injection may be useful.[65] In this particular report, steroids were prescribed only for patients in the "rush" and "anaphylactoid" categories; those in the "vasomotor" category received no steroids but were monitored closely throughout. Only 4 mild reactions were seen in 124 patients. Diphenhydramine hydrochloride (Benadryl) either intravenously immediately or orally one hour prior to the procedure may also be useful.[49] Combination of steroids and antihistamines has also been described.[39] This is the approach most used in our institution, although patients are individualized, and consultation with an allergist is commonly obtained. Where a large bolus of contrast medium is to be injected, a preliminary intravenous test dose of 5 ml is used. During selective angiography, involving only small quantities of contrast, the first intra-arterial injection is regarded as the test dose, and prior intravenous administration is omitted. To date no severe problems have been encountered using this sequence. However, this neither infers absolute safety in this technique nor precludes other techniques that may be in vogue elsewhere. The ethical problem can only be treated by full disclosure. Fortunately, this disclosure can include the facts just presented.

Treatment of adverse reactions occurring either de novo or after repeat exposure depends on their severity. Rashes or mild vasomotor reactions require no therapy or merely the administration of an antihistaminic drug. A severe anaphylactic reaction, however, must be treated swiftly and aggressively. This reaction may be manifested by respiratory distress or by severe hypotension and syncope, and may be expiratory due to bronchospasm or inspiratory due to laryngeal edema. The pharmacologic mainstays of this treatment are epinephrine and steroids as detailed in standard medical texts.[26] Endotracheal intubation and ventilation may be required, as may cardiopulmonary resuscitation if cardiac arrest supervenes.

REFERENCES

1. Ahlgren, P.: Amipaque myelography, the side effects compared with Dimer x, Neuroradiol. 9:197, 1975.
2. Adidinis, S. J., Zimmerman, R. A., Shapiro, H. M., Bilanuick, L. T., and Broennle, A. M.: Anesthesia for brain computer tomography, Anesthesia 44:420, 1976.
3. Aird, R. B.: Experimental encephalography with anesthetic gases, Arch. Surg. 32:193, 1936.
4. Bachman, D. S., Hodges, F. J., and Freeman, J. M.: Computerized axial tomography in neurologic disorders, Pediatrics 59:352, 1977.
5. Campkin, T. V.: General anaesthesia for neuroradiology, Br. J. Anaesth. 48:783, 1976.
6. Campkin, T. V., and Turner, J. M.: Blood pressure and cerebrospinal fluid pressure studies during lumbar air encephalography, Br. J. Anaesth. 44:849, 1972.
7. Coleman, F. C., Schenken, J. R., and Abbott, W. D.: Air embolism during pneumoencephalography, Am. J. Clin. Pathol. 20:966, 1950.
8. Corssen, G., Groves, E. H., Gomez, S., and Allen, R. J.: Ketamine: its place in anesthesia for neurosurgical diagnostic procedures, Anesth. Analg. 48:181, 1969.
9. Crnic, D. N., Seifert, F. C., and Ranniger, K.: Arterial injury in dogs after multiple percutaneous catheterizations at the same site of entry, Radiology 108:295, 1973.
10. Dallas, S. H., and Moxon, C. P.: Controlled ventilation for cerebral angiography, Br. J. Anaesth. 41:597, 1969.
11. Davidoff, L. M., and Dyke, C. G.: The normal encephalogram, Philadelphia, 1951, Lea & Febiger.
12. DiChiro, G., and Werner, L.: Angiography of the spinal cord, a review of contemporary techniques and applications, J. Neurosurg. 39:1, 1973.
13. Djindjian, R.: Angiography of the spinal cord, Baltimore, Md., 1970, University Park Press.
14. Doppman, J. L., Albertson, K., Ramsey, R., and

Saltzstein, M. D.: Intra-arterial valium—its safety and effectiveness, Neuroradiology 106:335, 1973.
15. Doppman, J. D., Brown, W. E., and Dichiro, G.: Angiographic demonstration of increased spinal cord blood flow following administration of a pressor amine, Radiology 92:239, 1969.
16. du Boulay, G., Edmonds-Seal, J., and Bostick, T.: The effect of intermittent positive pressure ventilation upon the caliber of cerebral arteries in spasm following subarachnoid haemorrhage—a preliminary communication, Br. J. Radiol. 41:46, 1968.
17. Edmonds-Seal, J., du Boulay, G., and Bostick, T.: The effect of intermittent positive pressure ventilation upon cerebral angiography with special reference to the quality of the films—a preliminary communication, Br. J. Radiol. 40:957, 1967.
18. Edwards, J. C., and Flowerdew, G. D.: Diazepam and local analgesia for lumbar air encephalography, Br. J. Anaesth. 42:999, 1970.
19. Elwyn, R. A., Ring, W. H., Loeser, E., and Myers, G. G.: Nitrous oxide encephalography: five year experience with 475 pediatric patients, Anesth. Analg. 55:402, 1976.
20. Evans, J., Rosen, M., Weeks, R. D., and Wise, C.: Ketamine in neurosurgical procedures, Lancet 1:40, 1971.
21. Feild, J. R., Robertson, J. T., and DeSaussure, R. L.: Complications of cerebral angiography in 2000 consecutive cases, J. Neurosurg. 19:775, 1962.
22. Ferrer-Brecher, T., and Winter, J.: Anesthetic considerations for cerebral computer tomography, Anesth. Analg. 56:344, 1977.
23. Fischer, H. W., and Doust, V. L.: An evaluation of pretesting in the problem of serious and fatal reaction to excretory urography, Radiology 103:497, 1972.
24. Gardner, A. E., Olsen, B. E., and Lichtiger, M.: Cerebrospinal fluid pressure during dissociative anesthesia with ketamine, Anesthesia 35:226, 1971.
25. Gordon, E., and Greitz, T.: The effect of nitrous oxide on the cerebrospinal fluid pressure during encephalography, Br. J. Anaesth. 42:2, 1970.
26. Harrison, T. R., editor: Principles of internal medicine, ed. 8, New York, 1977, McGraw-Hill Book Co.
27. Jacoby, J., Jones, J. R., Ziegler, J., Claassen, L., and Garvin, J. P.: Pneumoencephalography and air embolism: simulated anesthetic death, Anesthesia 20:336, 1959.
28. Jain, K. K.: Use of diazepam in carotid angiography, Can. J. Neurolog. Sci. 1:141, 1974.
29. Kerber, C., and Cromwell, L. D.: Pediatric pneumoencephalography with nitrous oxide, Childs Brain 2:309, 1976.
30. King, A. B., and Otenasek, F. J.: Air embolism occurring during encephalography: a report of two cases, J. Neurosurg. 5:577, 1948.
31. Laborit, T. H.: Reaction organique à l'agression, et choc, Paris, 1952, Masson et Cie.

32. Lewis, R. N., and Moore, B. A.: Some aspects of general anaesthesia for cerebral angiography, Br. J. Anaesth. **40**:37, 1968.

33. List, W. F., Crumrine, R. S., Cascorbi, H. F., Weiss, M. H.: Increased cerebrospinal fluid pressure after ketamine, Anesthesia **36**:98, 1972.

34. Lundevold, A., and Engeset, A.: Recordings of EEG, ECG, EMG and intra-arterial blood pressure during cerebral angiography, Acta Radiol. (suppl.) **270**:198, 1967.

35. Margolis, G., Griffin, A. T., Kenan, P. D., Tindall, G. T., Riggins, R., and Fort, L.: Contrast-medium injury to the spinal cord, the role of altered circulatory dynamics, J. Neurosurg. **16**:390, 1959.

36. Margolis, G., Tarazi, A. K., and Grimson, K. S.: Contrast medium injury to the spinal cord produced by aortography; pathologic anatomy of the experimental lesion, J. Neurosurg. **13**:349, 1956.

37. Margolis, G., Tindall, G. T., Phillips, R. L., Kenan, P. D., and Grimson, K. S.: Evaluation of roentgen contrast agents used in cerebral arteriography. I. A simple screening method, J. Neurosurg. **15**:30, 1958.

38. Margolis, G., and Yerasimides, T. G.: Vasopressor potentiation of neurotoxicity in experimental aortography—implications regarding pathogenesis of contrast medium injury, Acta Radiol. (Diagn) **5**:388, 1966.

39. Miller, W. L., Doppman, J. L., and Kaplan, A. P.: Renal arteriography following systemic reaction to contrast material, J. Allergy Clin. Immunol. **56**:291, 1975.

40. Newman, H.: Encephalography with ethylene, J.A.M.A. **108**:461, 1937.

41. Newton, T. H., and Potts, D. G.: Angiography, St. Louis, 1974, The C. V. Mosby Co.

42. Paxton, R., and Ambrose, J.: The EMI scanner; a brief review of the first 650 patients, Br. J. Radiol. **47**:530, 1974.

43. Perry, B. J., and Bridges, C.: Computerized transverse axial scanning (tomography). III. Radiation dose considerations, Br. J. Radiol. **46**:1048, 1973.

44. Ramsay, M. A. E., Colvin, M. P., Taylor, T. H., Gil-Rodriguez, J. A., Morris, J. L., and Wylie, I. G.: Cardio-respiratory changes during pneumoencephalography, Anaesthesia **31**:1179, 1976.

45. Raudzens, P., and Cole, A. F. D.: Thiopentone/lidocaine anaesthesia for pneumoencephalography, Can. Anaesth. Soc. J. **21**:1, 1974.

46. Samuel, J. R., Grange, R. A., and Hawkins, T. D.: Anaesthetic technique for carotid angiography, Anaesthesia **23**:543, 1968.

47. Saidman, L. J., and Eger, E. I., II: Change in cerebrospinal fluid pressure during pneumoencephalography under nitrous oxide anesthesia, Anesthesia **26**:67, 1965.

48. Saidman, L. J., and Moya, F.: Complications of anesthesia, Springfield, 1970, Charles C Thomas, Publisher.

49. Schatz, M., Patterson, R., O'Rourke, J., Nickelsen, J., and Northup, C.: The administration of radiographic contrast media to patients with a history of a previous reaction, J. Allergy Clin. Immunol. **55**:358, 1975.

50. Shapiro, H. M., and Aidinis, S. J.: Neurosurgical anesthesia, Surg. Clin. North Am. **55**:913, 1975.

51. Shapiro, H. M., Wyte, S. R., and Harris, A. B.: Ketamine anaesthesia in patients with intracranial pathology, Br. J. Anaesth. **44**:1200, 1972.

52. Shehadi, W. H.: Adverse reactions to intravascularly administered contrast media; a comprehensive study based on a prospective survey, Am. J. Roentgenol. Radium Ther. Nucl. Med. **124**:145, 1975.

53. Smith, A. L.: Barbiturate protection in cerebral hypoxia, Anesthesia **47**:285, 1977.

54. Smith, R. M.: Anesthesia for infants and children, St. Louis, 1968, The C. V. Mosby Co.

55. Welborn, S. G.: Anesthesia of EMI scanning in infants and small children, South. Med. J. **69**:1294, 1976.

56. Whittier, J. R.: Deaths related to pneumoencephalography during a six year period, Arch. Neurol. Psychiatr. **65**:463, 1951.

57. Wilson, G. H., Fotias, N. A., and Dioon, J. B.: Ketamine: a new anesthetic for use in pediatric neurorentgenologic procedures, Am. J. Roentgenol. Radium Ther. Nucl. Med. **106**:434, 1969.

58. Wilson, R. D., Overton, M. C., Waldron, R. L., and Snodgrass, S. R.: Abrupt postural changes in patients undergoing air contrast studies, J.A.M.A. **198**:970, 1966.

59. Wolfson, B., Kielar, C. M., Shenoy, N. R., and Hetrick, W. D.: Analgesic "cocktails" for pneumoencephalography: ketamine, diazepam, alphaprodine and droperidol, Anesth. Analg. **52**:779, 1973.

60. Wolfson, B., Siker, E. S., and Gray, G. H.: Postpneumoencephalography headache, a study of incidence and an attempt at therapy, Anaesthsia **25**:328, 1970.

61. Wolfson, B., Siker, E. S., Wible, L., and Dubansky, J.: Pneumoencephalography using neuroleptanalgesia, Anesth. Analg. **47**:14, 1968.

62. Wyte, S. R., Shapiro, H. M., Turner, P., and Harris, A. B.: Ketamine-induced intracranial hypertension, Anesthesia **36**:174, 1972.

63. Yerasimides, T. G., Margolis, G., and Ponton, H. J.: Prophylaxis of experimental contrast medium injury to the spinal cord by vasodepressor drugs, Angiology **14**:394, 1963.

64. Youngberg, J. A., Kaplan, J. A., and Miller, E. D.: Air embolism through a ventriculoatrial shunt during pneumoencephalography, Anesthesia **42**:487, 1975.

65. Zweiman, B., Mishkin, M. M., and Hildreth, E. A.: An approach to the performance of contrast studies in contrast material-reactive persons, Ann. Intern. Med. **83**:159, 1975.

8

Anesthesia for supratentorial tumor

STANLEY I. SAMUELS

In 1918 Harvey Cushing wrote the following:

During the shaving of the head, possibly an hour before the patient's turn will come, a sedative is given, a third of a grain of omnopon usually being sufficient, though this may be repeated if the patient is very restless or obstreperous. Then fifteen or twenty minutes before the operation, in the lines of proposed incision, the scalp is infiltrated with a 1 per cent novocain and adrenalin (15 drops to 30 c.cm.) solution, injected in the sub-aponeurotic layer.

There exists a difference of opinion regarding the relative merits of a general *versus* local anesthesia for cranial operations. The writer confesses to an original prejudice in favour of inhalation narcosis, but experience has led him completely to alter this view.

General narcosis increases intracranial tension, which exaggerates the difficulties of an operation already difficult enough. It increases bleeding from the scalp, which, with the adrenalin-novocain solution, is rendered negligible. It encourages the use of rougher methods, which a patient under local anesthesia would not tolerate, and which therefore are in all likelihood harmful. It encourages speed, which is to be decried if employed at the expense of delicacy. It leaves many patients, particularly those with threatened respiratory difficulties, in a condition in which inhalation troubles are prone to occur.

Until recovery from a general anesthetic is complete every patient should be under close observation, and this, at a casualty clearing station at least, is an impossibility. It is very rare, and then only in the case of semiconscious patients or those with restless irritability, that the operation cannot be carried through under local anesthesia, though this necessitates more gentle manipulations than those usually employed, particularly during the process of removing the area of cranial involvement.[12]

In the 60 years since the above words were written we have seen many changes in the practice of neuroanesthesia. Despite Dr. Cushing's warning, local anesthesia has given way to general anesthesia. Because of the improved operating conditions associated with hyperventilation, spontaneous ventilation as an anesthetic technique has virtually disappeared.

The use of hypothermia has decreased in the last decade. A recent symposium in the *British Journal of Anaesthesia* on neurosurgical anesthesia makes little or no mention of hypothermia.[37] The popularity of halothane has fluctuated over the past few years. The increasing use of intracranial pressure monitoring, especially in patients with brain tumors and head injuries, has led many anesthetists to reevaluate the role of halothane during neurosurgical procedures and to use it mainly as an adjunctive agent, not as the primary anesthetic drug. Intracranial pressure monitoring devices have moved from being research tools to being useful agents in the operating rooms and in intensive care units. Evidence from animal studies[34,45] seems to show that barbiturates have a protective effect on the brain. In the next decade we may see increasing use of barbiturate infusions both in the operating room and during the postoperative period so that postoperative neurosurgical patients may be returned to the intensive care unit, with their tracheas intubated and a barbiturate infused intravenously for many hours following surgery.

PRESSURE VOLUME CURVES

As a supratentorial mass expands, it produces certain well-defined effects, as may be seen on a pressure-volume compliance curve (Fig. 8-1). The cranium may be regarded as a semiclosed, nondistensible box. This box contains brain matter, cerebrospinal fluid (CSF), and blood, all of which are relatively incompressible. As the mass gradually enlarges, CSF is shifted from within the skull into the spinal subarachnoid space, thus preventing an increase in intracranial pressure (ICP) from its normal value of 10 to 15 torr. The ICP increase is further compensated for by increased absorption of CSF. This situation may be seen in the compli-

ance curve diagram as the change from 1 to 2. Point 2 on the curve represents decreased intracranial compliance. At point 3 (increased ICP) even small increases in volume result in marked increases in intracranial pressure (point 4). It is at any point on the curve, but especially points 3 and 4, that anesthetic agents and techniques that affect cerebral blood volume can alter intracranial pressure to the patient's detriment.

The clinical implication is that patients with supratentorial lesions may lie somewhere along a compliance curve such as this one. Between points 1 and 2 there may be minimal clinical signs or symptoms. Patients whose pressure-volume status is between points 2 and 4 may present with the classic signs and symptoms of increased ICP, that is, increasing drowsiness, headache, nausea, and papilledema.

If the intracranial pressure continues to increase, cerebral perfusion pressure (CPP) decreases. Cerebral perfusion pressure is defined as mean arterial blood pressure minus intracranial pressure (MAP − ICP). Should cerebral perfusion pressure decrease, there is a compensatory increase in blood pressure that maintains perfusion pressure. Ultimately this compensatory mechanism

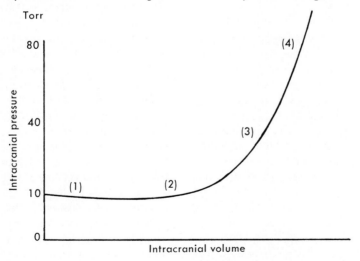

Fig. 8-1. Schematic representation of the cerebral pressure volume curve. Relatively flat part of curve *(1-2)* represents compensatory phase. Steep part of curve *(3-4)* indicates that a small change in volume will cause a steep increase in ICP. (From Shapiro, H. M.: Anesthesiology **43**:445, 1975.)

fails, and cerebral ischemia occurs. Quite apart from focal or global ischemia, an increase in ICP may lead to brain shifts, either across the midline or through the foramen magnum or tentorium. Cerebral blood flow and intracranial pressure are influenced by many factors, some of which are under the control of the anesthesiologist. These include changes in arterial carbon dioxide tension (Pa_{CO_2}) and arterial oxygen tension (Pa_{O_2}), changes in blood pressure, both arterial and venous and, of major importance, the effect of anesthetic agents and techniques.

FACTORS INFLUENCING CEREBRAL BLOOD FLOW AND INTRACRANIAL PRESSURE
Carbon dioxide

Carbon dioxide is a potent physiologic mediator of cerebrovascular tone. Put simply, an increase in arterial carbon dioxide partial pressure (Pa_{CO_2}) to 80 torr will double cerebral blood flow; a decrease in Pa_{CO_2} to 20 torr will decrease cerebral blood flow by one-half with consequent lowering of intracranial pressure.[85] This hypocapnic lowering of the intracranial pressure forms the basis of present-day neuroanesthesia.

Several authors have pointed out the similarity between extreme hyperventilation (Pa_{CO_2} below 25 torr) and arterial hypoxemia. The evidence that low Pa_{CO_2} levels lead to cerebral tissue hypoxia is indicated by functional changes, such as alterations in the critical flicker fusion frequency and in reaction time, by EEG changes, and by metabolic abnormalities.[10,65] Recommendations of "safe" limits for hyperventilation have been made by Harp and Wollman.[21] They point out that normal humans can tolerate hyperventilation to a Pa_{CO_2} of 20 torr for several hours with no cerebral metabolic decompensation. Tolerance to hypocarbia appears to depend on two major reserve mechanisms: first, the presence of cerebral blood flow sufficient to maintain adequate cerebral tissue P_{O_2} levels and also to remove products of metabolism; second, the ability of the brain to generate energy by anaerobic mechanisms. However, blood flow may be abnormal in and around brain tumors. It has been known for many years that vasomotor paralysis may occur in and around tumor areas or areas of cerebral infarction. Acid metabolites from the tumor diffuse into the surrounding tissues. The low pH engendered causes vasodilatation and an increase in blood flow. This has been termed "luxury perfusion."[31] Vasomotor paralysis may occur within focal ischemic areas, and these vessels then lose their reactivity to CO_2.

If Pa_{CO_2} is allowed to increase, blood will be shunted away from the ischemic area (vessels already maximally dilated) to the nonischemic area. This phenomenon has been termed the intracerebral steal syndrome. The inverse steal, or Robin Hood, phenomenon is seen in response to hypocarbia. Here, as CO_2 is lowered, the normal vessels constrict and blood is diverted to the already maximally dilated diseased area.[32]

Having considered the effects of CO_2 on normal and abnormal brain, what clinical recommendations can be made for patients who are to be ventilated? It can be said that hyperventilation is beneficial in that oxygenation and CO_2 removal are assured, cerebral blood flow and ICP are decreased, and a "slack" brain is produced. However, it may be prudent to keep Pa_{CO_2} at levels of 30 torr in patients whose cerebral circulation is bordering on the inadequate. These include elderly patients with cardiovascular disease and those patients in whom deliberate hypotension is to be instituted. In patients whose cerebral circulation is normal, Pa_{CO_2} levels of 25 to 30 torr are commonly used in neuroanesthetic practice and would appear to be safe levels.

Finally what can one say about the importance of the steal phenomena. It seems clear from clinical evidence that steal and inverse steal do occur, but that these effects may be rare. In the absence of regional cerebral blood flow measurements it is not known if any individual patient will respond physiologically or paradoxically to alteration in Pa_{CO_2}. Hence, the rationale of treating focal ischemia with hypocarbia or hypercarbia is doubtful, and the best course of action may be to maintain Pa_{CO_2} at the level of 25 to 35 torr.

Oxygen

The importance of adequate oxygenation is self-evident. If Pa_{O_2} is lowered while Pa_{CO_2} is maintained constant in awake humans, CBF is unaffected until Pa_{O_2} decreases below 50 torr. At this point cerebral vasodilatation occurs and CBF increases[10] (Fig. 8-2). It should be noted that hypoxia and hypercapnia produce synergistic effects and increase CBF more than either factor alone.[61]

Blood pressure

The ability of the brain to maintain its perfusion pressure over a wide range of blood pressure is known as autoregulation (Fig. 8-2). Autoregulation is in the nature of an active vascular response in that arteriolar constriction results from an increase in perfusion pressure and arteriolar dilatation from a decrease in perfusion pressure. Upper and lower limits for autoregulation have been defined. Below a mean blood pressure of 60 torr; CBF decreases; that is, autoregula-

tion is lost and CBF becomes entirely pressure-dependent.[78] At a mean pressure of 40 to 55 torr, symptoms of cerebral ischemia appear in the form of nausea, dizziness, and slow cerebration. In the normal brain the upper limit of autoregulation is 125 to 140 torr. Autoregulation "breakthrough" occurs at high arterial pressure and the blood-brain barrier is disrupted, which leads to forced vasodilatation with focal plasma leakage and consequent cerebral edema.[63,71]

In addition to the change produced by variations in Pa_{CO_2} levels, the tumor circulation may respond abnormally to variations in arterial blood pressure. Normally CBF would not alter with moderate increase or decrease in blood pressure if autoregulation is normal. However, autoregulation may be impaired in tumor circulation and increase in blood pressure may lead to increase in CBF and vice versa. The failure of autoregulation in tumor circulations may be due to local tissue acidosis around the tumor, leading to maximum vasodilation of the tumor vessels so that flow becomes dependent on perfusion pressure (analogous to the cause of steal and reverse steal conditions).

The ability of the brain to autoregulate may be lost in a variety of other conditions. Apart from cerebral tumors and infarcts,

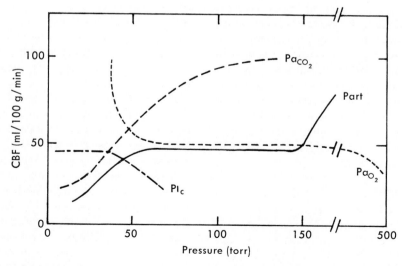

Fig. 8-2. Schematic control of cerebral blood flow. *Part* shows limits of autoregulation, Pa_{CO_2}, Pa_{O_2}, and chemical control of CBF. PI_c represents intracranial pressure.

these include hematoma, and hypoxia, or hypercapnia.[15,50]

In hypertensive patients both the lower and upper thresholds of autoregulation are set higher. Patients with chronic hypertension may have a shift to the right in their autoregulation curve so that a blood pressure at 60 torr does not provide adequate CBF. Mean blood pressure values of 80 to 90 torr or greater may be necessary to maintain adequate CBF.[14]

As can be seen from the above discussion the cerebral circulation may be abnormal in many conditions and thus not able to compensate for lowering of blood pressure, either induced or unexpected. Consequently, moderate hypotension may lead to cerebral ischemia. In fact, if deliberate hypotension is to be used as an anesthetic technique, it may be in this instance that the use of hypothermia may provide some protection against inadequate cerebral perfusion.[41] Conversely, as we have seen, sudden hypertension should be guarded against as this may lead to sudden increases in CBF, cerebral blood volume, ICP, and cerebral edema. If anesthesia is deepened, the hypertensive response may be attenuated.

The clinical lesson that should be learned is that blood pressure should be maintained at or near normal values during anesthesia in patients with abnormalities of cerebral circulation unless, of course, induced hypotensive anesthesia is to be carried out. Hypertensive incidents may occur during the conduct of any anesthetic, but they are commonest during laryngoscopy and intubation, when the skin is incised, and during extubation and recovery from surgery.[20,24,33,34,56] Hypertensive episodes should be guarded against especially zealously in patients with disturbed autoregulation.

Venous pressure

Venous pressure is usually low in the supine and erect positions. Arterial pressure is then the effective perfusion pressure. Should cerebral blood flow increase, venous pressure may also increase due to the guarding of the venous exits by either bony orifices or the rigidity of the dural layers surrounding the intracranial venous sinuses.[38a]

Increase in central venous pressure is directly transmitted to the intracranial veins and may also increase CSF pressure secondarily to pressure changes in the vertebral canal[82] as well as cause an increase in bleeding. Such incidents as coughing or straining on the endotracheal tube, excessive flexion or extension of the neck, the head-down position, securing the endotracheal tube by overzealous bandaging may increase intracranial pressure by obstructing cerebral venous outflow. Every effort should be made to avoid causing the above incidents.

Anesthetic drugs

Of primary concern to anesthetists is the effect of anesthetic agents on the cerebral circulation. Failure to appreciate the effects of anesthetic drugs on cerebral blood flow may have disastrous consequences for the patient. At best they may lead to poor operating conditions due to a bulging brain; at worst they may lead to sudden death from brain herniation.

With regard to their effect on cerebral blood flow (and ICP) anesthetic drugs may be classified into two groups. In the first group are those that cause cerebral vasodilatation, including the inhalation agents. In the second group are the intravenous anesthetic agents, which, with the exception of ketamine, curare, and succinylcholine, cause cerebral vasoconstriction (Table 8-1).

As has been mentioned previously, patients with brain tumors may have abnormal cerebral circulations. Effects of acute brain disease may be manifested as brain tissue acidosis and loss of autoregulation, metabolic control of tissue perfusion (the luxury perfusion syndrome), and reactivity to CO_2.

Volatile anesthetic agents can modify the autoregulatory response. With a progressive increase in dose of the volatile agent the plateau portion of the autoregulatory curve diminishes and higher cerebral blood flow occurs at the same perfusion pressure.[45a] If autoregulation is disturbed, the anesthetic drugs that produce inadvertent hypotension

Table 8-1. Effect of anesthetic agents on intracranial pressure and cerebral blood flow

Agent	CBF change	ICP change
Induction		
Thiopental	↓	↓
Althesin	↓	↓
Ketamine	↑	↑
Muscle relaxants		
Succinylcholine	?	↑
Tubocurarine	↑	↑
Pancuronium	0 or ↓	0 or ↓
Inhalational agents		
Nitrous oxide	↑	↑
Halothane	↑	↑
Enflurane	↑	↑
Intravenous		
Narcotics	↓	↓

may lead to episodes of global or regional ischemia.[13] On the other hand, if anesthetic drugs are allowed to increase CO_2, not only will ICP increase (an undesirable effect), but an intracerebral steal may shunt blood away from diseased areas to more normal areas of the brain. It should be emphasized that steals and loss of autoregulation do not invariably occur.[22,87] Ischemic brain may show only autoregulatory impairment, only steal (intracerebral or inverse), or any combination thereof.

Inhalation agents

Halothane, which will be discussed as a prototype of the inhalational agents, has been shown in many studies to be a cerebral vasodilator.[84] The effect of inhalation agents on patients with space-occupying lesions as opposed to patients with normal ICP is important. Normally an increase in ICP is compensated for by displacement of CSF from the cranium. In patients with chronically increased ICP this mechanism may fail and ICP may increase dramatically. Agents such as halothane, methoxyflurane, and trichlorethylene produce slight increases in the ICP in patients with normal CSF pathways; however, marked increases in ICP may occur in patients with space-occupying

lesions.[29] This increase in ICP may be attenuated either by hyperventilation (introduced prior to the inhalational agents) or by barbiturates.[1,58] It should be noted that the halothane effect on ICP is dose related and is minimal at 0.5 minimal alveolar concentration (MAC) or less. From a clinical point of view it should be realized that despite these maneuvers, intracranial compliance may not be improved. This situation may occur when the blood-brain barrier is disrupted or when CO_2 responsiveness is lost. Typically this situation is seen in and around brain tumors.

The newer agent enflurane increases ICP. In fact, like halothane, enflurane could cause sudden large increases in ICP with patients with space-occupying lesions.[46] Again, as with halothane, hypocapnia does not always protect against an increase in ICP. Another drawback to the use of enflurane in neurosurgical anesthesia is its ability to cause convulsions and spike wave EEG activity. These may be caused by a combination of high concentrations of enflurane together with marked hyperventilation.[7,70]

In summary, all the commonly used inhalational agents, including nitrous oxide, cause increases in ICP. The clinical lesson to be learned seems to indicate that in the presence of increased intracranial pressure these agents should not be used or used in limited doses (e.g., > 0.5 MAC for halothane). The rationale for not wishing to use such useful agents as these is that attenuation of the ICP increase with barbiturates and hyperventilation prior to the introduction of the inhalational agent may fail and the ICP may increase markedly. Such an increase in ICP may lead to cerebral ischemia from decreased perfusion pressure or even to brain herniation.

Intravenous agents

Barbiturates. It has been known for many years that barbiturates produce a pronounced dose-dependent cerebral vasoconstriction in humans. During normocapnia, thiopental anesthesia causes a decrease in cerebral oxygen consumption ($CMRO_2$) and

CBF. If hypocapnia is instituted, CBF decreases even more.[49] More importantly, recent animal studies indicate that barbiturates may decrease acute ischemic and hypoxic brain damage.[45,64] In animal studies, doses varied from thiopental 40 mg/kg or pentobarbital 55 mg/kg in the dog and 14 mg/kg pentobarbital in the Java monkey.

Michenfelder and Theye[44] believe that the protective effects of barbiturates lie in their ability to decrease $CMRO_2$ in actively functioning neurons. Hypothermia, on the other hand, is believed to protect cerebral function by its ability to decrease the energy requirements of all cerebral functions. Smith proposes that barbiturates protect primarily by decreasing cerebral blood flow, cerebral blood volume and, hence, ICP. Metabolic depression is of secondary importance. If this theory is correct, it might be expected that protection from acute ischemia is produced by other agents that cause decrease in CBF and ICP. Such drugs as the neuroleptic drugs, opiates, and steroid anesthetics cause a decrease in either CBF or ICP.

The clinical implications are obvious. If protection of the brain in acute ischemia can be afforded by drugs that decrease CBF or ICP, perhaps the agents of choice for maintenance of anesthesia should be either barbiturates, narcotics (see below), or neuroleptic agents. Hunter has recommended continuous intravenous barbiturate infusion as a suitable anesthetic technique in patients with intracranial tumors.[26]

Althesin. This recently (1971) introduced drug is a steroid induction agent and may well prove a useful agent in neuroanesthesia. Unfortunately it is not released for use in the United States. It decreases CBF, $CMRO_2$, and ICP in much the same way as thiopental does.[48,73] Its distinct advantages are that rapid recovery is usual and the incidence of postoperative vomiting is low. Althesin can be used as an induction agent or, more logically, as a constant infusion for maintenance of anesthesia.

Ketamine. This drug probably has no useful part to play in neuroanesthesia. It causes marked increases in CBF with increase in ICP both in normal and abnormal brain.[59,75] These effects can be attenuated with prior doses of thiopental.[86] However, the effect of ketamine on ICP may not be totally blocked and so may still increase ICP. Ketamine also has a stimulant effect on the CNS as evidenced in EEG studies. One other major drawback is that in the epileptic patient it can initiate seizures.[5] For all these reasons it is not recommended for neuroanesthesia.

Muscle relaxants. Succinylcholine hydrochloride has been in use as a muscle relaxant since 1949. Although a most useful agent, it has several disadvantages in neuroanesthesia. It is not uncommon to have to administer anesthesia to patients with muscle wasting disease or spinal cord injuries. Succinylcholine, if given during the early weeks of paresis, may lead to cardiac arrest. This is presumed to be due to potassium release from denervated muscle.[77] Another disadvantage of succinylcholine lies in the substantial increase in ICP it causes.[19,66] This increase in ICP is presumed to be due to the rapid and massive muscular twitching that increases both intra-abdominal and intrathoracic pressures. It could be expected that pretreatment with a nondepolarizing drug may diminish the increase in ICP. However, in patients with an increased ICP, it may be better to avoid the use of succinylcholine altogether.

Curare has also been implicated in the causation of increased ICP accompanied by a decrease in blood pressure and CPP. It is believed that histamine release is responsible for the increase in ICP.[76] The recently introduced muscle relaxant pancuronium bromide now appears to be the muscle relaxant of choice in neuroanesthesia. It has rapid onset of action, provides excellent relaxation for intubations and causes little histamine release. Unlike curare, it appears to cause little or no increase in ICP. A disadvantage is its penchant for causing an increase in pulse rate and blood pressure with perhaps an increase in ICP.

Narcotics. One of the main disadvantages of the inhalation agents is their propensity for causing increases in CBF and ICP, especially in patients with space-occupying lesions. It is of interest, therefore, that we do have drugs in our armamentarium that do not cause increases in CBF and ICP provided PCO_2 and blood pressure are kept within normal limits.

Morphine and meperidine both cause a progressive and parallel decrease in $CMRO_2$ and CBF.[39,81] In dogs, fentanyl causes a marked and short-lasting decrease in CBF and $CMRO_2$. Droperidol was found to be a more potent and longer acting cerebral vasoconstrictor than fentanyl.[44] For the purposes of anesthesia these agents may be administered either singly or in combination (Innovar). It has been demonstrated that in patients with both normal and abnormal CSF pathways, neuroleptanesthesia can lead to a decrease in ICP, probably due to a fall in CBF.[16]

As we have seen, control of CBF and ICP can be influenced by the anesthetic drugs and techniques. As clinicians, how best can we use the agents and techniques to achieve the maximum benefit for the neurosurgical patient?

First, agents that cause an increase in CBF should be avoided because of their tendency to increase ICP and cause a steal. Second, hypotension and hypertension should be avoided. If autoregulation is disturbed, hypotension may lead to cerebral ischemia; conversely, hypertension can cause further disruption of the blood-brain barrier and consequent hyperemia and cerebral edema. Third, deep barbiturate anesthesia may cause brain tissue to become more tolerant of moderate degrees of oligemia or hypoxemia. Finally, as we have noted previously, it may be possible to improve the perfusion of ischemic areas of the brain by inducing vasoconstriction (the inverse steal).

Hence, to sum up, the anesthetic technique chosen should encourage moderate cerebral vasoconstriction. Blood pressure should be maintained at normal or just below normal levels. Hypertension should be guarded against.

Among the drugs we have today the bar-biturates are perhaps the most suitable, as they cause proportional decreases in cerebral metabolism and flow. Other useful agents are the neuroleptic drugs. Inhalation agents such as halothane should only be used if hyperventilation is instituted prior to its introduction, CO_2 levels are kept at 25 to 30 torr, and dosage levels are kept below 0.5 MAC.

MONITORING OF THE NEUROSURGICAL PATIENT

The neurosurgical patient requires the same monitoring devices as are used during routine surgery. However, more sophisticated monitoring techniques may provide a greater margin of safety for the patient during complicated operative procedures. Induced hypotension, surgery near the vital centers of the brain, the sitting position, and the removal of vascular tumors provide examples of situations in which patient care may be improved by more elaborate monitoring.

Cardiovascular system

The esophageal stethoscope provides a simple, safe, and inexpensive monitor. Heart tones and breath sounds are easily heard, and arrhythmias can be detected. Continuous monitoring of breath sounds is particularly important because the upper torso and head are covered by drapes, making visualization of the connections of the breathing circuit to the patient difficult. The first sign of a disconnection would be a loss of breath sounds. Blood pressure measurements may be taken using a sphygmomanometer or, more usual in neurosurgical cases, directly using an intra-arterial catheter. The indications for the use of direct or arterial line vary with the individual anesthetist. It is extremely useful to monitor blood pressure beat by beat during the removal of vascular tumors or during induced hypotension. In these cases should therapeutic intervention be required it can be done with minimum delay. Another advantage of an indwelling arterial line is that blood gas measurements can be easily measured. The

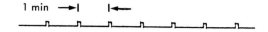

Fig. 8-3. Effect of hyperventilation at *H*. Hyperventilation commences at 0. End-tidal CO_2 decreases to approximately 21 torr after six breaths. (From Whitcher, C. E.: CO_2 monitoring in anesthesia: an audio-visual program, presented at the American Society of Anesthesiologists' meeting, October 1977.)

dorsalis pedis artery is particularly suitable for neuroanesthesia as it is easy to cannulate and readily accessible.[67]

The electrocardiogram (ECG) is useful not only for the detection (and treatment) of arrhythmias but for several other reasons. Patients with brain tumors (and other CNS lesions) sometimes show various ECG abnormalities. It is possible that these are due to centrally mediated increase in sympathetic tone, possibly due to the increased ICP.[27] However, transient cerebral ischemia may be due to cardiac arrhythmias. Whatever the cause it certainly is appropriate to monitor these patients with an ECG. In the detection of venous air embolism the ECG is extremely useful. Any alteration in rate or rhythm in the semirecumbent patient should alert one to the likelihood of air being entrained and the surgeon should be notified immediately and steps taken to remove the air. Finally surgically induced arrhythmias are not uncommon during brain surgery. They are usually secondary to stimulation of vital centers or cranial nerves. It would be extremely difficult to diagnose and treat these potentially life-threatening arrhythmias without the use of an ECG.

Ventilation

Nowadays the lungs of most neurosurgical patients are mechanically ventilated. Arterial blood gas values are regularly monitored, as are inspired oxygen concentration, tidal and minute volume, frequency of respiration, and the pressure within the anesthetic system. End-tidal CO_2 ($ETCO_2$) monitoring is now relatively easy using an infrared analyzer. In patients with no evidence of cardiorespiratory disease it gives a good reflection of Pa_{CO_2}. The end-tidal CO_2 monitor is of particular value during neurosurgical procedures to maintain the required degree of hypocapnia (Fig. 8-3). In the detection of venous air embolism, capnography provides a somewhat less sensitive indicator than the Doppler method (Fig. 8-4). However, unlike the Doppler method it is unaffected by the electrosurgical unit. Air in the right side of the heart may cause mechanical obstruction to the pulmonary outflow with consequent decrease in Pa_{CO_2} caused by an increase in dead space. Brechner and Bethune view any decrease in end-tidal CO_2 as presumptive evidence of air embolism.[6]

Urinary output

A satisfactory urinary output (over 60 ml/ hour) gives some evidence of the adequacy of renal perfusion. In patients undergoing induced hypotension or in patients in whom blood loss may be extensive the urinary output provides a good monitor of renal per-

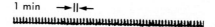

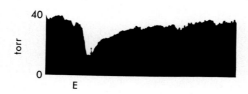

Fig. 8-4. Effect of air embolism. At *E* air embolism occurred with reduction of end-tidal CO_2 to approximately 14 torr. (From Whitcher, C. E.: CO_2 monitoring in anesthesia: an audio-visual program, presented at the American Society of Anesthesiologists' meeting, October 1977.)

fusion pressure. Following the use of osmotic diuretic agents the use of a urinary catheter is helpful to avoid undue bladder distension (1 to 2 liters of urine can be passed within an hour). Once diuretic agents are used, urinary output will no longer be a suitable monitor of renal perfusion.

Temperature

Decreases in body temperature are common during craniotomy. Cold operating rooms, cold intravenous fluids, and heat loss from the craniotomy site can cause a marked decrease in temperature. The effects of hypothermia may not be altogether beneficial. It may lead to increased peripheral resistance and increased myocardial work. The effect of the depolarizing muscle relaxants may be potentiated. Shivering in the postoperative patient leads to increased oxygen consumption. For the above reasons it is useful to monitor temperature and be able to take remedial action if necessary. The reverse situation can occur, and temperature may increase to high levels. Again this may be iatrogenic, due in part to warm operating rooms or heavy surgical draping. However, sudden increase in temperature may herald the onset of malignant hyperthermia. Finally, it should be remembered that small children lose heat easily and that temperature can decrease rapidly in these small

patients. Here again temperature monitoring should be performed routinely, and methods should be available to prevent undue hypothermia.

Muscle relaxation

It is vitally important that neurosurgical patients do not move, cough, or buck during surgery, and many anesthetists use muscle relaxants as an integral part of their anesthetic technique. The use of a peripheral nerve stimulator is a simple way to monitor muscle relaxation and rather more elegant than the cookbook approach of "2 mg of pancuronium every 40 minutes."

Intracranial pressure monitoring

Lundberg described three pressure waves in patients with brain tumors. Of the three, the plateau or A wave is the most significant.[35] These plateau waves are characterized by a sudden increase in ICP up to 80 to 100 torr, which lasts for 10 to 20 min. Following the wave, ICP decreases rapidly to below its previous level.[51] During the sustained increase in pressure, patients are symptomatic and may hyperventilate. The importance of plateau waves lies in the fact that they may be initiated by anxiety, pain, and the induction of anesthesia.[40] Patients exhibiting plateau waves may have little intracerebral compensatory space left. As mentioned previously and reiterated, the danger of increased intracranial pressure lies in the decrease in cerebral perfusion pressure that occurs when ICP increases. At first, increased blood pressure will compensate. If ICP continues to increase, cerebral ischemia may ensue. Increase in ICP may decrease flow through poorly perfused areas of the brain, or, of more importance, herniation of brain tissue may occur through the foramen magnum or through the tentorium. Intracranial pressure monitoring is now available in the operating room and intensive care units. Measurements are commonly made with a catheter placed in the ventricular system or in the epidural, subdural, or subarachnoid spaces and connected to an extracranial transducer. With ICP monitoring the conduct of anesthesia and surgery can be made safer. The disaster of increases in ICP and consequent decreases in CPP may be guarded against more easily and the end result may be to decrease mortality and morbidity preoperatively, intraoperatively, and postoperatively.

PREOPERATIVE ASSESSMENT AND MEDICATION OF THE PATIENT WITH BRAIN TUMOR
Assessment

The preoperative assessment of patients with brain tumor differs in several ways from that made during routine surgical procedures. The special aspects of preoperative evaluation of neurosurgical patients lie in the importance of detecting preoperative evidence of increased ICP. The importance of not allowing ICP to increase during anesthesia has been stressed—it should be remembered that inappropriate premedication may cause a dramatic increase in ICP due to hypoventilation, which may manifest itself as a deepening of the level of unconsciousness. From the surgeon's point of view this may pose a problem in diagnosis as it could be attributed to an intracranial bleed. Cerebral ischemia due to vascular disease (such as hypertension) should be a warning that the brain may tolerate hypotension poorly as autoregulation may be disrupted. Again, every effort should be made not to bring hypertensive patients to the operating room with their "pressure in their boots." The use of alpha adrenergic receptor blocking agents may be an inappropriate choice in such patients. Pneumoencephalography may not only disturb cerebral hemodynamics preoperatively but also intraoperatively. Saidman and Eger have shown that if air is used as the contrast medium, the use of intraoperative nitrous oxide will lead to significant increases in ICP. It may take several days for air to be absorbed from the ventricles,[54] and this fact should be remembered during the preoperative visit.

Patients with disorders of the pituitary gland present various problems in preoperative assessment. These problems are manifested in two ways: as pressure effects from the tumor or as abnormalities in endocrine production.

As a tumor of the anterior pituitary increases in size it may cause signs and symptoms ranging from visual defects to hydrocephalus. These tumors may encroach on third, fourth, and fifth cranial nerves as well as on the third ventricle. Perhaps of more immediate importance is the endocrine abnormalities that may be caused by the tumor. Should endocrine production be excessive, Cushing syndrome may result from the excessive secretion of adrenocorticotrophic hormone (ACTH). If increase in growth hormone (GH) occurs, gigantism or acromegaly results. If endocrine production is deficient, secondary hypothyroidism may occur due to deficiency in thyroid stimulating hormone (TSH). Similarly, should ACTH production be decreased, secondary adrenal failure may occur. If deficiency of antidiuretic hormone (ADH) occurs, diabetes insipidus may ensue.

Every effort should be made to correct endocrine abnormalities before surgery. Of particular importance is the correction in patients with minimal adrenal reserves. Should this not be possible or should unexplained hypotension occur during or following surgery, treatment with intravenous steroids should be instituted.

The physical characteristics of acromegalic

patients pose problems. The large head, mandible, and tongue may make mask ventilation, laryngoscopy, and intubation extremely difficult. It should also be remembered that diabetes mellitus, coronary artery disease, and cardiomyopathies are common among this group.

In the absence of ICP monitoring (and this may be the situation faced by many anesthetists in their practice) signs of increased ICP should be looked for during the preoperative visit. The symptoms and signs that should be looked for include history of nausea and vomiting or alterations in the level of consciousness. Eye signs such as dilatation of the pupils and decreased reactivity to light may be synonomous with increasing ICP, as are papilledema, bradycardia, hypertension, and disturbances in respiration. X-ray evidence and computerized axial tomography (CAT or EMI scan) may provide evidence of brain shift.

Premedication

The purpose of premedication in surgery is to allay anxiety, help smooth the induction and maintenance of anesthesia, and to protect the patient from potentially undesirably vagal reflexes. Neurosurgical patients differ from other patients in that they usually have either increased intracranial pressure or disturbances of cerebral autoregulation. Hence any drug given to the neurosurgical patient must take into account not only the drug effect on the patient's cardiorespiratory system but also the consequent secondary effects on cerebral perfusion.

It must be remembered that patients with intracranial pathology may be extremely sensitive to central nervous system depressants. The narcotics, useful agents that they are, have three main drawbacks in the premedication of the neurosurgical patient. First, by causing hypoventilation they may lead to increased CBF and consequent increase in ICP. Second, they may cause a decrease in the patient's level of consciousness. The third main disadvantage of the narcotic drugs is their propensity for causing nausea and vomiting, two of the common

presenting complaints in patients with brain tumors. The iatrogenic occurrence of these symptoms is not readily appreciated by patient, surgeon, or anesthetist immediately prior to surgery.

If narcotics are to used in premedication, they should only be used in small doses and in those patients who show little or no signs of increased ICP. Antiemetic drugs may be a useful addition, for example, a drug such as hydroxyzine, which has sedative and antiemetic effects and has little effect on the cardiorespiratory system. To protect against excessive upper and lower airway secretions and vagal reflexes, atropine is commonly used.

To sum up, in the lethargic, obviously obtunded patient no premedication or atropine only is given. In the patient with no or minimal symptoms of increased ICP, a narcotic antiemetic combination may be useful. This should be given in small doses, and atropine is commonly added. In the gray area between these two extremes, premedication depends to a large extent on the experience of the anesthetist. One drug that may play some part in this gray zone in the extremely anxious patient is diazepam. This drug causes little respiratory depression, promotes amnesia, and has little effect on ICP. In cases of doubt no premedication is the safest premedication.

Induction and intubation

There is no ideal anesthetic agent in the conduct of neuroanesthesia. Each individual agent has its advantages and disadvantages and a drug that may be suitable for one neurosurgical patient may be entirely unsuitable for another.

The principles underlying the conduct of anesthesia can be summed up as follows. The drugs used should have little effect on intracranial pressure and cause little in the way of depressive effects on cardiovascular, respiratory, or other organ systems. Blood pressure swings should be avoided as autoregulation may be lost or impaired in patients with brain tumors.

Induction should be rapid and smooth

and endotracheal intubation attempted only when total paralysis of skeletal muscles has occurred. No coughing or movements should be allowed to occur during induction and maintenance of anesthesia. Finally, emergence and extubation of the trachea should be as smooth as induction of anesthesia and intubation of the trachea. The reasons for smoothness in anesthetic technique are clear. Any movement in a patient undergoing abdominal surgery is of little importance. In patients undergoing craniotomy such movement can lead to disastrous increases in ICP, excessive bleeding into the wound, and perhaps most serious of all, a brain that continues to bulge from the wound, making surgical exposure virtually impossible. With these principles in mind and with an awareness of the deficiencies in the drugs available and the cerebral pathophysiology involved, the anesthesic agents and techniques should be planned for each individual patient.

When the patient arrives in the operating suite, an intravenous infusion is started. Simple monitoring devices such as a sphygmomanometer and ECG are attached. Following preoxygenation and spontaneous hyperventilation, anesthesia is induced with thiopental in sufficiently large doses to produce unconsciousness and narcotic as needed. This is followed by pancuronium bromide in an intubating dose of 0.12 mg/ kg. As previously mentioned, pancuronium is probably the relaxant of choice, as both succinylcholine and curare can cause an increase in intracranial pressure. At this stage respiration is controlled with moderate hyperventilation. The use of an end-tidal CO_2 monitor can make controlled hyperventilation extremely easy (Fig. 8-3). When the patient is totally relaxed, as evidenced by little or no neuromuscular response to peripheral nerve stimulation, intubation of the trachea is carried out using a flexometallic tube. To help prevent any increase in ICP and blood pressure, a bolus of sodium thiopental is given prior to intubation. This, together with muscle relaxation, an adequate dose of narcotics, and

topical anesthesia to the lower airway, helps diminish the hypertensive response to laryngoscopy.[58] Following intubation, bilateral breath sounds are listened for, nitrous oxide is added to the inspired gas mixture, and mechanical ventilation of the lungs is carried out by means of a respirator. If added before hyperventilation, nitrous oxide may, like all other inhalational agents, lead to an increase in ICP.[23] As noted previously, nitrous oxide may be contraindicated following pneumoencephalography. Ventilation is controlled to set a Pa_{CO_2} of 25 to 35 torr. Application of benzoin solution to the skin will help secure the endotracheal tube so that it will not become loosened by secretions. It is mandatory that the endotracheal tube be secure as it is a major disaster if dislodged during surgery. A flexometallic tube may be useful if kinking of the tube is likely to occur. This may happen if the neck is well flexed during posterior fossa surgery or cervical laminectomy surgery. Craniotomy for supratentorial tumors is usually carried out with the patient supine and the head elevated 10 to 15 degrees to facilitate venous drainage. As in any surgical procedure, attention to detail may help prevent peripheral nerve and eye injuries. Anesthesia should be deep enough to prevent coughing or straining on the tube during shaving and positioning of the head. At this stage an arterial catheter may be inserted if deemed necessary, as well as a second intravenous catheter if heavy blood loss is anticipated. Fluid therapy is of particular importance in the neurosurgical patient as inappropriate therapy may lead to brain edema and increase in ICP. Such a situation might occur if solutions such as dextrose 5% in water are given. Glucose and water solution is rapidly distributed through total body water. Blood glucose may decrease more rapidly than brain glucose, so that brain water becomes relatively hyperosmolar and the brain tissue accumulates water, which leads to brain edema.[83] Hypertonic salt solutions such as dextrose 5% in lactated Ringer solution appear to be the fluid of choice. An added advantage is that it will initially decrease brain water. It is particularly easy to overload patients with fluid during the induction of anesthesia, and care should be taken to avoid overhydrating neurosurgical patients.

Maintenance and recovery from anesthesia

One of the major advances in neuroanesthesia was the institution of controlled ventilation of the neurosurgical patient. From the surgeon's point of view, the relaxed brain facilitates operative exposure of the deeper cerebral structures. The benefits to the anesthesiologist and, of course, the patient lie in satisfactory oxygenation and carbon dioxide removal, the elimination of bucking and straining during surgery, and a decrease in intracranial pressure. As mentioned previously, hyperventilation should be moderate (25 to 35 torr). Pa_{CO_2} can be monitored by means of a previously placed intra-arterial line or on a breath-to-breath basis by an end-tidal CO_2 monitor.

The anesthetic technique chosen should be one that will have minimal effect on ICP. Hence, a popular technique is one that combines nitrous oxide and narcotic agents with moderate hyperventilation. If necessary, small amounts of halothane (less than 0.5%) may be added to prevent any undesirable increases in blood pressure. As always when scrupulous attention is paid to the patient's vital signs, increases in pulse and blood pressure will alert the anesthetist to deepen anesthesia. Painful stimuli may lead to cerebral vasodilation, and increase in CBF and ICP and should be prevented by adequate anesthesia. Muscle relaxation should be monitored with a peripheral nerve stimulator.

Once the dura is closed, preparations should be made to ensure that the patient awakens from anesthesia smoothly, without coughing in response to the endotracheal tube. This may be extremely difficult to achieve. Resorting to small doses of thiopental or succinylcholine immediately before bandaging the head may allow smooth emergence and extubation. Suctioning of the mouth and pharynx should be carried out before reversing the muscle relaxant. Occasionally naloxone may be required to reverse narcotic effects. All too often a smooth anesthetic is marred by coughing, straining, breath holding, and blood pressure variations in the immediate postoperative period, usually before or following extubation. It may be that the current neurosurgical practice of having the patient awake on the table might be a disservice to the patient and that a period of postoperative ventilation would be more appropriate therapy. The necessity for always having patients awake at the end of the operative procedure is certainly questionable. Other methods of determining what is happening in and to the postoperative brain include measuring evoked potentials, compressed spatial analysis of EEG, CAT scan, and, of course, ICP monitoring. It may be that using some of these (admittedly sophisticated) monitoring tools in the intensive care unit would make it feasible and perhaps desirable to maintain sedation and ventilate patients postoperatively. With monitoring of this caliber it should be possible to diagnose the dreaded complication of postoperative bleeding early rather than relying on later signs of pupillary dilatation or deepening levels of unconsciousness.

SPECIAL TECHNIQUES USED TO DECREASE INTRACRANIAL PRESSURE
Hyperosmotic agents

As has been noted previously, hyperventilation, avoidance of drugs that increase ICP, and smooth anesthetic technique may all help in producing a slack brain and thus help the surgical exposure immeasurably. However, the presence of a large space-occupying lesion may make dural opening and approach to deeper structures extremely difficult. Hence, special techniques may be called into play in order to decrease ICP and facilitate surgical exposure. The year 1919 saw the initial use of hyperosmotic agents in an effort to decrease brain mass.[80] The mechanism of action of these agents is to increase intravascular osmotic pressure, drawing water from the interstitial space and decreasing brain mass. These agents, in order to exert their maximum effect, require an intact blood-brain barrier. If the blood-brain barrier is disrupted, the osmotic agents may pass into the brain and cause cerebral edema with increase in brain size.

Urea (1 to 1.5 g/kg) and mannitol (1 to 1.5 g/kg) are the agents most often used in hyperosmolar therapies. Urea causes a rebound increase in ICP following initial decrease in ICP. This is due to the penetration of urea molecules into the brain when the blood urea level begins to decrease. The initial decrease in ICP occurs in about 30 minutes with a rebound increase in ICP occurring in 3 to 7 hours, lasting another 12 hours, and returning to normal values in 12 hours more. Quite apart from its rebound effect, urea may cause venous thrombosis, and if it infiltrates the tissues, it may lead to tissue necrosis.

Mannitol has replaced urea in most centers as it has less tendency to cause rebound phenomena and causes little venous thrombosis or tissue damage. It is given rapidly (over 30 minutes), and its action begins within 20 minutes, is maximal between one to two hours, and wears off in six hours. Urine production may reach 1 to 2 liters within the hour. At this dose, about 100 ml of water is expected to be removed from the brain.[62,69] Both of these agents cause an initial increase in cerebral blood volume and an increase in intracranial pressure. Therefore hyperosmotic agents should be administered slowly to patients who have increases in ICP. Likewise, both agents cause a transitory increase in circulating blood volume and so should be given slowly and with appropriate monitoring to patients with limited cardiac reserve.

Steroids and diuretics

A variety of pathologic conditions, including brain tumors, may lead to a disruption of the blood-brain barrier resulting in the leakage of a fluid similar to plasma into the brain tissue.[69] This leads to local increase in ICP and diminution of regional cerebral blood flow with local lactic acidosis, vasoparalysis, loss of autoregulation, and CO_2 reactivity of the cerebral vessels.[53] The steroids, in partic-

ular dexamethasone, are helpful in treating cerebral edema associated with brain tumors, although their mode of action is in doubt. Steroids may be used before surgery to improve the patient's preoperative status or they may be used following surgery to diminish postoperative reactive edema. Patients with metastatic brain tumors and glioblastomas respond best to steroids.[38,53] The response to more slowly growing tumors is less dramatic. Neurologic signs improved in patients treated with steroids who had brain tumors. Signs of increased ICP such as headache, nausea, and vomiting improved or disappeared in 12 to 36 hours.[38] In a study of mortality following operation and removal of supratentorial brain tumors, mortality was considerably decreased in that group of patients pretreated with dexamethasone two to five days before surgery and for five to seven days following surgery compared to a group not receiving dexamethasone.[53]

It has also been shown that diuretic agents such as ethacrynic acid (100 to 150 mg/day) and furosemide (250 mg infusion) may suppress brain edema. Of the two types of agents (steroids and diuretics) it appears that the steroid is the more effective drug. A study in patients with brain tumor showed a more marked decrease of perifocal edema and improved neurologic deficit in those patients on dexamethasone as compared to those on ethacrynic acid.[52]

Cerebrospinal fluid drainage

One of the oldest methods for decreasing ICP is the removal of cerebrospinal fluid, usually from the lumbar subarachnoid space. This method is useful when surgical approach to the tumor is difficult, as it is with tumors situated near the base of the skull or pituitary tumors. Should the ICP be increased, lumbar drainage of CSF may lead to tonsillar herniation if the fluid is allowed to escape too quickly. Cerebrospinal drainage is usually combined with hyperventilation and osmotic dehydration in order to decrease brain volume maximally. A combination of these techniques is usually used in order to produce optimal operating conditions.

In conclusion one can end no better than

to quote from McDowall in a recent editorial in the *British Journal of Anaesthesia*[37]: . . . The challenge that neurosurgical anaesthesia presents is that only meticulous and continuous attention to technical detail and to physiological and pharmacological principles allows optimal surgical conditions.

REFERENCES

1. Adams, R. W., Gronert, G. A., Sundt, T. M., and others: Halothane, hypocapnia and cerebrospinal fluid pressure in neurosurgery, Anesthesiology **37**:510, 1972.
2. Alexander, S. C., and Lassen, N. A.: Cerebral circulatory response to acute brain disease; implications for anesthetic practice, Anesthesiology **32**:60, 1970.
3. Alexander, S. C., Smith, T. C., Strobel, G., and others: Cerebral carbohydrate metabolism of man during respiratory and metabolic acidosis, J. Appl. Physiol. **24**:66, 1968.
4. Bakay, I., Crawford, J. D., and White, J. C.: The effects of intravenous fluids on cerebrospinal fluid pressure, Surg. Gynecol. Obstet. **99**:48, 1954.
5. Bennett, D. R., Madsen, J. A., Jordan, W. S., and others: Ketamine anesthesia in brain-damaged epileptics: electroencephalographic and clinical observations, Neurology **23**:449, 1973.
6. Brechner, V. I., and Bethune, R. W.M.: Recent advances in monitoring pulmonary air embolism, Anesth. Analg. (Cleve) **50**:255, 1971.
7. Burchiel, K. J., Stockard, J. J., Rowe, M. J., and others: EEG abnormalities following enflurane anesthesia; abstracts of scientific papers of the American Society of Anesthesiologists Annual Meeting, p. 309, 1975.
8. Burney, R. G., and Winn, R.: Increased cerebrospinal fluid pressure during laryngoscopy and intubation for induction of anesthesia, Anesth. Analg. (Cleve) **54**:687, 1975.
9. Cohen, P. J.: The effects of decreased oxygen tension on cerebral circulation, metabolism, and function; proceedings of the international symposium on the cardiovascular and respiratory effects of hypoxia, Karger, Basel, 1966, pp. 81-104.
10. Cohen, P. J., Alexander, S. C., Smith, T. C., and others: Effects of hypoxia and normocarbia on cerebral blood flow and metabolism in man, J. Appl. Physiol. **23**:183, 1967.
11. Cotev, S., and Shalit, M. N.: Effects of diazepam on cerebral blood flow and oxygen uptake after head injuries, Anesthesiology **43**:117, 1975.
12. Cushing, H.: Br. Med. J. p. 221, Feb. 23, 1918.
13. Dahlgren, B. E., Gordon, E., and Steiner, L.: Evaluation of controlled hypotension during surgery for intracranial arterial aneurysms; Progress in anaesthesiology, International congress series No. 200. In Boulton, T. B., Bryce-Smith, R., Sykes, M. K., and others, editors: Amsterdam, 1970, Excerpta Medica p. 1232.
14. Farbat, S. M., and Schneider, R. C.: Observations on the effect of systemic blood pressure on intracranial circulation in patients with cerebrovascular insufficiency, J. Neurosurg. **27**:441, 1967.
15. Fieschi, C., Agnoli, A., Battistini, N., and others: Derangement of regional cerebral blood flow and it regulatory mechanisms in acute cerebrovascular disease, Neurology **18**:1166, 1968.
16. Fitch, W., Barker, J., Jennett, W. B., and others: The influence of neuroleptanalgesic drugs on cerebrospinal fluid pressure, Br. J. Anaesth. **41**:800, 1969a.
17. Freeman, J., and Ingvar, D. H.: Elimination by hypoxia of cerebral blood flow autoregulation and EEG relationship, Exp. Brain Res. **5**:61, 1968.
18. Galicich, J. H., and French, L. A.: Use of dexamethasone in the treatment of cerebral edema resulting from brain tumors and brain surgery, Am Practit. **12**:169, 1961.
19. Gordon, E., editor: A basis and practice of neuroanesthesia. Amsterdam, 1975, Excerpta Medica, p. 178.
20. Greenbaum, R., Cooper, R., Hulme, A., and others: The effect of induction of anaesthesia on intracranial pressure; recent progress in anaesthesiology and resuscitation. In Arias, A., Llaurado, R., Nalda, M. A., and Lunn, J. N., editors: Amsterdam, 1975, Excerpta Medica, p. 794.
21. Harp, J. R., and Wollman, H.: Cerebral metabolic effects of hyperventilation and deliberate hypotension, Br. J. Anaesth. **45**:256, 1973.
22. Heiss, W. D.: Drug effects on regional cerebral blood flow in focal cerebrovascular disease, J. Neurol. Sci. **19**:461, 1973.
23. Hendricksen, H. T., and Jorgensen, P. B.: The effect of nitrous oxide on intracranial pressure in patients with intracranial disorders, Br. J. Anaesth. **45**:486, 1973.
24. Hulme, A., and Cooper, R.: Changes in intracranial pressure and other variables during the induction of general anaesthesia, Proc. R. Soc. Med. **65**:883, 1972.
25. Hunter, A. R.: The present position of anaesthesia for neurosurgery, Proc. R. Soc. Med. **45**:472, 1952.
26. Hunter, A. R.: Thiopentone supplemented anaesthesia for neurosurgery, B. J. Anaesth. **44**:506, 1972.
27. Jachuck, S. J., Ramani, P. S., Clark, F., and others: Electrocardiographic abnormalities associated with raised intracranial pressure, Br. Med. J. **1**:242, 1975.
28. Jelsma, R., and Buch, P. C.: The treatment of glioblastoma multiforme of the brain, J. Neurosurg. **27**:388, 1967.
29. Jennett, W. B., Barker, J., Fitch, W., and others: Effect of anesthesia on intracranial pressure in patients with space-occupying lesions, Lancet **1**:61, 1969.
30. Lassen, N. A.: Cerebral blood flow and oxygen consumption in man, Physiol. Rev. **39**:183, 1959.
31. Lassen, N. A.: The luxury-perfusion syndrome and

its possible relation to acute metabolic acidosis localized within the brain, Lancet Nov. 19, 1966, p. 1113.

32. Lassen, N. A., and Palvolgyi, R.: Cerebral steal during hypercapnia and the inverse reaction during hypocapnea observed by the "Xenon" technique in man, Scand. J. Lab. Clin. Invest. (suppl 102 XIV), 1968.

33. Leech, P., Barker, J., and Fitch, W.: Changes in intracranial pressure and systemic arterial pressure during the termination of anaesthesia, Br. J. Anaesth. **46**:315, 1974.

34. Leech, P., Barker, J., and Fitch, W.: Changes in intracranial pressure and systemic arterial pressure during the termination of anaesthesia. In Lundberg, N., Ponten, U., and Brock, M., editors: Intracranial pressure II, Berlin, 1975, Springer-Verlag, p. 342.

35. Lundberg, N.: Continuous recording and control of ventricular fluid pressure in neurosurgical practice, Acta Psychiatr. Scand. **36**(suppl. 149): 1, 1960.

36. Mackawa, T., Sakabe, T., and Takeshiko, H.: Diazepam blocks cerebral metabolic and circulatory responses to local anesthetic induced seizures, Anesthesiology **41**:389, 1974.

37. McDowall, D. G., and Norman, J. B., editors: Symposium on neurosurgical anesthesia, Br. J. Anaesth. **48**:8, 1976.

38. Maxwell, R. E., Long, D. M., and French, L. A.: The clinical effects of a synthetic glucocorticoid used for brain edema in the practice of neurosurgery. In Reulen, H. J., and Schurmann, K., editors: Steroids and brain edema. Berlin, Springer-Verlag, 1972, p. 219.

38a. Larson, C. P., Jr.: Anesthesia and the control of the cerebral circulation. In Wyler, E. J., and Ehrenfeld, W. K., editors: Extracranial occlusive cerebral vascular disease, Philadelphia, 1970, W. B. Saunders Co., pp. 152-183.

39. Messick, J. M., and Theye, R. A.: Effects of pentobarbital and meperidine on canine cerebral and total oxygen consumption rates, Can. Anaesth. Soc. J. **16**:321, 1969.

40. Michenfelder, J. D.: Anesthesia for intracranial surgery: physiologic considerations. In Hershey, S. G., editor: Refresher courses in anesthesiology, Philadelphia, 1975, J. B. Lippincott Co.

41. Michenfelder, J. D., Gronert, G. A., and Rehder, K.: Neuroanesthesia, Anesthesiology **30**:65, 1969.

42. Michenfelder, J. D., and Milde, J. H.: Influence of anesthetics on metabolic functional and pathological responses to regional cerebral ischaemia, Stroke **6**:405, 1975.

43. Michenfelder, J. D., Milde, J., and Smith, T.: Cerebral protection by barbiturates, Anaesth. Neurol. **33**:345, 1976.

44. Michenfelder, J. D., and Theye, R. A.: Effects of fentanyl, droperidol and innovar on canine cerebral metabolism and blood flow, Br. J. Anaesth. **43**:630, 1971.

45. Michenfelder, J. D., and Theye, R. A.: Cerebral protection by thiopental during hypoxia, Anesthesiology **39**:510, 1973.

45a. Morita, H., Bleyarnt, A. L., Stezoski, S. W., and others: The effect of halothane anesthesia on cerebral blood flow, autoregulation and cerebral metabolism of oxygen and glucose; abstracts of scientific papers, American Society of Anesthesiologists annual meeting, 1974, pp. 63-64.

46. Murphy, F. L., Kennell, E. M., Johnson, R. E., and others: The effects of enflurane, isoflurane, and halothane in cerebral blood flow and metabolism in man; abstracts of scientific papers, American Society of Anesthesiology, p. 61, 1971.

47. Olesen, J., Skinhoj, E., and Lassen, N. A.: Autoregulation of brain circulation in severe arterial hypertension, Br. Med. J. **1**:507, 1973.

48. Pickerodt, V. W. A., McDowall, D. G., Coroneos, N. J., and co-workers: Effect of Althesin on cerebral perfusion, cerebral metabolism and intracranial pressure in the anaesthetized baboon, Br. J. Anaesth. **44**:751, 1972.

49. Pierce, E. C., Lambertsen, C. J., Deutsch, S., and others: Cerebral circulation and metabolism during thiopental anaesthesia and hyperventilation in man, J. Clin. Invest. **41**:1664, 1962.

50. Plum, F., Posner, J. B., and Troy, B.: Cerebral metabolic and circulatory responses to induced convulsions in animals, Arch. Neurol. **18**:1, 1968.

51. Risberg, J., Lundberg, N., and Ingvar, D. H.: Regional cerebral blood volume during acute transient rises of the intracranial pressure (plateau waves), J. Neurosurg. **31**:303, 1969.

52. Reulen, H. J., Hadjidimos, A., and Schurmann, K.: The effect of dexamethasone on water and electrolyte content and on rCBF in perifocal brain edema in man. In Reulen, H. J., and Schurmann, K., editors: Steroids and brain edema, Berlin, 1972, Springer-Verlag, p. 239.

53. Reulen, M. J., Hajidimos, A., and Hase, U.: Steroids in the treatment of brain edema. In Advances in neurosurgery, Berlin, 1973, Springer-Verlag, p. 92.

54. Saidman, L. J., and Eger, E. I., II: Change in cerebrospinal fluid pressure during pneumoencephalography under nitrous oxide anesthesia, Anesthesiology **26**:61, 1965.

55. Schettini, A., Cook, A. W., and Owre, E. S.: Hyperventilation in craniotomy for brain tumor, Anesthesiology **28**:363, 1967.

56. Shapiro, H. M., and Galindo, A.: Acute intraoperative intracranial hypertension in neurosurgical patients: mechanical and pharmacological factors, Anesthesiology **37**:399, 1972.

57. Shapiro, H. M., Galindo, A., Wyte, Sr. R., and others: Europ. Neurol. **8**:118, 1972.

58. Shapiro, H. M., Galindo, A., Wyte, S. R., and others: Rapid intraoperative reduction of intracranial pressure with thiopentone, Br. J. Anaesth. **45**:1057, 1973.

59. Shapiro, H. M., Wyte, S. R., and Harris, A. B.:

Ketamine anaesthesia in patients with intracranial pathology, Br. J. Anaesth. **44:**1200, 1972.

60. Shapiro, H. M., Wyte, S. R., Harris, A. B., and others: Acute intraoperative intracranial hypertension in neurosurgical patients: mechanical and pharmacologic factors, Anesthesiology **37:**399, 1972.

61. Shapiro, W., Wasserman, A. J., and Patterson, J. L.: Human cerebrovascular response to combined hypoxia and hypercapnia, Circ. Res. **19:**903, 1966.

62. Shenkin, H. A., and Bouzarth, W. F.: Clinical methods of reducing intracranial pressure: role of the cerebral circulation, N. Engl. J. Med. **282:**1465, 1970.

63. Skinhoj, E., and Strandgaard, S.: Pathogenesis of hypertensive encephalopathy, Lancet **1:**461, 1973.

64. Smith, A. L., Hoff, J. T., and Nielsen, S. L.: Barbiturate protection in acute focal cerebral ischemia, Stroke **5:**1, 1974.

65. Smith, A. L., and Wollman, H.: Cerebral blood flow and metabolism: effects of anesthetic drugs and techniques, Anaesthesiology **36:**378, 1972.

66. Sondergard, W.: Intracranial pressure during general anaesthesia, Dan. Med. Bull. **8:**18, 1961.

67. Spoerel, W. E., Deimling, P., and Aitken, R.: Direct arterial pressure monitoring from the dorsalis pedis artery, Can. Anaesth. Soc. J. **22:**91, 1975.

68. Stern, W. E.: The cerebral edemas. In Mcritckey, J. L., O'Leary, and Jennett, B., editors: Scientific foundations of neurology, Philadelphia, 1972, F. A. Davis Co., pp. 289-296.

69. Stern, W. E., Abbott, M. L., and Cheseboro, B. W.: A study of the role of osmotic gradients in experimental cerebral edemas, J. Neurosurg. **24:**57, 1966.

70. Stockard, J. J., Burchiel, K. J., Smith, N. T., and others: The effects of nitrous oxide and carbon dioxide on epileptiform EEG activity produced by enflurane; abstracts of scientific papers, American Society of Anesthesiologists Annual Meeting, p. 309, 1975.

71. Strandgaard, S., MacKenzie, E. T., Sengupta, D., and others: Upper limit of autoregulation of cerebral blood flow in the baboon, Circ. Res. **34:**435, 1974.

72. Strandgaard, S., Olesen, J., Skinhoj, E., and others: Autoregulation of brain circulation in severe arterial hypertension, Br. Med. J. **1:**507, 1973.

73. Takahashi, T., Takasaki, M., Namiki, A., and others: Effects of Althesin on cerebrospinal fluid pressure, Br. J. Anaesth. **45:**179, 1973.

74. Takeshija, H., Michenfelder, J. D., and Theye, R.: The effects of morphine and N-allylnormop on canine cerebral metabolism and circulation, Anesthesiology **37:**605, 1972.

75. Takeshija, M., Okuda, Y., and Sari, A.: The effects of ketamine on cerebral circulation and metabolism in man, Anesthesiology **36:**69, 1972.

76. Tarkkanen, L., Laitnen, L., and Johansson, G.: Effects of d-tubocurarine on intracranial pressure and thalamic electrical impedance, Anesthesiology **40:**247, 1974.

77. Tobey, R. E., Jacomsen, P. M., Kable, C. T., and others: Serum potassium response to muscle relaxants in neural injury, Anesthesiology **37:**337, 1972.

78. Waltz, A. G.: Effects of blood pressure on blood flow in ischemic and non-ischemic cerebral cortex, Neurology **18:**613, 1968.

79. Ward, R. J., Allen, G. D., Deveny, L. J., and others: Halothane and the cardiovascular response to endotracheal intubation, Anesth. Analg. (Cleve) **44:**248, 1965.

80. Weed, L. H., and McKibben, P. S.: Experimental alteration of brain bulk, Am. J. Physiol. **48:**531, 1919.

81. Weitzner, S. W., McCoy, G. T., and Binden, L. S.: Effects of morphine levallorphan and respiratory gases on increased intracranial pressure, Anesthesiology **26:**291, 1963.

82. Williams, B.: The distending force in the production of syringomyelia, Lancet **2:**41, 1970.

83. Wise, B. I.: Fluids and electrolytes in neurological surgery, Springfield, Ill., 1965, Charles C Thomas, Publisher, p. 117.

84. Wollman, H., Alexander, S. C., Cohen, P. J., and others: Cerebral circulation of man during halothane anesthesia: effects of hypocarbia and of d-tubocurarine, Anesthesiology **25:**180, 1964.

85. Woolman, H., Smith, T. C., Stephen, G. W., and others: Effects of extremes of respiratory and metabolic alkalosis of cerebral blood flow in man, J. Appl. Physiol. **24:**60, 1968.

86. Wyte, S. R., Shapiro, H. M., Turner, P., and others: Ketamine-induced intracranial hypertension, Anesthesiology **36:**174, 1972.

87. Yamamoto, Y. L., Phillips, K. M., and Hodge, C. P.: Microregional blood flow changes in experimental cerebral ischemia, J. Neurosurg. **35:**155, 1971.

9

Anesthesia for posterior fossa procedures

PHILIPPA NEWFIELD

Exploration of the posterior cranial fossa is performed for resection of mass lesions, clipping of aneurysms, microvascular decompression of cranial nerves, and implantation of electrodes for cerebellar stimulation. Successful surgical intervention depends upon adequate exposure and minimal trauma. The sitting position is used most frequently, which provides excellent surgical access, improves venous and cerebrospinal fluid (CSF) drainage, facilitates hemostasis, and exposes the face for monitoring response to cranial nerve stimulation.

Some special circulatory problems occur, however, in the sitting position. Air embolization is a significant hazard in every patient undergoing surgery in the sitting position. Cardiac output and systemic arterial pressure can fall significantly.[5,6,91] Cerebral ischemia may result, depending upon the level of blood pressure, intracranial pressure, and venous pressure. For these reasons, the lateral or prone position may be more desirable in patients with significant preexisting cardiovascular disease.

Cardiac arrhythmias caused by retraction or manipulation of the brain stem or cranial nerves are seen in as many as 51% of adults[148] and 14% of children.[87] Significant bradycardia has been described in 25% of cases; ventricular asystole may occur as well.[6,94] Manipulation of the pons or brain stem can cause bradycardia, ventricular premature beats, or ventricular tachycardia. Bradycardia and hypertension may follow trigeminal (V) sensory root manipulation. Bradycardia and hypotension are seen with vagus nerve stimulation or traction. During spontaneous breathing, traction on vagal rootlets often produces a gasp, cough, or period of rapid breathing. Facial nerve (VII) stimulation causes facial twitch, and trigeminal nerve (V) motor root stimulation causes jaw jerk. Accessory nerve (XI) stimulation produces shoulder or sternomastoid movement.[54]

MICROVASCULAR DECOMPRESSION OF CRANIAL NERVES

Trigeminal neuralgia[65] and hemifacial spasm[64] are symptoms of disordered function of cranial nerves V and VII, respectively. As suggested originally by Dandy[37] and Jannetta,[62] a combination of arteriosclerotic elongation of the arteries of the cerebellopontine angle and venous compression associated with "sagging" of the hindbrain produces a vascular cross-compression of cranial nerves at their brain stem root entry zone into the posterior fossa. The lower cranial nerves are most vulnerable, since they are surrounded by many vessels that frequently impinge upon them. This mechanism may explain the increased incidence of these

168

symptom complexes in older population groups.[63]

Increased frequency or severity of trigeminal neuralgia and hemifacial spasm probably correlates with progressive elongation of a vascular loop. Decreased pain and remission may result from neural accommodation or a combination of neural denervation and reinnervation. Phenytoin and carbamazepine may produce symptomatic relief because they depress neuronal transmission.[63] Surgery is indicated for those individuals who have developed drug toxicity or who are refractory to treatment.

Microvascular nerve decompression is accomplished through a suboccipital craniectomy.[63] The procedure involves vascular mobilization and insertion of Gelfoam sponge, muscle, or fat between the nerve and the compressing vessel. Repeated Valsalva maneuvers are performed by the anesthetist after placement of tissue buffer to verify the relationship between nerve, vessel, and prosthesis. Basilar artery aneurysms and acoustic neuromas may produce hemifacial spasm[64] and tic douloureux by indirect neurovascular compression as well as by direct neural involvement.

CHRONIC CEREBELLAR STIMULATION

Chronic stimulation of the cerebellar cortex by implanted electrodes has been employed for alleviation of symptoms of cerebral palsy[27] and epilepsy.[26] This treatment is effective because of the cerebellar cortex's powerful inhibitory action on motor function. Since the entire efferent discharge of Purkinje cells of the cerebellar cortex is inhibitory, Purkinje cell inhibition can be prosthetically induced to modify neurologic activity abnormally heightened by pathologic facilitation or disinhibition.

A plate of silicone-coated mesh with platinum disc electrodes is inserted onto the superior surface of the cerebellum bilaterally through suboccipital craniectomies in the upright sitting position. The leads are directed through the craniectomy openings subcutaneously along the neck to a radio receiver implant. Stimulation occurs from radiofrequency pulses transmitted to the receiver.

Patients with cerebral palsy demonstrate improvement in spasticity, athetosis, speech, and functional status as well as psychometric testing and behavior with cerebellar stimulation. Intractable seizures may be modified or inhibited for periods of up to three years. Complications are related to air embolization, postoperative hemorrhage,[28] cerebellar edema, CSF leakage along the electrode tracks, minor CSF accumulations, infection and rejection, and hydrocephalus.

PREOPERATIVE EVALUATION

Patients with posterior fossa lesions may have altered levels of consciousness secondary to increased intracranial pressure from obstructive hydrocephalus. Brain stem compression with cranial nerve palsies and impairment of protective reflexes also occurs.

A preoperative history of hypertension is significant, since autoregulation is altered so that both upper and lower limits of cerebral perfusion pressure to which the brain will respond are elevated.[24,140] Hypotension in the sitting position may be especially detrimental. Mean arterial pressure during controlled hypotension should be maintained at a higher level than for the normotensive patient.[48]

Assessment of the patient's volume status immediately before surgery is important. Volume replacement with crystalloid or colloid (Albumisol or blood) before induction and positioning and application of compression bandages to the lower limbs to prevent hypotension may be necessary.

Air is frequently used as the contrast medium for pneumoencephalography, which is performed to elucidate brain stem tumors, and for gas myelography, which is used for superior cervical cord lesions. If a pneumoencephalogram with air has been performed within seven days before surgery, nitrous oxide cannot be used as part of the anesthetic technique for definitive surgery because of the differential solubility of nitrous oxide and its resultant expansion of intracranial air collections.[120] Either 100% oxygen, air, or an air-oxygen mixture is indicated in conjunction with neuroleptic analgesia or inhalation anesthesia.[13] This severe limitation of choice of anesthetic technique is completely avoidable, however, when neuroradiologists use oxygen, nitrous oxide, or a combination of the two[69] for gas contrast studies.

MONITORING

Thorough beat-to-beat monitoring provides essential information about the patient's course and should therefore be instituted before induction whenever possible and continued into the postanesthetic period.

Monitoring includes:
1. Esophageal stethoscope
2. ECG with oscilloscope display
3. Intra-arterial blood pressure
4. Venous pressure via central venous catheter
5. Precordial ultrasonic Doppler transducer
6. Esophageal, nasopharyngeal, or tympanic thermistor
7. Urinary catheter
8. $F_{I_{O_2}}$ analyzer
9. Intermittent measurement of arterial blood gases, hematocrit, and serum osmolarity and electrolytes (especially potassium)

Central venous catheters are important primarily for diagnosis and treatment of venous air embolism. Routes for insertion of central catheters include the basilic vein in the antecubital fossa, internal and external jugular veins, and subclavian vein in order of preference based on relative morbidity of each approach.

Advancement of the catheter into the basilic vein with the patient's arm in abduction and ear touching the ipsilateral shoulder usually prevents entry into the jugular vein. Turning the patient's head toward the site of catheter insertion is insufficient. If the antecubital route fails, internal jugular vein catheterization provides reliable access to the right heart. Complications from this method are less frequent than for the subclavian route but do include carotid or subclavian artery puncture and hematoma, inadvertent arterial catheterization, pneumothorax, and hemothorax. An intracranial procedure is not a contraindication to the use of neck veins for insertion of the right atrial catheter.

To facilitate aspiration of the greatest amount of air, the tip of the right atrial catheter should be placed at the junction of the right atrium and the superior vena cava. Position is verified by chest roentgenogram, transduced pressure wave form, or P wave configuration on ECG with the saline-filled catheter functioning as a unipolar ECG lead. Since the tip of the catheter now provides a direct conducting pathway to the heart, electroconduction may result when faulty equipment is used. Other electrical equipment must not be connected to the patient during positioning of the central catheter by this method. The location of the catheter should be checked again after the patient is moved to the operative position.

While delays and difficulties with central venous line placement are occasionally encountered, surgery, especially with patients in the sitting position, should not be undertaken until access to the right atrium is secured. Insertion of the catheter on the night before surgery is inadvisable because of the possibility of fluid overload, arrhythmia, thromboembolism, infection, or occlusion of the catheter. If the patient develops a fever as a result of the line, surgery may be cancelled, causing unnecessary expense and delay.

Doppler ultrasound is the most sensitive method currently available for detection of venous air embolism.[78] A precordial transducer is placed over the right heart and its position ascertained by injection of 10 ml of crystalloid through the right atrial catheter. The resultant turbulence provides a signal similar to air inflow.[144] (See discussion of venous air embolism, p. 173.) Because air embolism can also occur in the lateral, supine, and prone positions, the Doppler unit should be used for all neurosurgical cases in conjunction with a right atrial catheter.

ECG monitoring is particularly important. Alterations in heart rate and rhythm are immediate indicators of brain stem and cranial nerve compromise, the initial treatment

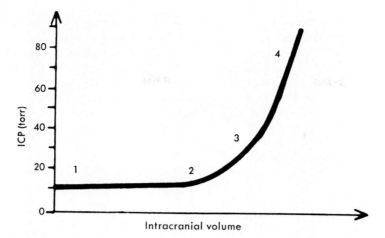

Fig. 9-1. Intracranial volume-pressure relationships. As we move along the curve from points 1 to 4, compliance decreases so that further volume expansion will result in a progressive increase in ICP. When ICP is already elevated, even small increments in intracranial volume cause marked intracranial hypertension (point 3).

of which is cessation of manipulation or release of retraction pressure. The use of chest leads to obtain a precordial ECG pattern offers a more sensitive index of ischemia than monitoring of the standard lead II since this tracing may remain unaffected in the presence of ST segment and T wave changes in the precordial leads.

Intravascular monitoring of arterial blood pressure is essential for posterior fossa procedures in view of the hemodynamic sequelae of positional changes and brain stem and cranial nerve manipulation. While indirect methods are useful, beat-to-beat knowledge is more conducive to rapid therapeutic intervention, especially since wide swings in blood pressure can be detrimental.

With an arterial cannula in place, cerebral perfusion pressure may be calculated as the difference between the mean arterial pressure when the transducer is at head level and the central venous pressure in patients without intracranial hypertension or the intracranial pressure in those with some elevation (Fig. 9-1).

POSITIONING

To avoid hypotension with position change, patients should have an adequate circulating blood volume. Legs are wrapped from toes to groin to facilitate venous return. The sitting position is achieved gradually with constant monitoring of blood pressure and ECG. Bolsters are placed under the patient's buttocks and the table flexed to its full extent, after which the foot section is lowered to flex the knees. The back of the table is then elevated so that the patient is actually semireclining with a 45- to 60-degree angle between body axis and the horizontal of the operating table (Fig. 9-2). Knees are flexed and maintained at the level of the heart. The patient's head is supported in a three-point pin head-holder[82] with neck flexed so that the chin is at least 1 inch from the sternum during inspiration. The support bar for the head rest should clear the abdomen. A soft bite block or small oropharyngeal airway is used to avoid macroglossia from obstruction of venous and lymphatic drainage of the tongue.[42,84]

The lateral position offers wide exposure of the back of the head for resection of acoustic neuromas and cerebellopontine angle tumors and for microvascular decompression of the cranial nerves. A roll is inserted through the dependent axilla to prevent brachial plexus injury. Care must be taken to avoid formation of an acute angle between the neck and down shoulder since this will cause jugu-

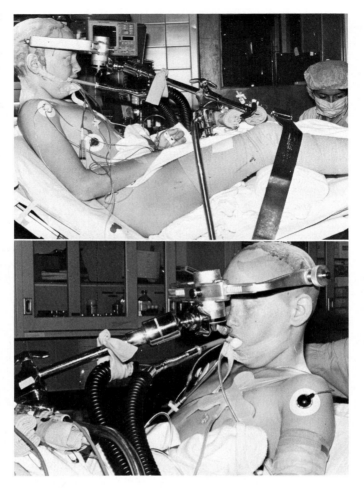

Fig. 9-2. Young patient in the sitting position for posterior fossa exploration with hips and knees flexed, adequate space between chin and sternum, and arms supported in lap (not dependent). Eyes are closed and protected with clear tape and legs wrapped from toes to groin. Clover leaf transducer of the Doppler ultrasound air bubble detector is taped over precordium. Arterial and central venous pressure transducers rest on knees at heart level. Blood pressure cuff, esophageal thermistor and stethoscope, ECG, and oral gastric tube are in place. (Courtesy Joyce McKinney.)

lar compression, impeding venous return, and increasing blood loss and intracranial pressure.

The prone position provides access to midline and lateral structures, but venous congestion may be a problem. The incidence of air embolism is less in the lateral and prone positions than the sitting position,[8] although fatalities have been reported.[129] Despite support from two abdominal bolsters, ventilation should be controlled since spontaneous respiration is usually inadequate and hyperventilation desirable.

ANESTHETIC TECHNIQUE

See Chapter 8 on anesthetic technique for supratentorial tumors.

Although armored endotracheal tubes rarely kink in positions other than supine, there have been reports of intraluminal obstruction of these tubes during surgery.[57,106] For this reason, red rubber or disposable

Table 9-1. Incidence of air embolism in sitting, lateral, supine, and prone positions*

Position	No. patients	Detectable air	Amount air aspirated (ml)	Gradient (cm)
Sitting	400	100	2.0->500	20.0-65.0
Lateral	26	5†	3.0-200	5.0-18.0
Supine	40	8‡	2.0-150	5.0-18.0
Prone	8	1§	45	7.5

*From Albin, M. S., Carroll, R. G., Tung, A., and others: Venous air embolism in the sitting, lateral, supine, and prone positions, International Anesthesia Research Society, 51st Congress, Hollywood, Florida, 1977.
†Two cases tic douloureux, two cases hemifacial spasm, one tumor.
‡Three cases transsphenoidal hypophysectomy, three intracranial tumors, and two cases tic douloureux, where air was detected after application of pin head holder in supine position prior to putting patient in sitting position or continuing after head holder was removed in supine position.
§Case of ependymoma of spinal cord.

soft-cuffed endotracheal tubes are used in some centers, although these have also kinked with flexion of the head in the sitting and supine positions. Since positioning may displace the tube, proper location of the endotracheal tube should be verified after intubation and again following achievement of the operative position.

VENOUS AIR EMBOLISM

A potentially serious and not infrequent complication of posterior fossa surgery is venous air embolism. The reported incidence of air embolism in the sitting position varies between 25%[5] and 39%.[74] Air has, however, been detected in the lateral, supine, and prone positions[7] as well, because entrainment of air may occur whenever a gradient of more than 5 cm exists between the right heart and the upper pole of the wound[81] (Table 9-1).

Scientists have long been cognizant of the occurrence of intravascular air and its pathophysiologic sequelae.[75] Three hundred and ten years ago, Francisco Redi noted that animals died after air had been blown into their veins. In 1821, Magendie described the use of a cannula to remove intravenous air after reporting a fatality due to air embolism in 1819. In 1830, Barlow reported the first death from air embolism in a patient undergoing surgery in the sitting position. Changes in heart sounds upon entrance of air into the right heart were described by Erichsen in 1844. Experimental and clinical studies by Senn in the 1880s prompted his recommendation of aspiration of air from the right side of the heart using a catheter inserted into the heart through the jugular vein.

Wolffe and Robertson[152] noted that air embolism causes pulmonary outflow obstruction. Morbidity attendant upon air embolism is proportional to the rate of air entry rather than the volume of air entering.[117] In support of this, Durant and his colleagues[40] demonstrated that while a dog might tolerate 1000 ml of air injected over 50 to 100 minutes, 100 ml given rapidly would be fatal. Stallworth[135] used a transthoracic needle to aspirate air from the heart while Ericsson[43] described the usefulness of closed-chest cardiac massage to force air out of the right heart in six instances of cardiac arrest secondary to air embolism.

Air enters veins in which there is subatmospheric or negative pressure. Several venous sinuses are noncollapsable because of their dural attachments; the walls of diploic veins are also fixed. Emissary veins and veins in cervical muscles and the spinal epidural space may entrain air too. During posterior fossa surgery, air may come from puncture sites of the pin head-holder,[5,150] from soft tissue, bone, the dural edge, the cut edge of the bone, dural sinuses, or bridging veins over the cerebellum.

While this situation frequently occurs during neurosurgery, air embolism has also been observed during operations involving veins in the neck, thorax, abdomen, and pelvis, open heart procedures,[51] repair of liver and vena caval lacerations, total hip replacement,[107] delivery with placenta previa, induction of pneumothorax and pneumperitoneum, pneumatic otoscopic air insufflation, and pneumorbitography.

Pathophysiologically, when air enters the heart, air and blood in the right ventricle prevent effective cardiac output. The mixture produces the characteristic but late-occurring "mill-wheel murmur."[19] Pulmonary edema and reflex bronchoconstriction may also result from the movement of air into the pulmonary circulation.[23] Signs preceding cardiovascular collapse include hypotension, tachycardia, arrhythmia, neck vein congestion, and cyanosis. With slow entry of air into the venous circulation, larger volumes of air are necessary to produce cardiovascular depression than are required with rapid entry.[136]

Death is secondary to acute cor pulmonale and anoxia from obstruction of the pulmonary circulation. Air may also pass through the pulmonary vessels in small amounts to reach the coronary and cerebral circulation while large quantities travel directly to the systemic system through intracardiac right-to-left shunts. Death in these instances results from air obstruction of the coronary arteries with ventricular fibrillation. Neurologic damage follows cerebral artery occlusion.

Early detection of air embolism is essential to its successful treatment. Since the "mill-wheel murmur" heard through an esophageal stethoscope is a late and catastrophic sign of a large amount of intracardiac air,[115] more sensitive methods of diagnosis were needed. The sudden decrease in end-expiratory CO_2 concentration during controlled ventilation is an early sign of air embolism.[16] This alteration in CO_2 excretion occurs because of a reduction in blood flow through the lungs. The decrease in end-expiratory CO_2 occurring with shock, hypovolemia, and cardiac arrhythmia is more gradual than that from air embolism. A Swan-Ganz catheter has also been used to monitor pulmonary artery pressure during air embolism[103] with the increase in pulmonary artery pressure corresponding to changes in end-expiratory CO_2 concentration at the time of embolization.

It was not until the Doppler ultrasonic transducer was introduced into clinical practice by Maroon[78] in 1968, however, that very small quantities of air could be detected. His[79] and others'[41,91] studies confirmed that cardiac auscultation with Doppler ultrasound is the most sensitive method of identifying venous air embolism, permitting diagnosis before the occurrence of pathophysiologic changes. Therapeutic measures may thus be instituted immediately to avoid cardiorespiratory collapse.

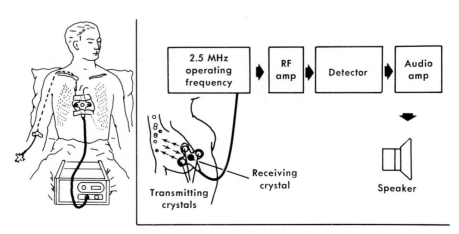

Fig. 9-3. Correct placement of clover leaf transducer over the precordium with illustration of the electronic processing for air embolism detection (inset).

The Doppler transducer generates a continuous 2.5 mHz ultrasonic signal that is reflected by moving red blood cells and cardiac structures. This reflected signal is electronically converted to sounds of audible frequency (Fig. 9-3): the high-pitched swishing of intracardiac blood flow and the thumping produced by heart wall and valve motion. Variation of Doppler tone intensity occurs with the respiratory cycle because of movement of cardiac structures away from the anterior chest wall during inspiration.

When intravascular air passes through the ultrasonic field, a louder "roaring" noise is generated. Its intensity is dependent upon the size of the embolism and the time it remains in the ultrasonic field. Air is "heard" because the air-blood interface is a much better acoustical reflector than red blood cells alone. The acoustical Doppler shift is greater, producing a characteristic frequency. Amounts as small as 0.25 ml can be detected (Fig. 9-4).

Accordingly, blood flow through the right heart is monitored intraoperatively by an ultrasound air embolism detector. The criteria for optimal Doppler transducer design include adequate depth of field, broad beam coverage across the right atrium, and internal rejection circuitry to silence the radiofrequency interference from electrocautery units.[80] Cardiac sounds are amplified and transmitted by speaker for monitoring by both anesthetists and surgeons throughout the procedure, all of whom are constantly attuned to changes in Doppler tone as well as alterations in heart rate and rhythm.

The Doppler multicrystal, flexible, cloverleaf transducer (Fetasonde, Roche Medical Electronics, Cranbury, N.J.) is placed on the chest over the right heart to the right of the sternum between the third and sixth interspaces. Position is verified by rapid injection of a bolus of crystalloid solution into the right atrial catheter. The turbulence and micro-air bubbles created alter the reflected ultra-

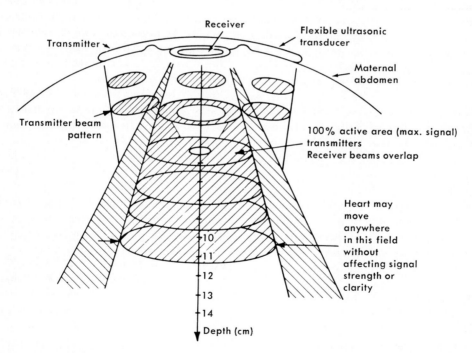

Fig. 9-4. Depth beam pattern for the wide beam ultrasonic multicrystal flexible transducer originally designed to monitor fetal heartbeat. Maximum breadth and depth of field are important in neurosurgery to ensure clarity of signal despite alterations in location of the heart in relation to the chest wall secondary to position change or ventilation.

sound and produce a signal similar to that caused by air.

While the Doppler technique has been criticized for being overly sensitive and not quantitative, the essential aspect of treatment of air embolism is early detection *before* cardiac arrest. In one large series, only 3% of patients with air embolism developed ECG, blood pressure, or oxygenation changes due to rapid institution of therapy.[4]

As soon as a change in the Doppler signal occurs, the right atrial catheter is aspirated and the surgeons alerted to identify and occlude sites of air entry by irrigating the field with saline, applying Gelfoam and cottonoids, and waxing all bone edges. Nitrous oxide is discontinued to avoid increasing the size of the air embolism[101] and the patient ventilated with 100% oxygen. Supplemental intravenous drugs may be given at this time. Elimination of nitrous oxide from the inspired gas following air embolism decreases pulmonary artery pressure and deadspace and increases cardiac output.[102] A Valsalva maneuver is performed or positive endexpiratory pressure (PEEP) applied to elevate mean intrathoracic pressure. PEEP has not, however, been found to be of prophylactic value in the prevention of air embolism.[3]

Complications of air embolism relate to the amount of air entrained with few problems occurring when less than 50 ml have been aspirated from the right atrial catheter.[5] These include hypotension, arrhythmias, hypoxia secondary to reflex bronchoconstriction and pulmonary edema, and cardiac arrest, which may require supportive management. Massive air embolism or inability to arrest air entry necessitates placement of the wound site at or below heart level and termination of surgery. This has rarely been reported to be necessary.

Technetium pertechnitrate macroaggregated albumin (T_EMAA) lung scans performed in patients after air embolism reveal a pathognomonic pattern of peripheral decortication crossing segmental lines.[22] Distribution of defects is in accordance with the effects of gravity on air bubbles and the rate of air entry. When air enters rapidly in moderate amounts (20 to 40 ml), segmental lesions occur that mimic pulmonary thromboemboli. Large quantities of air (50 to 75 ml) entering slowly produce a peripheral decortication pattern. Moderate amounts of air entrained over an intermediary period of time result in lesions of the apex and posterior superior portions of both lungs. These defects clear within 12 to 14 days without anticoagulant therapy, confirming their pneumatic rather than thromboembolic origin.

IMMEDIATE POSTOPERATIVE PROBLEMS

Edema, hematoma, and infarction of the brain stem and cerebellum following surgical trauma or devascularization in the posterior fossa are extremely serious because of the proximity of respiratory and cardiovascular control centers. Patients with severe compromise, previously awake and talking, will suddenly become unresponsive with systemic hypertension, bradycardia, and irregular or absent respirations. This triad, secondary to brain stem compression, is an indication for reintubation and immediate reexploration to relieve pressure on the brain stem through evacuation of hematoma or resection of infarcted areas.

Other patients, however, neither awaken nor resume spontaneous ventilation despite reversal of narcotic and muscle relaxant. Reexploration in such cases reveals no clot or infarction. These rare patients do awaken 12 to 24 hours after reoperation without neurologic deficit (Albin and Jannetta, personal communication). Delayed brain stem infarction may also occur up to a week after surgery, possibly due to vasospasm. Since hypotension is implicated in the development of vasospasm, dehydration and syncope are to be avoided, especially in the immediate postoperative period.

Patients are frequently hypertensive in the recovery room after posterior fossa surgery despite absence of a premorbid history of high blood pressure. Because of the danger of hematoma or hemorrhagic infarction, hypertension must be treated immediately. If analgesics in small doses are not effective, vasodilatation with nitroglycerin or nitro-prusside is indicated for rapid control. It is usually unnecessary to place previously normotensive patients on long-term therapy with α-methyldopa or hydralazine since the postoperative hypertension resolves within 12 hours after surgery. Ectopic beats, both atrial and ventricular, occur with increased frequency in the first 24 hours, especially in patients with a history of ectopy. Full monitoring of heart rate and rhythm as well as blood pressure is essential for at least 24 hours after surgery.

Serum electrolytes, osmolarity, and urinary volume and specific gravity should be measured as soon as patients reach the recovery room, since mannitol may decrease serum potassium and increase serum osmolality. Additionally, ADH levels rise with stress, resulting in dilutional hyponatremia. This is treated with fluid restriction and diuretics. Hypertonic saline (3%) is indicated for sodium levels below 120 mEq or the occurrence of changing levels of consciousness or seizures.

It is common for patients to develop temperatures to 39°C shortly after posterior fossa exploration. This febrile response is attributed to the presence of blood in the subarachnoid space. The incidence of temperature elevation is less in patients after supratentorial craniotomy.

POSTOPERATIVE COMPLICATIONS

Certain postoperative complications occur specifically after posterior fossa surgery because of manipulation of the brain stem and cranial nerves. Gastrointestinal hemorrhage (Cushing ulcer[36]) is seen with increased frequency, especially following dissection around the floor of the fourth ventricle. Ulcers are also exacerbated by steroids, which alter volume and mucopolysaccharide constituents of gastric mucus, leading to reduction of resistance to peptic and tryptic proteolysis. Steroids also prolong gastric cell regeneration time, perhaps leading to greater susceptibility to injury.[86]

Tenth nerve damage may depress reflexes and result in aspiration, requiring caution when patients are first fed after surgery. Complete inability to swallow or cough effectively may necessitate tracheotomy and gastrostomy. Patients usually compensate for unilateral paralysis of the vagus over days or months.

Compromise of trigeminal (V) and facial (VII) nerve function following surgery in the cerebellopontine angle may cause lid paralysis and loss of corneal reflexes and lid closing. Prevention of drying and local trauma by elevated patch or tarsorrhaphy is indicated. Abnormalities in eye muscle movement are produced by damage to the nuclear or internuclear apparatus or to the oculomotor nerves themselves. Treatment includes eye muscle surgery or temporary or permanent occlusion of one eye. Acoustic (VIII) nerve damage results in hearing impairment.

Hydrocephalus may persist when operation fails to correct CSF obstruction. A shunting procedure is required to relieve the blockage. Communicating hydrocephalus after posterior fossa surgery is due to interference with the absorptive system by blood, cisternal and subarachnoid adhesions, arachnoiditis, or leptomeningeal inflammation from infection.[137] Signs of increased intracranial pressure may not appear until 6 or 8 weeks after surgery for which a permanent shunt is indicated.

Spinal fluid fistulas occur with imperfect dural closure and elevation of intracranial pressure. Those that do not respond to simple suturing require reduction in spinal fluid pressure by either ventricular or lumbar subarachnoid drainage and head-up tilt to decrease the hydrodynamic pressure at the site of leakage.

Aseptic meningitis with meningismus, fever, malaise, and headache is associated with spillage of blood into the subarachnoid space. The response appears more often in infants and children and with increased frequency after posterior fossa surgery.[21] Sterile meningeal reactions also occur following exposure, manipulation, and excision of large blocks of tissue in which necrosis rather than blood is the likely mechanism. On lumbar puncture, CSF is bloody with increased protein content. CSF white cell count is elevated, but cultures are sterile and there is no peripheral leukocytosis. Patients with sterile meningeal responses remain alert without the aggravation of neurologic deficit seen with bacterial infection. Duration of illness is about 3 weeks with complete resolution and no sequelae.

Bacterial meningitis occurs in patients with CSF rhinorrhea, CSF fistula,[76] or following operations that impinge on barriers between meninges and contaminated spaces such as mastoid air cells during acoustic (VIII) nerve resection. *Staphylococcus, Pneumococcus, Enterococcus, Pseudomonas,* and *Klebsiella* are frequently encountered. While established meningitis with an identified organism usually responds to systemic antibiotics, operations that violate the barrier between infected site and intradural space, such as posterior fossa exploration with active mastoiditis, should include perioperative antibiotic coverage.

Although normal intellect is usually preserved in patients with cerebellar and brain stem damage, compromise of brain stem mechanisms involved in consciousness and emotions may produce prolonged coma ("akinetic mutism") as well as bizarre emotional states including euphoria and severe depression. Patients have been described who have recovered fully after being in a state of "akinetic mutism" for three months or longer. This comatose state results more often from brain stem strokes than from surgery, however.

REFERENCES

1. Adams, R. D., Fisher, C. M., Hakin, S., and others: Symptomatic occult hydrocephalus with normal cerebrospinal fluid pressure, N. Engl. J. Med. **273:**117, 1965.
2. Adams, R., Gronert, G., Sundt, T., and others: Halothane, hypocapnia, and cerebrospinal fluid pressure in neurosurgery, Anesthesiology **37:**510, 1972.
3. Albin, M. S.: Unpublished data.
4. Albin, M. S., Jannetta, P., Newfield, P., and others: Anesthetic considerations for patients in the sitting position; scientific manuscripts, American Association of Neurological Surgeons, Annual Meeting, New Orleans, April, 1978.
5. Albin, M. S., Jannetta, P. J., Maroon, J. C., and others: Anesthesia in the sitting position, Proc. IV Eur. Congr. Anaesth., Amsterdam, 1974, Excerpta Medica, p. 775.
6. Albin, M. S., Babinski, M., Maroon, J. C., and others: Anesthetic management of posterior fossa surgery in the sitting position, Acta Anaesth. Scand. **20:**117, 1976.
7. Albin, M. S., Carroll, R. G., Tung, A., and others: Venous air embolism in the sitting, lateral, supine, and prone positions, International Anesthesia Research Society, 51st Congress, Hollywood, Fla., March, 1977.
8. Albin, M. S., Chestnut, J. S., Gonzalez-Abola, E., and others: Clinical and experimental evaluation of intravenous nitroglycerin for induced hypotension, J. Neurosurg. **48:**704, 1978.
9. Albin, M. S., and Figallo, E.: Delayed postprandial solid food emesis in the postoperative patient, Proc. VI World Congr. Anaesth. Amsterdam, 1977, Excerpta Medica, p. 456.
10. Albin, M. S., Chestnut, J. S., Newfield, P. and others: Effects of anticholinergics and pre-induction oral sodium citrate on gastric pH and volume in the neurosurgical patient; scientific manuscripts, American Association of Neurological Surgeons, Annual Meeting, New Orleans, April, 1978.
11. Albright, L., and Reigel, D. H.: Management of hydrocephalus secondary to posterior fossa tumors, J. Neurosurg. **46:**52, 1977.
12. Apfelbaum, R. I.: A comparison of percutaneous radiofrequency trigeminal neurolysis and microvascular decompression of the trigeminal nerve for treatment of tic douloureux, Neurosurgery **1:**16, 1977.
13. Artru, A., Sohn, Y., and Eger, E.: Increased intracranial pressure from nitrous oxide five days after pneumoencephalography, Anesthesiology **49:**136, 1978.
14. Bailey, P., Buchanan, D. N., and Bucy, P.: Intracranial tumors of infancy and childhood, Chicago, 1939, University of Chicago Press.
15. Baringer, J. R., and Sworeland, P.: Recovery of herpes-simplex virus from human trigeminal ganglions, N. Engl. J. Med. **288:**648, 1973.
16. Bethune, R. W. M., and Brechner, V. L.: Detection of venous air embolism by carbon dioxide monitoring, Anesthesiology **29:**178, 1968.
17. Bleyaert, A. L., Nemoto, E. M., Stezoski, H., and others: Thiopental therapy after 16 minutes of global brain ischemia, Crit. Care Med. **4:**130, 1976.
18. Bloom, H. J. G.: Concepts in the natural history and treatment of medulloblastoma, Crit. Rev. Radiol. Sci. **2:**89, 1971.
19. Brechner, V. L., Bethune, W. M., and Soldo, N. J.: Pathological physiology of air embolism, Anesthesiology **28:**240, 1967.
20. Buhrley, L. E., and Reed, D. J.: The effect of furosemide on sodium-22 uptake into cerebrospinal fluid and brain, Exp. Brain Res. **14:**503, 1972.

21. Carmel, P. W., Fraser, R. A. R., and Stein, B. M.: Aseptic meningitis following posterior fossa surgery in children, J. Neurosurg. **41:**44, 1974.

22. Carroll, R., Albin, M. S., and Maroon, J.: Intraoperative air embolism, follow-up of 8 documented cases, Crit. Care Med. **4:**97, 1976.

23. Chandler, W., Demcheff, S., and Taren, J.: Acute pulmonary edema following venous air embolism during a neurosurgical procedure, J. Neurosurg. **40:**400, 1974.

24. Cherniak, J. S., and Longobardo, G. S.: Cheyne-Stokes breathing; an instability in physiologic control, N. Engl. J. Med. **288:**952, 1973.

25. Christensen, M., Holdt-Rasmussen, K., and Lassen, N.: Cerebral vasodilatation by halothane anaesthesia in man and its potentiation by hypotension and hypercapnia, Br. J. Anaesth. **39:**927, 1967.

26. Cooper, I. S. Amin, I., Riklan, M., and others: Chronic cerebellar stimulation in epilepsy; clinical and anatomical studies, Arch. Neurol. **33:**559, 1976.

27. Cooper, I. S., Riklan, M., Amin, I., and others: Chronic cerebellar stimulation in cerebral palsy, Neurology **26:**744, 1976.

28. Cooper, I. S., Amin, I., Upton, A., and others: Safety and efficacy of chronic stimulation, Neurosurgery **1:**203, 1977.

29. Cooperman, L. H., Strobel, G. E., and Kennell, E. M.: Massive hyperkalemia after administration of succinylcholine, Anesthesiology **32:**161, 1970.

30. Cottrell, J. E., Robustelli, A., Post, K., and others: Furosemide- and mannitol-induced changes in intracranial pressure and serum osmolarity and electrolytes, Anesthesiology **47:**28, 1977.

31. Cucchiara, R., Theye, R., and Michenfelder, J.: The effects of isoflurane on canine cerebral metabolism and blood flow, Anesthesiology **40:**571, 1974.

32. Cullen, D. J.: The effect of pre-treatment with non-depolarizing muscle relaxants on the neuromuscular blocking action of succinylcholine, Anesthesiology **35:**572, 1971.

33. Cushing, H.: Tumors of the nervus acousticus and the syndrome of the cerebellopontine angle, Philadelphia, 1917, W. B. Saunders Co.

34. Cushing, H.: Experiences with cerebellar medulloblastomas: a critical review, Acta Pathol. Microbiol. Scand. **7:**1, 1930.

35. Cushing, H.: Experiences with cerebellar astrocytomas; a critical review of seventy-six cases, Surg. Gynecol. Obstet. **52:**129, 1931.

36. Cushing, H.: Peptic ulcers and the interbrain, Surg. Gynecol. Obstet. **55:**1, 1932.

37. Dandy, W. E.: Concerning the cause of trigeminal neuralgia, Am. J. Surg. **24:**447, 1934.

38. Davis, R. M., Cullen, R. F., Flitter, M. A., and others: Control of spasticity and involuntary movements, Neurosurgery **1:**205, 1977.

39. Demopoulos, H., Flamm, E., Seligman, M., and others: Anti-oxidant effects of barbiturates in mod-

40. Durant, T. M., Long, J., and Oppenheimer, M. J.: Pulmonary (venous) air embolism, Am. Heart J. **33:**269, 1947.

41. Edmonds-Seal, J., Prys-Roberts, C., and Adams, A. P.: Transcutaneous Doppler ultrasonic flow detectors for diagnosis of air embolism, Proc. Roy. Soc. Med. **63:**831, 1970.

42. Ellis, S. C., Bryan-Brown, C. W., and Hyderally, H.: Massive swelling of the head and neck, Anesthesiology **42:**102, 1975.

43. Ericsson, J. A., Gottlieb, J. D., and Sweet, R. B.: Closed chest cardiac massage in the treatment of air embolism, N. Engl. J. Med. **270:**1353, 1964.

44. Fieschi, C., Agnoli, A., Battistini, N., and others: Derangement of regional cerebral blood flow and its regulatory mechanisms in acute cerebrovascular disease, Neurology **18:**1166, 1968.

45. Fitch, W., Barker, J., Jennett, W. B., and others: The influence of neuroleptanalgesic drugs on cerebrospinal fluid pressure, Br. J. Anaesth. **41:**800, 1969.

46. Fitch, W., McDowall, D. G.: Hazards of anesthesia in patients with intracranial space occupying lesions, Internat. Anesth. Clin. **7:**639, 1969.

47. Fitch, W., MacKenzie, E. T., Jones, J. V., and others: Effect of halothane on the autoregulation of cerebral blood flow in chronically hypertensive baboons, In Cerebral blood flow VIII, Acta Neurol. Scand. **56:**66, 1977.

48. Fitch, W., and McDowall, D. G.: Effect of halothane on intracranial pressure gradients in the presence of space-occupying lesions, Br. J. Anaesth. **43:**904, 1971.

49. Flamm, E., Demopoulos, M., Seligman, L., and others: Possible molecular mechanism of barbiturate-mediated protection in regional cerebral ischemia, Acta Neurol. Scand. **66:**150, 1977.

50. Forster, A., Van Horn, K., Marshall, L. F., and others: Influence of anesthetic agents on blood-brain barrier function during hypertension. In Cerebral blood flow VII, Acta Neurol. Scand. **56:**60, 1977.

51. Gallagher, E. G., and Pearson, D. J.: Ultrasonic identification of sources of microemboli during open heart surgery, Thorax **28:**295, 1973.

52. Gallon, S.: Controlled respiration in neurosurgical anaesthesia, Anaesthesia **14:**223, 1959.

53. Gordon, E.: Action of drugs on the intracranial contents. Proc. IV World Congr. Anaesth. Amsterdam, 1968, Excerpta Medica, p. 60.

54. Gronert, G. A.: Anesthesia for intracranial tumors, 24th Annual Refresher Course Lectures, American Society of Anesthesiologists, 1973, p. 107.

55. Gronert, G., and Theye, R.: Pathophysiology of hyperkalemia induced by succinylcholine, Anesthesiology **43:**89, 1975.

56. Hakim, A., and Moss, G.: Cerebral effects of barbiturate shift from "energy" to synthesis metab-

el membranes undergoing free radical damage, Acta Neurol. Scand. **66:**152, 1977.

olism for cellular viability, Surg. Forum **27:**497, 1976.

57. Hedden, M., Smith, R. B. F., and Torpey, D. J.: A complication of metal spiral-imbedded latex endotracheal tubes, Anesth. Analg. **51:**859, 1972.

58. Henriksen, H., and Jorgensen, P.: The effect of nitrous oxide on intracranial pressure in patients with intracranial disorders, Br. J. Anaesth. **45:**486, 1973.

59. Hoff, J. T., Smith, A. L., Hankinson, H. L., and others: Barbiturate protection from cerebral infarction in primates, Stroke **6:**28, 1975.

60. Hunter, A. R.: Discussion on the value of controlled respiration in neurosurgery, Proc. Roy. Soc. Med. **53:**365, 1960.

61. Hunter, A. R.: Neurosurgical Anaesthesia, ed. 2, Oxford, 1975, Blackwell Scientific Publications, p. 251.

62. Jannetta, P. J.: Arterial compression of the trigeminal nerve in patients with trigeminal neuralgia, J. Neurosurg. **26:**159, 1967.

63. Jannetta, P. J.: Microsurgical approach to the trigeminal nerve for tic douloureux, Prog. Neurol. Surg. **7:**180, 1976.

64. Jannetta, P. J., Abbasy, M., Maroon, J. C., and others: Etiology and definitive micro-surgical treatment of hemifacial spasm; operative techniques and results in 47 patients, J. Neurosurg. **47:**321, 1977.

65. Jannetta, P. J.: Treatment of trigeminal neuralgia by suboccipital and transtentorial cranial operations, Clin. Neurosurg. **24:**538, 1977.

66. Jared, M., Gilboe, D., and Cesano, T.: The rebound phenomenon and hypertonic solutions, J. Neurosurg. **21:**1059, 1964.

67. Jennett, W. B., Barker, J., Fitch, W., and others: Effects of anaesthesia on ICP in patients with intracranial space-occupying lesions, Lancet **1:**61, 1969.

68. Kaufman, B., Weiss, M. H., Young, H. F., and others: Effects of prolonged cerebrospinal fluid shunting on the skull and brain, J. Neurosurg. **38:**288, 1973.

69. Kerber, C., and Cromwell, L. D.: Pediatric pneumoencephalography with nitrous oxide, Child Brain **2:**309, 1976.

70. Kricheff, I. I., Becker, M., Schneck, S. A., and others: Intracranial ependymomas; a study of survival in 65 cases treated by surgery and irradiation, Am. J. Roentgenol. **91:**167, 1964.

71. Lall, N. G., and Jain, A. P.: Circulatory and respiratory disturbances during posterior fossa surgery, Br. J. Anaesth. **41:**447, 1969.

72. Langfitt, T. W., Weinstein, J. D., Kassell, N. F., and others: Transmission of increased ICP. I. Within the craniospinal axis, J. Neurosurg. **21:**989, 1964.

73. Lassen, N. A.: The luxury perfusion syndrome and its possible relation to acute metabolic acidosis localized within the brain, Lancet **2:**1113, 1966.

74. Lassen, N. A.: Control of the cerebral circulation in health and disease, Circ. Res. **34:**749, 1974.

75. Lesky, E.: Notes on the history of air embolism, Ger. Med. **6:**159, 1961.

76. MacGee, E. E., Cauthen, J. C., and Brackett, C. E.: Meningitis following acute traumatic cerebrospinal fluid fistula, J. Neurosurg. **33:**312, 1970.

77. Magendie, F.: Sur l'entree accidentelle de l'air dans les veines, J. Physiol. Exper. **1:**190, 1821.

78. Maroon, J. C., Goodman, J. M., and Horner, T. G.: Detection of minute venous air emboli with ultrasound, Surg. Gynecol. Obstet. **127:**1236, 1968.

79. Maroon, J. C., Edmonds-Seal, J., and Campbell, R. L.: An ultrasonic method for detecting air embolism, J. Neurosurg. **31:**196, 1969.

80. Maroon, J. C., and Albin, M. S.: Air embolism diagnosed by Doppler ultrasound, Anesth. Analg. **58:**399, 1974.

81. Maroon, J. C., Albin, M. S., and Carroll, R.: Venous air embolism in neurosurgery; scientific manuscripts, American Association of Neurological Surgeons, Annual Meeting, Toronto, April, 1977.

82. Martin, J. T.: Neuroanesthetic adjuncts for surgery in the sitting position. I. Introduction and basic equipment, Anesth. Analg. **49:**577, 1970.

83. Matson, D. D.: Neurosurgery of infancy and childhood, Springfield, Ill., 1969, Charles C Thomas, Publisher.

84. McAllister, R. G.: Macroglossia—a positional complication, Anesthesiology **40:**199, 1974.

85. McQueen, J., and Jones, L.: Dehydration and rehydration of the brain with hypertonic urea and mannitol, J. Neurosurg. **21:**118, 1964.

86. Menguy, R., and Masters, Y.: Effect of cortisone on mucoprotein secretion by gastric antrum of dogs, Surgery **54:**19, 1963.

87. Meridy, H. W., Creighton, R. E., and Humphreys, R. P.: Complications during neurosurgery in the prone position in children, Can. Anaesth. Soc. J. **21:**445, 1974.

88. Michenfelder, J. D., Terry, H. R., Daw, E. F., and others: Air embolism during neurosurgery, Anesth. Analg. **45:**390, 1966.

89. Michenfelder, J. D., Gronert, G. A., and Rehder, K.: Neuroanesthesia, Anesthesiology **30:**65, 1969.

90. Michenfelder, J. D., and Theye, R. A.: Effects of fentanyl, droperidol, and Innovar on canine cerebral metabolism and blood flow, Br. J. Anaesth. **43:**630, 1971.

91. Michenfelder, J. D., Miller, R. H., and Gronert, G. A.: Evaluation of an ultrasonic device (Doppler) for the diagnosis of venous air embolism, Anesthesiology **36:**164, 1972.

92. Michenfelder, J. D.: The interdependence of cerebral function and metabolic effects following massive doses of thiopental in the dog, Anesthesiology **41:**231, 1974.

93. Michenfelder, J. D., and Sundt, T. M.: Cerebral protection by barbiturate anesthesia and intensive care for 48 hours following permanent middle cere-

bral artery occlusion in Java monkeys. In Harper, A. M., Jennett, B., Miller, D., and others, editors: Blood flow and metabolism, Edinburgh, 1975, Churchill Livingston, p. 12.

94. Millar, R. A.: Neuroanesthesia in the sitting position, Br. J. Anaesth. **44:**495, 1972.

95. Miller, J. D., and Barker, J.: The effect of neuroleptanalgesic drugs on cerebral blood flow and metabolism, Br. J. Anaesth. **41:**554, 1969.

96. Miller, J. D., Stanek, A. E., and Langfitt, T. W.: A comparison of autoregulation to changes in intracranial and arterial pressure in the same preparation, Eur. Neurol. **6:**34, 1971.

97. Miller, J. D., and Leech, P.: Effects of mannitol and steroid therapy on intracranial volume-pressure relationships in patients, J. Neurosurg. **42:** 274, 1975.

98. Miller, R. D., and Way, W. L.: Inhibition of succinylcholine induced increased intragastric pressure by non-depolarizing muscle relaxants and lidocaine, Anesthesiology **34:**185, 1971.

99. Misfeldt, B., Jorgensen, P., and Rishoj, M.: The effect of nitrous oxide and halothane upon the intracranial pressure in hypocapneic patients with intracranial disorders, Br. J. Anaesth. **46:**853, 1974.

100. Moyer, J. H., Pontius, R. P., Morris, G., and others: Effect of morphine and n-allylnormorphine on cerebral hemodynamics and oxygen metabolism, Circulation **15:**379, 1957.

101. Munson, E. S., and Merrick, H. C.: Effect of nitrous oxide on venous air embolism, Anesthesiology **27:**783, 1966.

102. Munson, E. S.: Effect of nitrous oxide on the pulmonary circulation during venous air embolism, Anesth. Analg. **50:**785, 1971.

103. Munson, E. S., Paul, W. L., Perry, J. C., and others: Early detection of venous air embolism using a Swan-Ganz catheter, Anesthesiology **42:** 223, 1975.

104. Murphy, F. L., Kennell, E. M., Johnstone, R. E., and others: The effects of enflurane, isoflurane, and halothane on cerebral blood flow and metabolism in man; abstracts of scientific papers, American Society of Anesthesiologists Annual Meeting, Washington, D.C., 1974, p. 62.

105. Nasson, S. I., and Mount, L. A.: Papillomas of the choroid plexus, J. Neurosurg. **29:**73, 1968.

106. Ng, T. Y., and Kirimli, B. I.: Hazards in use of anode endotracheal tube; a case report and review, Anesth. Analg. **54:**710, 1975.

107. Ngai, S. H., Stinchfield, F. E., and Triner, L.: Air embolism during total hip arthroplasties, Anesthesiology **40:**405, 1974.

108. North, J. B., and Jennett, S.: Abnormal breathing patterns associated with acute brain damage, Arch. Neurol. **31:**338-344, 1974.

109. Olivecrona, H.: Acoustic tumors, J. Neurosurg. **16:** 6, 1967.

110. Pherman, J., and Shapiro, H.: Modification of ni-

trous oxide-induced intracranial hypertension by prior induction of anesthesia, Anesthesiology **46:** 150, 1977.

111. Phillips, T. L., Sheline, G. E., and Boldrey, E.: Therapeutic considerations in tumors affecting the central nervous system: ependymomas, Radiology **83:**98, 1964.

112. Pierce, E. C. Jr., Lambertsen, C. J., Deutsch, S., and others: Cerebral circulation and metabolism during thiopental anesthesia and hyperventilation in man, J. Clin. Invest. **41:**1664, 1962.

113. Plum, F.: Hyperpnea, hyperventilation and brain dysfunction, Ann. Intern. Med. **76:**328, 1972.

114. Pollay, M.: Formation of CSF; relation of studies of isolated choroid plexus to the standing gradient hypothesis, J. Neurosurg. **42:**665, 1975.

115. Proakis, A., and Harris, G.: Comparative penetration of glycopyrrolate and atropine across blood brain and placental barrier in anesthetized dogs, Fed. Proc. **36:**996, 1977.

116. Reulen, H. J., and Kreysch, H. G.: Measurement of brain tissue pressure in cold-induced cerebral edema, Acta Neurochir. (Wein) **29:**29, 1973.

117. Richardson, H. F., Coles, B. C., and Hall, G. E.: Experimental gas embolism. I. Intravenous air embolism, Can. Med. Assoc. J. **36:**584, 1937.

118. Roberts, B., and Smith, P.: Hazards of mannitol infusions, Lancet **2:**421, 1966.

119. Rosomoff, H. L.: Adjuncts to neurosurgical anaesthesia, Br. J. Anaesth. **37:**246, 1965.

120. Saidman, L. J., and Eger, E. I: Changes in cerebrospinal fluid pressure during pneumoencephalography under nitrous oxide anesthesia, Anesthesiology **26:**67, 1965.

121. Sakabe, T., Kuramoto, T., Inuoue, S., and others: Cerebral effects of nitrous oxide in the dog, Anesthesiology **48:**195, 1978.

122. Salem, M., Wong, A., Mani, M., and others: Premedicant drugs and gastric juice pH and volume in pediatric patients, Anesthesiology **44:**216, 1976.

123. Savarese, J. J., and Kitz, R. J.: Pharmacology of relaxants; Refresher Courses Anesth. **3:**153, 1975.

124. Sayers, M. P., and Hunt, W. E.: Posterior fossa tumors. In Youmans, J. R., editor: Neurological surgery, Philadelphia, 1973, W. B. Saunders Co., p. 1485.

125. Shapiro, H. M., Galindo, A., Wyte, S. R., and others: Rapid intra-operative reduction of intracranial hypertension with thiopentone, Br. J. Anaesth. **45:**1057, 1973.

126. Shapiro, H. M.: Intracranial hypertension: therapeutic and anesthetic considerations, Anesthesiology **43:**445, 1975.

127. Shapiro, W.: Chemotherapy of primary malignant brain tumors in children, Cancer **35:**965, 1975.

128. Sheline, G.: Radiation therapy of tumors of the central nervous system in childhood, Cancer **35:** 957, 1975.

129. Shenkin, H., and Goldfedder, P.: Air embolism

from exposure of posterior cranial fossa in the prone position, J.A.M.A. **210**:726, 1969.

130. Shepard, D.A.E.: Harvey Cushing and anaesthesia, Can. Anaesth. Soc. J. **12**:431, 1965.

131. Smith, A. L., and Wollman, H.: Cerebral blood flow and metabolism, Anesthesiology **36**:378, 1972.

132. Smith, A. L., Hoff, J. T., Nielsen, S. L., and others: Barbiturate protection in acute focal cerebral ischemia, Stroke **5**:1, 1974.

133. Smith, A. L., and Marque, J. J.: Anesthetics and cerebral edema, Anesthesiology **45**:64, 1976.

134. Sondergaard, N.: Intracranial pressure during general anesthesia, Dallas Med. Bull. **8**:18, 1961.

135. Stallworth, J. M., Martin, J. B., and Postelthwait, R. W.: Aspiration of the heart in air embolism, J.A.M.A. **43**:1250, 1950.

136. Steffey, E. P., Gauger, G. E., and Eger, E. I.: Cardiovascular effects of venous air embolism during air and oxygen breathing, Anesth. Analg. **53**:599, 1974.

137. Stein, B. M., Tenner, M. S., and Fraser, R. A. R.: Hydrocephalus following removal of cerebellar astrocytomas in children, J. Neurosurg. **36**:763, 1972.

138. Stone, W. A., Beach, T. P., and Hamelberg, W.: Succinylcholine—danger in the spinal cord injured patient, Anesthesiology **32**:168, 1970.

139. Strandgaard, S., Oleson, J., Skinhoj, E., and others: Autoregulation of brain circulation in severe arterial hypertension, Br. Med. J. **159**:507, 1973.

140. Strandgaard, S., MacKenzie, E. T., Sengupta, D., and others: Upper limits of autoregulation of cerebral blood flow in the baboon, Circ. Res. **34**:435, 1974.

141. Sturdee, D. W.: Diazepam: routes of administra-tion and rate of absorption, Br. J. Anaesth. **48**:1091, 1976.

142. Tarkkanen, L., Laitenen, L., and Johansson, G.: Effects of d-tubocurarine on intracranial pressure and thalamic electrical impedance, Anesthesiology **40**:247, 1974.

143. Tateishi, H.: Prospective study of air embolism, J.A.M.A. **43**:1306, 1972.

144. Tinker, J., Gronert, G., Messick, J., and others: Detection of air embolism: a test for positioning right atrial catheter and Doppler probe, Anesthesiology **43**:104, 1975.

145. Trowbridge, W. V., and French, J. D.: Benign arachnoid cysts of the posterior fossa. J. Neurosurg. **9**:398, 1952.

146. Waldman, T. A., Levin, E. H., and Baldwin, M.: The association of polycythemia with a cerebellar hemangioblastoma; the production of an erythropoiesis stimulating factor by the tumor, Am. J. Med. **31**:318, 1961.

147. Weintraub, H. D., Heisterkamp, D. V., and Cooperman, L. H.: Changes in plasma potassium concentration after depolarizing blockers in anaesthetized man, Br. J. Anaesth. **41**:1048, 1969.

148. Whitby, J. D.: Electrocardiography during posterior fossa operations, Br. J. Anaesth. **35**:624, 1963.

149. Whitehouse, S.: Acoustic neuroma: anaesthesia in acoustic neuroma, Otolaryngology **88**:628, 1969.

150. Wilkins, R. H., and Albin, M. S.: An unusual entrance site of venous air embolism during operations in the sitting position, Surg. Neurol. **7**:71, 1977.

151. Wilson, C. B.: Diagnosis and surgical treatment of childhood brain tumors, Cancer **35**:950, 1975.

152. Wolffe, J. B., and Robertson, F. H.: Experimental air embolism, Ann. Intern. Med. **9**:162, 1935.

10

Management of severe head injury

DEREK A. BRUCE

Only a small percentage of head injuries are seen by the specialist in critical care medicine or neurosurgery. The majority of patients injuring their heads do not seek medical attention because the effects of the injury are transient. Of those seeking medical attention, approximately 80% have scalp lacerations and require only minor therapy[11]; and, even of those admitted to hospital, two thirds are discharged within 48 hours.[18] Thus, it is a small percentage of head injuries that require the intensive therapy that will be discussed. In actual numbers, however, the problem is large, and approximately 600,000 patients per year sustain a severe head injury associated with epidural or subdural hematoma or cerebral laceration.[11] The mortality reported for patients following head injury varies markedly depending on the admission policies of the hospital from 5% for all head injury patients admitted to a general hospital[38] to 40% if only persons with severe head injuries are admitted.[31] Sevitt reported that 50% of deaths related to head injury following road traffic accidents occurred within the first two hours, 60% within 24 hours, and 75% within 48 hours.[50] This implies that up to 50% of the mortality from head injury occurs in patients who never reached a hospital. This early mortality includes the most severe primary brain injuries. If the patient survives long enough to reach the hospital, the primary injury has been insufficient to cause death

and, theoretically, therapy can control secondary injury and death should be preventable.

The concept of primary and secondary head injury is important to those involved in the care of patients who have sustained major head trauma. The primary head injury results from the biomechanical effect of the forces applied to the skull and brain at the time of the traumatic insult and is manifested within milliseconds of the injury. In its mildest form, this is represented as concussion, a transient but reversible loss of consciousness associated with pupillary dilatation, loss of corneal responses, bradycardia, and bradypnea. In its most severe form, physical disruption of the brain stem at the pontomedullary junction occurs with sudden death. The effect of the initial injury on neurons, axons, and glia is very poorly understood at present. If the patient survives the initial head injury long enough to reach the hospital, this implies that the biomechanical injury has not been sufficiently severe to cause death. If death occurs later, this must be due to a second series of events that may have been triggered by the initial trauma but that have progressed from the time of injury to cause secondary damage and, thus, death. This series of events is described as the secondary head injury and may be due to intracranial or systemic factors. Theoretically, the second head injury can be avoided by medical care and, thus, death can be prevented. Unfortunately, although death may be preventable, sufficiently severe injury may have occurred to the central nervous system to make a functional recovery impossible. At the present time, we have no treatment for the primary biomechanical brain damage and all our therapy is directed to preventing secondary injury due to hypoxia, hypercapnia, hypotension, or increased intracranial pressure (ICP). It is obvious that to be maximally effective therapy to prevent secondary head injury should begin immediately at the site of the accident. It is vitally important for the practitioner dealing with head injuries to distinguish in his or her mind clearly these two sets of events, the primary and secondary head injury, since therapy is based on a clear appreciation of these concepts.

One other major obstruction to the aggressive treatment of all severe head injuries has been the concept of primary brain stem injury. This diagnosis is frequently made in patients rendered unconscious at the time of injury and presenting with clinical signs of mesencephalic or pontine dysfunction. It has been generally accepted that this pattern is due to a select primary injury to the brain stem and that treatment to prevent the secondary head injury will not be beneficial, and death or poor outcome is inevitable. The pathologic studies of Adams and Graham[1] have demonstrated that in the population of patients seen in a neurosurgical unit, primary, isolated injury to the brain stem is extremely uncommon. The pathology seen in the brain of patients rendered immediately unconscious is that of diffuse injury to the white matter of the hemispheres, corpus callosum, and brain stem. Adams and Graham[1] reported an incidence of 50% or more of secondary ischemia lesions even in patients dying within a few hours with diffuse cerebral injury. Thus, most of the patients categorized as having brain stem injury do, in fact, have diffuse cerebral injury and 50%[44] to 80%[10] of these patients develop an elevated ICP that requires active therapy. As many as 80% may make a good recovery, especially younger patients.

If the primary mechanical injury is insufficient to kill the patient within the first minutes to hours following head injury, death, if it occurs, is due to the second head injury. Potentially, all the factors invoking the secondary head injury are treatable and, therefore, death should be preventable. This does not mean, however, that recovery will occur, since sufficient damage may have occurred to make recovery impossible and the patient may be left severely disabled or vegetative. The risk of salvaging many severely disabled patients has been a concern for those units treating head injuries. However, recent studies suggest that a significant decrease in mortality can be achieved without increasing the number of patients surviving in a vegetative or severely disabled state in both children and adults.[9,10,16,23]

One of the major difficulties in trying to evaluate the outcome from severe head injury has been the lack of a standard scale for defining the degree of neurologic impairment early in the course of injury. In an effort to remedy this, Teasdale and Jennett[56] introduced a coma score based on three separate sets of function: eye opening, speech, and motor function (see p. 185). This scale has been tested in four separate centers in Scotland, Holland, and the United States. This scaling system is quite constant from observer to observer and seems to be the best system available at present. Jennett and co-workers[31] have shown that mortality in the several centers is very closely related to the initial score on the coma scale and that the results are remarkably similar from unit to unit despite large differences in the incidence of hematomas, time of admission, and therapy. It is important for those taking care of the severely head-injured patient to be familiar with this simple grading system to make future reports of outcome meaningful and, hopefully, to allow the effects of different modalities of therapy to be evaluated.

In most intensive care units the Glasgow Coma Scale will not function adequately as a neurologic minute-to-minute checksheet since it does not include lower brain stem reflexes, such as corneals or calorics, and

---

GLASGOW COMA SCALE[31]

Eye opening
4 Spontaneous
3 To speech
2 To pain
1 None

Best verbal response
5 Oriented
4 Confused
3 Inappropriate
2 Incomprehensible
1 None

Best motor response
6 Obey commands
5 Localized pain
4 Withdraws
3 Flexion to pain
2 Extension to pain
1 None

---

does not include respiratory pattern, pulse, or blood pressure. Nonetheless, a progressively declining Glasgow Coma Scale will rapidly alert the clinician to a deteriorating level of consciousness. By the time changes in the midbrain and pontine reflexes have occurred it may be too late to obtain a satisfactory outcome from decompression (i.e., mass lesion) or from lowering the ICP. Thus, the Glasgow Coma Scale can serve as an adequate indicator of deteriorating neurologic state when combined with other physiologic parameters.

NEUROLOGIC EXAM

The purposes of the acute neurologic exam in the severely head-injured patient can be defined as follows: (1) to permit the clinician to estimate the degree and location of cerebral injury, (2) to establish a baseline neurologic state to which all future examinations will be referred in order to identify improvement or deterioration, (3) to establish the presence or absence of mass lesion that might require surgical intervention, and (4) to allow some estimate of prognosis for recovery to be made at the earliest possible time. This examination is intimately associated with the general systemic examination for evidence of other injuries.

As in other medical emergencies, a rapid history should be obtained if possible. The points to be gleaned are the time the injury occurred, the possible mechanisms of injury, since a blow to the fixed or static head is much more likely to result in local skull fracture and hematoma or contusion of the brain, whereas an accleration/deceleration injury to the head without impact is more likely to produce acute subdural hematomas and diffuse cerebral injury with multifocal contusions of the brain and cervical spine. A record of the level of consciousness of the patient at the earliest possible time following injury is extremely important if it can be obtained and may define whether the patient's level of consciousness is deteriorating and suggest the possibility of an expanding intracranial mass or whether unconsciousness occurred immediately following impact with the suggestion of diffuse cerebral injury. Was there a lot of blood at the accident suggesting the possibility of shock? Was there any observed period of apnea or cyanosis suggesting the possibility of secondary anoxic injury? Finally, it is important to endeavor to establish if anything is known of the patient's past medical history.

The neurologic exam must be rapid yet adequate to define the extent of injury and must not delay resuscitation. If the patient is comatose (defined as no eye opening, no verbal responses, and the inability to obey command), the purpose of the exam is to define the degree of dysfunction of the cortex, diencephalon, mesencephalon, pons, and medulla and to identify evidence of unilateral neurologic abnormalities that might indicate the presence of a mass lesion. The important aspects of the neurologic exam are the best motor response, which will define how well the brain is still relating to its environment (i.e., purposeful or nonpurposeful movements); the size and response of the pupils to light; the presence or absence of corneal reflex; oculomotor function defined by oculovestibular testing; gag response; respiratory and pulse patterns and blood pressure. If the patient has been conscious following injury, this strongly suggests that the primary biomechanical injury was insufficient to cause severe brain dysfunction and that secondary deterioration is occurring. This secondary deterioration is assumed to be due to an expanding mass lesion until proven otherwise. Increasing severity of headache followed by progressively deteriorating level of consciousness following head injury has to be assumed to be due to secondary intracranial hypertension even when no mass lesion is present and measurement and control of the ICP becomes vital.

If the patient is awake, alert, and oriented, specific testing for complex functions can be performed. Here we will discuss only those patients who are either unconscious or show signs of deteriorating consciousness. The definition of a severely head-injured patient is presented by Jennett and co-workers[31] and includes lack of eye opening and no verbal response or response to commands. For inclusion in this series of patients[31] this state has to exist for at least six hours. Although patients with surgical lesions will hopefully be operated upon within this six-hour period, the time limit excludes patients whose initial neurologic exam appears worse than the actual degree of cerebral injury sustained. This apparently poor examination is usually due to the presence of alcohol or drugs, systemic hypoxemia, or systemic shock.

Level of consciousness

In a patient who has speech or who can obey commands, any loss of these functions represents a significant deterioration in the patient's neurologic state and should be taken as an indication for the patient to be studied to rule out a progressing mass lesion. In the patient who is too irritable to follow commands but has some spontaneous speech, any loss of the limited speech ability should again be taken as a sign of deterioration. These patients frequently exhibit cyclic excitation and depression, and it is necessary to apply a sufficiently severe stimulus to overcome the depressed state when each examination is made; otherwise, an apparent deterioration will be recorded. In patients with no speech and who do not obey commands, a change in the level of consciousness is difficult to measure. A decrease in spontaneous activity or diminished response to pain may be the only change and, if not carefully sought and recorded, may easily be overlooked. The response to pain can be graded as purposeful, nonpurposeful, decortication, decerebration, and no response. A change in the level of pain response may be the only way of identifying a change in the neurologic state and is just as important or more important than the loss of speech function since the next stage in deterioration once pain responses are absent will be respiratory changes with progressive loss of brain stem reflexes and death. With the majority of surgically treated lesions following acute head injury, there is an excellent correlation with the neurologic state at the time of surgery and the final outcome. The worse the neurologic state, the worse the outcome. Thus, it is extremely important to identify evidence of an expanding lesion at the earliest possible time. Unfortunately, our ability to grade the degree of neurologic disturbance becomes increasingly less accurate as the patients have increasing degrees of neurologic damage. Because of this, once decerebration is present, we monitor the ICP and use changes in that to identify a deteriorating state.

Motor response

In the Glasgow Coma Score there is a section on best motor response, although there is an overlap between this and the estimate of level of consciousness as discussed above. The importance of including motor response as a separate category is that there is a good correlation between final outcome and best motor response within the first six hours. When coma is sufficiently deep for a nonpurposeful pain response to be elicited, the only measure available to grade further deterioration is a gradation of abnormal motor responses from abnormal flexion or

Table 10-1. Outcome following severe head injury with bilateral unreactive pupils

	Jennett et al.[31]	Becker et al.[3]	Bruce et al.[9]*
Pupils reactive	55%	28%	5%
Bilateral unreactive	91%	85%	29%
Outcome category	Dead/PVS/SD†	Dead/PVS/SD	Dead/PVS/SD

*Children 0 to 19 years.
†PVS, persistent vegetative state; SD, severely disabled.

decortication through abnormal extension or decerebration to flaccidity. The mortality and severe morbidity in patients with severe head trauma and no abnormal motor posturing varies from 0%,[9] 19%,[2] 25%,[5] and 52%[33]; that for patients with abnormal posturing is 23%,[9] 68%,[2] 72%,[5] and 90%.[33] The stimulus used to induce the response should be standard and intense; any change in response has the same importance as any other measure of a deteriorating state. We have found children with decerebrate posturing on admission to have a much better prognosis (17% mortality) than adults with a similar picture. Bricolo,[5] however, found no difference between adults and children and reported a mortality rate of 71%.

Pupillary responses

The examination of the size of the pupils and their response to light gives information about the mesencephalon and about the function of the third nerve. When transtentorial herniation occurs, dilatation of the pupil (usually on the ipsilateral side) is frequently seen. This is due to compression of the third nerve and since the pupillary fibers run superficially in the nerve they are involved early and enlargement of the pupil occurs due to interference with the parasympathetic supply. The compression probably occurs between the tentorial edge and the herniating uncus of the temporal lobe. Compression between the superior cerebellar and posterior cerebral arteries has also been implicated as a mechanism for third nerve dysfunction during progressive rostral caudal displacement of the brain stem. If the enlarged pupil is due to third nerve com-

pression, which is progressive, paresis of eye movement will also occur.

When bilateral pupillary dilatation is present, it is due either to bilateral third nerve compression secondary to uncal herniation or to local injury in the mesencephalon. If the eye movements are full and there is no history of progressive deterioration, the picture is most likely due to local mesencephalic injury but a mass lesion must always be kept in mind and ruled out by the appropriate studies. When sufficient herniation has occurred, bilateral pupillary dilatation due to secondary compression of the mesencephalon with secondary ischemia may be seen. When the examination of the pupils is performed, it is important to rule out local eye trauma, which not infrequently will give rise to either a locally large or small pupil that has nothing to do with disturbances in the intracranial space.

The prognosis for patients with acute, bilateral unreactive pupils is significantly worse than for those with preserved pupillary responses (Table 10-1). Once again, it can be seen that the outcome in children is more optimistic than that for adults.

Corneal responses

The anatomic pathway for this reflex is an afferent limb via the fifth cranial nerve and the motor limb via the seventh cranial nerve. This reflex is lost in experimental traumatic unconsciousness and is frequently absent in patients admitted with traumatic unconsciousness. The presence or absence of this reflex is not felt to be very beneficial either in defining the level of injury or as a prognostic indicator. The importance of

Table 10-2. Outcome correlated with presence or absence
of oculocephalic or oculovestibular reflex

	Jennett et al.[31]	Becker et al.[3]	Bruce et al.[9*]
Oculocephalic/vestibular intact	51%	19%	3%
Oculocephalic/vestibular impaired	86%	73%	33%
Outcome category	Dead/PVS/SD†	Dead/PVS/SD	Dead/PVS/SD

*Children 0 to 19 years.
†PVS, persistent vegetative state; SD, severely disabled.

recording the response is mainly related to the nursing needs of the unconscious patient and the need to lubricate the cornea frequently to avoid drying and scarring and to tape the eyes closed if necessary.

Ocular muscle function

The coordinated reflex eye movements are mediated through connections between the third, fourth, and sixth cranial nerves and their interconnecting tract, the medial longitudinal fasciculus, which runs from the pons to the mesencephalon in the periaqueductal area. In a comatose patient, no voluntary eye movements may be elicited and, therefore, the eye movements must be triggered using some reflex stimulus. Head turning (oculocephalic or doll's eye response) or instilling cold water into the ear (oculovestibular response) are the two simplist ways to stimulate the vestibular apparatus and obtain the desired information. We have restricted our examination in patients to the use of cold water stimulation of the ears because of the potential hazards of moving the head from side to side (doll's eye maneuver), since at the time the initial exam is performed a cervical spinal injury may also be present and could be aggravated by head movement. To perform the oculovestibular test, a standard volume of cool water or saline should be used. Before instillation of any water, the ear canal and drum should be inspected. If there is evidence of CSF leakage or fresh rupture of the eardrum, no stimulation is performed on that side. Clots or wax in the canal may well interfere with the test and, therefore, should be carefully removed if time permits. The head should be in the mid position and

flexed slightly. However, when initially performing the oculovestibular testing, we keep the neck in the neutral position until spinal bony injury has been ruled out. At least one minute should be allowed for evidence of function to be seen. In the unconscious patient with an intact brain stem, there should be tonic deviation of the eyes to the side of the cooling with no nystagmus. Two abnormal patterns are most frequently seen. In one, the abducting eye moves well laterally, but the adducting eye does not cross the midline. This suggests a lesion in the medial longitudinal fasciculus that may be present unilaterally or bilaterally. The other common pattern is of no response to stimulation either unilaterally or bilaterally and suggests a larger area of involvement of the periaqueductal gray or pontine areas. The finding of impaired oculovestibular or oculocephalic responses carries a poor prognosis (Table 10-2). The outcome is better in children than in adults.

Respiratory function

When no spontaneous ventilation is present on admission, the prognosis appears to be close to zero for any useful functional recovery unless the patient is seen within minutes post trauma. In this case, the apnea may be part of the early traumatic unconsciousness and may not be a measure of cerebral injury. Even in children we have seen no recovery better than the severely disabled category if apnea has been present on admission.[9]

In reporting outcome, the categories described by Jennett and Bond[30] will be used. These categories are (1) good recovery (a patient who can lead a full and independent life with or without minimal neurologic deficit); (2) moderately disabled (a patient with neurologic or intellectual impairment but who is independent; (3) severely disabled (a patient who is conscious but totally dependent on others to get through the activities of the day); (4) vegetative survival; and (5) death.

EMERGENCY THERAPY

Emergency therapy is begun at the site of the accident, if possible, in the ambulance, or certainly immediately upon admission to the emergency room. The primary concern is to secure an open airway and ensure adequate ventilation. The first step is simply to clean out the mouth and nasopharynx using a sponge and then to suction. An oral airway can then be inserted and ventilation by mask performed, if necessary. Hypercarbia and hypoxemia are almost constant findings in patients with severe head injuries admitted to hospitals. Cleaning the airway usually corrects the hypercarbia, and spontaneous hyperventilation is common. The hypoxemia remains, and supplemental oxygen (50%) is usually required. If the patient is not breathing spontaneously and artificial ventilation is necessary, great care must be used not to hyperextend the neck, since cervical injury may also be present. In children it is not usually necessary to hyperextend the neck, and an oral airway and mask and bag should be adequate to ensure ventilation. Gentle pressure on the cricoid cartilage prevents air from entering and distending the stomach and abdomen, raising the diaphragm, and interfering with respiration. It also prevents regurgitation of stomach contents. Even in adults, the jaw can usually be held forward and an open airway secured without hyperextending the neck. Once the airway is secured, a nasogastric tube can be inserted and the stomach contents evacuated.

As soon as the patient is stable, a lateral cervical spine x-ray is obtained. If this is normal, the patient now can be given pentothal and pancuronium (Pavulon), and careful endotracheal intubation can be performed under the best possible circumstances with the least rise in ICP. From this point until the CAT scan is completed and the patient is in the ICU or operating room, the muscle paralysis is continued. Efforts to intubate a patient who is struggling or gagging on the tube are more likely to cause harm than to do good. The only patients in whom the general approach described above cannot be used are those with severe maxillofacial trauma in whom an emergency tracheostomy may be necessary. As an airway is being secured, a pulse and blood pressure are recorded. With severe head injury either tachycardia or bradycardia may be present, and frequently there is marked sinus arrhythmia. Hypotension caused by the cerebral injury itself is seen only when respirations are agonal and marked bradycardia is present, suggesting imminent death. Thus, when a low blood pressure is recorded, a careful search for multiple fractures and abdominal or thoracic trauma is required. If there has been severe bleeding from the scalp or the ears, systemic hypotension can occasionally result. Abdominal lavage may be necessary to identify hemorrhage, and rapid x-ray of the abdomen and chest may be required. It is vital to exclude occult sources of blood loss. If there is no evidence of perineal trauma, a urinary catheter is carefully placed and the urine examined for evidence of blood. Before obtaining the abdominal films, an injection of Renografin may be given to identify the kidneys on film, thus obtaining an IVP. If severe perineal trauma is suspected, a urethrogram may be necessary to ensure there is no urethral injury before catheterization.

Long bone fractures should be immobilized. A large peripheral IV is begun and blood is drawn for CBC, clotting studies, electrolytes, type and cross match and any other indicated studies. Blood gases should always be checked once an airway is secured to ensure that the ventilation is adequate.

All comatose children with Glasgow coma scores of 6 or less and all adults with severe injury and coma scores of 8 or less receive an immediate dose of dexamethasone, 1 to 1.5 mg/kg IV. This steroid is continued through the first several days in doses of 1.5 mg/kg/day and then is gradually tapered, depending on the clinical course of the patient and the intracranial pressure. This dosage schedule is based on the work of Faupel[16] and Gobiet and co-workers.[23] These reports are the only ones as yet to show a significant beneficial effect of corticosteroids in patients with acute severe head trauma. Both studies showed no beneficial effect of the low more standard doses of corticosteroids.

The normal ICP is a pulsatile pressure whose upper limit is 15 mm Hg. An ICP of 15 to 20 torr is considered mildly elevated, and any pressure over 20 torr we regard as significant hypertension requiring therapy. During emergency resuscitation we assume that intracranial hypertension is present and, thus, the ventilatory support is designed to produce moderate hypocarbia to 25 torr, and all precautions are taken to avoid inducing large changes in systemic arterial pressure (SAP) by overreplacement of fluids in an effort to avoid further aggravating the ICP. Coughing or straining against the endotracheal tube or intermittent decerebration are treated with muscle paralysis to avoid elevations of central venous pressure that might further increase the ICP. It is a simple and brief procedure to insert an ICP monitor[27] in the subarachnoid space in the emergency room. Once this is done, the ICP is measured and, if it is elevated, rational therapy can be given. It is particularly important to insert the ICP monitor in the emergency room if a long period of resuscitation from shock is likely or if there is an abdominal catastrophy (i.e., ruptured spleen) producing hypotension and if, therefore, immediate surgery is required for splenic resection. Miller[44] has shown that some degree of elevated ICP is present in almost all patients with a mass lesion early in the course of their injury.

The use of osmotic agents to decrease the ICP during the period of resuscitation is viewed differently in adults and children.[7] Mannitol has been shown[8] to increase the CBF in patients with head injury regardless of the initial ICP and may do so without lowering the ICP. In adult patients with head injury, the CBF is usually markedly reduced[8] and, therefore, the routine use of mannitol to increase CBF and lower ICP would seem reasonable. Despite this, we do not routinely give mannitol during emergency resuscitation unless there is either a history of deteriorating level of consciousness or progressive deterioration occurring in the emergency room. We prefer to hold off on such therapy until the pathophysiology of the head injury is better defined. However, if an expanding mass lesion is suspected or if signs of transtentorial herniation are present (decreasing level of consciousness, enlarging homolateral pupil, and/or contralateral weakness or decerebration) mannitol in a dosage of 0.5 to 1 g/kg is given IV over five minutes. This therapy may result in dramatic improvement in the neurologic picture. It is then vital to obtain a special study, CAT scan, or arteriogram to identify the presence and location of a surgically treatable lesion, since the mannitol will give only temporary relief from the increased ICP. In children, we try to avoid the use of mannitol during the emergency resuscitation. We have observed[10] that 50% of severely head-injured patients have a CAT scan pattern of diffuse swelling of the brain with markedly diminished amounts of intracranial cerebral CSF. The evidence thus far suggests that this is not due to cerebral edema but to acute cerebrovascular dilatation with an increased cerebral blood flow (CBF) and cerebral blood volume (CBV).[9,57] Unlike adults 18 and older, the cerebral blood flow in children with head injury appears to be normal or increased[35,46] despite a low cerebral metabolism. Since mannitol increases CBF and also CBV, it is at least possible that mannitol could worsen the intracranial state before having any beneficial effect. Because of this, we use controlled hyperventilation to a Pa_{CO_2} of 20 to 25 torr as a major initial therapy in children. If, however, the child shows a rapid downhill clinical course with evidence of focal cerebral herniation suggesting an epidural hematoma, mannitol is not withheld as it may be life saving in this specific situation. We feel it is safer to give the mannitol once hypocapnia is established.

DIAGNOSIS

Following the clinical exam and emergency stabilization the underlying pathophysiology of the disease must be identified. The cervical spine, chest, and abdomen roentgenograms have already been discussed. At the time of x-ray of the cervical spine the skull is included and, thus, fractures can readily be identified. We do not feel that, if a CAT scan is available, there is any point in moving the patient to obtain a full set of skull films. Any information relative to the brain or skull that becomes visible on the skull films should be identified on the CAT scan with the possible exception of linear fractures. The only importance of the linear fracture is whether it is associated with any intracranial hemorrhage from the middle meningeal artery or the dural sinuses; both of these events will be better delineated on the CAT scan than plain skull films. If no CAT scan is available, an AP film of the skull may demonstrate a shift of the pineal gland and help make the decision about arteriography. We shall also see that in the case of epidural hematomas the skull films may be quite helpful.

The variety and magnitude of the information available through the CAT scan make it the study of choice in patients with acute head injury. It is rapid to perform, noninvasive, and requires few personnel. Focal pathology such as acute epidural, subdural, or intracerebral hemorrhages and their relative size are easily identified. Cerebral edema and hemorrhagic contusion can readily be differentiated from true focal hematomas and unnecessary surgery avoided. The large number of patients without a surgically accessible or treatable lesion can readily be identified and not subjected to exploratory surgery. Many children with the clinical picture of rapid deterioration or who present in deep coma[9] show no mass lesion but a pattern of diffuse brain swelling on the CAT scan. When this is seen the patients can be taken immediately to the critical care area for intensive monitoring without the need for exploratory burr holes. The incidence of surgically treatable lesions in both adults and children is quite low.[7] A similar pattern of diffuse swelling of the brain may be seen in adults in association with small hemorrhages in the white matter of the hemispheres, the corpus callosum, and the periventricular areas. This seems to represent a diffuse shearing injury of the brain and is associated with a poor prognosis.[22] Unilateral swelling of the brain underlying a small, acute subdural hematoma is frequently seen in adults and this too seems to indicate a rather poor prognosis. Table 10-2 shows that only a small percentage of children with acute severe head injury have surgically treatable lesions and that even in adults, if chronic subdural hematomas are excluded, surgical lesions account for only a small percentage.

In patients with acute trauma we routinely perform an unenhanced CAT scan. If, however, an isodense subdural hematoma is suspected because of displacement of the ventricles or from clinical history, Conray 60 is injected IV and the scan repeated. An isodense subdural hematoma is one in which the fluid in the subdural collection has the same CAT density as the brain and, therefore, can only be distinguished by displacement of the midline, compression of the ventricles, or following contrast enhancement of the lining membranes or displacement of the cortical veins. Plain skull films may be all that can be obtained in a patient with acute epidural hematoma and signs of a rapidly deteriorating neurologic condition. If a skull fracture is seen, it may be sufficient to define the center of the surgical craniotomy.[28] If a CAT scan is not available, the most useful diagnostic test is the arteriogram. This requires more time and personnel than the CAT scan and may take some hours to set up. Nonetheless, we feel that except in extreme circumstances, exploratory burr holes are less reliable and expose the patient to as much risk as the slight delay necessary to obtain an arteriogram. What patients need arteriography? In our opinion, all patients who have significantly disturbed consciousness with evidence of a focal neurologic abnormality, all patients who show signs of clinical deterioration, and all patients who are in deep coma require study. The third group should be studied because it may be impossible to distinguish between a patient in coma because of a mass and herniation and one with diffuse cerebral injury and no herniation. Jamieson[28] has shown that one third of patients with acute epidurals will be unconscious from the time of injury. Thus, if the patients are not studied, a treatable lesion may be missed. If in addition to the clinical exam the ICP is high, this is further strong indication of a potentially treatable surgical mass.

I am not convinced that the routine radionuclide brain scan is useful in acute trauma. Echoencephalography may indicate a shift of a midline and aid in the decision for or against arteriography, but unless performed by a knowledgeable technician it is filled with potential error. Becker and co-workers[3] have advocated the use of a ventricular cannula to measure the ICP and at the same time insert a small bolus of air to examine the position of the midline ventricular structures. This can be accomplished rapidly without danger to the patient but, unfortunately, the procedure does not define whether the displacement is due to swelling of the brain or to a hematoma. Since the introduction of the CAT scan, Becker and co-workers[3] have stopped using this technique, but it remains a potentially useful tool in selected patients.

In conclusion, the CAT scan is the ideal diagnostic test for the study of patients following acute head trauma. If no scan is available, arteriography is the next most satisfactory investigative procedure. Even if no mass lesion is seen on the initial CAT scan, a delayed rise in the ICP may indicate the need for repeat study. This is particularly true following removal of acute subdural hematomas since it is not at all uncommon to see the midline shift increased rather than decreased following surgery and to find residual blood still present.

TREATMENT OF SURGICAL LESIONS
Depressed skull fracture

If the depressed fracture is closed, the rationale for surgical correction is to evacuate any local mass if present (subdural, epidural, or intracerebral hematoma); repair any dural lacerations to prevent cerebral herniation through the defect; and to correct any cosmetic disfigurement caused by the depression. In general, if the depression on tangential views of the skull is greater than the thickness of the skull, there is a high chance that the dura is lacerated and surgery is recommended. Depression of lesser degree, unless over the forehead, rarely requires surgical exploration. In children, however, we have always found that the degree of disruption of bone and dura is greater than could be predicted by the roentgenogram. Generally, these patients have a good level of consciousness, and a CAT scan frequently eliminates the need for surgical exploration by showing minimal changes in the inner table with no hematoma and a normal-appearing brain. The surgical technique we use is described below.

All compound depressed skull fractures require surgical debridement. This is the commonest cause for surgical intervention in pediatric head injuries in our institution. If the injury has been caused by a blow to the static head, the level of consciousness is frequently well preserved, even though focal neurologic findings may be present. When the blow has been sustained to the moving head, consciousness may be impaired. With the majority of compound depressed skull fractures, we have not routinely obtained a CAT scan before surgery because our hospital used an EMI Mark I scanner with water bag and we wish to avoid compression of the fractured bone and herniating brain. With the newer scanners, no bag is present, and it is quite a simple procedure to scan this group of patients and to evaluate the state of the underlying brain.

The surgical technique we have used in children is also applicable to adults and is the same for both open and closed depressed fractures. A skin incision is made separate from the laceration already present and the fracture exposed. A burr hole is placed at some distance from the center of the depression where the dura is expected to be intact. A circular craniectomy is then performed using the air drill with the area of depression in the center of the bone flap. The flap can then be elevated essentially intact. If any fragments have penetrated the dura and brain and bleeding occurs, good exposure is immediately available and the bleeding can be controlled. The bone flap and fragments are then washed well and soaked in gentamycin solution, 1 mg/ml. The dura is then explored. If it is already lacerated, it is opened further and any necrotic brain or hematoma evacuated and careful debridement of the brain performed with the aspirator. The dura is then closed using a temporalis or pericranial graft, if necessary, to ensure that the brain cannot herniate through the defect. This we believe to be very important, since if brain swelling occurs a large cerebral fungus can occur with venous infarction and functional loss that could have been avoided had the dura been repaired. The pieces of bone are then remolded to make a normal curvature to the bone flap and are wired together and reinserted. The skin is closed after excision of the wound edges of the initial laceration. The patients are placed on antistaphylcoccal penicillin for five days, and tetanus toxoid is given as defined by the patient's vaccination status. We have treated 15 patients with compound fractures in this fashion over the last three years with no infection, and none of the children have required delayed cranioplasty. At the time of surgery, an ICP monitor is inserted through a separate stab wound in patients with a significant disturbance of consciousness preoperatively or in those who exhibit evidence of brain swelling at surgery.

Epidural hematoma

Epidural hematomas are the most readily correctible surgical lesions seen following trauma and it is to avoid missing an expanding epidural hematoma that the practice of hospitalizing all patients with transient unconsciousness is based. In fact, epidural hematomas are uncommon and we have found them present in only 5% of 317 consecutive adults and children admitted to our hospital following head injury.

The textbook description of a patient with an epidural hematoma is of transient loss of consciousness, recovery with a lucid interval during which the patient's neurologic state returns to normal, and the secondary onset of headache and a decreasing level of consciousness. The initial injury tears the middle meningeal vessels and causes traumatic unconsciousness. Spasm and clot occur in the middle meningeal artery and the bleeding stops. Over the next several hours the artery gradually bleeds, forming a hematoma stripping the dura from the inside of the skull. Once headache and decreasing level of consciousness become obvious, a secondary rise in ICP has already occurred and distortion of the brain with significant mass effect is present. It must be realized that the compensatory abilities of the intracranial space have already been exhausted and that rapid deterioration may occur. Further downhill course with dilatation of usually the ipsilateral pupil (80%)[19] due to third nerve compression by the herniating mesial temporal structures, progressive unconsciousness with weakness or decerebration of either the contralateral extremity (50%) or the ipsilateral extremities, Cheynes-Stokes respiration and, if no therapy is given, loss of pupillary response, caloric responses, bradycardia, and death. It is extremely important to identify the epidural hematoma at the earliest possible time (i.e., when the headache and drowsiness are the only complaints). This classic history and clinical progression is seen in only one third of patients with epidural hematomas. Another one third are unconscious from the time of injury, and a final one third are never unconscious.[28] In children, bradycardia and early papilledema may be the only warning signs. Finally, the rare but easily missed venous epidural hematoma, which is usually associated with fractures crossing the sinuses, may be silent and may present as late as two weeks post injury with classic signs and symptoms of elevated ICP, papilledema, headache, and vomiting.

The best diagnostic test is the CAT scan, if available. We have had no false-negative or -positive scan for epidural hematomas. The advantage of the CAT scan is that it demonstrates not only the location of the clot but also defines any other lesions within the cranium. These other findings have important prognostic implications. Plain skull films can be helpful in the patient who is showing signs of rapid deterioration and when a CAT scan is not readily available. Jamieson,[28] in a large series of acute epidural hematomas, stated that the clot is usually under the area of maximal fracture and suggested that arteriography is rarely necessary. In children, there is frequently no fracture seen on skull x-ray films,[18] and the location of the lesion is frequently high parietal rather than in the more typical anterior temporal region. Despite the ready availability of the CAT scan, 15% of our patients have had surgery without any special diagnostic study other than the skull film because of the rapidity of the downhill course. The most rapid presentation was in a 12-year-old child who had only a headache one and one-half hours post injury. By three hours, he was flaccid with fixed dilated pupils. This child had a massive epidural and took many months to recover, but one and one-half years after surgery he has a mild left hemiparesis and his functional IQ is 105.

The treatment of an epidural hematoma is surgical evacuation. Medical management to control rapidly progressive intracranial hypertension may be necessary to gain time to reach the operating room and evacuate the clot. Endotracheal intubation, muscle paralysis, sodium pentothal, hyperventilation, and osmotic agents may all be necessary. Frequently, under the influence of these measures, the pupil will return to more normal size and decorticate posturing may disappear long enough for definitive surgery to be carried out. In the temporal region, the classic small craniectomy is usually adequate to evacuate the hematoma and control bleeding. If the hematoma is over the convexity of the brain, we prefer to rapidly decompress through a burr hole, then lift a craniotomy flap. This avoids the need for second operation for cranioplasty. We always insert an ICP monitor in the opposite frontal area postoperatively.

Postoperative CAT scan usually shows rapid return of the midline structures with resolution of the epidural blood. The ICP is generally not elevated postoperatively, and in 80% of our patients no further need for therapy to control ICP was necessary. In the other 20%, severe postoperative intracranial hypertension is seen. These were the patients who had had the worst preoperative neurologic exams. Repeat CAT scan revealed severe cerebral edema frequently not confined to the side of the lesion. These patients required intensive therapy for ICP control for many days and recovered slowly.

The need for early diagnosis of epidural hematomas has been frequently stressed, and Hooper stressed that the mortality should not exceed 10%.[26] Recently, Becker[3] and Jamieson[28] both reported an 8% mortality for patients with epidural hematomas. Since the introduction of the CAT scan allowing even earlier diagnosis, our mortality is zero in 15 cases. Eight of these cases had associated lesions on CAT scan (i.e., subdural or hemorrhagic contusion). Previously, it has been reported[27] that the mortality rate for epidural hematomas when associated with other cerebral lesions is considerably higher than the 8% reported above, and in the presence of an epidural, subdural, and intracerebral hematoma a mortality rate as high as 80% is reported.[19,28] The majority of patients with epidural hematomas make a rapid recovery following evacuation of the clot, but some will require intensive therapy in the intensive care unit followed by active rehabilitation. While the initial neurologic state has a bearing on the final outcome, surgery should not be denied a patient with an epidural hematoma since excellent recovery can frequently occur despite a very poor initial neurologic state.[3]

Acute subdural hematomas

Collections of blood in the subdural space that are identified within the first 72 hours following trauma are arbitrarily classified as acute subdural hematomas. Jamieson[29] classified acute subdural hematomas in two main types: simple—collections of blood, liquid or solid, in the subdural space but not apparently associated with underlying cerebral contusion or laceration and complicated—liquid or clotted blood in the subdural space associated with obvious contusion or laceration of the surface of the brain. The bleeding in the simple subdurals probably arises from torn bridging veins; whereas, in the complicated subdurals the bleeding is frequently arterial from a contused or lacerated brain. The distribution in Jamieson's series was approximately 50/50.[29] Acute complicated subdurals are invariably associated with severe underlying cerebral injury, and it is probably this injury that has a greater effect on the outcome than the hematoma per se. We have found acute subdural hematomas to be approximately three times as common as epidural hematomas, with an incidence of 8% in children and 18% in adults who had CAT scan following head injury.[7]

The clinical presentation of patients with acute subdural hematomas is that of unconsciousness without a lucid period and frequently with signs suggestive of a mass lesion, hemiparesis, unilateral decerebration, or pupillary enlargement. However, patients with acute subdurals may never become unconscious or may show a typical lucid interval. Only 15% of patients with

acute subdurals appear to have a typical lucid interval, and another 29% never become unconscious.[29] These are usually the patients with simple subdurals.

It is necessary to obtain a special diagnostic study on this group of patients because there are frequently multiple lesions (84%).[7] The identification of multiple lesions helps in the decision for or against surgery and has definite prognostic implications. The mortality rate ranges between 60% and 100% when either bilateral subdural hematomas or single subdural hematoma with multiple lacerations are present.[17,29,45,55] Once again, the CAT scan is the ideal test since it will define the size and location of the hematoma, the degree of any midline displacement, the presence of significant cerebral edema, and the presence and location of other lesions (i.e., epidural or intracerebral hematomas). If no CAT scan is present, arteriography must be performed, initially on the side of the suspected mass. Frequently, a cross-compression injection is adequate to define the presence or absence of a bilateral extracerebral lesion. However, arteriography will not supply as useful information on the presence of intracerebral hematomas or contusions.

The best treatment of patients with acute subdurals is controversial. There are two separate but related pathophysiologic problems. One is the cerebral injury and associated contusion and edema. The second is the presence of blood in the subdural space. If the major problem contributing to the patient's poor neurologic condition is the mass of the hematoma, then that should be removed. If the main reason for the patient's state is the underlying cerebral injury, then treatment should be directed against that. This suggests that patients with simple subdurals with little cerebral injury and a deteriorating or poor level of consciousness, in whom the CAT scan shows a localized hematoma, will benefit from removal of the mass. Similarly, the patient who is immediately rendered unconscious with a diffuse small subdural over most of one hemisphere with the midline shift larger than the hematoma with or without other lesions (i.e., intracerebral hematomas or bilateral subdurals) is unlikely to be helped by surgery and needs intensive medical therapy to correct the elevated ICP and control the brain edema and swelling. In a patient with a moderately large but diffuse subdural hematoma with a midline shift larger than the hematoma and evidence of cerebral edema, it is more difficult to decide for or against surgery and the correct treatment of this patient remains the biggest area of controversy. We frequently do not operate on this patient but aggressively control the ICP.

If surgery is performed, we and others recommend a large frontotemperoparietal craniotomy flap so that the brain can be well visualized, the hematoma removed, and any bleeding controlled both from the surface of the brain and the bridging veins. At surgery an ICP monitor is always inserted, either an intraventricular cannula or subarachnoid screw, on the side contralateral from surgery. Postoperatively the management of these patients is the same of those patients not having surgical treatment. It is a mistake to believe that surgical evacuation of even a large acute subdural hematoma will necessarily be followed by continuous low ICP. Intracranial hypertension is extremely common following mass evacuation. The patients who are not operated upon are returned to the ICU following CAT scan, and an ICP monitor is also inserted.

The further treatment of both these groups of patients is with intensive medical therapy to maintain an ICP of less than 20 torr using corticosteroids, muscle paralysis, hyperventilation, mannitol, and barbiturates as necessary.[7] If the ICP is difficult to control, it is necessary to repeat the CAT scan or angiogram to reevaluate the amount of midline shift and to seek evidence of delayed hematoma formation. We have performed followup CAT scans within the first week of injury in 17 of the 44 patients with acute subdurals. Six of the 12 surgically treated patients showed evidence of increased midline shift,

some residual subdural blood, and increased focal edema. Clinically, two had improved, two were unchanged, and two were worse. Five patients treated without surgery showed increased local edema but in only one was there evidence of an increased midline shift and in none was the hematoma larger. The patient with the increased midline shift was the only one who had clinically deteriorated.[15] It is quite clear that when the subdural mass lesion associated with underlying cerebral injury and edema is present, evacuation of the mass will not result in a rapid return of the midline structures to their normal location and that continued intracranial hypertension may be present. Miller[44] has shown that 58% of patients operated on for evacuation of acute subdural hematomas developed increased ICP greater than 20 torr in the postoperative period and that approximately half of these patients die because of uncontrolled intracranial hypertension. Thus, a major part of the treatment of acute subdural hematomas is the control of the brain swelling, edema, and elevated ICP whether or not surgical decompression is performed. The major reason for surgical decompression is to correct the brain displacement and herniation.[44] However, the CAT scan has shown that this does not occur rapidly following surgery for subdural hematomas, whereas it does appear to happen in most patients operated upon for epidural hematomas. Again, we believe this is a reflection of the degree of primary cerebral injury associated with the former pathology.

The results of treatment of acute subdural hematomas have been poor, with mortality rates ranging from 63% to 42%.[17,29,45,44] The level of consciousness at the time of surgery correlates well with the final outcome and ranges from 1% to 2% for those patients conscious just prior to surgery to 78% for those unconscious and bilaterally decerebrate.[29] The timing of surgery, whether within the first 24 hours or within 48 hours, seems to have little effect on the mortality rate,[17] and surprisingly the age of the patient

Table 10-3. Mortality after surgery for acute subdural hematoma

Study	Mortality (%)
Miller et al.[44]	42
Fell et al.[17]	48
Moiel and Caram[45]	48
Jamieson and Yelland[29]	63
Talalla and Morin[55]	76
Bruce, Gennarelli, and Langfitt[7]	23

has not been shown to effect mortality until the eighth decade, when the mortality rate increases. Although Fell and co-workers[17] found little difference in mortality between subtemporal decompression with multiple burr holes and craniotomy, this was not a randomized study and we and most authors are now in favor of large craniotomy flaps if surgery is performed.[3] Despite early surgery, not only has the mortality remained around 50%, but the quality of survival has been poor. Only two authors have reported results of follow up. Fell and co-workers[17] noted that only 9% of survivors returned to work; McKissock,[39] although reporting 56% of patients doing well, did not specify whether or not they were employed. Our own results in a small series of 44 patients with acute subdural hematomas are shown in Table 10-3. Only half the patients were operated on, but all had aggressive therapy to control the ICP. The overall mortality is 23%—21% in those operated and 24% in those not. Eighty-four percent of the patients had evidence on CAT scan of some other lesion (i.e., contusion, a second subdural, or an intracerebral hematoma), and this combination of lesions supposedly carries a high mortality.[29] We have been encouraged by the low mortality, and we are presently evaluating the degree of disability in these patients.

Acute subdural hematomas are classified as simple or complicated. Complicated subdurals are always associated with underlying cerebral injury, contusion, or laceration, and it is frequently difficult to be sure what effect a relatively small hematoma is playing.

Surgical evacuation remains the treatment of choice when a large localized hematoma is present. However, there is controversy over the treatment of the more diffuse, smaller subdural. The rationale for surgery is to correct the displacement and herniation of the brain and to restore normal ICP. We have found on serial CAT scan that surgery rarely restores the midline to its normal position. Indeed, in approximately half the patients, an increased midline shift occurs over the following several days despite surgical decompression and mass evacuation. Miller and co-workers[44] have demonstrated that evacuation of the mass is followed by significant intracranial hypertension in at least 50% of the cases and that half of these will die because of uncontrollable intracranial hypertension. We are forced to conclude that all patients with acute subdural hematomas require ICP monitoring with careful control of the ICP and that surgery is not necessary or helpful in a significant number of patients.

Intracerebral hematoma

Intracerebral hematomas are readily identified on CAT scan and have been found in 6% of 146 children and 13% of 171 adults studied after head trauma—essentially the same frequency with which we see hemorrhagic contusions (Table 10-4). The clinical picture may vary from no neurologic deficit to deep coma. Two clinical patterns, however, should be emphasized. Patients with slowly accumulating frontal or temporal pole hematomas frequently demonstrate a rather slowly deteriorating level of consciousness with minimal focal signs over 24 to 48 hours. These hematomas must be identified because a sudden change in ICP precipitated by seizure or suctioning may produce an acute herniation and death. The second unusual clinical pattern is seen in patients with delayed hemorrhage.[2] These patients show progressive recovery of level of consciousness over 10 to 14 days and then suddenly develop headache followed by rapid neurologic deterioration. CAT scan or ar-

Table 10-4. Frequency of mass lesions on CAT scan in 146 children and 171 adults following head trauma (%)

	Children	Adults
Epidural hematoma	4	5
Acute subdural hematoma	8	18
Chronic subdural hematoma	0	30
Hemorrhagic contusion	6	15
Intracerebral hematoma	6	13
Diffuse cerebral swelling	35	5

teriography shows an intracerebral hematoma. The exact pathology of this delayed hemorrhage is not clear, but it probably is fresh hemorrhage and not the sudden expression of a preexisting hematoma.

The only way to identify posttraumatic intracerebral hematomas is by special study of the brain. The CAT scan is excellent at identifying acute hemorrhage and is superior to an arteriogram because of the ease of defining the size of the hematoma relative to any surrounding edema, its ability to distinguish hematoma from contusion, and to identify other lesions scattered throughout the brain. Large solitary intracerebral hematomas should be evacuated, as should the delayed hemorrhage discussed above. It is not our practice to evacuate medium or small hematomas or multiple hematomas. The mortality following surgery for traumatic intracerebral hematoma has been reported at 42%.[44] Once again, the main problem in these patients is usually the degree of cerebral injury and intensive monitoring, and management of the patient is the mainstay of therapy.

Chronic subdural hematoma

Not infrequently, a chronic subdural hematoma is identified (Table 10-4) following acute head injury. Occasionally on CT scan one sees fresh bleeding into the chronic lesion. We have never identified a chronic subdural hematoma in a child following acute trauma. However, we see the lesion in ap-

proximately 30% of adults. Once again, the initial study of choice is the CAT scan. However, if a subdural hematoma of the same density as the brain is suspected (isodense subdural), a repeat CAT scan with contrast injection or an angiogram or both may be necessary to identify the lesions, particularly if they are located bilaterally. The treatment of chronic subdural hematomas following acute head injury is burr hole drainage. Occasionally, if a lot of solid clot is found, craniotomy may be necessary. The outcome depends on the level of consciousness at the time of surgery more than any other single factor.

Cerebral contusions

Cerebral hemorrhagic contusions are seen frequently in patients, particularly adults, following head injury, and 75% of patients who die from head injury are found to have contusions at autopsy.[14] The frequency with which these lesions are seen is shown in Table 10-4. In children, hemorrhagic contusions are infrequently seen, but areas of localized decreased density on CAT scan may represent nonhemorrhagic contusions or possibly areas of focal ischemia. The diagnosis is most easily made on the CAT scan. Arteriography can only diagnose contusion by inference based on displacement of blood vessels, draping of blood vessels, sluggish capillary flow, and the general pattern of displacement. It may be impossible to differentiate the local contusion from a localized hematoma.

In general, there is no question of surgical treatment for cerebral contusions, since the removal of brain that may potentially recover is not acceptable and certainly cannot be done in the areas of major motor, sensory, or visual portions of the brain. However, when contusion occurs over the frontal or temporal poles, it is feasible to remove the contused brain surgically to make more room within the intracranial space and remove a focus for edema formation. When a temporal lobe contusion is present and signs of uncal herniation are found, surgical excision of 5 cm of the temporal lobe with removal of the herniating mesial structures has been performed. The purpose of surgery in the past was frequently to rule out the presence of a localized temporal tip hematoma and to decompress the uncus. With the CAT scan it is quite possible to differentiate hematoma from contusion the majority of the time, and it has not been our practice over the last few years, either in adults or children, to resect potentially recoverable areas of brain. We treat patients with contusions by controlling the ICP as described below. The group of patients with signs of herniation from temporal lobe swelling are at a great risk should a sudden change in the intracranial dynamics occur due to ventilatory problems, seizure activity, and so on, and these patients must be very carefully monitored with strict control of ICP, blood gases, and motor activity. If this monitoring cannot be performed, it may indeed be safer to remove the offending temporal contusion and open the tentorial notch, even though the portion of brain removed might recover since if the herniation continues and the patient dies, obviously none of the brain will recover. The decision for or against surgical intervention is one that must be made by the individual neurosurgeon in light of the diagnostic and monitoring facilities available.

Surgery for decompression of raised ICP

Generalized brain injury with edema or contusion is a common finding in head-injured patients, both in those who have acute subdural hematomas and in those with no mass lesion. The clinical picture varies from a moderately obtunded patient with progressive deterioration to immediate deep coma. CAT scan may show multiple parenchymal and extraparenchymal lesions, diffuse loss of CSF spaces with compression of the ventricles and mesencephalic cisterns, or multifocal areas of cerebral edema. We treat these patients by careful control of the ICP by medical means as outlined below. How-

ever, recurrently suggestions are put forward for either internal decompression by removal of a frontal or temporal lobe or external decompression by large bilateral or unilateral bony decompressions. We have neither been convinced of the need nor the efficacy of such procedure.[12,13] We do not recommend them and have not found a need to perform decompressive craniectomies in any patient over the last three years.

MONITORING

All patients with severe head injuries are treated with endotracheal intubation, muscle paralysis, and continuous monitoring of arterial pressure (SAP), central venous pressure (CVP), urine output, temperature, and ECG. Other specific monitoring techniques (i.e., ICP, CBF, cerebral metabolism [CMR], evoked responses, and Swan-Ganz catheters) play a role in defining the response to injury and in helping in the selection of therapy.

Intracranial pressure monitoring (ICP)

A normal ICP is a pulsatile pressure that varies with cardiac impulse and respirations. The mean ICP should remain below 15 torr. The occurrence of increased ICP following head injury has been a source of debate, but recent studies in which continuous recording of ICP has been performed have demonstrated quite clearly that in most patients with mass lesions[44] and from 30%[44] to 80%[9] of those with no mass lesions, an elevated ICP occurs at some time during the course of the disease. It has been frequently observed that alterations in the ICP may not be reflected by any change in the neurologic exam or in vital signs.[34] This is especially true in patients who have marked impairment of consciousness in whom the first evidence of increased ICP may be precipitate and associated with bilateral pupillary dilatation caused by transtentorial herniation and associated with the risk of secondary brain stem hemorrhage. If the increased pressure is treated at this time, no recovery may occur because secondary brain stem hemorrhages have already taken place and converted a potentially reversible injury into an irreversible one. Waves of elevated pressure or steady state elevated ICP can only be consistently identified if a continuous record of ICP is obtained. As a result of monitoring, therapy can be started early whenever a change occurs. The results of therapy can be seen, and the need for repeating therapy or changing modality of therapy is clearly indicated. We believe that the use of therapies that make it difficult or impossible to monitor the neurologic exam (i.e., muscle paralysis or barbiturate coma) can only be used safely when the ICP is continuously recorded. The various methods of recording ICP have been discussed in Chapter 4 and will not be reiterated here. We use a subarachnoid bolt[26] in almost all children and either the subarachnoid bolt or an intraventricular cannula in adults, depending on ventricular size.[8]

Ideally, the ICP should be recorded from the earliest possible time following injury. In practice we usually insert the ICP monitor within one to two hours from admission after the CAT scan has been obtained. In the meantime, the patient is treated with steroids, moderate (marked in children) hyperventilation, and careful positioning of the head as if elevated ICP were present. If a long resuscitation is envisaged or if a delay in obtaining the CAT scan is foreseen, we insert the subarachnoid bolt in the ER. We monitor the ICP in all adult patients who have no eye opening, no verbal response, and nonpurposeful motor responses. In children, we always monitor those with no eye opening, no verbal response, and decerebration or flaccidity and occasionally monitor those with lesser degrees of motor impairment. All patients who are operated upon have an ICP monitor inserted. If the monitor is inserted prior to the CAT scan, it must be placed in the region of the coronal suture and not more than 2 inches from the midline. This position will avoid the creation of artifacts on CAT scan.

Very high levels of ICP (greater than 40 torr) from the time of insertion of the monitor carry a poor prognosis.[3,35,57] A high ICP occurring later in the course of the disease also carries a poor prognosis in adults[44] but not in children.[10] A low ICP while associated with a relatively low mortality[35] may well be associated with a poor degree of functional recovery. In patients with mass lesions, the correlation between ICP and outcome is not very good.[3] However, in adults the correlation between pressure and outcome in those with no mass lesion is positive: the higher the ICP, the higher the mortality.[44] In children we have not found this to be true if patients in whom ICP was equal to SAP at the time of insertion of the recording are excluded.[9] Primary deaths are frequently associated with a rising ICP, and Becker and co-workers[3] reported that 50% of deaths occurred as a result of uncontrollable intracranial hypertension. Recent data suggests that the use of high doses of barbiturate may significantly decrease the mortality in this group of patients by bringing the intracranial hypertension under control.[41] Although normal brain has the ability to maintain adequate cerebral blood flow (CBF) at even quite high cerebral perfusion pressures (CPP), there is good evidence that when the brain is injured, particularly when edema is present, there is a poor correlation between CPP and local CBF in the injured areas.[8,40] Because of this unpredictable relationship we arbitrarily endeavor to keep the ICP below 20 torr in this severely ill group of patients. A protocol for this has been outlined.[7,9] In children there is more emphasis in the early stages (first 24 to 48 hours) of therapy to use marked hyperventilation, 23 to 25 torr, and little or no mannitol; whereas in adults only moderate hyperventilation is used, 28 to 30 torr, with mannitol being a main standby of therapy. The reason is a rather marked difference in blood flow found in these two groups of patients. We and others are convinced of the usefulness of ICP monitoring in the severely head-injured patient but would point out that it is not the monitoring that is beneficial but the response of the physician to the information presented by the monitoring system.

Cerebral blood flow

Ideally, we would like to know the local cerebral blood flow and metabolism in each small area of brain and then use various therapeutic measures to ensure that there is an adequate match between flow and metabolism (i.e., to ensure that no area of brain has a substrate delivery that is inadequate to meet its metabolic demands). At present, this is still impossible, but the improved resolution and availability of positron emission CAT scanning may make this possible within a few years. Until the last few years the information on CBF and head injury has been obtained by the intracarotid injection of xenon = 133 and recording of its clearance curve from the brain using a series of collimated sodium iodide scintillation detectors. This technique generally showed a decrease in CBF in both the fast and slow components of the clearance curves, usually to values above 50% of normal CBF. When no focal brain injury was seen on the angiogram, the CBF values were similar throughout both hemispheres, with flow and metabolism apparently being reduced in concert.[8] When a mass lesion was present or had been surgically evacuated, marked variability of CBF was found from area to area, sometimes higher than the surrounding brain and sometimes lower. The ability of the blood vessels to respond normally to changes in transmural pressure (pressure autoregulation) was well preserved in over 50% of the cases studied and seems to have little bearing on the outcome. Finally, the response of the cerebral circulation to drug therapy has been evaluated. Mannitol has been shown to increase the CBF in patients irrespective of whether or not the ICP was lowered and in a number of patients to also increase the value for cerebral metabolic rate from oxygen ($CMRO_2$).[8] The major limitation of the technique is that repeat CBF studies over an extended period of time could not be performed because of the dangers of an indwelling carotid artery catheter. Some longitudinal studies have been performed using intermittent carotid artery cannulation and have suggested that the delayed occurrence

of a hyperemia (increased CBF relative to metabolic need) carries a poor prognosis.[48]

Obrist[46] has derived a method of using inhalation or intravenous injection of ^{133}Xe to measure the regional blood flow serially in humans. The arterial clearance curve is monitored by sampling the end-tidal air. Thus, an arterial curve that can be used to calculate the amount of recirculation of xenon is obtained. The clearance curves from the head can then be corrected for recirculation,[46] and an analysis of just the clearance from the cranium obtained. Unlike the intracarotid technique, blood flow is detected in the scalp, muscles, and bone as well as in the brain and, although these extracerebral flows are slow compared to normal CBF when a generalized decrease in CBF occurs, errors in the calculations of the CBF are introduced by the contamination of this third compartment and have to be taken into account when interpreting the data. This methodology allows serial measurements of CBF to be made during the course of head injury. Thus far, studies in adults have shown a low initial CBF as described with the intracarotid methods but have shown also that, as recovery progresses, there is a concomitant increase in CBF, whereas in patients who are deteriorating, the CBF falls further, suggesting in both cases prime processes occurring within the brain itself as the cause of improvement or deterioration.[36] The response of the cerebral blood vessels to changes in Pa_{CO_2} is preserved until close to death, and preliminary evidence suggests that the decrease in CBF induced by hypocarbia remains present for several days in the brain-injured patient, whereas in normal volunteers, the CBF rises to almost control values within six hours despite continued hypocapnia.[47,49] Studies are underway to examine the effects of barbiturate-induced coma on CBF and $CMRO_2$. At present, a significant effect on CBF seems to occur with a lesser change in $CMRO_2$. In adolescents, a pattern of normal or high blood flow is seen in the face of a markedly decreased $CMRO_2$. This CBF pattern is seen in association with a CAT scan that frequently shows minimal-to-absent ventricles and perimesencephalic cisterns and has been described by us as diffuse cerebral swelling.[9,58] This pattern is found in over 50% of severe pediatric head-injured patients. The brain density on CAT scan is higher than normal in the white matter, and we believe the whole picture is due to intraparenchymal vasodilatation and hyperemia and that only after 24 hours or more does true cerebral edema occur.

Further development of continuous rCBF techniques are required since we believe that the detrimental effects of elevated ICP are mediated via decreased blood flow and ischemia. As discussed in the section on ICP, we do not know in any given patient whether a given CPP is adequate to ensure perfusion to all parts of the brain or not and have somewhat arbitrarily chosen an ICP above 20 torr as requiring therapy. If we could correlate CPP, CBF, and rCMRO$_2$ in each patient, we would have a more rational basis for therapy and might be able to tailor therapy to the exact situation in any given patient.

Intermittent noninvasive measurements of rCBF can now be made in the ICU. The data may be helpful in deciding what initial therapy is required (low flow versus hyperemia). There is certain prognostic information to be had from the flow trends, and beneficial effects of therapy can readily be measured. More information is required on the match between flow and metabolism in small areas of the brain and what the effects of such therapy as barbiturates are on this match. It is unlikely that either positron scanning with rCBF measurements or stable xenon and transmission CAT scannings will be applicable to the ICU for some time to come because of the size and complexity of the equipment.

Cerebral metabolism

The importance of measuring CBF to the brain is to further our understanding of the relationships between blood flow and cerebral metabolism. If the prime cause of unconsciousness following head injury is neuronal depression, the CBF will be reduced (metabolic autoregulation) pari passu with the decreased tissue substrate demand. If, however, the primary effect of head injury is to decrease CBF, then areas of brain may lack sufficient substrate delivery to fulfill their metabolic demands and will be secondarily ischemic. At present, we believe that the former explanation is the most frequently valid in head injury. However, if SAP falls or ICP rises (i.e., CPP falls), a primary decrease in CBF can occur and secondary ischemia may result. Thus, it would be ideal to be able to measure the rCBF and rCMRO$_2$ in each small area of brain and to be able to manipulate therapy to keep all regions adequately perfused. At present, this is not possible. However, rapid advances in the positron emission scanning techniques have put this goal within our reach in the foreseeable future.

In general, the CMRO$_2$ ([AVDO$_2$ × CBF] /100; normal 3-3.5 ml O$_2$/100g/min) is reduced, and the arteriovenous difference for oxygen (AVDO$_2$) is normal or slightly reduced, suggesting that no global ischemia is present. A CMRO$_2$ of less than 1 ml O$_2$/100g/ min on initial measurement or of 1.2 ml O$_2$/ 100 g/min at seven days has been reported to be incompatible with survival.[25,51] We have not found this to be true[8,36] but have noted that in adult patients a low AVDO$_2$ carries a poor prognosis for recovery.[6] In adolescents, it appears that the the CMRO$_2$ is equally as depressed as in adults, yet the CBF is higher. Thus, a small AVDO$_2$ in children cannot be interpreted as a poor prognostic sign.

If the metabolic rate is constant, changes in jugular bulb oxygenation will give an indication of changing CBF. Thus, when ICP rises and global changes in flow occur, a lowered jugular oxygen content is an indicator of a decrease in CBF. Unfortunately, this sort of change is not very helpful when regional damage is present because the damaged area with initially reduced flow will contribute little to the total outflow and, thus, even if a further decrease in CBF occurred in this small region, it would not be readily identified in the jugular venous blood. At the present time, monitoring cerebral metabolism has two practical implications in patient management. If the $AVDO_2$ is normal or low and no focal pathology is present, there appears to be no need for therapy to increase CBF. When a therapeutic modality is used, it is possible to compare whether the match between CBF and metabolism has improved or not. It is also possible that small changes in metabolism could be used as indicators for a need for the treatment of elevated ICP, and the level at which therapy was required could be individually measured in each patient. There are also several important research questions that can only be answered by the use of metabolic measurements combined with other measurements. What are the effects of the new therapies (i.e., barbiturates) on CBF/CMR match? What prognostic information, if any, can be obtained early in the course of management? What is the interrelationship of CMR to evoked potential responses? Is it possible to establish in each patient a CBF, CMR, CPP threshold which might be used to define a threshold CPP at which no ischemia occurred and therapy directed to maintaining this CPP?

Evoked potentials

The standard EEG has not proved to be a helpful diagnostic or prognostic tool in head injury largely because of the insensitivity of standard reading techniques and the fact that the EEG is generally diffusely abnormal in traumatic unconsciousness. The use of fast Fourrier transfer to define the power spectrum of the EEG is a more sensitive technique to measure differences in the amplitude and frequency of the EEG and may prove to be a useful method of EEG interpretation in head-injured patients. This is particularly so if a continuous write-out of EEG power could be compared with changes in ICP, CPP, blood gases, and possibly evoked potential responses. Decrease in amplitude of the EEG appears to be the first change seen with alterations in blood flow and, thus, it may be possible to use

the EEG power spectrum and height as an indicant of the need to treat a given change in ICP or CPP.

The recent use of cortical far field and short latency evoked potentials on the visual, auditory and somatosensory systems has increased the amount of information that can be obtained about the functional state of the brain in comatose patients. Reports suggest a good correlation between the pattern of the evoked response, particularly the auditory evoked response (BER) and the degree of persisting neurologic disability post coma.[21,24] Following prolonged coma the evoked responses may show recovery days to weeks before neurologic function improves and may, therefore, help predict recovery.[24] BER has been most extensively used in head injury because of the proximity of the ascending pathways of the auditory system to the ascending reticular system. The presence of a normal BER suggests a nonstructural lesion of the brain stem while the absence of BER is associated with structural brain stem damage.[52-54] Thus, in head-injured comatose patients an absent BER suggests secondary or primary brain stem hemorrhage and recovery is most unlikely. However, the preservation of BER does not necessarily imply a good prognosis, since there may be diffuse white matter injury of such severity as to preclude functional recovery but without secondary hemorrhage and, therefore, a normal BER.[22] The continuous recording of evoked responses, particularly if several systems are included, may well indicate early changes in cerebral function in association with increases in ICP, decreases in CBF, edema, or herniation. However, we have seen the BER take as long as three days to disappear in a patient with complete cessation of cortical flow. Thus, those responses may not be as sensitive to changes as we would like. Much more needs to be done in defining the exact role of evoked responses in the monitoring of severely head-injured patients.

The use of evoked potentials in the ICU as part of the routine monitoring of severely head-injured patients is really in its infancy.

So far, it appears possible to distinguish coma with and without structural brain stem lesions. It is possible that continuous recordings of evoked potentials in association with the EEG will enable us to identify the very first signs of deterioration of CBF and/or herniation and allow therapy to be used at the earliest possible moment. Whether or not the evoked potential profile will add to the accuracy of early estimate of prognosis requires further study.

Control of intracranial hypertension

As we have seen above, a large number of patients with severe head injuries develop elevated ICP. One major cause of the second head injury is cerebral ischemia produced by disturbance of the cerebral circulation secondary to changes in CPP (usually changes in the ICP). At present, we do not possess adequate monitoring techniques to be certain in any single patient whether a given level of ICP is interfering with rCBF or not and, therefore, have rather arbitrarily used a level of 20 torr as the point at which we begin therapy. Frequently, the base pressure may be less than 20 torr, but waves of ICP may rise to 25 torr or higher. We feel that these should also be treated since they also suggest an unstable intracranial situation with low compliance. The various techniques and drugs used to control ICP will only be briefly described since they are treated extensively elsewhere in this book (see Chapter 5).

The first simple consideration is the patient's position. Overflexion of the chin or rotation of the head to one side or the other may obstruct the jugular veins and restrict venous return from the brain. Moderate elevation of the head to 30 degrees will encourage venous return, reduce jugular venous pressure, and lower ICP if the CSF pathways are still patent.

Hyperventilation is an effective and rapid way to lower ICP. We have seen above that in children a relatively high CBF is frequently present early in the course of their injury and that increased ICP is probably due to vasodilatation. Thus, we instigate hyper-

ventilation to a Pa_{CO_2} of 20 to 25 torr during emergency resuscitation and maintain it at that value for several days. In adults, less hyperventilation is used to maintain Pa_{CO_2} of 25 to 30 torr because of the theoretical risk of lowering the CBF too far and, in fact, producing cerebral ischemia. At a Pa_{CO_2} over 20 torr this does not seem to be a problem, and what evidence we have suggests that rather than decreasing the $CMRO_2$ an increase may occur,[20] possibly due to more homogenous tissue perfusion at the lower ICP. We also have limited evidence that in children the continued low Pa_{CO_2} is associated with continuously lowered CBF, a situation not found in normal volunteers where the CBF rises towards normal within six hours.[49]

Corticosteroids are routinely used in all severe adult head injury and in all children with focal CAT lesions, decerebration, or flaccid coma. The doses used are 1 to 1.5 mg/kg/24 hours of dexamethasone or the equivalent dose of methyl prednisolone with an equal immediate IV loading dose. This schedule is continued for at least five days, depending on the ICP, and then gradually tapered. Until recently there has been no firm data showing improved outcome with the use of steroids in head-injured patients. Two recent studies, however, have shown a marked decrease in mortality, 50% to 20%, with an increased rate of good recovery with the use of high doses of steroids.[16,23] In older patients the blood glucose must be monitored carefully. We have not seen any increase in chest infections or gastrointestinal hemorrhages with the use of these large doses of steroids either acutely or on a chronic basis.[43]

Diuretics, particularly furosemide and ethacrynic acid, have been used to promote systemic dehydration and have been shown to have an ICP-lowering effect. Bourke and co-workers[4] have experimental data suggesting that the beneficial effect may not be purely via renal mechanisms but by some direct effect on astroglial metabolism. We use these agents sparingly following acute head trauma. When high pulmonary artery pressures with evidence of pulmonary shunting are seen, furosemide is frequently helpful in decreasing the pulmonary pressures, improving interstitial pulmonary edema, improving systemic oxygenation, and concomitantly lowering the ICP. We most frequently use this form of therapy in children within the first 24 hours of trauma if the ICP is elevated and in adult patients who appear to have some increased vascular volume. We have not seen any consistent ICP lowering effect of these diuretics when no increased vascular volume or pulmonary congestion has been present, and we do not put any great reliance on them as agents to lower the ICP.

There are several agents that act directly to remove brain water via a mechanism of increased plasma osmolality. The agent we use most commonly is mannitol in a standard dose of 0.5 mg/kg IV over a three- to five-minute period. Doses up to 1.5 mg/kg can be used, but a recent study by Marshall and co-workers[42] suggests that there is little difference in the ICP-lowering effect between the lower and higher per kilogram dosage. The effect of the larger doses may last slightly longer. We prefer the smaller dosage schedule because less volume is needed and the effects on serum osmolality are less prolonged and less dramatic. Urea may be the agent of choice when there is concern about the ability of the patient to tolerate a volume load because urea, being a smaller molecule, manifests a greater effect per gram weight of compound and, therefore, less volume of fluid needs to be given. We have no experience with the use of IV glycerol. Because of the potential rebound effect of urea and the fact that it does seem to enter across a normal blood-brain barrier, we have preferred to use mannitol under most circumstances. The dangers of hyperosmolar therapy are of dehydration with electrolyte disturbances, renal shutdown, and cardiac effects of prolonged high levels of osmolality. We endeavor to withhold osmolar therapy if the serum osmolality is greater than 320 mOsm/l, but occasionally there may be no other choice because of a rising ICP that will respond to no other

therapy. We have seen mannitol lower the ICP even with initial serum osmolalities of 340 mOsm/l. We use mannitol frequently in adult patients, since we have shown that there is an increase in CBF produced by the mannitol. In children we are reluctant to use mannitol in the first 24 hours because of the frequent presence of cerebral hyperemia described previously.[9] It is possible that mannitol would, by increasing CBF and CBV, raise the ICP before lowering it and cause deterioration rather than improvement. After 24 hours, when the ICP is known, we do use mannitol in pediatric patients and then in the smallest doses that are effective, usually 0.5 mg/kg. In children with a rapidly progressing deficit with evidence of tentorial herniation in whom an epidural hematoma is suspected, mannitol should not be withheld as it may be lifesaving. Even in this situation, however, we prefer to insert an endotracheal tube and hyperventilate the patient before the mannitol is given. In adults, though not in children, we have used continuous mannitol infusion to maintain a normal ICP and keep the serum osmolality elevated. Very careful attention has to be given to maintain an adequate fluid and electrolyte balance. The purpose of mannitol or other hyperosmolar therapy is not to dehydrate the patient but to draw fluid from the brain down an osmotic gradient. It is a mistake not to replace some of the urine output, since when large doses of mannitol are required, failure to maintain an adequate circulating volume may lead to renal shutdown.

The most recent family of drugs to be used to control increased ICP is the barbiturates. In the clinical setting we do not feel that we are using barbiturate-induced coma to "protect" the brain but to lower the ICP and maintain an adequate CPP. The most commonly used barbiturate has been pentobarbital. The usual loading dose is 5 mg/kg IV followed by a constant infusion of 1 to 5 mg/kg/hour. The aim of therapy is to maintain an ICP below 20 torr without pressure waves. To achieve this goal, the necessary blood levels vary from 1.5 to 6 mg/

100 ml depending on the individual patient. If there is doubt whether the levels are adequate, it is preferable to monitor the EEG. When a burst suppression pattern or flat EEG is obtained, there seems to be no value to increasing the barbiturate levels further. We have had no major problems associated with the use of barbiturates, but the potential problems seem to be different in adults and children. In adults the systemic blood pressure is usually markedly decreased to a mean of around 70 torr and, especially in older patients, toxic effects on the heart can lead to pulmonary edema and acute vascular collapse. In children, our experience is that the blood pressure remains quite high, frequently greater than 100 torr. Monitoring of the cardiovascular parameters at this time frequently shows a high systemic resistance with a low cardiac index and normal or slightly increased pulmonary pressures with a normal or low CVP. These findings are more markedly deranged if the patients are also hypothermic. If the cardiac index is below an acceptable range and therapy is necessary, we have used a combination of peripheral vasodilatation, usually initially with sodium nitroprusside and careful volume replacement. This has proved to be a most successful line of therapy leading to decrease in pulmonary and systemic resistance, decreased cardiac work, improved cardiac index, and lower blood pressure. It also has proved possible with this regimen to avoid elevating the ICP.

Since the use of high doses of barbiturates completely abolishes the neurologic exam, the monitoring throughout this period has to be perfect. All instrumentation has to be constantly checked to ensure accuracy of the recording, since any malfunction in the catheters (SAP, ICP, Swan-Ganz, and so on) could be catastrophic for the patient. Eventually, pupillary responses, corneal responses, and oculovestibular responses are abolished, and the only signs of continued brain function are the preservation of the BER and occasionally the deep tendon reflexes. Once 48 hours have passed with no signs of increased ICP or waves, the bar-

biturates are discontinued. If waves recur or the ICP rises, therapy is reinstigated. The average duration of barbiturate coma has been five days, but this period varies from 2 to as long as 25 days. The rate of recovery from the iatrogenic coma also varies, and several days may be required before signs of spontaneous cerebral activity return.

The barbiturate mechanism that results in a lower ICP is not known, but we believe there is a direct constrictor action on cerebral blood vessels and that the decreased neuronal metabolism induced by the barbiturates leads to a further decrease in CBF and CBV through metabolic autoregulation. Marshall and Shapiro[41] reported on 25 patients with ICP over 20 torr that could not be controlled by a combination of the standard methods. Nineteen patients responded to barbiturates, and six did not. The mortality rate was 21% in the former group and 83% in the latter. We have used barbiturates in 20 children with Glasgow coma scores of 3 or 4 (decerebrate or flaccid) in whom the ICP could not be maintained below 20 torr by the usual methods (hyperventilation, steroids, mannitol, and position). The ICP responded and was maintained below 20 torr in 19 patients. Three patients died, two of secondary problems after consciousness had been regained, 2 were left in a vegetative or severely disabled state, and 15 made a good recovery.[9] There is no question in our minds as to the usefulness of high doses of barbiturates in controlling an elevated ICP after head injury. However, these agents can only be used when adequate monitoring facilities are available, especially for the ICP.

OUTCOME

Several recent reviews of the outcome following severe head injury are available.[32,36] In a large series of severe head injuries evaluated six hours after injury, the mortality rate was 50%.[31] Using more intensive therapy and strict control of ICP to less than 40 torr, Becker and co-workers[3] reported a mortality of 32% for a similar group of patients. Using the criteria (Fig.

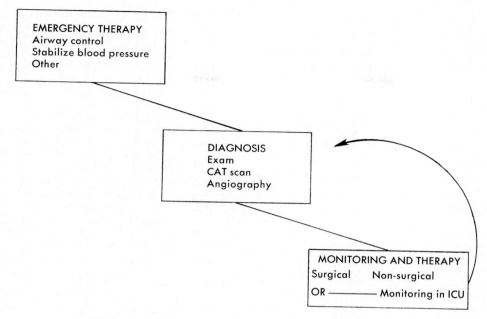

Fig. 10-1. Stepwise management of severe head trauma.

10-1) for therapy outlined above, we report a mortality of 19% in 132 severely head-injured patients. The biggest therapeutic difference in our patients is the control of ICP to less than 20 torr. We must point out that the mean age of our 132 patients is 20.5 years; 7 years and 14 years, respectively, younger than the patients in the series of Becker and co-workers[3] and Jennett and co-workers.[31] The mortality in patients in our series under 19 years is 9% and for those greater than 20 years, 36%. In neither Becker and co-workers[3] nor our own series[7] was there any significant increase in vegetative survival, suggesting that the intensive therapy for severely head-injured patients, especially children, is well worth the time and money since dramatic recovery can occur in a majority of patients.

SUMMARY

The acceptance of the concept of the primary and secondary head injury and the conceptual abandonment of the primary brain stem injury have set the stage for a more aggressive approach to the treatment of severely head-injured people. The neurologic exam can be rapid and uncomplicated, providing the physician understands the purpose of that exam. Serial exams are most important in defining the patient's course and the need for therapy. Therapy is aimed at preventing secondary injury and establishing the ideal milieu for recovery. The use of the CAT scan early in the course of the disease process has helped to diagnose surgically treatable lesions at the earliest possible time before unconsciousness is too greatly impaired, thereby improving the surgical results. Equally important has been the ability of the CAT scan to rule out a surgically remediable lesion and thereby remove the need for exploratory and frequently negative intervention. Secure in the knowledge that there is no surgically treatable mass lesion, the patient can be admitted to the ICU, where aggressive control of the ICP can be performed and any systemic problems cared for. A multimodality approach using steroids, hyperventilation, muscle paralysis, osmoltherapy, and barbiturates usually results in adequate control of the ICP at levels less than 20 torr. Therapy is designed to prevent any secondary injury to the brain and to establish, at the earliest possible time, a good milieu for recovery.

Along with other physiologic systems, we feel that the ICP should be continuously monitored. Only by knowing the ICP can rational therapy be given, and such therapy as muscle paralysis with hyperventilation or barbiturates can only be used if the ICP is recorded, since the clinical neurologic exam is obliterated by the therapy. We feel that this is acceptable since at the time barbiturates or paralysis and hyperventilation are instigated unconsciousness is already present with abnormal motor responses. Thus, we feel that the accuracy of the neurologic examination is no longer adequate to pick up impending severe changes in the intracranial pressure. The outcome from severe head injury has been improved using the approaches described in this chapter, and the number of patients surviving in a vegetative or severely disabled state has not been increased. As the ability to clinically investigate the pathophysiology improves still further (emission computerized tomography, EEG spectroanalysis, evoked responses), it is to be hoped that further improvements in outcome may result. There is no doubt that there will always be a number of patients in whom even the most active therapy will not result in recovery because of the severity of the underlying injury. The large mortality that occurs before hospitalization obviously will not be influenced by the approaches described above and may only be influenced by a decrease in the number of accidents. In children, it would appear that the mortality and severe morbidity may be able to be limited to 10% to 12%,[9] while in adults, it is not yet clear whether the mortality rate can be consistently lowered to less than 25%. The results of the intensive care of head-injured patients is extremely encouraging, and we feel that this positive attitude should be passed on to all personnel involved in the ICU care of this very large group of patients.

REFERENCES

1. Adams, H., and Graham, D. I.: The pathology of blunt head injuries. In Critchley, M., O'Leary, J. L., and Jennett, B., editors: Scientific foundations of neurology, Philadelphia, 1972, F. A. Davis Co., pp. 478-491.
2. Baratham, G., and Dennyson, W. G.: Delayed traumatic intracerebral hemorrhage, J. Neurol. Neurosurg. Psychiatr. 35:698-706, 1972.
3. Becker, D. P., Miller, J. D., Ward, J. D., Greenberg, R. P., and others: The outcome from severe head injury with early diagnosis and intensive management, J. Neurosurg. 47:491-502, 1977.
4. Bourke, R. S., Kimelberg, H. K., Daze, M. A., and Popp, A. J.: Studies on the formation of astroglial swelling and its inhibition by clinically useful agents. In Popp, A. J., Bourke, R. S., Nelson, L. R., and Kimelberg, H. K., editors: Neural trauma, New York, 1979, Raven Press, pp. 95-113.
5. Bricolo, A., Turazzi, S., Alexandre, A., and Rizzuto, N.: Decerebrate rigidity in acute head injury, J. Neurosurg. 47:680-698, 1977.
6. Bruce, D. A., and Langfitt, T. W.: The prognostic value of ICP, CPP, CBF and $CMRO_2$ in head injury. In McLaurin, R. L., editor: Head injuries, New York, 1976, Grune & Stratton, Inc., pp. 23-25.
7. Bruce, D. A., Gennarelli, T. A., and Langfitt, T. W.: Resuscitation from coma due to head injury, Crit. Care Med. 6:254-269, 1978.
8. Bruce, D. A., Langfitt, T. W., Miller, J. D., and others: Regional cerebral blood flow, intracranial pressure and brain metabolism in comatose patients, J. Neurosurg. 38:131-144, 1973.
9. Bruce, D. A., Raphaely, R. C., Goldberg, A. I., Zimmerman, R. A., Bilaniuk, L. T., Schut, L., and Kuhl, D. E.: The pathophysiology, treatment and outcome following severe head injury in children, Child Brain 5:174-191, 1979.
10. Bruce, D. A., Schut, L., Bruno, L. A., Wood, J. H., and Sutton, L. N.: Outcome following severe head injury in children, J. Neurosurg. 48:679-688, 1978.
11. Caveness, W. F.: Incidence of craniocerebral trauma in the United States, 1970-75, Abstr. Ann. Neurol. 1:507, 1977.
12. Clark, K., Nash, T. M., and Hutchison, G. C.: The failure of circumferential craniotomy in acute traumatic cerebral swelling, J. Neurosurg. 29:367, 1968.
13. Cooper, P. R., Rovit, R. L., and Ransohoff, J.: Hemicraniectomy in the treatment of acute subdural hematoma: a re-appraisal, Surg. Neurol. 5:25, 1976.
14. Courville, C. B.: Contre coup injuries of the brain in infancy, Arch. Surg. 90:157-165, 1965.
15. Dolinskas, C., Bilaniuk, L. T., Gennarelli, T. A., and Zimmerman, R. A.: Cranial computed tomography of post-traumatic extracerebral hematomas:

correlation with clinical examination and neuropathology, J. Trauma **19**:163, 1979.

16. Faupel, G., Reulen, H. S., Muller, D., and Schurmann, K.: Double blind study on the effect of steroids on severe closed head injury. In Pappius, H. M., and Feindel, W., editors: Dynamics of brain edema, New York, 1976, Springer-Verlag, pp. 337-343.

17. Fell, D. A., Fitzgerald, S., Moiel, R. H., and Caram, P.: Acute subdural hematomas; review of 144 cases, J. Neurosurg. **42**:37, 1975.

18. Galbraith, S. C.: Age distribution of extradural hemorrhage without skull fracture, Lancet **1**:1217-1218, 1973.

19. Gallagher, J. P., and Browder, E. J.: Extradural hematoma; experience with 167 patients, J. Neurosurg. **29**:1-12, 1968.

20. Gennarelli, T. A., Obrist, W. D., Langfitt, T. W., and Segawa, H.: Vascular and metabolic reactivity to changes in pCO$_2$ in head-injured patients. In Popp, A. J., Bourke, R. S., Nelson, L. R., and Kimelberg, H. K., editors: Neural trauma, New York, 1979, Raven Press, pp. 1-8.

21. Gennarelli, T. A., and Ommaya, A. K.: A neurophysiological assay of head injury severity; proceedings from the American Association of Neurological Surgeons, St. Louis, 1974, (in press).

22. Gennarelli, T. A., Zimmerman, R. A., and Bilaniuk, L. T.: Diffuse white matter shearing injury of the brain; proceedings of the American Association of Neurological Surgeons, New Orleans, 1978.

23. Gobiet, W., Bock, W. J., Liesegang, J., and Grote, W.: Treatment of acute cerebral edema with high dose of dexamethasone. In Beks, J. W. F., Bosch, D. A., and Brock, M., editors: Intracranial pressure III, New York, 1976, Springer-Verlag, pp. 231-235.

24. Greenberg, R. P., Becker, D. P., Miller, J. D., and Mayer, D. J.: Evaluation of brain function in severe human head trauma with multimodality evoked potentials, J. Neurosurg. **47**:163, 1977.

25. Hass, W. K.: Prognostic value of cerebral oxidative metabolism in head trauma. In McLaurin, R., editor: Head injuries, New York, 1977, Grune & Stratton, Inc., pp. 35-37.

26. Hooper, R.: Observations on extradural haemorrhage, Br. J. Surg. **47**:71, 1959.

27. James, H. E., Bruno, L. A., and Schut, L.: Intracranial subarachnoid pressure monitoring in children, Surg. Neurol. **3**:313, 1975.

28. Jamieson, K. G., and Yelland, J. D. N.: Extradural hematoma; report of 167 cases, J. Neurosurg. **29**: 13, 1968.

29. Jamieson, K. G., and Yelland, J. D. N.: Surgically treated traumatic subdural hematomas, J. Neurosurg. **37**:137, 1972.

30. Jennett, B., and Bond, M. R.: Assessment of outcome after severe brain damage, Lancet **1**:480, 1975.

31. Jennett, B., Teasdale, G., Galbraith, S., and others: Severe head injuries in three countries, J. Neurol Neurosurg. Psychiatr. **40**:291, 1977.

32. Jennett, B.: Injuries of the brain and skull. In Vinken, P. J., and Bruyn, G. W., editors: Handbook of clinical neurology, vol. 24, New York, 1975, American Elsevier Pub. Co., Inc., pp. 669-681.

33. Jennett, B., Teasdale, G., Braakman, R., Minchenhoud, J., and Knell-Jones, R.: Predicting outcome in individual patients after severe head injury, Lancet **1**:1031, 1976.

34. Johnston, I. H., and Jennett, B.: The place of continuous intracranial pressure monitoring in neurosurgical practice, Acta. Neurochir. **29**:53, 1973.

35. Johnston, I. H., Johnston, J. A., and Jennett, B.: Intracranial pressure changes following head injury, Lancet **2**:433, 1970.

36. Langfitt, T. W., Obrist, W. D., Gennarelli, T. A., O'Connor, M. J., and ter Weeme, C. A.: Correlation of cerebral blood flow with outcome in head injured patients, Ann. Surg. **186**:411, 1977.

37. Langfitt, T. W.: Measuring the outcome from head injuries, J. Neurosurg. **48**:673-678, 1978.

38. Lewin, V.: Planning for head injuries, Br. Med. J. **1**:131-134, 1959.

39. McKissock, W., Richardson, A., and Bloom, W. H.: Subdural hematomas; a review of 389 cases, Lancet **1**:1365, 1960.

40. Marshall, L. F., Bruce, D. A., Graham, D. I., and Langfitt, T. W.: Alterations in behaviour, brain electrical activity, cerebral blood flow and intracranial pressure produced by triethyl tin induced cerebral edema, Stroke **7**:21-25, 1976.

41. Marshall, L. F., and Shapiro, M. R.: Barbiturate control of intracranial hypertension in head injury and other conditions: iatrogenic coma. In Ingvar, D. H., and Lassen, N. A., editors: Cerebral function, metabolism and circulation, Copenhagen, 1977, Munksqaard, pp. 156-157.

42. Marshall, L. F., Smith, R. W., Rauscher, L. A., and Shapiro, H. M.: Mannitol dose requirements in brain-injured patients, J. Neurosurg. **48**:169-172, 1978.

43. Marshall, L. F., King, J., and Langfitt, T. W.: The complications of high-dose corticosteroid therapy in neurosurgical patients; a prospective study, Ann. Neurol. **1**:201-203, 1977.

44. Miller, J. D., Becker, D. P., Ward, J. D., Sullivan, H. G., and others: Significance of intracranial hypertension in severe head injury, J. Neurosurg. **47**:503, 1977.

45. Moiel, R. H., and Caram, P. C.: Acute subdural hematoma; a review of 84 cases, a six year evaluation, J. Trauma **7**:660, 1967.

46. Obrist, W. D., Thompson, H. K., Wang, H. S., and Wilkinson, W. E.: Regional cerebral blood flow estimated by Xenon[133] inhalation, Stroke **6**:245, 1975.

47. Obrist, W. D., Langfitt, T. W., ter Weeme, C., and others: Non-invasive, long-term serial studies of rCBF in acute head injury. In Ingvar, D. H., and Lassen, N. A., editors: Cerebral function, metabolism and circulation, Copenhagen, 1977, Munksgaard, pp. 178-181.
gaard, pp. 178-181.

48. Overgaard, J., and Tweed, W. A.: Cerebral circulation after head injury. I. Cerebral blood flow and its regulation after closed head injury with emphasis on clinical correlations, J. Neurosurg. **41**:531-541, 1974.

49. Raichle, M. E., Posner, J. B., and Plum, F.: Cerebral blood flow during and after hyperventilation, Arch. Neurol. **23**:394, 1970.

50. Sevitt, S.: Fatal road accidents in Birmingham: times to death and their cause, Injury **4**:281-293, 1973.

51. Shalit, M. N., Beller, A. S., Feinsod, N. M., Zeigler, M., and Coteu, S.: Critical values for cerebral oxygen utilization in man. In Russel, R., editor: Brain and blood flow, London, 1971, Pitman, pp. 130-135.

52. Starr, A., and Achor, J. L.: Auditory brain stem responses in neurological disease, Arch. Neurol. **32**:761, 1975.

53. Starr, A., and Hamilton, A. E.: Correlation between confirmed sites of neurological lesions and abnormalities of far field auditory brain stem responses, Electroenceph. Clin. Neurophysiol. **41**:595, 1976.

54. Stockard, J. J., and Rossiter, V. S.: Clinical and pathological correlates of brain stem auditory response abnormalities, Neurol. **27**:316, 1977.

55. Talalla, A., and Morin, M. A.: Acute traumatic subdural hematoma; a review of 100 consecutive cases, J. Trauma **11**:771, 1971.

56. Teasdale, G., and Jennett, B.: Assessment of coma and impaired consciousness, a practical scale, Lancet **2**:81-84, 1974.

57. Troupp, H.: Intraventricular pressure in patients with severe brain injuries, J. Trauma **5**:373, 1965.

58. Zimmerman, R. A., Bilaniuk, L. T., Bruce, D. A., Dolinskas, C., Obrist, W., and Kuhl, D.: Computed tomography of pediatric head trauma: acute general cerebral swelling, J. Radiol. **126**:403-408, 1978.

11

Peripheral sequelae of acute head injury

MARTHA JANE MATJASKO

"Peripheral" refers to the nonneurosurgical, direct and indirect, multisystem sequelae of head trauma. Some of these conditions are extremely rare, but this effort is intended to be a compilation of the recognized sequelae of acute head injury and a bibliographical source for those managing such patients on a day-to-day basis. A certain degree of expertise in management of the critically ill is assumed. This chapter is not meant to be an exhaustive manual of diagnosis and therapeutics, but approaches to and controversies in pathophysiology, diagnosis, and management are included. Where indicated, supplementary reading material is suggested.

Head trauma, alone or in combination with multisystem trauma, is the most common injury among the victims of motor vehicle accidents.[3] In the United States, 33,000 people die each year following motor vehicle–related head injury.[35] In Britain, one third of trauma unit admissions are because of head trauma; this accounts for 16% of the mortality in males age 15 to 40 years.[11] Since airway management was recognized as a necessary adjunct to the successful therapy of head injury,[19] efforts have been directed to earlier recognition and more aggressive management of intracranial hypertension and various associated nonintracranial disturbances in the hope that this approach would

lead to more useful survival. Cerebral compression, hypoxia, and ischemia—the so-called "second injury"—negatively influence the outcome of severe head injury.[19] Mortality approaches 50% in many comparable large series.[15,23,25,28] Becker and colleagues[2] have been able to significantly reduce mortality to 36% with uniform and aggressive surgical and medical therapy without increasing the number of vegetative survivals, which remains stable at about 10%. Patients with intracranial mass lesions have a poorer prognosis than those with diffuse brain injuries; the presence of abnormal posturing, impaired or absent oculocephalic responses, and bilaterally fixed pupils alone or in combination is associated with increased mortality. Early surgical decompression, continuous intracranial pressure monitoring, early mechanical ventilation, steroids, osmotic diuretics, and meticulous attention to cardiopulmonary and metabolic derangements have been shown to be instrumental in reducing mortality.

In a series of 116 patients known to have talked before dying from severe head injury, one or more avoidable factors could be identified in 74%. In 54% an avoidable factor was judged certainly to have contributed to death; most common avoidable factors were delay in the treatment of an intracranial hematoma, poorly controlled

211

epilepsy, meningitis, hypoxia, and hypotension.[16,26,27]

Thirty percent of head-injured patients have associated injuries, 8% of them serious.[11] Up to 40% of head-injured patients may be under the influence of alcohol at the time of injury.[14,24] Experimental CNS injuries are more extensive when animals are pretreated with ethanol.[6] In the unconscious or confused patient the mental status may be incorrectly attributed to ethanol intoxication[7,36] or the patient may not complain of neck, chest, or abdominal pain, which leads

---

PERIPHERAL SEQUELAE OF ACUTE HEAD INJURY

Cardiopulmonary
Abnormal breathing patterns
Airway obstruction
Hypoxemia
Shock
Adult respiratory distress syndrome (ARDS)
Neurogenic pulmonary edema (NPE)
Fat embolism
Venous thromboembolism
Electrocardiographic changes
Diaphragmatic paralysis

Hematologic
Inhibition of neutrophil phagocytosis
Trauma and coagulation
Disseminated intravascular coagulation
  (DIC)

Endocrinologic
Anterior pituitary insufficiency
Posterior pituitary dysfunction
  Diabetes insipidus (DI)
  Syndrome of inappropriate ADH
  (SIADH)

Metabolic
Metabolic response to head injury
Cerebrospinal fluid metabolic changes
Nonketotic hyperosmolar hyperglycemic
  coma (NHHC)

Gastrointestinal

Skeletal
Cervical spine injuries
Maxillofacial injuries

---

to delay in diagnosis and treatment of associated injuries.[36] Osmotic diuretics used to reduce intracranial pressure may mask the oliguric sign of hypovolemia.[4] Patients with apparently minor head injuries may require general anesthesia for laparotomy or fracture reduction.[11] During this anesthetic there may be natural evolution of the intracranial process or volatile anesthetic-induced increases in intracranial pressure leading to cerebral edema and herniation.* Repeated pupil examination is essential in such a patient, and if deterioration occurs, diagnostic burr holes and/or craniotomy may be life saving. Smith[32,33] suggests that thiobarbiturate anesthesia is superior to a volatile agent in the head-injured patient. Significant increases in ICP and systemic arterial pressure may occur at the termination of anesthesia, caused by sympathetic stimulation, increases in Pa_{CO_2} and intrathoracic pressure; this may be particularly damaging in the absence of cerebral autoregulation.[18]

The commonly recognized nonneurosurgical sequelae of acute head injury are listed opposite. Appropriate management of these disorders as well as attention to aggressive comprehensive care protocols can significantly reduce mortality following head injury.

CARDIOPULMONARY SEQUELAE OF ACUTE HEAD INJURY

Many "sinking spells" in head-injured patients can be directly related to inattention to the principles of airway management. This is true at the scene of the accident and during diagnostic studies, particularly computerized axial tomography. Enlisting the services of an anesthesiologist early following severe head injury can buy time for adequate neurodiagnostic studies and at the same time allow necessary airway protection, hyperventilation, and resuscitation to proceed simultaneously and without delay.

Initial pulmonary findings

At the time of concussion, acute elevations in intracranial pressure may tempo-

---

*References 1, 5, 8-10, 12, 13, 17, 20-22, 29-32, 34.

rarily or permanently affect the respiratory center, leading to apnea.[16] Perhaps this mechanism accounts for a certain percentage of immediately fatal head injuries.

Abnormal breathing patterns were recorded at some time in 60% of 227 patients with head injury, intracranial tumor, or subarachnoid hemorrhage.[56] Periodic, irregular, and rapid breathing occurred equally commonly in all groups; tachypnea (>25 per minute) and hyperventilation ($Pa_{CO_2} < 30$ torr) were associated with a poorer prognosis when they were combined; however, the breathing patterns observed did not correlate anatomically with the site of the lesion.

The unconscious state predisposes to upper airway obstruction, hypoxemia, and respiratory acidosis. At the time of injury, laryngeal and pharyngeal reflexes may be acutely depressed,[16] allowing silent or overt aspiration of blood, mucus, foreign body or gastric contents, and the development of atelectasis, pulmonary edema, and secondary bronchopneumonia.

In the absence of airway obstruction, 30% to 50% of acutely head-injured patients demonstrate hypoxemia and spontaneous hyperventilation.* Elevated cerebrospinal fluid lactic acid or severe dysfunction of medial pontine structures[58] may be the stimulus for such a picture.[37,50] Supplemental oxygen often corrects the hypoxemia without terminating the hyperventilation. Brain-injured patients may have a low cerebrospinal fluid pH and bicarbonate and high lactic acid levels correlating with the severity of injury[37,50]; hyperventilation will return CSF pH to normal.[13,63] Minute ventilation may be twice normal, particularly if carbon dioxide production is above normal as in the decerebrate patient. Severe refractory hypoxemia indicates a poor prognosis.[38,55] The increased dead space to tidal volume ratio (as high as 0.6) in the absence of shock and the large intrapulmonary shunt point to an ill-defined effect of acute intracranial hypertension on ventilation-perfusion relationships.[24,33,45,53]

---

*References 1, 24, 38, 40, 52, 62, 64.

Shock and the adult respiratory distress syndrome (ARDS)

Six percent to 39% of head-injured patients have thoracic and/or abdominal injuries leading to hypotension and shock.[9,15,71] Ten percent of head-injured patients have associated cervical spine injury. Spinal shock (hypotension and bradycardia) may be present on admission or develop following careless manipulation of the neck during resuscitation. Cardiogenic shock can compound hemorrhagic shock due to unknown effects of the protracted low-flow state on myocardial muscle function.

Neurogenic shock is rare.[34] In adults a fatal degree of cerebral compression usually develops before there is vasomotor center collapse. In young children with an expansile skull and relatively small blood volume, a significant proportion of the blood volume may accumulate intracranially and lead to hypotension. Also in young children, small scalp lacerations can lead to a significant reduction in blood volume. In Clark's[14] study of 721 head-injured patients, 49 had shock attributable to the head injury; these patients were neurologically moribund, and 46 did not survive.

Approximately 20% of head-injured patients develop acute respiratory failure[26,40]; that is, progressive hypoxemia resistant to oxygen therapy[5,45,52] and continuous positive airway pressure associated with measured reductions in functional residual capacity[40,52,60,62] and pulmonary compliance,[10,12,40] pulmonary hypertension,[39,76] and the typical radiologic infiltrates of "shock lung." Coincident shock and thoracic trauma predispose to respiratory failure and can significantly impair cerebral perfusion and oxygenation, leading to a greater compromise of the injured brain and perhaps extension of ischemia and edema to noninjured cerebral tissue.

Pathologically, the lungs are stiff and heavy with varying degrees of hemorrhagic edema throughout the airways, alveoli, and interstitium.[5,74] Platelet aggregation and microthrombosis of pulmonary capillaries may initiate the release of vasoactive substances (serotonin, histamine),[11] leading to increases in pulmonary vascular resistance (perhaps primarily venular).[3,54,69] Metabolic and respiratory acidosis, endogenous catecholamines, prostaglandins,[30] and alveolar hypoxia may all lead to increased pulmonary vascular resistance.[3,7,8,27,74] Damage to the capillary and epithelial cells permits movement of fluid, cells, and protein into the interstitium. When the transport capacity of the pulmonary lymphatics is exceeded, edema develops in the loose connective tissues surrounding the respiratory bronchiole and its accompanying arteriole, venule, and lymphatics.[67,68] Peribronchiolar edema leads to an increase in small airway resistance; alveolar interstitial edema reduces lung compliance. Later, alveolar edema occurs. Inspired gases tend to be diverted to more compliant alveoli, leading to an increased intrapulmonary shunt. Functional residual capacity and compliance fall. Atelectasis, hyaline membrane formation, and diffuse fibrosis develop with virtual cessation of gas exchange capability. As long as nitrogen is present in alveolar gas, alveoli with low ventilation-perfusion ratios tend to stay open. When the inspired oxygen tension is raised, the structurally important nitrogen tension decreases, and with continued uptake of oxygen from a partially obstructed but totally perfused alveolus, the intra-alveolar oxygen tension falls toward mixed venous levels; the alveolus tends to collapse.[17,47,73,75]

Early treatment (intubation, mechanical ventilation with end-expiratory pressure, careful fluid management) can abort or minimize the full-blown symptom complex. In many trauma centers, death from respiratory insufficiency has been reduced to less than 2% when expectant and preventive management is stressed.

Priorities in the management of hemorrhagic shock in the head-injured patient are airway control and volume replacement. Smooth intubation and hyperventilation (Pa_{CO_2} 25 torr) are indicated. High minute volumes may be needed to compensate for the cerebral lactic acidosis and increased dead space associated with head injury[24,33]

and the pulmonary hypoperfusion of the shock state.[20,23] Swift volume replacement with blood and appropriate crystalloid and/or colloid is necessary to restore adequate organ perfusion, maximize oxygen-carrying capacity and cardiac output, and minimize alveolar dead space.[23,57] Inspired oxygen tension must be adjusted serially, depending on the patient's response to therapy and recognizing that inspired tensions above .40 (PA_{O_2} 250 torr) can adversely affect pulmonary gas exchange in normal as well as traumatized patients.[47,73,75] In addition to microatelectasis, high inspired oxygen tensions may have ill-defined effects on pulmonary vasculature leading to ventilation-perfusion mismatching and increased right-to-left shunting.

Positive end-expiratory pressure[49,60,61,72] may restore functional residual capacity; improvement in ventilation-perfusion relationships may allow reductions in inspired oxygen concentration.[52] PEEP-induced increases in mean alveolar pressure[19] are transmitted to the pleural cavity, heart, and great vessels in direct relationship to the lung compliance; that is, as PEEP increases, the level at which cardiac output is depressed varies inversely with the lung compliance.[29,49] Alveolar pressure applied to the pulmonary capillary or the disease process itself may increase pulmonary vascular resistance,[61] while raising alveolar P_{O_2} may be instrumental in reversing hypoxic pulmonary vasoconstriction. When marked pulmonary hypertension exists, changes in airway pressure have little effect on pulmonary artery pressure, since in such patients a significant fraction of right heart output is perfusing nonaerated lung that is protected from the airway pressure. Theoretically, increases in transpulmonary pressure may be transmitted principally to normal alveoli and hence reduce perfusion in these areas, leading to a worsening of the shunt.[6,36,51] High levels of PEEP may reduce cardiac output below levels sufficient for oxygen consumption; greater peripheral venous desaturation occurs because of this reduction in oxygen availability, and alveolar-to-arterial

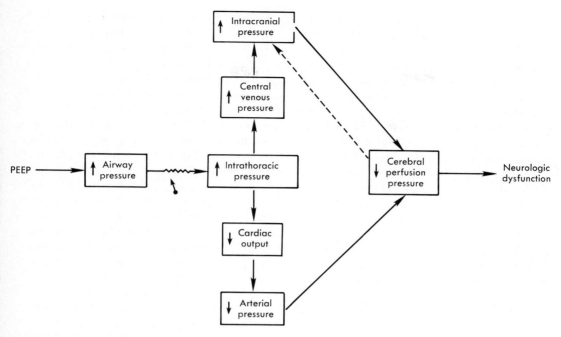

Fig. 11-1. Pathophysiologic effects of PEEP on intracranial dynamics and cerebral perfusion pressure in the presence of an intracranial mass lesion. (From Aidinis, S. J., and others: Anesthesiology 45:275, 1976.)

oxygen tension gradients can increase substantially in the presence of an unchanging venous admixture. In some patients improvement in shunting can be more than offset by a fall in cardiac output with a consequent reduction in oxygen availability to the tissues (available oxygen = oxygen content × cardiac output). Therefore, mechanical ventilation with positive end-expiratory pressure may improve shunting by increasing functional residual capacity and reducing hypoxic pulmonary vasoconstriction; it may also increase shunting by shifting pulmonary blood flow to nonventilated regions of the lung and by reducing cardiac output. Ideal management of these patients is best accomplished when serial functional residual capacity, cardiac output, oxygen consumption, oxygen availability, pulmonary vascular resistance, and blood gas measurements are available.[18,61,70] Extracorporeal membrane oxygenation may prove life-saving when conventional ventilatory care fails.[31]

Highly variable effects of PEEP on intra-cranial pressure and neurologic status have been noted in animals and humans. Aidinis and co-workers[2] demonstrated in cats with intracranial mass lesions that PEEP can initiate changes in intracranial pressure and systemic blood pressure leading to further neurologic dysfunction. Reductions in cerebral perfusion pressure (CPP) were particularly damaging in animals with impaired autoregulation; neurologic dysfunction may develop at cerebral perfusion pressures greater than 60 torr in patients with impaired or absent autoregulation. Fig. 11-1 is a schematic representation of the possible effects of PEEP on cerebral perfusion pressure. The authors caution that application and removal of PEEP may be particularly dangerous. PEEP removal may precipitate a sudden increase in central blood volume, a subsequent increase in blood pressure and cerebral perfusion pressure and lead to increased cerebral edema in patients with low intracranial compliance and loss of autoregulation. PEEP application and other clinical situations in which intrathoracic pressure is raised (intubation, coughing, suctioning, Valsalva maneuver) may adversely affect CPP and ICP.[42,43] Barbiturate therapy may be indicated to prevent and treat increases in intrathoracic and intracranial pressures.[46,66]

Variable effects of PEEP have been reported in severely head-injured patients. McAslan[48] exposed eight supine patients to increases in PEEP from 5 to 20 cm H_2O; no change in ventricular fluid pressure was observed until PEEP exceeded 15 cm H_2O. Cerebral perfusion pressure remained above normal in all but one patient, whose blood pressure fell at 20 cm H_2O PEEP. No specific deteriorations in neurologic status were noted. Frost[25] exposed 10 patients (30-degree head-up tilt) to varying PEEP levels and observed no changes in intracranial pressure despite increases in central venous pressure and pulmonary wedge pressure. PEEP of 35 cm H_2O applied for 10 minutes, however, did lead to pressure waves indicating reduced intracranial compliance. Apuzzo[4] applied 10 cm H_2O of PEEP in 25 severely head-injured patients (no mention of head position). In 12 of 13 patients with increased elastance (decreased compliance) PEEP caused increases in intracranial pressure at times greater than double the baseline level; of these 12 patients, 6 had cerebral perfusion pressures below 60 torr. In 12 of 12 patients with normal elastance, no change in intracranial pressure occurred with PEEP. Caution must be exercised in the individual patient. PEEP should not be withheld when it is essential for improvement of FRC and venous admixture. The lowest effective PEEP level should be applied with simultaneous observance of its effect on intracranial pressure, cardiac output, mean arterial pressure, cerebral perfusion pressure, and oxygen availability. This is important when high-dose barbiturate therapy is being used. Significant circulatory depression frequently occurs; continuous CPP measurement is mandatory.

Magnaes[44] measured ventricular fluid pressure during rapid postural changes. In some patients with elevated intracranial pressure, rapid sitting up or lying down led to clinical symptoms, which occurred concomitantly with large transient or stationary CSF pressure waves. Symptoms were aggravated when a craniospinal block developed in the sitting position and were reduced when tilting up or down was performed slowly over two to three minutes. Most neurosurgical patients are nursed in a slight head-up position (30 degrees) based on the clinical observation that this maneuver can reduce intracranial pressure by hydrostatic reductions in cerebral venous outflow pressure and ventricular fluid pressure. Most patients adjust to this postural change by a compensatory rise in peripheral vascular resistance, maintaining blood pressure and hence cerebral perfusion pressure. Patients moribund with elevated intracranial pressures and intracranial vasomotor paralysis may not be able to tolerate even transient small reductions in cerebral perfusion pressure without decompensation; in these patients head-up position may not be good and may even harm.

Frequent blood gases, cardiac output, pulmonary arterial and wedge pressures, ongoing neurologic assessment and intracranial pressure measurements are all necessary for intelligent management of this complex changing situation. The anesthetized, paralyzed patient presents a challenge. Normal minute ventilation in a patient with an increased alveolar dead space can lead to hypercarbia and increases in intracranial blood volume. Appropriate consideration must be given to the effects of ketamine[28] and volatile anesthetic agents[35] on intracranial blood volume and secondarily intracranial pressure, even in the patient who has sustained a relatively minor head injury. Equally damaging changes in ICP and mean arterial pressure can occur when anesthesia is terminated due to sympathetic activity or hypercarbia.[46]

Weaning from mechanical ventilation must be individualized, based on the severity of respiratory involvement and associated injuries; however, the usual criteria apply—vital capacity at least 10 ml/kg, maximum inspiratory force at least -20 to -30 cm H_2O,[21,32,59] dead space to tidal volume ratio less than 0.6,[65] $A - aDo_2$ less than 300 to 350 torr,[22] cardiovascular stability, and normal metabolic state.[41]

Neurogenic pulmonary edema (NPE)

Following a variety of central nervous system insults, fulminant pulmonary edema may develop characterized by marked pulmonary vascular congestion, intra-alveolar hemorrhage, and a protein-rich edema fluid. The syndrome most often occurs in the absence of underlying cardiopulmonary disease; traditional therapy for pulmonary edema of cardiac origin is ineffective and the outcome is frequently fatal.[70]

The association between central nervous system injury and pulmonary disease dates back to 1874 when Nothnagel[54] reported the death of a rabbit from pulmonary congestion following probing of the brain at unspecified points. In 1918, Moutier[52] noted the frequent occurrence of fatal, acute pulmonary edema associated with battle injuries, namely gunshot wounds to the head. Edema developed within one hour of injury and was associated with hypertension and bradycardia; deaths were attributed to overactivity of the suprarenal glands.

To date, neurogenic pulmonary edema has been reported following a variety of conditions: head trauma,[9,16,21,24,64] intracranial hemorrhage[15,73] and tumors,[9,28,43,72] strokes,[9] seizures,[8,30,38] Guillain-Barré syndrome,[33] meningitis,[9] poliomyelitis,[1] venous air embolism,[13] intrathecal hypertonic saline,[71] and insulin shock treatment of schizophrenia.[53]

Pulmonary edema has been produced in a variety of experimental animals, including primates, subsequent to an increase in intracranial pressure by means of gun impact,[2] wooden block blow,[46] inflation of an epidural balloon,* or infusion of saline,[7,23,32,35,59] blood[10] or fibrin[10,61,62] into the intracranial space. Electrolytic lesions of the hypothalamus,[47,58] low cervical spinal cord transection,[6] and bilateral cervical vagotomy[25,26]

---

* References 3, 4, 11, 12, 22, 23.

have led to neurogenic pulmonary edema.

The influence of raised intracranial pressure on circulatory dynamics was described by Harvey Cushing[18] in his classic study published in 1901. Dogs exposed to local and general cerebral compression developed an increase in intracranial pressure and a concomitant increase in systemic blood pressure, which tended to "find a level slightly above that of the pressure exerted against the medulla." This elevation in pressure apparently serves to spare medullary function. The systemic hypertension was not attenuated by cervical vagotomy but was totally abolished by cervical cord transection or topical cocainization of the medulla, implying a sympathetic nervous system–mediated mechanism. Cushing also exposed the small intestine and directly observed splanchnic vasoconstriction coincident with the systemic hypertension. Rhythmic variations in blood pressure (Traube-Hering waves) occurred during the intracranial hypertension; the crests of the waves were higher and the valleys lower than the intracranial pressure. By direct observation through a cranial window, the crests of the blood pressure waves were associated with hyperemia of the cortical vessels and Cheyne-Stokes respiration. The valleys were accompanied by anemia of the cortical surface vessels and concomitant respiratory arrest. Although no animal developed pulmonary edema, despite intracranial pressures greater than 200 torr, respiratory rate and volume were affected. He concluded that an increase in intracranial pressure to levels greater than blood pressure led to medullary ischemia and vasomotor center stimulation, prompting a rise in blood pressure slightly above the pressure exerted against the medulla. This increase in blood pressure led to medullary reflow and vasomotor center inhibition, prompting a fall in blood pressure below intracranial pressure and initiation of the cycle again.[19]

Over the next 70 years many investigators postulated humoral or neural mechanisms to account for the left ventricular failure and/or increased pulmonary capillary permeability of neurogenic pulmonary edema. Any pathophysiologic mechanism must account for the specific characteristic features of this syndrome[69,70]:

1. Rapid onset
2. Relationship to hypothalamic lesions
3. Prevention or attenuation by alpha blockers and central nervous system depressants
4. Specific sequence of hemodynamic changes
5. High protein content edema fluid
6. Resemblance to epinephrine-induced pulmonary edema

The rapid onset suggests a massive neural discharge from the injured brain secondary to intracranial hypertension. Weisman[73] performed autopsies in 686 patients following fatal intracranial hemorrhage. Eight of 13 patients who died immediately and two thirds of the patients who died within one hour had pulmonary edema. Small laboratory animals have been subjected to severe cerebral trauma and have been observed to die within a few minutes in fulminant pulmonary edema.[46] In Vietnam, patients with penetrating head injuries without associated injuries showed a high incidence of pulmonary edema. Seventeen of 20 patients who died within a few minutes following head injury had associated pulmonary edema. If cervical cord transection or massive hemorrhage accompanied the head injury, pulmonary edema did not occur.[64] Because of the rapid onset, conventional forms of heart failure are unlikely.

Specific hypothalamic electrolytic lesions in rats can produce pulmonary edema. Maire and Patton[47] postulate the existence of a hypothalamic "edemagenic center" whose impulses arise from postchiasmatic hypothalamic structures. This edemagenic center is normally inhibited by structures in the preoptic area; destructive preoptic lesions release this inhibition, leading to pulmonary edema. Vagotomy and cervical cord transection prevent edema after such lesions. Reynolds[58] offers an alternative interpretation: electrolytic lesions cause pulmonary edema on the basis of irritation of the sympathetic pathways in the hypothalamus and subsequent massive neural discharge. It is probable that the hypothalamus would be vulnerable to dysfunction by a variety of proximal or distal brain insults. Perhaps the massive neural discharge of neurogenic pulmonary edema is centrally mediated with an important hypothalamic component. However, Chen and co-workers[14] have reported that the hypothalamus is not essential for the development of pulmonary edema, since midbrain lesions producing decerebration in animals did not affect either the cardiovascular or pulmonary changes induced by cerebral compression.

Pretreatment with central nervous system depressants (phenobarbital, ether, chloral hydrate) and alpha adrenergic blocking agents prevented or attenuated the severity of pulmonary edema compared to untreated controls following the same head trauma.[2,5,46] Adrenalectomy offered no protection. Studies by Brown[7] suggest that neurogenic pulmonary edema is mediated largely through the sympathetic nervous system, specifically the alpha adrenergic system, and that the sympathetic nervous system response is centrally mediated because it is attenuated by central nervous system depressants. Dogs pretreated with Dibenzyline do not exhibit massive increases in systemic blood pressure or peripheral resistance following acute intracranial hypertension.[7] Elevated blood catecholamine levels occur during intracranial hypertension; peak levels are reached when systemic hypertension is greatest.[60]

A specific sequence of hemodynamic changes has been observed in susceptible animals.* Twenty percent of the time animals show massive increases in systemic arterial, pulmonary arterial, pulmonary venous, and superior vena caval pressures accompanied by a dramatic increase in total peripheral resistance. As a result of the increase in peripheral resistance, blood shifts from the peripheral to the pulmonary vascular bed documented by pressure and blood volume changes (increased size of left atrium, pulmonary venous engorgement). Within 15

---

*References 7, 22, 23, 48, 61, 62.

minutes the lungs become cyanotic and edematous. Eighty percent of animals tend to have decreasing systemic, pulmonary arterial, and pulmonary venous pressures over the next few minutes and no pulmonary edema.[23]

After an initial phase of increased pulmonary vascular pressure, pulmonary edema persists while this pressure returns to normal. In three patients, pulmonary wedge pressures were normal when pulmonary edema was well established. This observation suggests that pulmonary capillary membrane disruption has occurred.[31]

The electron microscopic picture of vascular wall rupture with leakage of red blood cells and amorphous material into the perivascular and intra-alveolar spaces and the clinical finding of high protein content in the edema fluid suggest that capillary membrane disruption is an important feature of NPE.[14,37,63] Even though the hemodynamic abnormalities that produce the capillary structural damage subside quickly, altered pulmonary capillary permeability may persist, requiring extreme caution in respiratory and fluid management.

The profound vasoconstriction that follows intravenous epinephrine[44,45,75] precipitates pulmonary edema, which can be prevented by pretreatment with alpha adrenergic blockers. These studies indicate that the immediate cause of neurogenic pulmonary edema is a sudden increase in pulmonary capillary pressure and eventual capillary membrane disruption. Left atrial and left ventricular end-diastolic pressures rise due to increased afterload and decreased left ventricular compliance. Therefore, changes in cardiac function are brief and based on an increase in cardiac work and not related to intrinsic cardiac failure.[70]

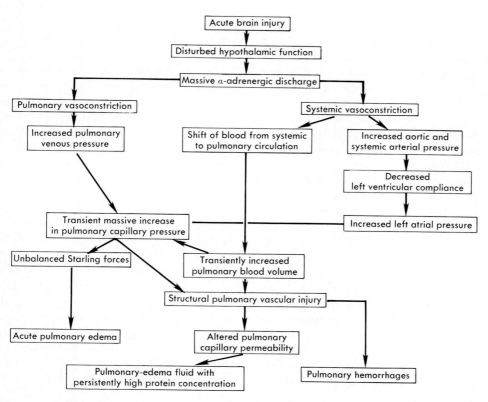

Fig. 11-2. Pathogenesis of neurogenic pulmonary edema. (From Theodore, J., and Robin, E. D.: Am. Rev. Resp. Dis. **113**:405, 1976.)

The current working hypothesis relative to the pathophysiology of this condition is illustrated in Fig. 11-2.

Therapy consists of immediate relief of intracranial hypertension pharmacologically and surgically, continuous positive pressure ventilation, careful fluid management, and perhaps sodium nitroprusside, which may be useful because of its ability to directly dilate peripheral and pulmonary vessels.[17]

Vigorous inspiratory effort against a closed glottis or totally obstructed airway can generate severe negative intra-alveolar pressures and lead to pulmonary edema. This mechanism may be operative in head-injured patients who are unconscious with upper airway obstruction.[56]

Various forms of noncardiac pulmonary edema—high altitude,[36,39,66] opiate-induced,[20,55] smoke inhalation, and pulmonary edema following decompression—have been explained on the basis of hypoxic pulmonary vasoconstriction leading to pulmonary hypertension,[27,41,57,67] arterial wall rupture, and leakage of protein-rich fluid into the interstitium and alveoli. An alternative theory is that damaged arterial walls attract fibrin and platelets, which form thrombi that may then shower the capillary and venous bed with microemboli, producing pulmonary capillary hypertension, capillary rupture, and edema formation.[42,65,74] Activated intravascular clotting or fibrinolysis may have an important role in high altitude pulmonary edema.[29,34,40]

There are striking similarities in the pathologic and clinical picture of shock lung and neurogenic pulmonary edema. Moss[49-51] has subjected dogs to hypoxic cerebral perfusion (Pa_{O_2} 35 ± 5 torr) without systemic ischemia, acidemia, hypercarbia, or hypotension. Within two hours the animals developed impaired pulmonary function pathologically similar to shock lung. He postulates that many respiratory distress syndromes have a common cerebral etiology; the initiating trauma interferes with hypothalamic cellular metabolism, which leads to autonomically mediated increased pulmonary venular resistance. This results in increased capillary pressures and vascular congestion, interstitial and intra-alveolar edema and hemorrhage, and right-to-left shunting. Lung denervation can prevent these changes.[68] The transudated plasma and resulting hyaline membrane formation inactivate surfactant and predispose to atelectasis. Systemic hypoxia should also produce this syndrome as in acute mountain sickness or high altitude pulmonary edema. This is an attractive unifying theory to explain posttraumatic pulmonary insufficiency and adult respiratory distress syndrome, as well as the varied forms of noncardiac pulmonary edema, including neurogenic pulmonary edema.

Fat embolism

Fat embolism may be associated with fractures of any bone containing marrow. Nearly all patients who die shortly after sustaining fractures have fat emboli in the lungs post mortem,[10] while only 1% to 2% of patients with fractures develop clinical features compatible with fat embolism.[9] Mortality has been reduced in recent years because of appropriate respiratory management.[4]

Clinical symptoms usually develop 24 to 48 hours post trauma; most frequent are changes in mental status from restlessness to coma. Accompanying findings are pyrexia, tachycardia, tachypnea, cyanosis, seizures, paralysis, and an evanescent petechial rash associated with thrombocytopenia best seen on the anterior axillary folds, neck, abdominal wall, and conjunctiva.[5] Thirty-seven of 45 patients reported by Ross had this classic petechial rash with or without other signs.[9] Failure to recover consciousness following general anesthesia may lead to suspicion of this diagnosis, particularly in the absence of head injury. Droplets lodging in the pulmonary circulation may lead to hypoxemia; they may be seen in sputum and, if they traverse the pulmonary capillary, they may be seen in retinal vessels and urine. It has been suggested that biochemical changes in the plasma during shock disrupt the lipid suspension system, allowing fatty acids and free fat to appear.[6] Free fat in the pulmonary capillary may cause a release of lipase, produced in the pulmonary parenchyma, with resultant breakdown of fat to free fatty acids.[1] Toxic free fatty acids may produce epithelial damage, platelet aggregation, inactivation of lung surfactant, increased capillary permeability, decreased lung compliance, and hypoxemia due to increased right-to-left shunting.[3,8] The associated anemia and thrombocytopenia in fat embolism have been accounted for on the basis of disseminated intravascular coagulation.[7] Differential diagnosis must include posttraumatic pulmonary insufficiency, shock, venous thromboembolism, and aspiration pneumonitis. Secondary deterioration in a head-injured patient may be due to fat embolism.

The chest roentgenogram may show the characteristic "snow storm" appearance or diffuse, fluffy, hazy infiltration. Other laboratory findings may be anemia, thrombocytopenia, and hypocalcemia due to the interaction between fatty acids and calcium. No laboratory test is pathognomonic. Treatment must primarily be directed to correction of hypoxemia. Pharmacologic steroid therapy and heparinization may be of value.[2,4,7]

Venous thromboembolism

The incidence of fatal pulmonary embolism in neurosurgical patients in general and head-injured patients in particular is unknown. In a group of 599 postoperative neurosurgical deaths (intracranial tumor, aneurysm), pulmonary embolism demonstrated at autopsy was judged to be the principal cause of death in 18 patients (3%), an incidence identical to that following other major surgical procedures.[12]

Twenty percent of patients who have deep vein thrombosis develop pulmonary embolism with an 18% mortality.[3] Joffe[6] recently reported a 43% incidence of postoperative deep thrombosis (Doppler,[10] [125]I fibrinogen[9]) in neurosurgical patients; 90% were asymptomatic and none developed clinical evidence of pulmonary embolism. Warlow reports a 13% incidence of pulmonary embolism in 30 patients following cerebrovascular

accidents; two of four patients with pulmonary embolism died.[11]

Barnett and co-workers[1] have shown that minidose heparin therapy (5000 units subcutaneously q 12 h as long as bedridden)[4,7,8] can be used safely following a variety of neurosurgical procedures; however it remains to be seen whether this approach can prevent deep vein thrombosis and pulmonary embolism in the neurosurgical population, including head-injured patients.

Brisman and Mendell[2] report a higher incidence of thromboembolic complications in patients with suprasellar tumors compared to nonsuprasellar tumors. Clinical and autopsy evidence of thromboembolic disease was present in 5 of 15 patients (33%) with suprasellar tumors and 15 of 223 (6.7%) of patients with brain tumors in nonsuprasellar locations. A relationship between suprasellar tumors and hypothalamic associated hypercoagulability is implied. Hypothalamic stimulation has been shown to result in an increase in factor VIII levels[5]; dehydration, obesity, and/or immobilization, which may be associated with hypothalamic malfunction, may themselves predispose to thromboembolism.[2]

Electrocardiographic changes

Jacobson and Danufsky[5] produced arrhythmias in mice after experimental head injury; atropine pretreatment prevented these arrhythmias, implying that vagal stimulation was responsible. Bradycardia, shortened QT interval, elevated ST segment, nodal rhythm, and increased T wave amplitude have been reported following experimental concussion in monkeys. Cardiac arrest may also occur.[8] Atrial fibrillation following head injury with and without intracranial hypertension has also been reported.[6,7] The pathogenesis of varied electrocardiographic abnormalities following head injury,[3,8] subarachnoid hemorrhage,[2,4,10] and cerebrovascular accidents[1] is obscure. Central autonomic stimulation at cortical, hypothalamic, or brain stem levels or interruption or spasm of deep perforating vessels to the hypothalamus could account for these observations.[4,9] There seems to be no correlation between intracranial hypertension or electrolyte imbalance and ECG changes in patients with subarachnoid hemorrhage, meningitis, or space-occupying lesions.[4]

Diaphragmatic paralysis

Transient diaphragmatic paralysis following head trauma has been reported infrequently.[2] In stroke and hemiplegic patients contralateral diaphragmatic paralysis has been observed.[1] When the brain injury is diffuse, a possible cause of transient phrenic nerve dysfunction may be hyperextension of the neck resulting in stretching, edema, or hemorrhage in the nerve without complete avulsion. Recovery occurred in one to six months in the cases reported by Prasad and Athreya.[2] Diaphragmatic paralysis may aggravate the respiratory problems of the head-injured patient and be responsible for difficulty in weaning because of inadequate lung expansion and poor coughing ability.

HEMATOLOGIC SEQUELAE
Inhibition of phagocytosis

Many disease states, including anoxic brain damage,[1,4,5] drug therapy,[7,9] and general anesthesia without coincident surgery, can inhibit the phagocytic function of neutrophilic granulocytes.[3] Van Woerkom and co-workers[11] exhibited a correlation between the severity of head injury and the degree of phagocyte inhibition; clinical improvement was accompanied by improvement in phagocytic function. Patients with head injuries and cerebrovascular accidents had an 80% and 52% incidence of nonphagocytosing granulocytes, respectively, compared to 6% in normal persons, 22% in surgical patients, and 13% in subacute and chronic neurologic disorders. Severe disturbances in phagocyte function have been observed in some head-injured patients with clear consciousness but with posttraumatic diabetes insipidus, implying a hypothalamic mechanism.[11] Head injury can lead to decreased platelet aggregation and an associated increase in cytoplas-

mic adenosine 3, 5 monophosphate (cyclic AMP)[12]; brain ischemia can produce changes in lymphocyte transplantation antigens.[10] Brain damage apparently has widespread influence on blood cells.[8]

Hypothalamic effects on the pituitary-adrenal axis and on the autonomic nervous system may be responsible for the observed alterations in phagocytosis. Plasma cortisol levels increase in proportion to the severity of trauma[6]; steroids inhibit phagocytosis in vitro.[7] Elevated cerebrospinal fluid serotonin levels in head-injured patients have been correlated with inhibition of phagocytosis.[11,13] Steroids also stimulate serotonergic metabolism in the brain.[2]

Trauma and coagulation

The severely traumatized patient displays a multitude of clotting abnormalities.[1-3,9] Among 42 patients with a wide variety of traumatic injuries reported by Innes and Sevitt,[10] hypercoagulable and fibrinolytic states existed in the first few hours post trauma, probably due to release of tissue thromboplastin presumably for hemostatic purposes. The duration of exaggerated fibrinolysis correlated with the severity of the injury. Hypocoagulability in these patients was probably related to clotting factor deficiencies (II, VII, platelets). Frequently these patients demonstrate an abrupt rebound antifibrinolysis, perhaps again a hemostatic mechanism. Adrenergic hyperactivity subsequent to trauma may trigger hypercoagulability.[5,6,12]

Good correlation exists between the severity of morbidity following massive trauma and a decrease in platelets, prothrombin (factor II), proaccelerin (factor V), and plasminogen and an increase in fibrin degradation products. When intravascular coagulation is present, increased clinical morbidity in the form of respiratory and other organ failure usually develops.[13] It is recognized that multiple transfusions, shock, sepsis, and unknown factors may influence coagulation.[7,8] Aspirin, phenylbutazone, chlorpromazine, penicillin, general anesthetics, furosemide, and many other drugs and head trauma have been shown to impair platelet aggregation in vitro and in vivo.[4,11,14,15]

Disseminated intravascular coagulation (DIC)

Disseminated intravascular coagulation is a physiologic response to a variety of underlying stimuli that provoke a generalized activation of the hemostatic mechanism leading to the intravascular consumption of clotting factors with subsequent thrombosis and/or bleeding diathesis. This syndrome reflects the interplay of two basic processes. The first is a complex sequence of events leading to the evolution of thrombin; the second is a series of protective mechanisms employed by the body to defend itself against the disseminated clotting that would occur in the presence of unchecked thrombin activity. Therefore, thrombin formation and fibrinolysis occur, leading to the clinical picture of simultaneous thrombosis and hemorrhage.[8] Etiologically, DIC can be the result of three processes: (1) endothelial cell injury, which activates Hageman factor and the intrinsic clotting system; (2) tissue injury, which activates the extrinsic clotting system; and (3) red cell or platelet injury, with the release of coagulant phospholipids.[7] These processes lead to the formation of thrombin, which in turn cleaves fibrinogen, activates factor XIII (fibrin stabilizing factor), aggregates platelets, releases platelet constituents, and triggers secondary fibrinolysis.[21] The fibrinolytic agent, plasmin, splits fibrinogen, producing fibrin degradation or split products that themselves have anticoagulant properties. Analysis of a series of 90 patients revealed that diagnostic criteria for DIC require the presence of at least three abnormal screening tests (prolonged prothrombin time, decreased fibrinogen, decreased platelets). If only two of the three are abnormal, a test for fibrinolysis (thrombin time, euglobulin clot lysis, or fibrinogen degradation products) should be abnormal to establish the diagnosis.[7]

In the head-injured patient several clotting

abnormalities may be present, and DIC has been reported following mild and severe cerebral trauma* and anoxic brain damage.[1]

Reduced platelet aggregation associated with elevated cytoplasmic adenosine 3, 5 monophosphate (cyclic AMP) has been reported following head injury.[24,27] Goodnight and co-workers[12] prospectively examined coagulation profiles in 26 head-injured patients. Twelve of 13 patients in whom no brain tissue destruction occurred had normal fibrinogen, factor VIII, and platelet levels. Fibrin degradation products were minimally elevated. In 9 of 13 patients with brain tissue destruction established by direct inspection, evidence of DIC was present, based on elevated fibrin degradation products, low factor V, VIII, and platelets. Many of these parameters returned to normal within hours, although occasionally the coagulation defect caused hemostatic difficulty during surgery.

Vecht and co-workers[28] noted activated clotting in a series of 34 patients with moderate-to-severe head injury; no DIC occurred. In another series of six patients with massive blunt head injury, Vecht[26] reports prolonged prothrombin and thrombin times, shortened partial thromboplastin time, reduced factor V levels, and enhanced fibrinolysis. No clinically detectable DIC was observed. It is interesting that while these patients were unconscious platelet aggregability remained decreased in the presence of normal platelet counts.

The pathogenesis of DIC in head injury is uncertain. The severity of coagulation abnormalities correlates with the severity of head injury and associated multiple injuries. Shock, sepsis, extensive surgery,[7,8,14] and fat embolism[16] have all been associated with the development of DIC and may be concurrent factors in the head-injured patient. Brain tumors are also known to predispose to DIC.[17,25]

The brain as a whole is rich in tissue thromboplastin and contains 50 units per gram of tissue; in fact, human brain thrombo-

---

*References 9, 10, 12, 15, 18, 20, 28.

plastin is used in the performance of the Quick prothrombin time. The lung is the only organ with higher thromboplastin levels than brain, up to 200 units per gram.[2] Takashima and co-workers[22] and Tovi[23] have shown that high levels of fibrinolytic activity are present in brain, primarily in the highly vascular connective tissue of the choroid plexus and meninges. Fibrinolytic activity is low in brain tissue itself and the amount of either substance liberated into the general circulation following head trauma is unknown.

Central nervous system mechanisms exist for the regulation of plasma levels of blood clotting factors. Gunn and Hampton[13] have reported that direct hypothalamic stimulation can lead to a decrease in factor VIII levels. Stimulation of permanent electrodes in subcortical areas of 12 dogs demonstrated that factor VIII levels were decreased by stimulation of ventral and lateral hypothalamic areas with its medial forebrain bundle overlying the optic tract, the ventral hippocampus, the nucleus supramammilaris, and the segmental fields of Forel. Factor VIII levels were increased by stimulation of the mesencephalic pontine reticular formation, central gray, lateral hypothalamic area, habenula, and the habenular interpeduncular tract. There is a relationship between peripheral autonomic function and blood coagulation. Stress,[5] splanchnic nerve stimulation,[6] and epinephrine[4] administration may lead to hypercoagulability.

The mortality in DIC associated with head injury is very high and may be due to intractable cerebral edema, intracerebral or intraventricular hemorrhage, multiple organ failure due to microthrombosis, or uncontrollable hemorrhage.

It is essential that appropriate coagulation studies be done early in the course of management of the head-injured patient. Therapy is directed primarily toward the underlying disease process. In the potentially salvageable patient, optimal correction of hemostatic defects after head injury may require administration of cryoprecipitate (fibrinogen, factor VIII), fresh frozen plasma (factor V), platelet concentrates, and fresh red cells. Such therapy is of doubtful validity in the deeply comatose patient with evidence of irreversible brain damage. Heparin therapy may produce dramatic effects within a few hours, raising fibrinogen levels to normal, shortening thrombin times, raising the plasminogen levels, and allowing resynthesis of consumed clotting factors. Heparin therapy may predispose the head-injured patient to intracranial hemorrhage. Caution should also be exercised in the use of aspirin and steroids in the immediate posttrauma period because of deleterious effects on platelet function[3,19,29] and possible precipitation or aggravation of gastrointestinal bleeding.[11]

ENDOCRINOLOGIC SEQUELAE
Anterior pituitary insufficiency

Anterior pituitary insufficiency following head trauma is reported approximately one dozen times in the literature and is certainly a rare clinical condition.[1,7,10,11,15] At autopsy, however, recognizable pituitary or hypothalamic damage following head trauma is common.[5] Crompton[3] reported a 42% incidence of anterior hypothalamic ischemia or hemorrhage in a series of 106 patients who died soon after closed head injury.

The pathogenesis of posttraumatic anterior pituitary insufficiency is not certain. Anterior lobe necrosis similar in extent and location to the infarcted area following section of the pituitary stalk in animals and humans has been observed in several autopsy series.[2,4,8] Pituitary infarction may be due to traumatic rupture of the stalk or interruption of the vascular supply at the time of head injury. Since interruption of the long hypophyseal portal veins may cause central anterior pituitary necrosis, Crompton[3] theorized that hypothalamic and stalk lesions were due to shearing of small portal vessels at the time of impact. Hypopituitarism may be secondary to vascular collapse in the head-injured patient with associated hemorrhagic shock[14] or to traumatic hemorrhage into the pituitary gland.[12] It is more likely to occur in the patient with a skull fracture, especially of the middle fossa, and is frequently accompanied by transient or permanent diabetes insipidus[5]; normal ADH function can be maintained after pituitary stalk section since ADH can be released from fibers ending in the median eminence.[9,13]

Dzur and Winternitz[5] reported anterior pituitary insufficiency in a patient who sustained massive facial trauma and exhibited transient diabetes insipidus. Decreased ACTH, growth hormone, and gonadotropin and elevated prolactin levels were observed. These findings are consistent with a lesion separating the hypothalamus functionally from the anterior lobe of the pituitary and the loss of hypothalamic inhibition leading to excessive prolactin secretion. Low or normal prolactin levels would be seen in conditions affecting the pituitary cells themselves since they are responsible for prolactin synthesis and release independent of the prolactin-inhibiting factor. Stimulation tests with synthetic thyrotropin releasing factor (TRF) may show subnormal thyroid-stimulating hormone (TSH) and supranormal prolactin release by the anterior pituitary compatible with pituitary rather than hypothalamic dysfunction. In the presence of hypothalamic dysfunction, TRF would be expected to promote a significant release of TSH from the pituitary.[6,11]

Anterior pituitary insufficiency should be considered in patients with basal skull fractures and/or posttraumatic diabetes insipidus who develop secondary amenorrhea, galactorrhea, regression of secondary sexual characteristics or in whom poor recovery, posttraumatic psychosis, or general malaise persists.[5] Appropriate replacement therapy is indicated when specific deficiencies are proven through endocrinologic testing. Prolactin levels may not drop after replacement therapy, since loss of hypothalamic inhibition may persist.

Posterior pituitary dysfunction

Diabetes insipidus (DI). Diabetes insipidus is a relatively common phenomenon after craniofacial trauma and basilar skull fracture[10,23] and can be permanent or transient, disappearing in a few days or weeks.

McLaurin[15] reports that 6% of all cases of diabetes insipidus are due to trauma. Hypoxic brain damage subsequent to cardiopulmonary arrest[25] and drug overdose[9] can cause DI. Hemorrhagic shock can predispose to necrosis of the posterior pituitary.[14,24] DI has occurred following fat embolization to the posterior pituitary.[11,26,28]

Antidiuretic hormone, vasopressin, is an octapeptide synthesized in the supraoptic nuclei of the anterior hypothalamus and transported along the neurohypophyseal pathway attached to a large carrier protein, neurophysine, to be stored in the posterior lobe of the pituitary. It is released in response to many stimuli, the most important being increased plasma osmolality, hypovolemia, pain, emotional stress, drugs (nicotine, barbiturates, morphine, carbamazepine (Tegretol), tricyclic antidepressants, chlorpropamide, vincristine), hormonal mediators (thyroxin, angiotensin, glucocorticoids), cholinergic and beta adrenergic stimulation, and positive airway pressure.[18,20,21,27,31] Head injury and acute intracranial hypertension can stimulate ADH production and release.[3,8] ADH secretion is inhibited by increased plasma volume, reduced plasma osmolality, alpha adrenergic stimulation, and by several drugs—ethanol, atropine, phenytoin, reserpine, and chlorpromazine.[7,13,20]

In the kidney, ADH attaches to the contraluminal side of the renal medullary tubular cell by means of a specific vasopressin receptor. It then activates renal medullary adenyl cyclase, which in turn stimulates production of cyclic AMP (cyclic adenosine monophosphate). Cyclic AMP activates a protein, kinase, on the luminal side of the cell, causing phosphorylation of membrane protein leading to increased permeability of the cell to water, facilitating its transport into the intercellular spaces, into the renal medullary circulation, and back into the general circulation.[12,20,22] Adrenocortical insufficiency in humans is associated with a subnormal diuretic response to hydration and plasma hypo-osmolality and sustained elevation of plasma ADH. Steroid replacement therapy lowers plasma ADH to normal and permits the normal diuretic response to hydration. Perhaps glucocorticoids inhibit the secretory activity of the supraoptic neurons.[1,29]

Clinical manifestations of ADH deficiency include polyuria (greater than 2 to 3 l/day), polydipsia, hypernatremia, high serum osmolality (320 to 330 mosmol/kg), dilute urine, and ratio of urine to serum osmolality of less than 1. The differential diagnosis of polyuria following trauma or surgery in the area of the pituitary and hypothalamus may be difficult due to a variety of causes. Solute diuresis may be the result of osmotic or loop diuretics, high urea levels, hyperglycemia, or inability to retain sodium due to mineralocorticoid deficiency. During solute diuresis urine specific gravity is between 1.009 and 1.035, urine osmolality is usually 250 to 320 mosmol/kg, the serum sodium is normal or slightly decreased, and thirst is not usually a complaint. Water and solute diuresis may be precipitated by too vigorous crystalloid therapy. During water diuresis the urine specific gravity is between 1.001 and 1.005, urine osmolality between 50 and 150 mosmol/kg, serum sodium is normal or increased, and thirst is usually a prominent feature.[30] The most commonly used diagnostic test is cautious fluid restriction with measurement of urine volume and osmolality.[17,20] A normal subject exposed to water deprivation can reduce urine flow to less than .5 ml/min and increase urine osmolality to greater than 800 mosmol/kg. Diagnosis can be confirmed by measurement of ADH levels in plasma and urine in relation to plasma osmolality. Response of the renal tubule can be tested by the administration of aqueous vasopressin intramuscularly or intravenously.[19,20,30]

Treatment in the recently traumatized or postsurgical patient cannot be long acting until the degree and duration of the disease process is apparent. Frequently, posttraumatic DI is transient; occasionally long-term therapy is necessary. Daily weights, careful intake and output, serum BUN, electrolytes, osmolality, urine specific gravity, and osmolality are essential in management. The patient's hourly urine output is replaced, plus the usual estimate for insensible loss with solutions containing water and little or no electrolytes. The administration of sodium-containing solutions is perhaps the commonest error in the management of diabetes insipidus. Saline solutions deliver a continuing solute load to the kidneys that aggravates the renal loss of water. Water intoxication (lethargy, confusion, seizures, and coma) can occur if excess vasopressin is administered.[2,30]

If the patient is awake and alert and able to take oral fluids, fluid balance can be maintained satisfactorily. If urinary output exceeds 250 ml/hr for two consecutive hours or 6 to 7 l/day, or the patient is unable to maintain fluid balance, aqueous vasopressin (5 to 10 international units IM or IV q 4 to 6 hours) is administered. When stable, vasopressin tannate-in-oil (5 international units IM every 24 to 72 hours) may be used.

Additional hormonal therapies include lysine vasopressin nasal spray and DDAVP (1-deamino-8-D-arginine vasopressin). Lysine vasopressin nasal spray is a synthetic preparation and less likely to cause allergic reactions. It is supplied in 5 ml bottles containing 50 international units per milliliter and can be administered by nasal instillation three to four times a day. Each spray delivers two international units. DDAVP is supplied in 2.5 ml bottles with 100 μg/ml; the usual dose is 10 to 20 μg intranasally every 12 to 24 hours.

Nonhormonal treatment methods include chlorpropamide and thiazide diuretics. Chlorpropamide, an oral hypoglycemic agent, is effective in reducing polyuria in hypothalamic but not nephrogenic diabetes insipidus. The drug is given in doses ranging from 50 to 250 mg/day. Chlorpropamide appears to act by potentiating the antidiuretic effect of low levels of endogenous ADH and is therefore most effective in mild cases.[4,16,32] Thiazide diuretics contract the extracellular fluid volume secondary to sodium loss and therefore reduce urine volume and raise urine osmolality by an indirect effect. The antidiuresis is enhanced by low sodium intake and diminished by a high sodium intake.

Supplemental potassium is usually required.[5,6]

Syndrome of inappropriate antidiuretic hormone secretion (SIADH). Schwartz[23] has described hyponatremia and renal salt-wasting unrelated to renal or adrenal disease in a variety of clinical conditions. The typical features of the inappropriate ADH syndrome are hyponatremia with corresponding hypo-osmolality of the serum and extracellular fluid, continued renal excretion of sodium, absence of clinical evidence of volume depletion (normal skin turgor and blood pressure), urine osmolality greater than serum osmolality, normal renal and adrenal function. The excessive water retention and renal sodium loss result in hypo-osmolality of the extracellular fluid and lead to the picture of water intoxication. Symptoms include anorexia, nausea, vomiting, irritability, personality changes, neurologic abnormalities (loss of reflexes, muscular weakness, bulbar or pseudobulbar palsy, positive Babinski sign, stupor, convulsions). The renal salt-wasting mechanism is obscure but is probably related to suppression of proximal tubular reabsorption of sodium in response to the expansion of extracellular fluid volume.[3] Aldosterone levels in patients with SIADH are in the normal range.[16,24]

Many CNS conditions including meningitis,[18] encephalitis,[22] head injury,* brain abscess,[18] tumor,[5,12] Guillain-Barré syndrome,[6] acute intermittent porphyria,[3,14,20] and subarachnoid hemorrhage[15] have been associated with inappropriate ADH secretion, previously known as "cerebral salt-wasting."

Anesthesia and surgery can cause elevations in blood ADH levels secondary to pain, stress, and various drugs.[8,19] In neurosurgical patients all the cardinal features of SIADH can be produced by the administration of vasopressin in water during the overvigorous therapy of diabetes insipidus.[17,23] Other hyponatremic syndromes may be differentiated primarily on clinical grounds. True sodium-depletion hyponatremia is accompanied by evidence of a contracted blood volume (low

blood pressure, decreased skin turgor, elevated hematocrit). In dilutional hyponatremia, edema is a prominent feature and there may be evidence of congestive heart failure or hepatic disease.[13]

In a prospective study of 15 patients with facial bone fractures and associated cerebral injury, three had unequivocal SIADH. Inappropriate ADH secretion following head trauma probably results from overproduction or release of ADH in response to irritation of the hypothalamic-pituitary axis; limbic structures may facilitate or fail to inhibit ADH release.[4] Increased ADH secretion may be enhanced by stimulation of the intrathoracic volume receptors when patients are nursed in the head-up position. The head-up position may exacerbate SIADH if it is present; fluid restriction, common in the head-injured patient, may prevent the full-blown syndrome.[2]

The syndrome of inappropriate ADH secretion usually begins 3 to 15 days post trauma and with appropriate therapy lasts no more than 10 to 15 days. Treatment includes, most importantly, water restriction, with or without hypertonic saline. In patients whose serum sodium is less than 110 meq/l, 5% saline containing 855 meq of sodium per liter, or 3% saline containing 513 meq/l can be used. Caution must be exercised in patients with heart disease, hypertension, or intracranial bleeding, and in the elderly. Phenytoin may be needed for control of seizures, and it has the desirable side effect of inhibiting ADH release in some patients with SIADH, although routine oral or intramuscular administration has no significant clinical effect.[10]

Fichman[11] measured elevated ADH levels in 25 nonedematous patients on long-term thiazide therapy. These patients resemble those with inappropriate ADH syndrome except that the low serum sodium is usually accompanied by hypokalemia and alkalosis. The potassium depletion of long-term diuretic therapy facilitates entry of sodium into cells, producing further extracellular fluid volume contraction; this may enhance a volume receptor–mediated release of vaso-

---

*References 4, 5, 10, 16, 21, 24.

pressin with resultant water retention and hyponatremia.

Hyponatremia can occur after prolonged mannitol diuresis if sodium losses are not replaced, but in these patients total osmolality is increased and circulatory volume is reduced.

Although glucocorticoid therapy reduces ADH secretion and promotes renal free water clearance,[1,7] dexamethasone has no significant effect on salt and water balance in SIADH.[9]

Metabolic sequelae

Water and electrolyte balance. The majority of head-injured patients have no clinically detectable abnormalities of water and electrolyte balance. Sodium retention is a normal response to bodily injury. Following head injury, sodium retention is related to the severity of injury, lasts two to four days, and appears to be related to aldosterone secretion and to hypothalamic stimulation and subsequent ACTH release. There is no relationship between the severity of sodium retention and the location of brain damage. Major trauma may lead to a mild degree of ADH-mediated water retention lasting two or three days. Prolonged retention is rare but does occur if inappropriate ADH secretion ensues. Despite sodium retention, head-injured patients may be mildly hyponatremic because of the concomitant water retention.[23] Negative water balance may be the result of diabetes insipidus. Fluid restriction, abnormal thirst mechanisms, high protein hyperalimentation or tube feedings,[11] and prolonged osmotic diuresis reduce circulating volume and stimulate aldosterone-mediated salt retention. The hypertonicity promotes vasopressin-mediated water retention.[31]

Glucose metabolism. Glucose intolerance is a common phenomenon after trauma.[17,22,31,39] High catecholamine levels diminish insulin release.[17,22] ACTH, serum cortisol, and growth hormone levels may be elevated post trauma.[16,23] Exogenously administered steroids are diabetogenic.[3] Serum immunoreactive insulin levels may be ele-

vated but to levels lower than expected in relation to blood sugar elevations. Catecholamines and growth hormone oppose insulin release and cellular activity.[23] Steroids promote glyconeogenesis, increasing hepatic glucose production; they may also stimulate pancreatic beta cell function with ensuing exhaustion and degranulation of these cells, and peripheral glucose utilization is impaired through an unknown mechanism.[19] Severe diabetes develops only in a few patients receiving steroids, and only with reduced insulin reserve (as in the adult-onset diabetic) is the diabetogenic action of steroids extreme.[1] Latent diabetes mellitus may be precipitated by trauma and may be detrimental to the patient's recovery if unrecognized.[23]

Cerebrospinal fluid metabolic changes. Cerebrospinal fluid acid-base status more closely reflects brain interstitial fluid acid-base status than does either arterial or venous blood values.[23] Brain injury results in cerebrospinal fluid lactic acidosis with low pH and bicarbonate concentration and systemic respiratory alkalosis.[15,23,40] The severity of CSF metabolic acidosis is related to the severity of the head injury and seems to be dependent on the amount of lactic acid produced by the injured and hypoxic brain tissue.[22] Persistently elevated CSF lactate would suggest continued cerebral ischemia and hypoxia.[23] Marked intracranial hypertension, causing a reduction in cerebral blood flow, is accompanied by long lasting but reversible cerebral tissue lactic acidosis. The acidosis may explain the reactive hyperemia commonly seen in experimental models when blood flow is restored following a period of intracranial hypertension.[18,40]

A low CSF pH promotes spontaneous hyperventilation; lowering CSF CO_2 restores the normal 20:1 ratio of bicarbonate to carbon dioxide and returns CSF pH toward normal levels.[6]

Serotonin levels in cerebrospinal fluid rise following head trauma; the higher the levels, the more severe the trauma.[34] CSF cyclic AMP levels were lowest in patients in the deepest grades of coma following head injury or spontaneous intracranial hemorrhage.[28] Other reports indicate that acute brain injury can cause a temporary increase in brain and spinal fluid cyclic AMP.[35,36] The subnormal levels in comatose patients may reflect a depletion of brain cyclic AMP uniquely associated with prolonged coma after trauma or intracranial hemorrhage.[28]

Nonketotic hyperosmolar hyperglycemic coma (NHHC)

Nonketotic hyperosmolar hyperglycemic coma (NHHC) has been observed as a complication of many primary illnesses both in diabetic and nondiabetic patients.[1,21,29] Park and co-workers[24] report a 10% incidence of this condition in seriously ill patients who died while in a neurosurgical intensive care unit over a three-year period. The patients had various neurosurgical conditions (transsphenoidal hypophysectomy for metastatic breast cancer, intracerebral hemorrhage, ischemic infarction, closed and penetrating head injury, brain tumor), and many had no previous history of diabetes mellitus.

Diagnostic criteria for NHHC are listed in the box below. Blood sugars may range from 400 to 2760 mg/100 ml, sodium from 119 to 188 meq/l, and plasma osmolality from 268 to 465 mosmol/kg; there may be severe potassium depletion and dehydration due to the osmotic diuresis. These patients may also exhibit leukocytosis, hemoconcentration, and azotemia with a BUN-to-creatinine ratio of 30:1 implying a prerenal extracellular fluid deficit; acute renal failure may develop.[21]

This condition has a 40% to 70% mortality rate. The average age of patients is 57 years. Two thirds of the patients have no previous history of diabetes mellitus; 50% have some precipitating event such as infection, dehydration due to increased losses or inadequate replacement, or ingestion of drugs known to aggravate glucose homeostasis (thiazides,[5] steroids,[4,32,38] phenytoin,[13,25] and glycerol[30]). Many patients are febrile, in shock and in coma, with or without focal neurologic signs.[20] Coma and subsequent death are usually attributed to total body sodium depletion or to cellular dehydration, particularly in the brain,[27] although this may not be apparent at autopsy.[26] Patients with a normal level of consciousness have a considerably higher survival rate, less severe associated illness, and smaller requirements for insulin and fluid replacement.[21] Because serum glucose levels are not paralleled by high levels of glucose in brain and spinal fluid, an osmotic shift of free water into the intravascular space may occur, leading to severe intracellular dehydration of the brain and resultant coma.[7,27]

In the neurosurgical patient many predisposing factors to NHHC are present: steroids,[4,32] prolonged mannitol therapy,[2,10,12] hyperosmolar tube feedings,[11,37] phenytoin,[13,25] and limited water replacement. Whether hypothalamic damage predisposes to this condition is unknown. In Park's series,[24] autopsies on many of the patients did not show evidence of cerebral edema, transtentorial herniation, or brain stem damage, which implies that the central nervous system lesions present were compatible with survival except for the presence of NHHC. The causes of death in these patients were renal failure, arrhythmias, cerebrovascular accidents, and systemic thromboembolic complications.[21,24]

The pathogenesis of NHHC is not clear, particularly in those patients without a history of diabetes mellitus and who require no insulin therapy following resolution of NHHC. The absence of ketosis may reflect the antiketogenic effects of severe hyperglycemia or may reflect the effect of insulin on fat and carbohydrate metabolism. At very low plasma insulin concentrations (reported in patients with NHHC and maturity-onset

---

DIAGNOSTIC CRITERIA FOR NHHC

Hyperglycemia
Glucosuria
Absence of ketosis
Posmol > 330 mosmol/kg
Dehydration
CNS dysfunction

diabetes mellitus), insulin has no effect on glucose uptake by cells, yet still can inhibit release of free fatty acids from adipose tissue.[19,21]

Steroids have long been recognized for their diabetogenic potential secondary to increased hepatic glucose production, exhaustion of pancreatic beta cells, and decreased peripheral glucose utilization.[19] The diabetogenic action of steroids is extreme only when there is a reduced insulin reserve as in the maturity-onset diabetic or in a patient with NHHC.[3,14] Hyperosmolar tube feedings may precipitate hypernatremia and hyperglycemia secondary to extracellular water deficits from osmotic diuresis or diarrhea. Thirst mechanisms are absent in the comatose patient leading to difficulty or inattention to the state of hydration. Mannitol therapy in patients with acute renal failure or hepatic disease can lead to hyperosmolar states associated with increased or decreased serum sodium concentrations. Toxic serum phenytoin levels result in delayed and subnormal insulin response to a glucose load; hyperglycemia following phenytoin therapy has been observed in the critically ill diabetic and nondiabetic patient. Phenytoin has been shown to decrease tissue uptake of glucose and to increase glycogenolysis in the liver.[13]

Prior to therapy, appropriate laboratory data must be obtained. Serum sodium may be high, low, or normal, depending on the state of hydration. Urine sodium may be in the range of 10 to 50 meq/l. Serum potassium is usually low due to the combined effects of the release of aldosterone stimulated by low extracellular fluid volume and to the continued delivery of sodium to the distal tubule sodium-potassium exchange site as a result of the glucose diuresis. If lactic acidosis is also present, hydrogen ion may enter cells in exchange for potassium and result in elevated serum potassium in spite of total body depletion. When blood glucose rises above the renal threshold, glucose will appear in the urine and prevent maximal urine concentration even in the presence of ADH. Serum osmolality must be high to make the diagnosis of NHHC. Serum osmolality measured

in an osmometer (freezing point depression) may be elevated because of the osmotic contribution of urea, which is free to move across the semipermeable cell membrane and therefore does not exert effective osmotic pressure in vivo. Effective osmolality can be calculated using the formula:

$$\text{Posmol} = 2\,(\text{Na}^+) + \frac{\text{Glucose}}{18}$$

In an azotemic patient this will be significantly lower than the osmolality measured in an osmometer, the difference representing the osmotic contribution of urea.

Hypovolemia and hypertonicity are the immediate threats to life. Hypotonic saline may not improve sodium and water deficits fast enough, therefore normal saline is used, unless a patient is hypertensive or edematous, until blood pressure and urine output are stabilized. If a patient is in hypovolemic shock, isotonic sodium chloride or plasma may be necessary regardless of the osmolality. Large amounts of insulin in such a patient may precipitate hypotension and shock and subsequent renal failure because the drop in blood sugar may remove a significant percentage of the already inadequate plasma water.[9,33] Diuretics may be necessary if oliguria persists after sodium repletion. If plasma osmolality is normal or low in a hyperglycemic hyponatremic patient, there is excess water present; removal of the osmotic contribution of glucose by administering insulin or hypotonic saline may precipitate water intoxication.

Serial laboratory data are essential. Once sodium deficits are replaced and blood pressure and urine output are stable, water deficits can be replaced with 0.45% saline. The volume of hypotonic fluid varies in individual patients but is usually greater than 5 l in the first 12 hours and averages 500 to 1300 ml/hr until plasma osmolality reaches 325 mosmol/l. Severe potassium losses may also have occurred due to the osmotic diuresis.

Hyperglycemia will usually respond dramatically to relatively small doses of insulin. Large doses of insulin, with rapid lowering of serum glucose, may increase mortality by decreasing plasma volume before there has been adequate fluid and salt replacement, by producing cerebral edema or hypoglycemia. McCurdy recommends not exceeding 25 units of insulin per hour until sodium deficits have been replaced. When the effective plasma osmolality approaches 325 mosmol/l, decreased glucosuria permits renal mechanisms for salt and water homeostasis to finally restore osmolality and plasma volume to normal levels.[21]

Intermittent furosemide (Lasix) therapy for cerebral edema may obviate severe hyperosmolar stresses, particularly in the elderly, the adult-onset diabetic, or in the patient with compromised renal function.[8]

GASTROINTESTINAL SEQUELAE

The relationship between intracranial disease and gastrointestinal bleeding has been known for over 100 years.[38] Since Cushing's[11] paper on the coincidence of peptic ulceration and intracranial pathology, Cushing ulcer is the term usually applied to all gastroduodenal ulcers coexisting with brain disease. In patients dying from intracranial disorders, the incidence of gastroduodenal ulceration and hemorrhage post mortem is twice that of those dying from all other causes (12.5% versus 6%). Esophageal ulceration seems to be more common in the neurologic population, while duodenal ulceration is more common in the nonneurologic population. The frequency of gastric lesions in both groups is approximately the same. There is no correlation between the type of neurosurgical disorder (diffuse or discrete) or intracranial hypertension and gastroduodenal hemorrhage or ulceration.[26]

In 433 patients with head injury of differing severity, the overall incidence of clinically detectable gastrointestinal bleeding (blood in gastric juice, melena, endoscopy) was 17%. There was a correlation between the severity of injury and the frequency of GI bleeding. In comatose and decerebrate patients the incidence was 30%. In severely injured patients receiving glucocorticoid therapy the incidence was higher than in the less severely injured receiving steroid ther-

apy. The existence of shock did not seem to predispose to bleeding.[25]

Cushing[11] felt that a diencephalic parasympathetic center stimulated vagal nuclei, inducing vagal hyperactivity and subsequent acid hypersecretion. French and co-workers[16] were able to produce prompt and excessive elevation of gastric acid secretion by direct anterior hypothalamic stimulation. Anterior hypothalamic ablative lesions frequently resulted in gastric mucosal and submucosal hemorrhages. Presumably the sympathetic center in the posterior hypothalamus was then unopposed and the hemorrhagic changes resulted from this imbalance. Prior sympathectomy protected animals from the hemorrhagic changes. Posterior hypothalamic lesions increased vagal tone and pure gastric erosions occurred that could be prevented by vagotomy.

Gastric mucosal barrier disruption may play a role in the pathogenesis of such ulcers.[42] As a group, patients with neurosurgical disease have normal gastric mucosal permeability. However, general surgical and neurosurgical patients who develop upper gastrointestinal bleeding have a significantly increased permeability and a higher incidence of sepsis, hypotension, respiratory failure, renal insufficiency, and jaundice than either of the groups with normal permeability.[19,43] Aspirin and ethanol increase gastric mucosal permeability.[31] Ethanol in combination with aspirin and acid is especially harmful and frequently produces mucosal bleeding.[12] Steroids do not alter gastric mucosal permeability but may enhance the effect of other agents that do.[1,7]

Watts and Clark[49] have reported gastric hyperacidity in patients comatose from head injury. Bleeding occurred in five of seven hypersecretors who were decerebrate with signs and symptoms of lower diencephalon or upper brain stem injury. Hyperacidity has not been demonstrated in patients with postburn (Curling) or postsurgical ulcers.[19]

The role of steroids in the production of gastroduodenal ulcerations is controversial. ACTH and cortisone[30] reduce the rate of renewal of surface epithelial cells and mucous secretion[31] in the canine gastric antrum. Gray and associates[20,21,22] have shown that human gastric acid and pepsin secretion increase after the administration of ACTH, cortisone, and the physical stress of surgery. In Davis'[13] series it was noted that neurosurgical patients with a previous history of GI symptomatology experienced a reactivation of symptoms and frequently disastrous episodes of hematemesis following surgery. Steroid ulcers are primarily antral and can effectively be prevented by antacid therapy.[18,39] Examination of several prospective studies suggests that the frequency of peptic ulceration is not increased by steroid treatment.[9] In these studies, however, the spectrum of neurosurgical diseases is not represented.

Evidence suggests that stress ulcers are not due to circulating endogenous steroids. Ulcers following steroid therapy have a longer time course (4 to 10 days or longer) and tend to occur in the gastric antrum or duodenum as opposed to the fundus.[17,39] In addition, Goodman and Osborne[18] were able to produce the typical fundal stress ulcer in adrenalectamized pigs. Long-term high-dose cortisone acetate therapy does not alter gastric antral or duodenal resistance to digestion by an acid pepsin stream.[51]

Stress ulcer has been loosely used to refer to upper gastrointestinal lesions following major medical illnesses, surgery, trauma, severe burns, frost bite, neurosurgical procedures, and steroid therapy. Goodman has shown in humans and in pigs that ulcers following shock and sepsis are different clinically and pathologically from postburn, postneurosurgical, and steroid ulcers.[18]

Hemorrhagic shock is a specific and sufficient stress to lead to superficial, linear erosions of the gastric fundus,[4,23,27] primarily on the crests of the rugal folds. Most patients with these lesions eventually die from severe and persistent hemorrhage superimposed upon their already grave clinical conditions. Perhaps these lesions are secondary to mucosal ischemia as suggested by Virchow.[48] Hemorrhagic shock leads to elevated catecholamine levels. It is not clear whether hypovolemia alone or in combination with increased sympathetic tone is responsible for the observed severe reductions in mucosal blood flow. Klemperer[27] and Baronofsky[2] were able to produce arteriolar vasospasm and gastric ulceration following adrenalin administration. Vasoconstriction and resultant ischemia are regularly followed by mucosal hemorrhage and ulceration. It is possible that ulceration could result from hypercoagulable, hyperviscous, or hypoxic[36] states associated with various disease processes. The hypovolemia, hemoconcentration, high peripheral resistance and reduced cardiac output in the immediate postburn period seem to predispose to decreased organ flow and may lead to gastric mucosal ischemia.[15,35,37]

The neurogenic ulcer tends to perforate due to esophagogastric malacia, whereas acute postshock ulcers rarely perforate.[11,18,46] Postburn ulcers are primarily located at the depths of the rugal folds of the gastric fundus and the duodenum.[18] They are round and deep with well-defined margins and may show bacterial colonies at their base.[35,37]

Goodman and Osborne[18] suggest a reclassification of stress ulcers: ulcers following head trauma and intracranial operations as neurogenic ulcers; postburn ulcers as Curling ulcers; ulcers following long-term steroid therapy as steroid ulcers; posttraumatic and postsurgical ulcers associated with shock and sepsis as stress ulcers.

Other sources of gastric irritation may be present in head-injured patients. Ethanol ingestion can produce hemorrhagic gastritis. Aspirin and phenylbutazone[30] cause shedding of gastric surface mucosal cells without a concomitant increase in the rate of cell renewal. They reduce antral mucous secretion, as do ACTH and cortisone.[14,31-33] Ethanol and aspirin increase gastric mucosal permeability.[44] Aspirin and phenylbutazone depress platelet aggregation[45,52,53] and may oppose prostaglandin regulation of gastric acid secretion.[47] Positive end-expiratory pressure and passive hyperventilation may lead to increased splanchnic vascular resistance and subsequent gastric mucosal ischemia.[24]

Signs and symptoms of gastrointestinal ulceration and/or perforation may include pain, abdominal distention, ileus, anemia, hypotension, hematemesis, and melena, depending on the level of consciousness of the patient. Steroid-induced bleeding into the GI tract may be painless. Antacid therapy administered orally or via nasogastric tube may be of value in preventing and treating postneurosurgical and steroid ulcers.[17] Anticholinergic drugs reduce acid secretion in comatose patients.[34,50] Maintaining gastric pH above 5 may be effective in reducing the need for surgical control of bleeding; however double-blind series are lacking.[40]

Bleeding is usually self-limiting and requires nasogastric suction (perhaps cold saline lavage), fluid replacement, and transfusion. When operative treatment is necessary for protracted hemorrhage, partial gastrectomy and vagotomy may be more effective operative treatment than vagotomy and pyloroplasty.[37,41]

Histamine appears to be the major, if not the only, stimulator of parietal cell hydrogen ion secretion.[8] The final common pathway appears to be an H_2 receptor at the base of the parietal cell.[3,5] H_2 receptor blockers (Metiamide, Cimetidine) inhibit all forms of gastric secretion. Clinical trials are not available; however this approach may prove to be effective in prophylaxis and therapy of a variety of stress ulcer syndromes.[28,29]

H_2 receptor blocking drugs can produce agranulocytosis.[10] Cimetidine treatment has been shown to stimulate prolactin secretion in humans but to have no effect on thyrotropin, growth hormone, or thyroxine levels. Perhaps histamine has an important function in the regulation of prolactin secretion in humans.[6]

SKELETAL SEQUELAE
Cervical spine injuries

Ten percent of patients with head injury have an associated cervical spine injury. Seven percent of motor vehicle accident victims have neck and cervical spine injuries.[2] Fifty percent of patients with cervical spine injury have concurrent evidence of head trauma.[8]

Failure to diagnose a cervical spine fracture may lead to serious medical and legal complications, particularly if subsequent neurologic deficit develops or progresses.[6,7] Head-injured patients should be considered to have cervical spine injury until proven otherwise.[5,7] Tenderness or crepitus of the spinous processes of the cervical vertebrae may point to the diagnosis. Hyperextension of the neck during laryngoscopy and endotracheal intubation may displace an unstable fracture leading to spinal cord compression. All diagnostic and therapeutic maneuvers must be done extremely cautiously until the stability of the cervical spine is established.[9]

High spinal cord transection (above C3) is most frequently incompatible with life due to the absence of diaphragmatic and intercostal muscle function and to subsequent hypoventilation and secondary infection.[1,3] Survival is possible with vigorous therapy and rehabilitation.

The absence of sympathetic tone leads to hypotension, bradycardia, (cardiac output may be high, low, or normal), and an increase in alveolar dead space due to a reduction in pulmonary perfusion. Mechanical ventilation may be indicated in the face of ventilation-perfusion abnormalities (atelectasis secondary to hypoventilation, infection, shock lung) and hypercarbia (increased alveolar dead space without compensation). Continuous positive pressure breathing may have severe negative effects on cardiac output by reducing venous return in a patient unable to increase venous tone.

Volume replacement, adequate hemoglobin levels, adjustment of minute volume, and positive end-expiratory pressure levels must be combined to achieve maximum acceptable cardiopulmonary function in the individual circumstance. Weaning of such patients must be individualized, although the usual criteria apply—vital capacity at least

10 ml/kg (or twice normal tidal volume), maximum inspiratory force at least -20 to -30 cm H_2O, dead space to tidal volume ratio less than 0.6, $A - aDo_2$ less than 300 to 350 torr, cardiovascular stability, and normal metabolic state.

Maxillofacial injuries

Blunt cervical trauma can lead to carotid artery injury. Compression or stretching of the vessel may lead to thrombosis, transient ischemic attacks, Horner syndrome, or lateral neck hematoma and airway obstruction. Mortality is 40%.[4]

Horner syndrome may develop following neck trauma due to pressure or direct injury to the sympathetic supply of the face. Unilateral pupillary constriction that results may lead to confusion and overtreatment of a suspected intracranial mass. A combination of relative miosis, slight ptosis (narrowing of the palpebral fissure), slight enophthalmus, increase in temperature and sweating on the affected side of the face, and preservation of normal reflexes to light and convergence should lead to the diagnosis.[10] For further discussion of the effects of trauma to the orbit and cranial nerves and their influence on pupillary findings, the reader is referred to standard neurology and neurosurgical texts.

Subcutaneous emphysema may result from frontal or ethmoid sinus fractures and has to be distinguished from that due to thoracic injury. Cribriform plate fractures may allow a nasogastric tube to enter the intracranial space.[11] In such circumstances, these tubes must be placed under direct vision through the mouth; gastrostomy may be indicated.

SUMMARY

Head injury cannot be considered an isolated, single-system injury. Head-injured patients frequently sustain other organ trauma. Equally important are the multisystem effects of trauma to any part of the body and the unique effects of head trauma on the hypothalamic-pituitary axis, which influences such diverse pansystemic functions as blood coagulation, pulmonary venular tone, gastric acid secretion, renal water conservation, and glucose metabolism.

Management of most head injuries is nonsurgical, and functional survival obviously depends on attention to these multisystem derangements.

REFERENCES

1. Adams, R. W., Gronert, G. A., Sundt, T. M., and Michenfelder, J. D.: Halothane, hypocapnia, and cerebrospinal fluid pressure in neurosurgery, Anesthesiology **37**:510-517, 1972.
2. Becker, D. P., Miller, J. D., Ward, J. D., and others: The outcome from severe head injury with early diagnosis and intensive management, J. Neurosurg. **47**:491-502, 1977.
3. Braunstein, P. W.: Medical aspects of automotive crash injury research, J.A.M.A. **163**:249-255, 1957.
4. Coleman, D. J., and Buckell, M.: The effect of urea and mannitol infusions on circulatory volume, Anaesthesia **19**:507-510, 1964.
5. Cucchiara, R. F., Theye, R. A., and Michenfelder, J. D.: The effects of isoflurane on canine cerebral metabolism and blood flow, Anesthesiology **40**:571-574, 1974.
6. Flamm, E. S., Demopoulos, H. B., Seligman, M. L., and others: Ethanol potentiation of central nervous system trauma, J. Neurosurg. **46**:328-335, 1977.
7. Galbraith, S. L.: Misdiagnosis and delayed diagnosis in traumatic intracranial hematoma, Br. Med. J. **1**:1438-1439, 1976.
8. Gardner, A. E., Dannemiller, F. J., and Dean, D.: Intracranial cerebrospinal fluid pressure in man during ketamine anesthesia, Anesth. Analg. **51**:741-745, 1972.
9. Gibbs, J. M.: The effect of intravenous ketamine on cerebrospinal fluid pressure, Br. J. Anaesth. **44**:1298-1301, 1972.
10. Henriksen, H. T., and Jorgensen, P. B.: The effect of nitrous oxide on intracranial pressure in patients with intracranial disorders, Br. J. Anaesth. **45**:486-491, 1973.
11. Horton, J. M.: The anaesthetist's contribution to the care of head injuries, Br. J. Anaesth. **48**:767-771, 1976.
12. Jennett, W. B., McDowall, D. G., and Barker, J.: The effect of halothane on intracranial pressure in cerebral tumors, J. Neurosurg. **26**:270-274, 1967.
13. Jennett, W. B., Barker, J., Fitch, W., and McDowall, D. G.: Effect of anaesthesia on intracranial pressure in patients with space-occupying lesions, Lancet **1**:61-64, 1969.
14. Jennett, B.: Some medicolegal aspects of the management of acute head injury, Br. Med. J. **1**:1383-1385, 1976.
15. Jennett, B., Teasdale, G., Braakman, R., and

others: Predicting outcome in individual patients after severe head injury, Lancet **1:**1031-1034, 1976.

16. Jennett, B.: Early complications after mild head injuries, N.Z. Med. J. **84:**144-147, 1976.

17. Johnston, I. H., Johnston, J. A., and Jennett, B.: Intracranial-pressure changes following head injury, Lancet **2:**433-436, 1970.

18. Leech, P., Barker, J., and Fitch, W.: Changes in intracranial pressure and systemic arterial pressure during the termination of anaesthesia, Br. J. Anaesth. **46:**315-316, 1974.

19. Lewin, W.: Changing attitudes to the management of severe head injuries, Br. Med. J. **2:**1234-1239, 1976.

20. McDowall, D. G., Barker, J., and Jennett, W. B.: Cerebro-spinal fluid pressure measurements during anaesthesia, Anaesthesia **21:**189-201, 1966.

21. Michenfelder, J. D., and Cucchiara, R. F.: Canine cerebral oxygen consumption during enflurane anesthesia and its modification during induced seizures, Anesthesiology **40:**575-580, 1974.

22. Misfeldt, B. B., Jorgensen, P. B., and Rishoj, M.: The effect of nitrous oxide and halothane upon the intracranial pressure in hypocapnic patients with intracranial disorders, Br. J. Anaesth. **46:**853-858, 1974.

23. Pagni, C. A.: The prognosis of head injured patients in a state of coma with decerebrated posture, J. Neurol. Sci. **17:**289-295, 1973.

24. Patel, A. R., Jennett, B., and Galbraith, S.: Alcohol and head injury, Lancet **1:**1369-1370, 1977.

25. Pazzaglia, P., Frank, G., Frank, F., and others: Clinical course and prognosis of acute post-traumatic coma, J. Neurol. Neurosurg. Psychiatr. **38:**149-154, 1975.

26. Reilly, P. L., Adams, J. H., Graham, D. I., and Jennett, B.: Patients with head injury who talk and die, Lancet **2:**375-377, 1975.

27. Rose, J., Valtonen, S., and Jennett, B.: Avoidable factors contributing to death after head injury, Br. Med. J. **2:**615-618, 1977.

28. Rossanda, M., Selenati, A., Villa, C., and others: Role of automatic ventilation in treatment of severe head injuries, J. Neurol. Sci. **17:**265-270, 1973.

29. Shapiro, H. M., Galindo, A., Wyte, S. R., and Harris, A. B.: Acute intracranial hypertension during anesthetic induction, Eur. J. Neurol. **8:**118-121, 1972.

30. Shapiro, H. M., Wyte, S. R., Harris, A. B., and Galindo, A.: Acute intraoperative intracranial hypertension in neurosurgical patients: mechanical and pharmacologic factors, Anesthesiology **37:**399-405, 1972.

31. Smith, A. L., Neigh, J. L., Hoffman, J. C., and others: Effects of general anesthesia on autoregulation of cerebral blood flow in man, J. Appl. Physiol. **29:**665-669, 1970.

32. Smith, A. L., and Wollman, H.: Cerebral blood flow and metabolism: effect of anesthetic drugs and techniques, Anesthesiology **36:**378-400, 1972.

33. Smith, A. L.: Barbiturate protection in cerebral hypoxia, Anesthesiology **47:**285-293, 1977.

34. Sondergard, W.: Intracranial pressure during general anesthesia, Dan. Med. Bull. **8:**18-25, 1961.

35. Tarlov, E.: Optimal management of head inuries, Int. Anesthesiol. Clin. **14:**69-94, 1976.

36. Trowbridge, A., and Giesecke, A. H.: Multiple injuries, Clin. Anesth. **11:**79-84, 1976.

Cardiopulmonary sequelae

1. Abrams, J. S., Deane, R. S., and Davis, J. H.: Pulmonary function in patients with multiple trauma and associated severe head injury, J. Trauma **16:**543-549, 1976.

2. Aidinis, S. J., Lafferty, J., and Shapiro, H. M.: Intracranial responses to PEEP, Anesthesiology **45:**275-286, 1976.

3. Allardyce, B., Hamit, H. F., Matsumoto, T., and Moseley, R. V.: Pulmonary vascular changes in hypovolemic shock: radiography of the pulmonary microcirculation and the possible role of platelet embolism in increasing vascular resistance, J. Trauma **9:**403-411, 1969.

4. Apuzzo, M. L. J., Weiss, M. H., Petersons, V., and others: Effect of positive end expiratory pressure ventilation on intracranial pressure in man, J. Neurosurg. **46:**227-232, 1977.

5. Ashbaugh, D. G., Bigelow, D. B., Petty, T. L., and Levine, B. E.: Acute respiratory distress in adults, Lancet **2:**319-323, 1967.

6. Ashbaugh, D. G., and Petty, T. L.: Positive end-expiratory pressure: Physiology, indications and contraindications, J. Thorac. Cardiovasc. Surg. **65:**165-170, 1973.

7. Aviado, D. M., Ling, J. S., and Schmidt, C. F.: Effects of anoxia on pulmonary circulation: reflex pulmonary vasoconstriction, Am. J. Physiol. **189:**253-262, 1957.

8. Aviado, D. M.: Adenosine diphosphate and vasoactive substances, J. Trauma **8:**880-890, 1968.

9. Beck, G. P., and Neill, L. W.: Anesthesia for associated trauma in patients with head injuries, Anesth. Analg. **42:**687-695, 1963.

10. Beckman, D. L., Bean, J. W., and Baslock, D. R.: Neurogenic influence in pulmonary compliance, J. Trauma **14:**111-115, 1974.

11. Blaisdell, F. W., Lim, R. C., and Stallone, R. J.: The mechanism of pulmonary damage following traumatic shock, Surg. Gynecol. Obstet. **130:**15-22, 1970.

12. Brueggemann, M. W., Loudon, R. G., and McLaurin, R. L.: Pulmonary compliance changes after experimental head injury, J. Trauma **16:**16-20, 1976.

13. Christensen, M. S.: Acid-base changes in cerebrospinal fluid and blood, and blood volume changes following prolonged hyperventilation in man, Br. J. Anaesth. **46:**348-357, 1974.

14. Clark, K.: The incidence and mechanisms of shock in head injury, South. Med. J. **55:**513-517, 1962.

15. Crighton, H. C., and Giesecke, A. H.: One year's experience in the anesthetic management of trauma, Anesth. Analg. **45**:835-842, 1966.

16. Denny-Brown, D., and Russell, W. R.: Experimental cerebral concussion, Brain **64**:93-164, 1941.

17. Déry, R., Pelletier, J., Jacques, A., and others: Alveolar collapse induced by denitrogenation, Can. Anaesth. Soc. J. **12**:531-544, 1965.

18. Downs, J. B., Klein, E. F., and Modell, J. H.: The effect of incremental PEEP on Pa_{O_2} in patients with respiratory failure, Anesth. Analg. **52**:210-215, 1973.

19. Dueck, R., Wagner, P. D., West, J. B.: Effects of positive end-expiratory pressure on gas exchange in dogs with normal and edematous lungs, Anesthesiology **47**:359-366, 1977.

20. Eckenhoff, J. E., Enderby, G. E. H., Larson, A., and others: Pulmonary gas exchange during deliberate hypotension, Br. J. Anaesth. **35**:750-758, 1963.

21. El-Naggar, M.: Weaning, Mid East J. Anaesth. **3**:401-406, 1972.

22. Feeley, T. W., and Hedley-Whyte, J.: Weaning from controlled ventilation and supplemental oxygen, N. Engl. J. Med. **292**:903-906, 1975.

23. Freeman, J., and Nunn, J. F.: Ventilation-perfusion relationships after haemorrhage, Clin. Sci. **24**:135-147, 1963.

24. Froman, C.: Alterations of respiratory function in patients with severe head injuries, Br. J. Anaesth. **40**:354-360, 1968.

25. Frost, E. A. M.: Effects of positive end-expiratory pressure on intracranial pressure and compliance in brain-injured patients, J. Neurosurg. **47**:195-200, 1977.

26. Fulton, R. L., and Jones, C. E.: The cause of post-traumatic pulmonary insufficiency in man, Surg. Gynecol. Obstet. **140**:179-186, 1975.

27. Geiger, J. P., and Gielchinsky, I.: Acute pulmonary insufficiency, Arch. Surg. **102**:400-405, 1971.

28. Gibbs, J. M.: The effect of intravenous ketamine on cerebrospinal fluid pressure, Br. J. Anaesth. **44**:1298-1301, 1972.

29. Harken, A. H., Brennan, M. F., Smith, B., and Barsamian, E. M.: The hemodynamic response to positive end-expiratory ventilation in hypovolemic patients, Surgery **76**:786-793, 1974.

30. Hedley-Whyte, J., Burgess, G. E., Feeley, T. W., and Miller, M. G.: Applied physiology of respiratory care, Boston, 1976, Little Brown & Co., p. 57.

31. Hill, J. D., O'Brien, T. G., Murray, J. J., and others: Prolonged extracorporeal oxygenation for acute post-traumatic respiratory failure (shock-lung syndrome), N. Engl. J. Med. **286**:629-634, 1972.

32. Hodgkin, J. E., Bowser, M. A., and Burton, G. G.: Respirator weaning, Crit. Care Med. **2**:96-102, 1974.

33. Huang, C. T., Cook, A. W., and Lyons, H. A.: Severe craniocerebral trauma and respiratory abnormalities, Arch. Neurol. **9**:545-554, 1963.

34. Illingworth, G., and Jennett, W. B.: The shocked head injury, Lancet **2**:511-514, 1965.

35. Jennett, W. B., Barker, J., Fitch, W., and McDowall, D. G.: Effect of anaesthesia on intracranial pressure in patients with space-occupying lesions, Lancet **1**:61-64, 1969.

36. Kanarek, D. J., and Shannon, D. C.: Adverse effect of positive end-expiratory pressure on pulmonary perfusion and arterial oxygenation, Am. Rev. Resp. Dis. **112**:457-459, 1975.

37. Katsurada, K., Sugimoto, T., and Onji, Y.: Significance of cerebrospinal fluid bicarbonate ions in the management of patients with cerebral injury, J. Trauma **9**:799-805, 1969.

38. Katsurada, K., Yamada, R., and Sugimoto, T.: Respiratory insufficiency in patients with severe head injury, Surgery **73**:191-199, 1973.

39. Kim, S. I., and Shoemaker, W. C.: Development of pulmonary hemodynamic and functional changes after operative and accidental trauma, Surg. Gynecol. Obstet. **133**:617-620, 1971.

40. Laver, M. B., and Lowenstein, E.: Lung function following trauma in man, Clin. Neurosurg. **19**:133-174, 1972.

41. Lecky, J. H., and Ominsky, A. J.: Postoperative respiratory management, Chest **62** (suppl.):50S-57S, 1972.

42. Leech, P., Barker, J., and Fitch, W.: Changes in intracranial pressure and systemic arterial pressure during the termination of anaesthesia, Br. J. Anaesth. **46**:315-316, 1974.

43. Lofgren, J.: Airway pressure—neurosurgical aspects, Anesthesiology **45**:269-272, 1976.

44. Magnaes, B.: Body position and cerebrospinal fluid pressure. I. Clinical studies on the effect of rapid postural changes, J. Neurosurg. **44**:687-697, 1976.

45. Markello, R., Schuder, R., and Border, J.: Arterial-alveolar N_2 differences documenting ventilation-perfusion mismatching following trauma, J. Trauma **14**:423-426, 1974.

46. Marshall, L. F., and Shapiro, H. M.: Barbiturate control of intracranial hypertension in head injury and other conditions: iatrogenic coma, Acta Neurol. Scand. (suppl.) **56**:156-157, 1977.

47. McAslan, T. C., Matjasko-Chiu, J., Turney, S. Z., and Cowley, R. A.: Influence of inhalation of 100% oxygen on intrapulmonary shunt in severely traumatized patients, J. Trauma **13**:811-821, 1973.

48. McAslan, T. C., Turney, S., Paul, R., and Polanco, O.: The effect of stepwise increase in airway pressure on ventricular fluid pressure in humans with severe head injury. Presented at Annual American Society of Anesthesiologists Meeting, San Francisco, Oct., 1976.

49. McIntyre, R. W., Laws, A. K., and Ramachandran, P. R.: Positive expiratory pressure plateau; improved gas exchange during mechanical ventilation, Can. Anaesth. Soc. J. **16**:477-486, 1969.

50. McLaurin, R. L., and King, L. R.: Recognition and

treatment of metabolic disorders after head injuries, Clin. Neurosurg. **19:**281-300, 1972.

51. Modell, J. H.: Ventilation/perfusion changes during mechanical ventilation, Dis. Chest **55:**447-451, 1969.
52. Monaco, V., Burdge, R., Newell, J., and others: Pulmonary venous admixture in injured patients, J. Trauma **12:**15-23, 1972.
53. Moseley, R. V., and Doty, D. B.: Hypoxemia during the first twelve hours after battle injury, Surgery **67:**765-772, 1970.
54. Murakami, T., Wax, S. D., and Webb, W. R.: Pulmonary microcirculation in hemorrhagic shock, Surg. Forum **21:**25-27, 1970.
55. Naeraa, N.: Blood-gas analyses in unconscious neurosurgical patients on admission to hospital, Acta Anaesthesiol. Scand. **7:**191-199, 1963.
56. North, J. B., and Jennett, S.: Abnormal breathing patterns associated with acute brain damage, Arch. Neurol. **31:**338-344, 1974.
57. Nunn, J. F., and Freeman, J.: Problems of oxygenation and oxygen transport during hemorrhage, Anaesthesia **19:**206-216, 1964.
58. Plum, F., and Swanson, A. G.: Central neurogenic hyperventilation in man, Arch. Neurol. Psychiatr. **81:**535-549, 1959.
59. Pontoppidan, H., Laver, M. B., and Geffin, B.: Acute respiratory failure in the surgical patient, Adv. Surg. **4:**163-254, 1970.
60. Powers, S. R., Burdge, R., Leather, R., and others: Studies of pulmonary insufficiency in non-thoracic trauma, J. Trauma **12:**1-14, 1972.
61. Powers, S. R., Mannal, R., Neclerio, M., and others: Physiologic consequences of positive end-expiratory pressure (PEEP) ventilation, Ann. Surg. **178:**265-272, 1973.
62. Ramachandran, P. R., and Fairley, H. B.: Changes in functional residual capacity during respiratory failure, Can. Anaesth. Soc. J. **17:**359-369, 1970.
63. Severinghaus, J. W., Mitchell, R. A., Richardson, B. W., and Singer, M. M.: Respiratory control at high altitude suggesting active transport regulation of CSF pH, J. Appl. Physiol. **18:**1155-1166, 1963.
64. Sinha, R. P., Ducker, T. B., and Perot, P.: Arterial oxygenation: findings and its significance in central nervous system trauma patients, J.A.M.A. **224:**1258-1260, 1973.
65. Skillman, J. J., Malhotra, I. V., Pallotta, J. A., and Bushnell, L. S.: Determinants of weaning from controlled ventilation, Surg. Forum **22:**198-200, 1971.
66. Smith, A. L.: Barbiturate protection in cerebral hypoxia, Anesthesiology **47:**285-293, 1977.
67. Staub, N. C.: The pathophysiology of pulmonary edema, Human Pathol. **1:**419-432, 1970.
68. Staub, N. C.: Pathogenesis of pulmonary edema, Am. Rev. Respir. Dis. **109:**358-372, 1974.
69. Sugg, W. L., Craver, W. D., Webb, W. R., and others: Pressure changes in the dog lung secondary to hemorrhagic shock: protective effect of pulmonary reimplantation, Ann. Surg. **169:**592-598, 1969.

70. Suter, P. M., Fairley, H. B., and Isenberg, M. D.: Optimum end-expiratory airway pressure in patients with acute pulmonary failure, N. Engl. J. Med. **292:**284-289, 1975.
71. Trowbridge, A., and Giesecke, A. H.: Multiple injuries, Clin. Anesth. **11:**79-84, 1976.
72. Uzawa, T., and Ashbaugh, D. G.: Continuous positive-pressure breathing in acute hemorrhagic pulmonary edema, J. Appl. Physiol. **26:**427-432, 1969.
73. Wagner, P. D., Laravuso, R. B., Uhl, R. R., and West, J. B.: Continuous distributions of ventilation-perfusion ratios in normal subjects breathing air and 100% O_2, J. Clin. Invest. **54:**54-68, 1974.
74. Webb, W. R.: Pulmonary complications of non-thoracic trauma: summary of the National Research Council Conference, J. Trauma **9:**700-711, 1969.
75. West, J. B.: New advances in pulmonary gas exchange, Anesth. Analg. **54:**409-418, 1975.
76. Zapol, W. M., and Snider, M. T.: Pulmonary hypertension in severe acute respiratory failure, N. Engl. J. Med. **296:**476-480, 1977.

Neurogenic pulmonary edema

1. Baker, A. B.: Poliomyelitis 16: A study of pulmonary edema, Neurology **7:**743-751, 1957.
2. Bean, J. W., and Beckman, D. L.: Centrogenic pulmonary pathology in mechanical head injury, J. Appl. Physiol. **27:**807-812, 1969.
3. Berman, I. R., and Ducker, T. B.: Pulmonary, somatic, and splanchnic circulatory responses to increased intracranial pressure, Ann. Surg. **169:**210-216, 1969.
4. Berman, I. R., and Ducker, T. B.: Changes in pulmonary, somatic, and splanchnic perfusion with increased intracranial pressure, Surg. Gynecol. Obstet. **128:**8-14, 1969.
5. Brashear, R. E., and Ross, J. C.: Hemodynamic effects of elevated cerebrospinal fluid pressure: alterations with adrenergic blockade, J. Clin. Invest. **49:**1324-1333, 1970.
6. Brisman, R., Kovach, R. M., Johnson, D. O., and others: Pulmonary edema in acute transection of the cervical spinal cord, Surg. Gynecol. Obstet. **139:**363-366, 1974.
7. Brown, F. K.: Cardiovascular effects of acutely raised intracranial pressure, Am. J. Physiol. **185:**510-514, 1956.
8. Bonbrest, H. C.: Pulmonary edema following an epileptic seizure, Am. Rev. Resp. Dis. **91:**97-100, 1965.
9. Cameron, G. R.: Pulmonary oedema, Br. Med. J. **1:**965-972, 1948.
10. Cameron, G. R., and De, S. N.: Experimental pulmonary edema of nervous origin, J. Pathol. Bacteriol. **61:**375-387, 1949.
11. Campbell, G. S., and Visscher, M. B.: Pulmonary lesions in guinea pigs with increased intracranial pressure, and the effect of bilateral cervical vagotomy, Am. J. Physiol. **157:**130-134, 1949.

12. Campbell, G. S., Haddy, F. J., Adams, W. L., and Visscher, M. B.: Circulatory changes and pulmonary lesions in dogs following increased intracranial pressure and the effect of atropine upon such changes, Am. J. Physiol. **158:**96-102, 1949.

13. Chandler, W. F., Dimcheff, D. G., and Taren, J. A.: Acute pulmonary edema following venous air embolism during a neurosurgical procedure, J. Neurosurg. **40:**400-404, 1974.

14. Chen, H. I., Sun, S. C., and Chai, C. Y.: Pulmonary edema and hemorrhage resulting from cerebral compression, Am. J. Physiol. **224:**223-229, 1973.

15. Ciongoli, A. K., and Poser, C. M.: Pulmonary edema secondary to subarachnoid hemorrhage, Neurology **22:**867-870, 1972.

16. Cohen, H. B., Gambill, A. F., and Eggers, G. W. N.: Acute pulmonary edema following head injury: two case reports, Anesth. Analg. **56:**136-139, 1977.

17. Cohn, J. N., and Franciosa, J. A.: Vasodilator therapy of cardiac failure, N. Engl. J. Med. **297:**254-258, 1977.

18. Cushing, H.: Concerning a definite regulatory mechanism of the vaso-motor centre which controls blood pressure during cerebral compression, Johns Hopkins Hosp. Bull. **12:**290-292, 1901.

19. Cushing, H.: Some experimental and clinical observations concerning states of increased intracranial tension, Am. J. Med. Sci. **124:**375-400, 1902.

20. Duberstein, J. L., and Kaufman, D. M.: A clinical study of an epidemic of heroin intoxication and heroin-induced pulmonary edema, Am. J. Med. **51:**704-714, 1971.

21. Ducker, T. B.: Increased intracranial pressure and pulmonary edema, I. Clinical study of 11 patients, J. Neurosurg. **28:**112-117, 1968.

22. Ducker, T. B., Simmons, R. L., and Anderson, R. W.: Increased intracranial pressure and pulmonary edema. III. The effect of increased intracranial pressure on the cardiovascular hemodynamics of chimpanzees, J. Neurosurg. **29:**475-483, 1968.

23. Ducker, T. B., and Simmons, R. L.: Increased intracranial pressure and pulmonary edema. II. The hemodynamic response of dogs and monkeys to increased intracranial pressure, J. Neurosurg. **28:**118-123, 1968.

24. Ducker, T. B., Simmons, R. L., and Martin, A. M.: Pulmonary edema as a complication of intracranial disease, Am. J. Dis. Child. **118:**638-641, 1969.

25. Farber, S.: Studies on pulmonary edema. II. The pathogenesis of neuropathic pulmonary edema, J. Exp. Med. **66:**405-411, 1937.

26. Farber, S.: Neuropathic pulmonary edema, Arch Pathol. **30:**180-197, 1940.

27. Gopiathan, K., Sajoja, J., Spears, R., and others: Hemodynamic studies in heroin induced acute pulmonary edema, Circulation (suppl. 3), vols. 61 and 63, pp. III-44, 1970.

28. Graf, C. J., and Rossi, N. P.: Pulmonary edema and the central nervous system: a clinico-pathological study, Surg. Neurol. **4:**319-325, 1975.

29. Gray, G. W., Bryan, A. C., Freedman, M. H., and others: Effect of altitude exposure on platelets, J. Appl. Physiol. **39:**648-652, 1975.

30. Greene, R., Platt, R., and Matz, R.: Postictal pulmonary edema, N.Y. State J. Med. **75:**1257-1261, 1975.

31. Harari, A., Rapin, M., Regnier, B., and others: Normal pulmonary-capillary pressures in the late phase of neurogenic pulmonary edema, Lancet **1:**494, 1976.

32. Harrison, W., and Liebow, A. A.: The effects of increased intracranial pressure on the pulmonary circulation in relation to pulmonary edema, Circulation **5:**824-832, 1952.

33. Haymaker, W., and Kernohan, J. W.: The Landry-Guillain-Barré syndrome, Medicine **28:**59-141, 1949.

34. Henton, E., Ross, A. M., Takeda, V. A., and others: Alterations in blood coagulation at high altitude, Adv. Cardiol. **5:**32-40, 1970.

35. Hoff, J. T., and Nishimura, M.: Experimental neurogenic pulmonary edema in cats, J. Neurosurg. **48:**383-389, 1978.

36. Houston, C. S.: Acute pulmonary edema of high altitude, N. Engl. J. Med. **263:**478-480, 1960.

37. Hücker, H., Frenzel, H., Kremer, B., and Richter, I. E.: Time sequence and site of fluid accumulation in experimental neurogenic pulmonary edema, Res. Exp. Med. **168:**219-227, 1976.

38. Huff, R. W., and Fred, H. L.: Postictal pulmonary edema, Arch. Intern. Med. **117:**824-828, 1966.

39. Hultgren, H. N., Spickard, W. B., Hellriegel, K., and others: High altitude pulmonary edema, Medicine **40:**289-313, 1961.

40. Hyers, T. M., Reeves, J. T., and Grover, R. F.: Effect of altitude on platelets, fibrinolysis and spirometry in man, Clin. Res. **25:**133A, 1977.

41. Karliner, J. S.: Noncardiogenic forms of pulmonary edema, Circulation **46:**212-215, 1972.

42. Kleiner, J. P., and Nelson, W. P.: High altitude pulmonary edema; a rare disease? J.A.M.A. **234:**491-499, 1975.

43. Lipinska, D., and Kurzaj, E.: Neurogenic pulmonary oedema in the course of increased intracranial pressure, J. Neurosurg. Sci. **18:**239-243, 1974.

44. Luisada, A. A.: Mechanism of neurogenic pulmonary edema, Am. J. Cardiol. **20:**66-68, 1967.

45. Mackay, E. M.: Experimental pulmonary edema IV. Pulmonary edema accompanying trauma to the brain, Proc. Soc. Exper. Biol. Med. **74:**695-697, 1950.

46. Mackay, E. M., Jordan, M. D., and Mackay, L. L.: Experimental pulmonary edema. II. Pathogenesis

of pulmonary edema caused by ammonium ion, Proc. Soc. Exp. Biol. Med. **72:**421-424, 1949.

47. Maire, F. W., and Patton, H. D.: Neural structures involved in the genesis of preoptic pulmonary edema, gastric erosions and behavior changes, Am. J. Physiol. **184:**345-350, 1956.

48. Malik, A. B.: Pulmonary vascular response to increase in intracranial pressure: role of sympathetic mechanisms, J. Appl. Physiol. **42:**335-343, 1977.

49. Moss, G., and Stein, A. A.: Cerebral etiology of the acute respiratory distress syndrome: diphenylhydantoin prophylaxis, J. Trauma **15:**39-41, 1975.

50. Moss, G., Staunton, C., and Stein, A. A.: Cerebral etiology of the shock lung syndrome; J. Trauma **12:**885-890, 1972.

51. Moss, G.: The role of the central nervous system in shock: the centroneurogenic etiology of the respiratory distress syndrome, Crit. Care Med. **2:**181-185, 1974.

52. Moutier, F.: Hypertension et mort par oedema pulmonaire aigu, Presse Medicale (Paris) **26:**108-109, 1918.

53. Nielsen, J. M., Ingham, S. D., and Von Hagen, K. O.: Pulmonary edema and embolism as complications of insulin shock in the treatment of schizophrenia, J.A.M.A. **111:**2455-2458, 1938.

54. Nothnagel, H. (quoted by Benassi, G.): Traumatismes cranio-encephaliques et oedema pulmonaire, Paris Med. **103:**525-532, 1937.

55. Osler, W.: Oedema of left lung—morphia poisoning, Montreal Gen. Hosp. Rev. **1:**291, 1880.

56. Oswalt, C. E., Gates, G. A., and Holmstrom, F. M. G.: Pulmonary edema as a complication of acute airway obstruction, J.A.M.A. **238:**1833-1835, 1977.

57. Penaloza, D., and Sime, F.: Circulatory dynamics during high altitude pulmonary edema, Am. J. Cardiol. **23:**369-378, 1969.

58. Reynolds, R. W.: Pulmonary edema as a consequence of hypothalamic lesions in rats, Science **141:**930-932, 1963.

59. Rodbard, S., Reyes, M., Mininni, G., and Saiki, H.: Neurohumoral transmission of the pressor response to intracranial compression, Am. J. Physiol. **176:**341-346, 1954.

60. Rossi, N. P., and Graf, C. J.: Physiological and pathological effects of neurologic disturbances and increased intracranial pressure on the lung; a review, Surg. Neurol. **5:**366-372, 1976.

61. Sarnoff, S. J., and Sarnoff, L. C.: Neurohemodynamics of pulmonary edema. II. The role of sympathetic pathways in the elevation of pulmonary and system vascular pressures following the intracisternal injection of fibrin, Circulation **6:**51-62, 1952.

62. Sarnoff, S. J., and Sarnoff, L. C.: Neurohemodynamics of pulmonary edema. I. Autonomic influence on pulmonary vascular pressures and the acute pulmonary edema state, Dis. Chest **22:**685-698, 1952.

63. Schäfer, U., Hücker, H., and Meinen, K.: Early morphological alterations of the rat lung with increased intracranial pressure. II. A scanning electron microscopic study using different fixation procedures, Res. Exp. Med. **165:**1-8, 1975.

64. Simmons, R. L., Martin, A. M., Heisterkamp, C. A., and Ducker, T. B.: Respiratory insufficiency in combat casualties. II. Pulmonary edema following head injury, Ann. Surg. **170:**39-44, 1969.

65. Singh, I.: High altitude pulmonary edema, Am. Heart J. **70:**435-439, 1965.

66. Singh, I., Khanna, P. K., Srivastava, M. C., and others: Acute mountain sickness, N. Engl. J. Med. **280:**175-184, 1969.

67. Steinberg, A. D., and Karliner, J. S.: The clinical spectrum of heroin pulmonary edema, Arch. Intern. Med. **122:**122-127, 1968.

68. Sugg, W. L., Craver, W. D., Webb, W. R., and others: Pressure changes in the dog lung secondary to hemorrhagic shock: protective effect of pulmonary reimplantation, Ann. Surg. **169:**592-598, 1969.

69. Theodore, J., and Robin, E. D.: Pathogenesis of neurogenic pulmonary oedema, Lancet **2:**749-751, 1975.

70. Theodore, J., and Robin, E. D.: Speculations on neurogenic pulmonary edema (NPE), Am. Rev. Respir. Dis. **113:**405-411, 1976.

71. Thompson, G. E.: Pulmonary edema complicating intrathecal hypertonic saline injection for intractable pain, Anesthesiology **35:**425-427, 1971.

72. Urabe, M., Segawa, Y., Tsubokawa, T., and others: Pathogenesis of the acute pulmonary edema occurring after brain operation and brain trauma, Jpn. Heart J. **2:**147-169, 1961.

73. Weisman, S. J.: Edema and congestion of the lungs resulting from intracranial hemorrhage, Surgery **6:**722-729, 1939.

74. Whayne, T. F., and Severinghaus, J. W.: Experimental hypoxic pulmonary edema in the rat, J. Appl. Physiol. **25:**729-732, 1968.

75. Worthen, M., Placik, B., Argano, B., and others: On the mechanism of epinephrine-induced pulmonary edema, Jpn. Heart J. **10:**133-141, 1969.

Fat embolism

1. Armstrong, H. J., Kuenzig, M. C., and Peltier, L. F.: Lung lipase levels in normal rats and rats with experimentally produced fat embolism, Proc. Soc. Exp. Biol. Med. **124:**959-961, 1967.

2. Ashbaugh, D. G., and Petty, T. L.: The use of corticosteroids in the treatment of respiratory failure associated with massive fat embolism, Surg. Gynecol. Obstet. **123:**493-500, 1966.

3. Bruecke, P., Burke, J. F., Lam, K. W., and others: The pathophysiology of pulmonary fat embolism, J. Thorac. Cardiovasc. Surg. **61:**949-955, 1971.

4. Dines, D. E., Linscheid, R. L., and Didier, E. P.: Fat embolism syndrome, Mayo Clin. Proc. **47:**237-240, 1972.

5. Evarts, C. M.: The fat embolism syndrome: a review, Surg. Clin. North Am. **50**:493-507, 1970.
6. Fuchsig, P., Brücke, P., Blümel, G., and others: A new clinical and experimental concept on fat embolism, N. Engl. J. Med. **276**:1192-1193, 1967.
7. Kieth, R. G., Mahoney, L. J., and Garvey, M. B.: Disseminated intravascular coagulation: an important feature of the fat embolism syndrome, Can. Med. Assoc. J. **105**:74-76, 1971.
8. Peltier, L. F.: A few remarks on fat embolism, J. Trauma **8**:812-820, 1968.
9. Ross, A. P. J.: The fat embolism syndrome: with special reference to the importance of hypoxia in the syndrome, Ann. R. Coll. Surg. Engl. **46**:159-171, 1970.
10. Sevitt, S.: The boundaries between physiology, pathology, and irreversibility after injury, Lancet **2**:1203-1210, 1966.

Venous thromboembolism

1. Barnett, H. G., Clifford, J. R., and Llewellyn, R. C.: Safety of mini-dose heparin administration for neurosurgical patients, J. Neurosurg. **47**:27-30, 1977.
2. Brisman, R., and Mendell, J.: Thromboembolism and brain tumors, J. Neurosurg. **38**:337-338, 1973.
3. Coon, W. W., and Coller, F. A.: Clinicopathologic correlation in thromboembolism, Surg. Gynecol. Obstet. **109**:259-269, 1959.
4. Gallus, A. S., Hirsch, J., O'Brien, S. E., and others: Prevention of venous thrombosis with small, subcutaneous doses of heparin, J.A.M.A. **235**:1980-1982, 1976.
5. Gunn, C. G., and Hampton, J. W.: CNS influence on plasma levels of factor VIII activity, Am. J. Physiol. **212**:124-130, 1967.
6. Joffe, S. N.: Incidence of post operative deep vein thrombosis in neurosurgical patients, J. Neurosurg. **42**:201-203, 1975.
7. Kakkar, V. V., Field, E. S., Nicolaides, A. N., and others: Low doses of heparin in prevention of deep vein thrombosis, Lancet **2**:669-671, 1971.
8. Kakkar, V. V., Corrigan, T., Spindler, J., and others: Efficacy of low doses of heparin in prevention of deep-vein thrombosis after major surgery: a double blind, randomized trial, Lancet **2**:101-106, 1972.
9. Kakkar, V.: The diagnosis of deep vein thrombosis using the I^{125} fibrinogen test, Arch. Surg. **104**:152-159, 1972.
10. Sigel, B., Felix, R., Popky, G. L., and others: Diagnosis of lower limb venous thrombosis by Doppler ultrasound technique, Arch. Surg. **104**:174-179, 1972.
11. Warlow, C., Ogston, D., and Douglas, A. S.: Venous thrombosis following strokes, Lancet **1**:1305-1306, 1972.
12. Wetzel, N., Anderson, M. C., and Shields, T. W.: Pulmonary embolism as a cause of death in the neurosurgical patient, J. Neurosurg. **17**:664-668, 1960.

Electrocardiographic changes

1. Fentz, V., and Gormsen, J.: Electrocardiographic patterns in patients with cerebrovascular accidents, Circulation **25**:22-28, 1962.
2. Galloon, S., Rees, G. A. D., Briscoe, C. E., and others: Prospective study of electrocardiographic changes associated with subarachnoid hemorrhage, Br. J. Anaesth. **44**:511-515, 1972.
3. Hersch, C.: Electrocardiographic changes in head injuries, Circulation **23**:853-860, 1961.
4. Hersch, C.: Electrocardiographic changes in subarachnoid hemorrhage, meningitis, and intracranial space-occupying lesions, Br. Heart J. **26**:785-793, 1964.
5. Jacobson, S. A., and Danufsky, P.: Marked electrocardiographic changes produced by experimental head trauma, J. Neuropathol. Exp. Neurol. **13**:462-466, 1954.
6. Marks, J.: Central nervous system influence in the genesis of atrial fibrillation, Ohio State Med. J. **52**:1054-1055, 1956.
7. Marshall, A. J.: Transient atrial fibrillation after minor head injury, Br. Heart J. **38**:984-985, 1976.
8. McLaurin, R. L., and King, L. R.: Recognition and treatment of metabolic disorders after head injuries, Clin. Neurosurg. **19**:281-300, 1972.
9. Weinberg, S. J., and Fuster, J. M.: Electrocardiographic changes produced by localized hypothalamic stimulations, Ann. Intern. Med. **53**:332-341, 1960.
10. Weintraub, B. M., and McHenry, L. C.: Cardiac abnormalities in subarachnoid hemorrhage: a resumé, Stroke **5**:384-392, 1974.

Diaphragmatic paralysis

1. Keltz, H., Kaplan, S., and Stone, D. J.: Effect of quadriplegia and hemidiaphragmatic paralysis on thoracoabdominal pressure during respiration, Am. J. Phys. Med. **48**:109-115, 1969.
2. Prasad, S., and Athreya, B. H.: Transient paralysis of the phrenic nerve associated with head injury, J.A.M.A. **236**:2532-2533, 1976.

HEMATOLOGIC SEQUELAE
Inhibition of phagocytosis

1. Alexander, J. W.: Host defense mechanisms against infection, Surg. Clin. North Am. **52**:1367-1378, 1972.
2. Azmitia, E. C., and McEwen, B. S.: Adrenocortical influence on rat brain tryptophan hydroxylase activity, Brain Res. **78**:291-302, 1974.
3. Cullen, B. F., Hume, R. B., and Chretien, P. B.: Phagocytosis during general anesthesia in man, Anesth. Analg. **54**:501-504, 1975.
4. Dodsworth, H., and Harris, R.: Granulocyte function in patients with brain damage and anoxia, Acta Haematol. **45**:350-355, 1971.
5. Douglas, S. D.: Analytic review: disorders of phagocyte function, Blood **35**:851-866, 1970.
6. King, L. R., McLaurin, R. L., Lewis, H. P., and

Knowles, H. C.: Plasma cortisol levels after head injury, Ann. Surg. **172:**975-984, 1970.

7. Kvarstein, B., and Stormorken, H.: Influence of acetylsalicylic acid, butazolidine, colchicine, hydrocortisone, chlorpromazine and imipramine on the phagocytosis of polystyrene latex particles by human leucocytes, Biochem. Pharmacol. **20:**119-124, 1971.

8. McLaurin, R. L., and King, L. R.: Recognition and treatment of metabolic disorders after head injuries, Clin. Neurosurg. **19:**281-300, 1972.

9. Miller, D. R., and Kaplan, H. G.: Decreased nitroblue tetrazolium dye reduction in the phagocytes of patients receiving prednisone, Pediatrics **45:**861-865, 1970.

10. Siebel, E. E., Geppert, H., Heumann, W., and others: Die Hirnischämie als ursache für die änderung der transplantationsantigene des hundes im zytotoxischen test, Res. Exp. Med. **166:**229-234, 1975.

11. Van Woerkom, T. C. A. M., Huijbers, W. A. R., Teelken, A. W., and others: Biochemical and ultrastructural aspects of the inhibited phagocytosis by neutrophil granulocytes in acute brain-damaged patients, J. Neurol. Sci. **31:**223-235, 1977.

12. Vecht, C. J.: Additional studies on platelet function. In Minderhoud, J. M., and Braakman, R., editors: Haemostasis in acute neurologic disorders (monographs on clinical neurology and neurosurgery), vol 2, Assen, The Netherlands, 1975, Van Gorcum, pp. 113-124.

13. Vecht, C. J., Van Woerkom, T. C. A. M., Teelken, A. W., and Minderhoud, J. M.: Homovanillic acid and 5-hydroxyindoleacetic acid cerebrospinal fluid levels, Arch. Neurol. **32:**792-797, 1975.

Trauma and coagulation

1. Attar, S., McLaughlin, J., Mansberger, A. R., and Cowley, R. A.: Prognostic significance of coagulation studies in clinical shock, Surg. Forum **17:**8-11, 1966.

2. Attar, S., Kirby, W. H., Masaitis, C., and others: Coagulation changes in clinical shock. I. Effect of hemorrhagic shock on clotting time in humans, Ann. Surg. **164:**34-50, 1966.

3. Attar, S., Boyd, D., Layne, E., and others: Alterations in coagulation and fibrinolytic mechanisms in acute trauma, J. Trauma **9:**939-965, 1969.

4. Barrer, M. J., and Ellison, N.: Platelet function, Anesthesiology **46:**202-211, 1977.

5. Cannon, W. B., and Gray, H.: Factors affecting the coagulation time of blood. II. The hastening or retarding of coagulation by adrenalin injections, Am. J. Physiol. **34:**232-242, 1914.

6. Cannon, W. B., and Mendenhall, W. L.: Factors affecting the coagulation time of blood. IV. The hastening of coagulation in pain and emotional excitement, Am. J. Physiol. **34:**251-261, 1914.

7. Colman, R. W., Robboy, S. J., and Minna, J. D.: Disseminated intravascular coagulation (DIC): an approach, Am. J. Med. **52:**679-684, 1972.

8. Deykin, D.: The clinical challenge of disseminated intravascular coagulation, N. Engl. J. Med. **283:**636-644, 1970.

9. Hardaway, R. M.: Disseminated intravascular coagulation in experimental and clinical shock, Am. J. Cardiol. **20:**161-173, 1967.

10. Innes, D., and Sevitt, S.: Coagulation and fibrinolysis in injured patients, J. Clin. Pathol. **17:**1-13, 1964.

11. O'Brien, J. R.: Effects of salicylates on human platelets, Lancet **1:**779-783, 1968.

12. Sevitt, S.: The boundaries between physiology, pathology, and irreversibility after injury, Lancet **2:**1203-1210, 1966.

13. String, T., Robinson, A. J., and Blaisdell, F. W.: Massive trauma: effect of intravascular coagulation on prognosis, Arch. Surg. **102:**406-410, 1971.

14. Vecht, C. J., and Smit Sibinga, C.T.: Head injury and defibrination, Lancet **2:**905, 1974.

15. Weiss, H. J., Aledort, L. M., and Kochwa, S.: The effect of salicylates on the hemostatic properties of platelets in man, J. Clin. Invest. **47:**2169-2180, 1968.

Disseminated intravascular coagulation

1. Anderson, J. M., and Brown, J. K.: Brain ischemia and disseminated intravascular coagulation, Lancet **1:**373-374, 1972.

2. Astrup, T.: Assay and content of tissue thromboplastin in different organs, Thromb. Diath. Haemorrh. **14:**401-416, 1965.

3. Barrer, M. J., and Ellison, N.: Platelet function, Anesthesiology **46:**202-211, 1977.

4. Cannon, W. B., and Gray, H.: Factors affecting the coagulation time of blood. II. The hastening or retarding of coagulation by adrenalin injections, Am. J. Physiol. **34:**232-242, 1914.

5. Cannon, W. B., and Mendenhall, W. L.: Factors affecting the coagulation time of blood. IV. The hastening of coagulation in pain and emotional excitement, Am. J. Physiol. **34:**251-261, 1914.

6. Cannon, W. B., and Mendenhall, W. L.: Factors affecting the coagulation time of blood. III. The hastening of coagulation by stimulating the splanchnic nerves, Am. J. Physiol. **34:**243-250, 1914.

7. Colman, R. W., Robboy, S. J., and Minna, J. D.: Disseminated intravascular coagulation (DIC): an approach, Am J. Med. **52:**679-684, 1972.

8. Deykin, D.: The clinical challenge of disseminated intravascular coagulation, N. Engl. J. Med. **283:**636-644, 1970.

9. Drayer, B. P., and Poser, C. M.: Disseminated intravascular coagulation and head trauma: two case studies, J.A.M.A. **231:**174-175, 1975.

10. Druskin, M. S., and Drijansky, R.: Afibrinogenemia with severe head trauma, J.A.M.A. **219:**755-756, 1972.

11. Glenn, F., and Grafe, W. R.: Surgical complications of adrenal steroid therapy, Ann. Surg. **165:**1023-1034, 1967.

12. Goodnight, S. H., Kenoyer, G., Rapaport, S. I., and others: Defibrination after brain tissue destruction; a serious complication of head injury, N. Engl. J. Med. **290:**1043-1047, 1974.

13. Gunn, C. G., and Hampton, J. W.: CNS influence on plasma levels of factor VIII activity, Am. J. Physiol. **212:**124-130, 1967.

14. Hardaway, R. M.: Disseminated intravascular coagulation in experimental and clinical shock, Am. J. Cardiol. **20:**161-173, 1967.

15. Keimowitz, R. M., and Annis, B. L.: Disseminated intravascular coagulation associated with massive brain injury, J. Neurosurg. **39:**178-180, 1973.

16. Keith, R. G., Mahoney, L. J., and Garvey, M. B.: Disseminated intravascular coagulation: an important feature of the fat embolism syndrome, Can. Med. Assoc. J. **105:**74-76, 1971.

17. Matjasko, M. J., and Ducker, T. B.: Disseminated intravascular coagulation associated with removal of a primary brain tumor, J. Neurosurg. **47:**476-480, 1977.

18. McGauley, J. L., Miller, C. A., and Penner, J. A.: Diagnosis and treatment of diffuse intravascular coagulation following cerebral trauma; case report, J. Neurosurg. **43:**374-376, 1975.

19. O'Brien, J. R.: Effects of salicylates on human platelets, Lancet **1:**779-783, 1968.

20. Preston, F. E., Malia, R. G., Sworn, M. J., and others: Disseminated intravascular coagulation as a consequence of cerebral damage, J. Neurol. Neurosurg. Psychiatr. **37:**241-248, 1974.

21. String, T., Robinson, A. J., and Blaisdell, F. W.: Massive trauma: effect of intravascular coagulation on prognosis, Arch. Surg. **102:**406-410, 1971.

22. Takashima, S., Koga, M., and Tanaka, K.: Fibrinolytic activity of human brain and cerebrospinal fluid, Br. J. Exp. Pathol. **50:**533-539, 1969.

23. Tovi, D.: Fibrinolytic activity of human brain; a histochemical study, Acta Neurol. Scand. **49:**152-162, 1973.

24. Van Woerkom, T. C. A. M., Huijbers, W. A. R., Teelken, A. W., and others: Biochemical and ultrastructural aspects of the inhibited phagocytosis by neutrophil granulocytes in acute brain-damaged patients, J. Neurol. Sci. **31:**223-235, 1977.

25. Vardi, Y., Streifler, M., Schujman, E., and Loewenthal, M.: Diffuse intravascular clotting associated with a primary brain tumour, J. Neurol. Neurosurg. Psychiatr. **37:**987-990, 1974.

26. Vecht, C. J., and Smit Sibinga, C. T.: Head injury and defibrination, Lancet **2:**905, 1974.

27. Vecht, C. J.: Additional studies on platelet function. In Minderhoud, J. M., and Braakman, R., editors: Haemostasis in acute neurologic disorders (monographs on clinical neurology and neurosurgery), vol. 2, Assen, The Netherlands, 1975, Van Gorcum, pp. 113-124.

28. Vecht, C. J., Smit Sibinga, C. T., and Minderhoud, J. M.: Disseminated intravascular coagulation and head injury, J. Neurol. Neurosurg. Psychiatr. **38:**567-571, 1975.

29. Weiss, H. J., Aledort, L. M., and Kochwa, S.: The effect of salicylates on the hemostatic properties of platelets in man, J. Clin. Invest. **47:**2169-2180, 1968.

Endocrinologic sequelae
Anterior pituitary insufficiency

1. Altman, R., and Pruzanski, W.: Post traumatic hypopituitarism, Ann. Intern. Med. **55:**149-154, 1961.

2. Ceballos, R.: Pituitary changes in head trauma (analysis of 102 consecutive cases of head injury), Ala. J. Med. Sci. **3:**185-198, 1966.

3. Crompton, M. R.: Hypothalamic lesions following closed head injury, Brain **94:**165-172, 1971.

4. Daniel, P. M., Prichard, M. M. L., and Treip, C. S.: Traumatic infarction of the anterior lobe of the pituitary gland, Lancet **2:**927-930, 1959.

5. Dzur, J., and Winternitz, W. W.: Posttraumatic hypopituitarism: anterior pituitary insufficiency secondary to head trauma, South. Med. J. **69:**1377-1379, 1976.

6. Frantz, A. G.: Prolactin, N. Engl. J. Med. **298:**201-207, 1978.

7. Goldman, K. P., and Jacobs, A.: Anterior and posterior pituitary failure after head injury, Br. Med. J. **2:**1924-1926, 1960.

8. Kornblum, R. N., and Fisher, R. S.: Pituitary lesions in craniocerebral injuries, Arch. Pathol. **88:**242-248, 1969.

9. Magoun, H. W., and Ranson, S. W.: Retrograde degeneration of the supraoptic nuclei after section of the infundibular stalk in the monkey, Anat. Rec. **75:**107-123, 1939.

10. McCullagh, E. P., and Schaffenburg, C. A.: Anterior pituitary insufficiency following skull fracture, J. Clin. Endocrinol. Metab. **13:**1283-1290, 1953.

11. Paxson, C. L., and Brown, D. R.: Post-traumatic anterior hypopituitarism, Pediatrics **57:**893-896, 1976.

12. Robertson, J. D., and Kirkpatrick, H. F. W.: Simmond's disease (hypopituitarism) in a man due to traumatic hemorrhage into the pituitary gland, Lancet **1:**1048-1051, 1951.

13. Sharkey, P. C., Perry, J. H., and Ehni, G.: Diabetes insipidus following section of hypophyseal stalk, J. Neurosurg. **18:**445-460, 1961.

14. Sheehan, H. L.: Post-partum necrosis of the anterior pituitary, J. Pathol. Bacteriol. **45:**189-214, 1937.

15. Weiss, S. R., Jacobi, J. D., Fishman, L. M., and Lemaire, W. J.: Hypopituitarism following head trauma, Am. J. Obstet Gynecol. **127:**678-679, 1977.

Posterior pituitary dysfunction
Diabetes insipidus

1. Ahmed, A. B. J., George, B. C., Gonzales-Auvert, C., and Dingman, J. F.: Increased plasma arginine vasopressin in clinical adrenocortical insufficiency and its inhibition by glucosteroids, J. Clin. Invest. **46:**111-123, 1967.

2. Bartter, F. C., and Schwartz, W. B.: The syndrome

of inappropriate secretion of antidiuretic hormone, Am. J. Med. **42:**790-806, 1967.

3. Chang, L. R., Chen, C. F., and Chai, C. Y.: The effect of head injury on antidiuretic hormone synthesis or release in rats, Arch. Int. Physiol. Biochimie **80:**679-684, 1972.

4. Cinotti, G. A., Stirati, G. and Ruggiero, F.: Abnormal water retention and symptomatic hyponatremia in idiopathic diabetes insipidus during chlorpropamide therapy, Postgrad. Med. **48:**107-112, 1972.

5. Crawford, J. D., and Kennedy, G. C.: Chlorthiazid in diabetes insipidus, Nature **183:**891-892, 1959.

6. Earley, L. E., and Orloff, J.: The mechanism of antidiuresis associated with the administration of hydrochlorthiazide to patients with vasopressin-resistant diabetes insipidus, J. Clin. Invest. **41:**1988-1997, 1962.

7. Fichman, M. P., Kleeman, C. R., and Bethune, J. E.: Inhibition of antidiuretic hormone secretion by diphenylhydantoin, Arch. Neurol. **22:**45-53, 1970.

8. Gaufin, L., Skowsky, W. R., and Goodman, S. J.: Release of antidiuretic hormone during mass-induced elevation of intracranial pressure, J. Neurosurg. **46:**627-637, 1977.

9. Glauser, F. L.: Diabetes insipidus in hypoxemic encephalopathy, J.A.M.A. **235:**932-933, 1976.

10. Griffin, J. M., Hartley, J. H., Crow, R. W., and Schatten, W. E.: Diabetes insipidus caused by craniofacial trauma, J. Trauma **16:**979-984, 1976.

11. Hansen, O. H.: Fat embolism and post-traumatic diabetes insipidus, Acta Chir. Scand. **136:**161-165, 1970.

12. Hays, R. M.: Antidiuretic hormone, N. Engl. J. Med. **295:**659-665, 1976.

13. Kleeman, C. R., Rubini, M. E., Lamdin, E., and Epstein, F. H.: Studies on alcohol diuresis. II. The evaluation of ethyl alcohol as an inhibitor of the neurohypophysis, J. Clin. Invest. **34:**448-455, 1955.

14. Machiedo, G., Bolanowski, P. J. P., Bauer, J., and Neville, W. E.: Diabetes insipidus secondary to penetrating thoracic trauma, Ann. Surg. **181:**31-34, 1975.

15. McLaurin, R. L., and King, L. R.: Recognition and treatment of metabolic disorders after head injuries, Clin. Neurosurg. **19:**281-300, 1972.

16. Miller, M., and Moses, A. M.: Mechanism of chlorpropamide action in diabetes insipidus, J. Clin. Endocrinol. Metab. **30:**488-496, 1970.

17. Moses, A. M., and Miller, M.: Urine and plasma osmolality in differentiation of polyuric states, Postgrad. Med. **52:**187-190, 1972.

18. Moses, A. M., and Miller, M.: Drug-induced dilutional hyponatremia, N. Engl. J. Med. **291:**1234-1239, 1974.

19. Moses, A. M., Miller, M., and Streeten, D. H. P.: Pathophysiologic and pharmacologic alterations in the release and action of ADH, Metabolism **25:**697-721, 1976.

20. Moses, A. M.: Diabetes insipidus and ADH regulation, Hosp. Prac. **12:**37-44, 1977.

21. Murdaugh, H. V., Sieker, H. O., and Manfredi, F.: Effect of altered intrathoracic pressure on renal hemodynamics, electrolyte excretion and water clearance, J. Clin. Invest. **38:**834-842, 1959.

22. Orloff, J., and Handler, J. S.: The cellular mode of action of antidiuretic hormone, Am. J. Med. **36:**686-697, 1964.

23. Porter, R. J., and Miller, R. A.: Diabetes insipidus following closed head injury, J. Neurol. Neurosurg. Psychiatr. **11:**258-262, 1948.

24. Robinson, R. O., and Pagliero, K. M.: Polyuria after cardiac surgery, Br. Med. J. **3:**265-266, 1970.

25. Rothschild, M., and Shenkman, L.: Diabetes insipidus following cardiorespiratory arrest, J.A.M.A. **238:**620-621, 1977.

26. Rottenberg, D. A., Bennett, W. M., and Wolpow, E. R.: Transient diabetes insipidus complicating systemic fat embolization, J. Trauma **12:**731-733, 1972.

27. Schrier, R. W., and Berl, T.: Nonosmolar factors affecting water excretion, N. Engl. J. Med. **292:**141-145, 1975.

28. Sevitt, S.: Fat embolism, London, 1962, Butterworths & Co..

29. Sharkey, P. C., Perry, J. H., and Ehni, G.: Diabetes insipidus following section of hypophyseal stalk, J. Neurosurg. **18:**445-460, 1961.

30. Shucart, W. A., and Jackson, I.: Management of diabetes insipidus in neurosurgical patients, J. Neurosurg. **44:**65-71, 1976.

31. Smith, H. W.: Salt and water volume receptors, Am. J. Med. **23:**623-652, 1957.

32. Webster, B., and Bain, J.: Antidiuretic effect and complications of chlorpropamide therapy in diabetes insipidus, J. Clin. Endocrinol. Metab. **30:**215-227, 1970.

Inappropriate ADH syndrome

1. Ahmed, A. B. J., George, B. C., Gonzalez-Auvert, C., and Dingman, J. F.: Increased plasma arginine vasopressin in clinical adrenocortical insufficiency and its inhibition by glucosteroids, J. Clin. Invest. **46:**111-123, 1967.

2. Auger, R. G., Zehr, J. E., Siekert, R. G., and Segar, W. E.: Position effect on antidiuretic hormone, Arch. Neurol. **23:**513-517, 1970.

3. Bartter, F. C., and Schwartz, W. B.: The syndrome of inappropriate secretion of antidiuretic hormone, Am. J. Med. **42:**790-806, 1967.

4. Becker, R. M., and Daniel, R. K.: Increased antidiuretic hormone production after trauma to the craniofacial complex, J. Trauma **13:**112-115, 1973.

5. Carter, N. W., Rector, F. C., and Seldin, D. W.: Hyponatremia in cerebral disease resulting from inappropriate secretion of antidiruetic hormone, N. Engl. J. Med. **264:**67-72, 1961.

6. Cooper, W. C., Green, I. J., and Wang, S.: Cerebral salt wasting associated with the Guillain-Barré syndrome, Arch. Intern. Med. **116:**113-119, 1965.

7. Davis, B. B., Bloom, M. E., Field, J. B., and

Mintz, D. H.: Hyponatremia in pituitary insufficiency, Metabolism 18:821-832, 1969.

8. Deutsch, S., Goldberg, M., and Dripps, R. D.: Postoperative hyponatremia with the inappropriate release of antidiuretic hormone, Anesthesiology 27: 250-256, 1966.

9. Fichman, M. P., and Bethune, J. E.: The role of adrenocorticoids in the inappropriate antidiuretic hormone syndrome, Ann. Intern. Med. 68:806-820, 1968.

10. Fichman, M. P., Kleeman, C. R., and Bethune, J. E.: Inhibition of antidiuretic hormone secretion by diphenylhydantoin, Arch. Neurol. 22:45-53, 1970.

11. Fichman, M. P., Vorherr, H., Kleeman, C. R., and Telfer, N.: Diuretic-induced hyponatremia, Ann. Intern. Med. 75:853-863, 1971.

12. Fox, J. L., Falik, J. L., and Shalhoub, R. J.: Neurosurgical hyponatremia: the role of inappropriate antidiuresis, J. Neurosurg. 34:506-514, 1971.

13. Haden, H. T., and Knox, G. W.: Cerebral hyponatremia with inappropriate antidiuretic hormone syndrome, Am. J. Med. Sci. 249:381-390, 1965.

14. Hellman, E. S., Tschudy, D. P., and Bartter, F. C.: Abnormal electrolyte and water metabolism in acute intermittent porphyria, Am. J. Med. 32:734-746, 1962.

15. Joynt, R. J., Afifi, A., and Harbison, J.: Hyponatremia in subarachnoid hemorrhage, Arch. Neurol. 13:633-638, 1965.

16. Knochel, J. P., Osborn, J. R., and Cooper, E. B.: Excretion of aldosterone in inappropriate secretion of antidiuretic hormone following head trauma, Metabolism 14:715-725, 1965.

17. Leaf, A., Bartter, F. C., Santos, R. F., and Wong, O.: Evidence in man that urinary electrolyte loss induced by pitressin is a function of water retention, J. Clin. Invest. 32:868-878, 1953.

18. Mangos, J. A., and Lobeck, C. C.: Studies of sustained hyponatremia due to central nervous system infection, Pediatrics 34:503-510, 1964.

19. Moran, W. H., Miltenberger, F. W., Shuayb, W. A., and Zimmerman, B.: The relationship of antidiuretic hormone to surgical stress, Surgery 56:99-108, 1964.

20. Nielsen, B., and Thorn, A.: Transient excess urinary excretion of antidiuretic material in acute intermittent porphyria with hyponatremia and hypomagnesemia, Am. J. Med. 38:345-358, 1965.

21. Richards, D. E., White, R. J., and Yashon, D.: Inappropriate release of ADH in subdural hematoma, J. Trauma 11:758-762, 1971.

22. Rovit, R. L., and Sigler, M. H.: Hyponatremia with herpes simplex encephalitis: possible relationship of limbic lesions and ADH secretion, Arch. Neurol. 10:595-603, 1964.

23. Schwartz, W. B., Bennett, W., Curelop, S., and Bartter, F. C.: A syndrome of renal sodium loss and hyponatremia probably resulting from inappropriate secretion of antidiuretic hormone, Am. J. Med. 23: 529-542, 1957.

24. Vogel, J. H. K.: Aldosterone in cerebral salt wasting, Circulation 27:44-50, 1963.

Metabolic sequelae

1. Arieff, A. L., and Carroll, H. J.: Nonketotic hyperosmolar coma with hyperglycemia: clinical features, pathophysiology, renal function, acid-base balance, plasma-cerebrospinal fluid equilibria and the effects of therapy in 37 cases, Medicine 51:73-94, 1972.

2. Aviram, A., Pfau, A., Czaczkes, J. W., and Ullman, T. D.: Hyperosmolality with hyponatremia, caused by inappropriate administration of mannitol, Am. J. Med. 42:648-650, 1967.

3. Bookman, J. J., Drachman, S. R., Schaefer, L. E., and Aldersberg, D.: Steroid diabetes in man: the development of diabetes during treatment with cortisone and corticotropin, Diabetes 2:100-111, 1953.

4. Boyer, M. H.: Hyperosmolar anacidotic coma in association with glucocorticoid therapy, J.A.M.A. 202:1007-1009, 1967.

5. Brenner, W. I., Lansky, Z., Engelman, R. M., and Stahl, W. M.: Hyperosmolar coma in surgical patients: an iatrogenic disease of increasing incidence, Ann. Surg. 178:651-654, 1973.

6. Christensen, M. S.: Acid-base changes in cerebrospinal fluid and blood, and blood volume changes following prolonged hyperventilation in man, Br. J. Anaesth. 46:348-357, 1974.

7. Clements, R., Prockop, L., and Winegrad, A.: Acute cerebral edema during treatment of hyperglycemia, Lancet 2:384-386, 1968.

8. Cottrell, J. E., Robustelli, A., Post, K., and Turndorf, H.: Furosemide- and mannitol-induced changes in intracranial pressure and serum osmolality and electrolytes, Anesthesiology 47:28-30, 1977.

9. Fitzgerald, M. G., O'Sullivan, D. J., and Malins, J. M.: Fatal diabetic ketosis, Br. Med. J. 1:247-250, 1961.

10. Flanigan, W. J., Thompson, B. W., Casali, R. E., and Caldwell, F. T.: The surgical significance of hyperosmolar coma, Am. J. Surg. 120:653-659, 1970.

11. Gault, M. H., Dixon, M. E., Doyle, M., and Cohen, W. M.: Hypernatremia, azotemia, and dehydration due to high-protein tube feeding, Ann. Intern. Med. 68:778-791, 1968.

12. Gipstein, R. M., and Boyle, J. D.: Hypernatremia complicating prolonged mannitol diuresis, N. Engl. J. Med. 272:1116-1117, 1965.

13. Goldberg, E. M., and Sanbar, S. S.: Hyperglycemic, non-ketotic coma following administration of Dilantin (diphenylhydantoin), Diabetes 18:101-106, 1969.

14. Henry, D. P., and Bressler, R.: Serum insulin levels in nonketotic hyperosmotic diabetes mellitus, Am. J. Med. Sci. 256:150-154, 1968.

15. Katsurada, K., Sugimoto, T., Onji, Y.: Significance of cerebrospinal fluid bicarbonate ions in the man-

agement of patients with cerebral injury, J. Trauma **9:**799-805, 1969.

16. King, L. R., McLaurin, R. L., Lewis, H. P., and Knowles, H. C.: Plasma cortisol levels after head injury, Ann. Surg. **172:**975-984, 1970.

17. King, L. R., Knowles, H. C., McLaurin, R. L., and Lewis, H. P.: Glucose tolerance and plasma insulin in cranial trauma, Ann. Surg. **173:**337-343, 1971.

18. Lassen, N. A.: The luxury-perfusion syndrome and its possible relation to acute metabolic acidosis localized within the brain, Lancet **2:**1113-1115, 1966.

19. Levine, R., and Mahler, R., R.: Production, secretion, and availability of insulin, Ann. Rev. Med. **15:** 413-432, 1964.

20. Maccario, M.: Neurological dysfunction associated with nonketotic hyperglycemia, Arch. Neurol. **19:** 525-534, 1968.

21. McCurdy, D. K.: Hyperosmolar hyperglycemic nonketotic diabetic coma, Med. Clin. North Am. **54:** 683-699, 1970.

22. McLaurin, R. L., and King, L. R.: Recognition and treatment of metabolic disorders after head injuries, Clin. Neurosurg. **19:**281-300, 1972.

23. McLaurin, R. L., and King, L. R.: Metabolic effects of head injury, Handbook Clin. Neurol. **23:**109-131, 1975.

24. Park, B. E., Meacham, W. F., and Netsky, M. G.: Nonketotic hyperglycemic hyperosmolar coma: report of neurosurgical cases with a review of mechanisms and treatment, J. Neurosurg. **44:**409-417, 1976.

25. Peters, B. H., and Samaan, N. A.: Hyperglycemia with relative hypoinsulinemia in diphenylhydantoin toxicity, N. Engl. J. Med. **281:**91-92, 1969.

26. Poser, C. M.: Hyperglycemic non-ketotic coma: role of sodium in the pathogenesis of the neurologic manifestations, Dis. Nerv. Sys. **33:**725-729, 1972.

27. Prockop, L.: Hyperglycemia, polyol accumulation and increased intracranial pressure, Arch. Neurol. **25:**126-140, 1971.

28. Rudman, D., Fleischer, A., and Kutner, M. H.: Concentration of 3'5' cyclic adenosine monophosphate in ventricular cerebrospinal fluid of patients with prolonged coma after head trauma or intracranial hemorrhage, N. Engl. J. Med. **295:**635-638, 1976.

29. Sament, S., and Schwartz, M. B.: Severe diabetic stupor without ketosis, S. Afr. Med. J. **31:**893-894, 1957.

30. Sears, E. S.: Nonketotic hyperosmolar hyperglycemia during glycerol therapy for cerebral edema, Neurology **26:**89-94, 1976.

31. Sevitt, S.: The boundaries between physiology, pathology, and irreversibility after injury, Lancet **2:**1203-1210, 1966.

32. Spenney, J. G., Eure, C. A., and Kreisberg, R. A.: Hyperglycemic, hyperosmolar, nonketoacidotic diabetes; a complication of steroid and immunosuppressive therapy, Diabetes **18:**107-110, 1969.

33. Taubin, H., and Matz, R.: Cerebral edema, diabetes insipidus, and sudden death during the treatment of diabetic ketoacidosis, Diabetes **17:**108-109, 1968.

34. Vecht, C. J., Van Woerkom, T. C. A. M., Teelken, A. W., and Minderhoud, J. M.: Homovanillic acid and 5-hydroxyindoleacetic acid cerebrospinal fluid levels, Arch. Neurol. **32:**792-797, 1975.

35. Watanabe, H., and Passonneau, J. V.: Cyclic adenosine monophosphate in cerebral cortex: alterations following trauma, Arch, Neurol. **32:**181-184, 1975.

36. Welch, K. M. A., Meyer, J. S., and Chee, A. N. C.: Evidence for disordered cyclic AMP metabolism in patients with cerebral infarction, Eur. Neurol. **13:** 144-154, 1975.

37. Wilson, W. S., and Meinert, J. K.: Extracellular hyperosmolarity secondary to high-protein nasogastric tube feeding, Ann. Intern. Med. **47:**585-590, 1957.

38. Woods, J. E., Zincke, H., Palumbo, P. J., and others: Hyperosmolar nonketotic syndrome and steroid diabetes; occurrence after renal transplantation, J.A.M.A. **231:**1261-1263, 1975.

39. Young, M. K., Seraile, L. G., and Brown, W. L.: Inhibition of glucose utilization following thermal injury: uptake studies by diaphragm in plasma from burned rats, Am. J. Physiol. **191:**119-123, 1957.

40. Zwetnow, N.: Effects of intracranial hypertension: acid base changes and lactate changes in CSF and brain tissue, Scand. J. Lab. Clin. Invest. Suppl. **102:**III:D, 1968.

Gastrointestinal sequelae

1. Aubrey, D. A., and Burns, G. P.: Topically administered prednisolone and the antral phase of gastric secretion, Arch. Surg. **105:**448-453, 1972.

2. Baronofsky, I., and Wangensteen, O. H.: Erosion or ulcer (gastric and/or duodenal) experimentally produced through the agency of chronic arterial spasm invoked by the intramuscular implantation of epinephrine or pitressin in beeswax, Bull. Am. Coll. Surg. **30:**59-60, 1945.

3. Black, J. W., Duncan, W. A. M., Durant, C. J., and others: Definition and antagonism of histamine H₂-receptors, Nature **236:**385-390, 1972.

4. Boles, R. S., Riggs, H. E., and Griffiths, J. O.: The role of the circulation in the production of peptic ulcer, Am. J. Dig. Dis. **6:**632-636, 1939.

5. Brimblecombe, R. W., Duncan, W. A. M., Durant, C. J., and others: Cimetidine-A non-thiourea H₂-receptor antagonist, J. Intern. Med. Res. **3:**86-92, 1975.

6. Carlson, H. E., and Ippoliti, A. F.: Cimetidine, an H₂-antihistamine, stimulates prolactin secretion in man, J. Clin. Endocrinol. Metab. **45:**367-370, 1977.

7. Chung, R. S. K., Field, M., and Silen, W.: Gastric permeability to H^+: effects of prednisolone and acetylsalicylic acid on the coefficient of H^+ diffusion, Gastroenterology **58:**1038, 1970.

8. Code, C. F.: Reflections on histamine, gastric secretion and the H$_2$-receptor, N. Engl. J. Med. **296:** 1459-1462, 1977.

9. Conn, H. O., and Blitzer, B. L.: Nonassociation of adrenocorticosteroid therapy and peptic ulcer, N. Engl. J. Med. **294:**473-479, 1976.

10. Craven, E. R., and Whittington, J. M.: Agranulocytosis four months after cimetidine therapy (letter), Lancet **2:**294-295, 1977.

11. Cushing, H.: Peptic ulcers and the interbrain, Surg. Gynecol. Obstet. **55:**1-34, 1932.

12. Davenport, H. W.: Gastric mucosal hemorrhage in dogs: effects of acid, aspirin, and alcohol, Gastroenterology **56:**439-449, 1969.

13. Davis, R. A., Wetzel, N., and Davis, L.: Acute upper alimentary tract ulceration and hemorrhage following neurosurgical operations, Surg. Gynecol. Obstet. **100:**51-58, 1955.

14. Desbaillets, L., and Menguy, R.: Inhibition of gastric mucous secretion by ACTH: an experimental study, Am. J. Dig. Dis. **12:**582-588, 1967.

15. Fletcher, D. G., and Harkins, H. N.: Acute peptic ulcer as a complication of major surgery, stress, or trauma, Surgery **36:**212-226, 1954.

16. French, J. D., Porter, R. W., von Amerongen, F. K., and others: Gastrointestinal hemorrhage and ulceration associated with intracranial lesions, Surgery **32:**395-407, 1952.

17. Glenn, F., and Grafe, W. R.: Surgical complications of adrenal steroid therapy, Ann. Surg. **165:**1023-1034, 1967.

18. Goodman, A. A., and Osborne, M. P.: An experimental model and clinical definition of stress ulceration, Surg. Gynecol. Obstet. **134:**563-571, 1972.

19. Gordon, M. J., Skillman, J. J., Zervas, N. T., and Silen, W.: Divergent nature of gastric mucosal permeability and gastric acid secretion in sick patients with general surgical and neurosurgical disease, Ann. Surg. **178:**285-294, 1973.

20. Gray, S. J., Benson, J. A., Reifenstein, R. W., and Spiro, H. M.: Chronic stress and peptic ulcer, J.A.M.A. **147:**1529-1537, 1951.

21. Gray, S. J., Benson, J. A., Spiro, H. M., and Reifenstein, R. W.: Effect of ACTH and cortisone upon the stomach: its significance in the normal and in peptic ulcer, Gastroenterology **19:**658-673, 1951.

22. Gray, S. J., Ramsey, C., Reifenstein, R. W., and Benson, J. A.: The significance of hormonal factors in the pathogenesis of peptic ulcer, Gastroenterology **25:**156-172, 1953.

23. Harjola, P. T., and Sivula, A.: Gastric ulceration following experimentally induced hypoxia and hemorrhagic shock: in vivo study of pathogenesis in rabbits, Ann. Surg. **163:**21-28, 1966.

24. Johnson, E. E.: Splanchnic hemodynamic response to passive hyperventilation, J. Appl. Physiol. **38:** 156-162, 1975.

25. Kamada, T., Fusamoto, H., Kawano, S., and others: Gastrointestinal bleeding following head injury: a clinical study of 433 cases, J. Trauma **17:**44-47, 1977.

26. Karch, S. B.: Upper gastrointestinal bleeding as a complication of intracranial disease, J. Neurosurg. **37:**27-29, 1972.

27. Klemperer, P., Penner, A., and Bernhein, A. I.: The gastro-intestinal manifestations of shock, Am. J. Dig. Dis. **7:**410-414, 1940.

28. MacDonald, A. S., Steele, B. J., and Bottomley, M. G.: Treatment of stress-induced upper gastrointestinal haemorrhage with metiamide, Lancet **1:**68-70, 1976.

29. Macdougall, B. R. D., Bailey, R. J., and Williams, R.: H$_2$-receptor antagonists and antacids in the prevention of acute gastrointestinal haemorrhage in fulminant hepatic failure, Lancet **1:**617-619, 1977.

30. Max, M., and Menguy, R.: Influence of adrenocorticotropin, cortisone, aspirin, and phenylbutazone on the rate of exfoliation and the rate of renewal of gastric mucosal cells, Gastroenterology **58:**329-336, 1976.

31. Menguy, R., and Masters, Y. F.: Effect of cortisone on mucoprotein secretion by gastric antrum of dogs: pathogenesis of steroid ulcer, Surgery **54:**19-28, 1963.

32. Menguy, R., and Masters, Y. F.: Effects of aspirin on gastric mucous secretion, Surg. Gyneol. Obstet. **120:**92-98, 1965.

33. Menguy, R., and Desbaillets, L.: Influence of phenylbutazone on gastric secretion of mucus, Proc. Soc. Exp. Biol. Med. **125:**1108-1111, 1967.

34. Norton, L., Greer, J., and Eiseman, B.: Gastric secretory response to head injury, Arch. Surg. **101:** 200-204, 1970.

35. O'Neill, J. A., Pruitt, B. A., Moncrief, J. A., and Switzer, W. E.: Studies related to the pathogenesis of Curling's ulcer, J. Trauma **7:**275-287, 1967.

36. Palmer, E. D., and Sherman, J. L.: Hypoxia of abnormal physiologic origin as the final common pathway in gastroduodenal ulcer genesis, Arch. Intern. Med. **101:**1106-1117, 1958.

37. Pruitt, B. A., Foley, F. D., and Moncrief, J. A.: Curling's ulcer: a clinical-pathology study of 323 cases, Ann. Surg. **172:**523-539, 1970.

38. Rokitansky, C.: A manual of pathologic anatomy, vol. 2, London, 1849-1854, The Sydenham Society.

39. Robert, A., and Nezamis, J. E.: Ulcerogenic property of steroids, Soc. Exp. Biol. Med. Proc. **99:**443-447, 1958.

40. Silen, W.: Stress ulcers, Viewpoints Dig. Dis. vol. 3, no. 5, 1971.

41. Skillman, J. J., Bushnell, L. S., Goldman, H., and Silen, W.: Respiratory failure, hypotension, sepsis, and jaundice, Am. J. Surg. **117:**523-530, 1969.

42. Skillman, J. J., and Silen, W.: Acute gastroduodenal "stress" ulceration: barrier disruption of varied pathogenesis? Gastroenterology **59:**478-482, 1970.

43. Skillman, J. J., Gould, S. A., Chung, R. S. K., and

Silen, W.: The gastric mucosal barrier: clinical and experimental studies in critically ill and normal man, and in the rabbit, Ann. Surg. **172:**564-584, 1970.

44. Smith, B. M., Skillman, J. J., Edwards, B. G., and Silen, W.: Permeability of the human gastric mucosa; alteration by acetylsalicylic acid and ethanol, N. Engl. J. Med. **285:**716-721, 1971.

45. Smith, J. B., and Willis, A. L.: Aspirin selectively inhibits prostaglandin production in human platelets, Nature (New Biol.) **231:**235-237, 1971.

46. Spencer, J. A., Morlock, C. G., and Sayre, G. P.: Lesions in upper portion of the gastrointestinal tract associated with intracranial neoplasms, Gastroenterology **37:**20-27, 1959.

47. Vane, J. R.: Prostaglandins and the aspirin-like drugs, Hosp. Prac. **7:**61-71, 1972.

48. Virchow, R.: Historisches, kritisches und positives zur lehre der unterleibsaffektionen, Arch. Pathol. Anat. **5:**281-375, 1853.

49. Watts, C. C., and Clark, K.: Gastric acidity in the comatose patient, J. Neurosurg. **30:**107-109, 1969.

50. Watts, C. C., and Clark, K.: Effects of an anticholinergic drug on gastric acid secretion in the comatose patient, Surg. Gynecol. Obstet. **130:**61-63, 1970.

51. Weinshelbaum, E. I., and Ferguson, D. J.: The effect of cortisone on mucosal resistance to ulceration, Gastroenterology **44:**52-56, 1963.

52. Weiss, H. J., Aledort, L. M., and Kochwa, S.: The effect of salicylates on the hemostatic properties of platelets in man, J. Clin. Invest. **47:**2169-2180, 1968.

53. Zucker, M. B., and Peterson, J.: Effect of acetylsalicylic acid, other nonsteroidal anti-inflammatory agents, and dipyridamole on human blood platelets, J. Lab. Clin. Med. **76:**66-75, 1970.

Skeletal sequelae

1. Bergsofsky, E. H.: Quantitation of the function of respiratory muscles in normal individuals and quadriplegic patients, Arch. Phys. Med. Rehab. **45:**575-580, 1964.

2. Braunstein, P. W.: Medical aspects of automotive crash injury research, J.A.M.A. **163:**249-255, 1957.

3. Bricker, D. L., Waltz, T. A., Telford, R. J., and Beall, A. C.: Major abdominal and thoracic trauma associated with spinal cord injury: problems in management, J. Trauma **11:**63-75, 1971.

4. Jernigan, W. R., and Gardner, W. C.: Carotid artery injuries due to closed cervical trauma, J. Trauma **11:**429-435, 1971.

5. Maull, K. I., and Sachatello, C. R.: Avoiding a pitfall in resuscitation: the painless cervical fracture, South. Med. J. **70:**477-478, 1977.

6. Rubsamen, D. S.: Head injury with unsuspected cervical fracture; a malpractice trap for the unwary physician, J.A.M.A. **229:**576-577, 1974.

7. Scher, A. T.: A plea for routine radiographic examination of the cervical spine after head injury, S. Afr. Med. J. **51:**885-887, 1977.

8. Shrago, G. G.: Cervical spine injuries; association with head trauma. A review of 50 patients, Am. J. Roentgenol. Radium Ther. Nucl. Med. **118:**670-673, 1973.

9. Tarlov, E.: Optimal management of head injuries, Int. Anesth. Clin. **14:**69-94, 1976.

10. White, P. R.: Horner's syndrome and its significance in the management of head and neck trauma, Br. J. Oral Surg. **14:**165-170, 1976.

11. Wyler, A. R., and Reynolds, A. F.: An intracranial complication of nasogastric intubation; case report, J. Neurosurg. **47:**297-298, 1977.

12

Barbiturate protection of the ischemic brain

EUGENE S. FLAMM
MYRON L. SELIGMAN
HARRY B. DEMOPOULOS

Because of the extent of cerebrovascular disease in our population and the devastating disability produced by stroke, a pharmacologic method of protecting the brain from cerebral ischemia would be of great benefit. Recent advances in cerebral revascularization and aneurysm surgery, as well as a better understanding and ability to control adherence and aggregation of platelets, have made cerebral ischemia and protection from it an important area of clinical investigation.[20,63] In addition to these microsurgical procedures, newer techniques for operative and intravascular obliteration of arteriovenous malformations would be greatly improved if an effective method of protecting patients from a major complication of these procedures, namely cerebral ischemia, could be developed.

The concept of protecting the brain against cerebral ischemia is not new. Thomas Willis was aware of the importance of collateral circulation to protect the brain from regional ischemia in the case of carotid artery occlusion.[78] He apparently envisioned a type of autoregulation to keep cerebral blood flow (CBF) constant. In a 1681 English translation of *Cerebri Anatome*, we find:

For inasmuch as the carotid arteries do communicate between themselves in various places, and

are mutually grafted; from thence a double benefit results, though of a contrary effect; because by this one and the same means care is taken, both lest the brain should be defrauded of its due watering of the blood, and also lest it should be overwhelmed by the too impetuous flowing of the swelling stream or torrent. As to the first, lest that should happen, one of the carotids perhaps being obstructed, the other might supply the provision of both; then lest the blood rushing with too full a torrent, should drown the channels and little ponds of the brain, the flood is chastised or hindered by an opposite emissary, as it were a floodgate, and so is commanded to return its flood, and haste backward by the same ways, and to return back with an ebbing tide.*

Many reports, both experimental and clinical, have discussed the use of hypothermia, steroids, hypertension, and low molecular weight dextran to offset the effects of reduced delivery of oxygen and glucose to the brain.[7,48,55,61] In reviewing these papers, it is necessary to differentiate between models that produced anoxia, hypoxia, or ischemia. Ischemic reduction of oxygen and substrate delivery to the brain is the most frequently encountered clinically in neurology and neurosurgery. A recent review has detailed the

---

*Willis, T.: The remaining medical works, London, 1681, Dring, Harper, Leigh and Martyn.

differences in the histopathologic changes in glia and neurons, between anoxic, hypoxic, or ischemic situations.[26]

Attempts to minimize the extent of tissue necrosis after arterial occlusion are not restricted to the brain. A number of animal studies involving a decrease in the size of acute myocardial infarcts following experimental coronary artery occlusion have been successful.[6,39] The pharmacologic agents employed included propanolol and hyaluronidase.[40]

BARBITURATE PROTECTION IN CEREBRAL ISCHEMIA

The administration of barbiturates as a means of protecting the brain against ischemia has recently been the subject of many investigations. Indications that barbiturates might mitigate the effects of cerebral hypoxia were suggested by Danish workers in the 1960s. Arnfred and Secher noted a greater tolerance of mice to hypoxia following barbiturate anesthesia.[1] Mice given thiopental (52 to 87 mg/kg) and exposed to 4% oxygen survived 10 times longer than nonanesthetized controls (45 as opposed to 4 minutes). These animals were studied at 24° C. Later, Wilhjelm and Arnfred compared survival of mice anesthetized with various anesthetics and placed in 100% nitrogen at 32° to 34° C. Thiopental prolonged survival more than halothane, ether, or cyclopropane.[77]

In 1972, Yatsu and his colleagues reported protection from brain ischemia in rabbits following the administration of methohexital. The model consisted of lowering arterial blood pressure and ventilating with 4% oxygen and 96% nitrogen. In methohexital-treated animals, a more rapid return of the EEG from an isoelectric state, as well as increased survival of the treated animals, was noted.[79]

Smith and co-workers studied the effects of several anesthetic techniques in a dog model of regional ischemia produced by occlusion of the middle cerebral and internal carotid arteries.[72] In three regimens that utilized pentobarbital or thiopental administered either before or shortly after the surgical occlusion was performed, the neurologic condition was normal in all but 1 of 18 animals. The size of the cerebral infarct produced was significantly smaller than in nontreated controls.

Similar models of focal cerebral ischemia have been developed in primates to study the effects of barbiturates. Hoff and co-workers reported a reduction in the size of infarcts in baboons pretreated for one hour with 60, 90, or 120 mg/kg of pentobarbital when compared to animals receiving only halothane anesthesia.[31] Statistical significance in the reduction of infarct size was seen in animals receiving 90 mg/kg or more, and there appeared to be a dose-dependent response.

In an experiment designed to simulate a clinical situation more closely, Michenfelder[47] sedated Java monkeys for 48 hours after middle cerebral artery occlusion while caring for the animals in a laboratory intensive care unit. Half of the animals received pentobarbital (14 mg/kg) 30 minutes after MCA occlusion and 7 mg/kg every 2 hours for the next 42 hours. The total dose was 100 mg/kg/24 hours. The control group was sedated with diazepam over a similar period of time. Both groups were paralyzed, intubated, and maintained on ventilators during sedation. After 48 hours the animals were allowed to awaken and were observed over the next five days. Animals treated with pentobarbital had fewer neurologic deficits during the week they were observed and at autopsy had fewer and smaller infarcts than the control group.

Barbiturates have also been reported to protect against ischemia, hypoxia, and cryogenic edema in other animals, such as dog, gerbil, cat.[3,9,42,51,52] Protection was achieved even when barbiturates were administered one hour after arterial occlusion.[12]

Several clinical studies have been reported in which beneficial effects have been attributed to the use of large doses of barbiturates. Marshall and Shapiro have treated 25 patients with uncontrollable, increased intracranial pressure (ICP) (>40 mm Hg) with barbiturates.[41] In 13 of these 25 patients, ICP was reduced below 15 mm Hg, thus maintaining cerebral perfusion pressure between 60 and 70 mm Hg. Ten of these severely injured, comatose patients made good functional improvement. Hoff and co-workers treated seven patients who had temporary or permanent occlusion of a major cerebral artery during aneurysm surgery with pentobarbital, 15 mg/kg/24 hours, over a 48-hour period.[32] Although not a controlled study, four of the seven patients did not develop neurologic deficits.

From this body of work, primarily of an experimental nature, considerable interest in the role of barbiturates in protection against cerebral ischemia has arisen. At the last Cerebral Blood Flow Meeting in Copenhagen in 1977, an entire section of the symposium was devoted to barbiturate therapy.[33]

POSSIBLE MECHANISMS OF BARBITURATE PROTECTION

Since several reports have indicated protective effects of barbiturates in cerebral ischemia, it is necessary to develop a good understanding of the possible mechanisms of action if a clinical protocol is to be developed. Most of the authors cited above have addressed themselves to this matter, but as yet there is no clear uniform explanation.

Another unknown step in the understanding of the effects of ischemia on the central nervous system is precisely how a reduction in blood supply initiates and produces the cellular changes leading to infarction. Although many reports of the changes produced by ischemia, seen by both light and electron microscopy, have appeared, no clear understanding of the pathologic events at a molecular level has emerged. It appears that phenomena such as major deprivation of oxygen in the brain, once thought to be immediately irrevocable, involve a sequence of pathologic changes, some of which are apparently reversible. If we are to gain an understanding of the mechanisms of protection by various physical and pharmacologic agents, we must first be able to answer the question of how reductions of the oxygen and glucose

supply lead to dissolution of cellular function and structure. The major emphasis, thus far, has been on the alterations in cerebral energy metabolism brought about by hypoxia.[69,70] The connection between the reduction of energy production and the development of autolytic changes has yet to be explained.

The mechanisms of barbiturate action that have been considered to explain protection against cerebral ischemia include reduction of cerebral blood flow (CBF), a decrease in utilization of oxygen ($CMRO_2$), an increase in activity of the hexose monophosphate shunt, production of hypothermia, reduction in cerebral edema, and control of pathologic free radical reactions initiated by reduced oxygen supply.*

A major paradox that exists in explaining the protective action of barbiturates is the observation that protection has not been seen with the use of other nonbarbiturate agents,[31,46] even though $CMRO_2$ is reduced by many types of anesthesia, including halothane. Halothane has actually increased the size of lesions produced.[72,73] Similarly, barbiturates also reduce CBF in addition to $CMRO_2$.[35,58] If an ideal drug were to be designed, one might expect that its actions would include a reduction in oxygen requirements, as well as an augmentation of cerebral blood flow, such as is seen with halothane. Several authors have addressed themselves to resolving this apparent conflict. Michenfelder has pointed out that the major brain effect of barbiturates rests not so much in the reduction of the oxygen requirement but in a decrease in the functional activity of the brain.[45] The reduction in $CMRO_2$ is a secondary response to decreased neuronal activity and is a reduction in oxygen requirement, rather than oxygen utilization. He studied this by anesthetizing dogs with increasing doses of thiopental until an isoelectric EEG was obtained. At this point, further increase in barbiturate dose failed to reduce $CMRO_2$ below a basal level, implying

---

*References 10, 23, 29, 44, 46, 47, 73.

that once functional activity had been halted, utilization of oxygen would not decline further.

A further problem in explaining the protective effect of barbiturates by reduction in $CMRO_2$ is the observation that much larger doses of barbiturates are required to protect the brain than are necessary to bring about a reduction in $CMRO_2$. This may indicate that the protective effect attributed to barbiturates is accomplished through some mechanism other than its action as an anesthetic as has been suggested in studies of radiation protection.[68] In several laboratories where the protective effects of large doses of barbiturates are under investigation, animals are anesthetized with barbiturates such as pentobarbital, 30 mg/kg; the large protective dose of barbiturate is then started at the time of, or shortly after, arterial occlusion. The nontreated controls reliably develop cerebral infarcts, in spite of anesthetic levels of barbiturates, whereas animals receiving large doses at or beyond "lethal" levels are protected.

Other mechanisms that have been invoked to explain the protective effect of barbiturates have included the production of an inverse intracerebral steal. The reduction in cerebral blood flow that accompanies high doses of barbiturates is brought about by vasoconstriction within nonischemic brain.[30] This does not occur in the ischemic area, since these vessels are maximally dilated as the result of the lesion, a situation described as vasomotor paralysis. As a result, blood may be preferentially shunted to the ischemic area with an overall reduction in cerebral blood flow and a concomitant decrease in intracranial pressure.

An alternate explanation has been a reduction in cerebral edema in the ischemic area. Barbiturates have been effective in the reduction of edema in cold injury models.[9] The difficulty in accepting this as the major protective mechanism is the inability of such potent antiedema agents, such as steroids and osmotic diuretics, to offer any substantial protection against cerebral ischemia.[60]

One of the effects of the administration of barbiturates in the dose range under consideration is reduction in body temperature. Since each degree Celsius of fall in temperature produces a 6% to 8% reduction in metabolic requirements, part of the protection seen may be related to hypothermia.[61,71] It has long been observed that any degree of ischemia even including total cardiac arrest is tolerated better at low body temperature. The original studies of Arnfred, Secher, and Wilhjelm were done at lowered body temperatures.[1,77]

For several years, we have considered the possibility that a variety of insults to the central nervous system, such as ischemia, direct trauma, and freeze lesions, may initiate a series of pathologic free radical reactions that may account for changes in biomembranes through alterations in molecular configuration and composition.[13-16,21-24,66] These pathologic changes in different types of cell membranes may then be responsible for defects in the functions of subcellular organelles, such as mitochondria and lysosomes, and in the barrier functions of plasma membranes of endothelial cells, glia, and neurons. To test this hypothesis, we have used both in vivo and in vitro models to study the effects of these conditions on various parameters. The studies discussed below indicated that cerebral ischemia in an experimental model utilizing transorbital microsurgical occlusion of the middle cerebral artery (MCAO) was capable of initiating free radical membrane damage within the distribution of the occluded vessel. We therefore investigated the possibility that protection reported by the administration of barbiturates in similar ischemia models might operate by inhibiting these pathologic free radical reactions in membranes.

EFFECTS OF BARBITURATES ON PATHOLOGIC FREE RADICAL REACTIONS

We first studied the effect of MCAO in cats on the content of the naturally occurring antioxidant, ascorbic acid, to determine the amount of available reduced ascorbic acid.[24] Ascorbic acid was extracted from brain in dimethyl sulfoxide (DMSO) and converted to its free radical state as monodehydroascorbic acid. This was assayed by electron paramagnetic resonance (epr) spectrometry.[15] By one hour after MCAO, we noted an approximate 25% decrease in ascorbic acid within the ischemic area compared to the contralateral middle cerebral artery territory. By five hours, this reduction was 50% of control. This has been a reliable indicator of free radical damage, as demonstrated by the consumption of this antioxidant within in vitro model systems, in which pathologic free radical reactions can be produced and quantitated. Ascorbic acid added to radical damaged liposomal model membrane systems disappears in a time course that parallels membrane free radical damage; nondamaged control liposomes show no consumption of the added ascorbic acid.[15] The implication of the MCAO experiments is that this ubiquitous antioxidant, ascorbic acid, present in higher concentrations in the central nervous system than anywhere except for the adrenals, is consumed in an attempt to control pathologic free radical reactions.[15] The CNS has efficient mechanisms in the choroid plexus to actively pump ascorbic acid from the plasma into the cerebrospinal fluid (CSF) to produce high CSF ascorbic acid levels; neural tissue cells also actively transport ascorbic acid into the cells and further increase the parenchymal ascorbic acid content.[74] These active ascorbic acid pumps explain the otherwise anomalous finding of very high levels of an aqueous-soluble substance in the most lipid-rich organ system. The turnover of CNS ascorbic acid is 2% per hour. Our findings of 25% decrease in ascorbic acid content after the first hour following MCAO and 50% after five hours cannot be explained by natural turnover coupled with a failure to deliver replacement supplies, since that explanation would account for only a 2% and 10% reduction, respectively.

The mechanism by which cerebral ischemia might initiate pathologic free radical mechanisms within membrane lipids centers

Table 12-1. Components of the respiratory chain

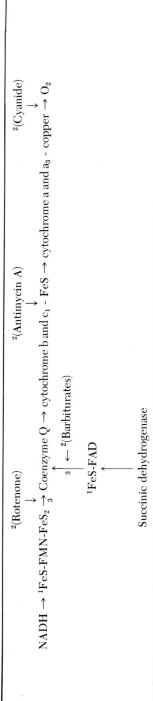

$$NADH \rightarrow {}^1FeS\text{-}FMN\text{-}FeS_2 \xrightarrow{3} Coenzyme\ Q \rightarrow cytochrome\ b\ and\ c_1 \text{-} FeS \rightarrow cytochrome\ a\ and\ a_3 \text{-} copper \rightarrow O_2$$

^{2}(Rotenone) ^{2}(Antimycin A) ^{2}(Cyanide)

^{2}(Barbiturates)

^{1}FeS-FAD

Succinic dehydrogenase

^{1}FeS = Nonheme iron and sulfur protein centers; several different FeS centers exist.
^{2}Inhibitors of specific points in respiration.
^{3}The interactions of the FeS centers, flavin moieties, and CoQ normally involve free radicals.

about changes in several members of the electron transport chain (Table 12-1).[75,76] Reduction of oxygen at the terminus of the electron transport chain favors the maintenance of members of the carrier system in a reduced state. Coenzyme Q (CoQ) or ubiquinone is normally found as a semiquinone free radical during active electron transport in mitochondria.[62] Under normal circumstances, it is well controlled by tight association with the electron transport system. When oxygen supplies are reduced, the electron transport factors disassociate and substances such as CoQ are no longer controlled.[37] Since Coenzyme Q is lipid soluble and lies within the lipoidal, hydrophobic portion of the inner mitochondrial membrane, the process of ischemia or hypoxia introduces an uncontrolled substance that readily assumes a radical configuration into that portion of the membrane that is most susceptible to free radical damage, i.e., the hydrophobic area with its many polyunsaturated fatty acids in phospholipids.[43] CoQ readily undergoes autoxidation when it dissociates from the other electron transport factors. There is sufficient O_2 to support this autoxidation, as well as the pathologic lipid free radical reactions that ensue, for two reasons: (1) the models of cerebral ischemia are *not* anoxic; oxygen content, brought in by collaterals, is about 20% to 30% of normal; (2) O_2 is seven times more soluble than water within nonpolar lipoidal environments.[36]

Additional evidence supports this hypothesis. Boveris has shown that high rates of production of hydrogen peroxide occur when electron transport is blocked by antimycin A.[4,5] He has localized this to the step between Coenzyme Q and cytochrome b. The interaction of the reduced CoQ (semiquinone) with oxygen leads to the production of the superoxide radical ($\cdot O_2^-$). The production of hydrogen peroxide is dependent on the presence of the superoxide radical and the enzyme superoxide dismutase.[34]

$$\cdot O_2^- + \cdot O_2^- + 2H^+ \rightarrow H_2O_2 + O_2 \qquad [1]$$

Of greater significance in terms of producing radical species that may damage membrane systems is the nonenzymatic Haber-Weiss reaction, which can generate both hydroxyl radicals ($\cdot OH$) and singlet oxygen ($^1O_2$), both felt to be likely initiators of lipid peroxidation in membranes.[34]

$$H_2O_2 + \cdot O_2^- \rightarrow OH + OH^- + {}^1O_2 \qquad [2]$$

Most of these studies have been carried out in vitro with mitochondria obtained from various organs. While there is no data to support these reactions in vivo within the central nervous system, there is a significant amount of data to indicate that these very reactions ([1] and [2]) form the basis for the killing of microorganisms by phagocytic cells.[2]

In support of the hypothesis that barbiturates act as antioxidants is the recent observation[68] that pentobarbitone directly protects against the acute effects of ionizing radiation, a modality known to induce major lipid free radical reactions within membranes.[57] The amelioration of radiation injury by pentobarbitone was beyond the protective effect that could be expected as a result of the vasospastic and hypothermic properties of barbiturates.[68] Significantly, other workers[56,57] have shown that ionizing radiation leads to the production of $\cdot O_2^-$ and that the administration of superoxide dismutase will protect against radiation injury by blocking formation of the $\cdot O_2^-$-related radicals ($\cdot OH$, $^1O_2$). Furthermore, lysosomal membranes can be damaged and labilized by $\cdot OH$ and $\cdot O_2^-$ radicals and result in leakage of their hydrolytic enzymes.[25] This offers yet another mechanism by which free radical reactions, once initiated, might contribute to cellular autolysis. In addition to producing structural changes leading to autolysis in biomembranes by free radical reaction, the release of lysosomal enzymes themselves may further the intracellular pathology.

What interactions of the barbiturates with these molecular events within organelles and membranes are known? The fact that barbiturate-phospholipid interactions occur has been demonstrated by Novak and Swift with nuclear magnetic resonance (NMR) studies.[53] A close hydrophobic and ionic association between the barbiturate and the membrane phospholipids was demonstrated by a decrease in the different NMR signals that can be ascribed to the various parts of the phospholipid molecule.[53]

Barbiturates, as well as other anesthetics, have been shown in many studies to block electron transport.[8,19] How important this is to the overall mechanism of anesthesia has been the subject of many studies. Of particular interest is the observation that barbiturates like Rotenone block electron transport between the flavins (FMN and FAD), and coenzyme Q (Table 12-1).[8,19,37] Such a locus of interaction of barbiturates would favor the maintenance of electron carriers beyond this point of blockade in a nonreduced state. This would prevent the formation of the semiquinone and maintain CoQ in its nonradical configuration in spite of a reduction in available oxygen. It is our hypothesis that prevention of free radical reactions may represent an important mechanism by which barbiturates mitigate the effects of cerebral ischemia.

We have examined the interaction of methohexital with CoQ in vitro by epr spectrometry.[23] By dissolving CoQ in alkaline ethanol with tetrahydrofuran (THF) to enhance CoQ solubility, a multiline spectrum characteristic of the CoQ radical was obtained. Under these conditions the decay of the epr signal was 45 minutes. Addition of equimolar amounts of methohexital resulted in an immediate loss of signal, indicating a quenching effect of methohexital upon the CoQ radical (Fig. 12-1).

To study the interaction of barbiturates with free radicals occurring in membrane phospholipids, an in vitro system of lipid peroxidation in liposomes was utilized.[64] Liposomes were prepared with ovolecithin according to the method of Pietronigro and co-workers.[59] Peroxidation was induced by exposure to ultraviolet irradiation for up to 90 minutes.[16] Thiopental, in concentrations of 1.08×10^{-2}, 1.08×10^{-3}, and 1.08×10^{-4} M was added to separate liposomal suspensions prior to irradiation. At various time intervals, samples were removed and the

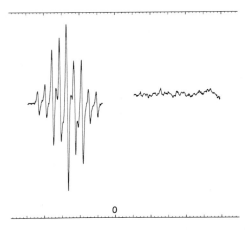

Fig. 12-1. The free radical epr signal of coenzyme Q is displayed on the left. It is the typical multiline spectrum of CoQ in an alkaline ethanol solution with tetrahydrofuran added. Under the conditions of the experiment, the signal had a decay time of 45 minutes. However, when equimolar amounts of methohexital were added, the CoQ signal was immediately eliminated, as shown on the right.

thiobarbituric acid (TBA) test was used to detect malonaldehyde, an indicator of lipid peroxidation in polyunsaturated fatty acids.[65] As the concentration of thiopental was increased, there was a proportional decrease in the production of malonaldehyde for any given time period of irradiation (Fig. 12-2). This suppression of malonaldehyde production in liposomes undergoing peroxidation suggests that barbiturates, in this case thiopental, may serve as an antioxidant in a manner similar to such normally occurring substances as ascorbic acid and alpha tocopherol.[38] Both of these latter agents have been shown to be effective in preventing peroxidative damage to polyunsaturated fatty acids.[11,15]

To study the effects of barbiturates on cerebral ischemia, we carried out two sets of experiments in cats undergoing MCAO by a transorbital microsurgical approach to eliminate any manipulative trauma to the brain. The first group of experiments consisted of analyses by gas chromatography–mass spectroscopy of cell membrane components,

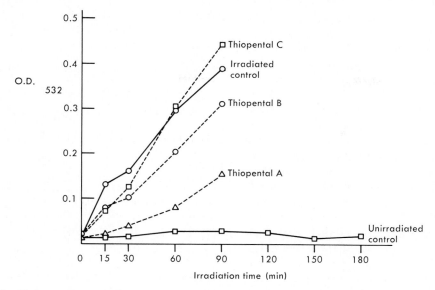

Fig. 12-2. Liposomes in aqueous suspension were exposed to ultraviolet light and the resultant amount of malonaldehyde, a free radical product, measured by the TBA reaction. Graded amounts of thiopental were added to identically treated aliquots and the rates of free radical damage compared to irradiated liposomes *without* thiopental. A nonirradiated control showed no TBA reaction. A dose-response is indicated, in that smaller amounts of thiopental conferred less protection: $C = 1.08 \times 10^{-4}$ M, $B = 1.08 \times 10^{-3}$ M, and $A = 1.08 \times 10^{-2}$ M.

cholesterol, and phospholipid fatty acids. In addition to this, ascorbic acid content was measured. The second group of experiments was designed to examine brain and vessels within the parenchyma following MCAO by scanning electron microscopy (SEM).

Treated animals received a continuous infusion of methohexital (25 mg/kg/hr) beginning at the time of the middle cerebral artery occlusion and continuing up through the time of sacrifice, one, three, or five hours after occlusion. This particular barbiturate was selected because of its high lipid solubility.[67] If the site of action of barbiturates in protecting the brain from ischemia is at the membrane level, the drug should theoretically have a high degree of lipid solubility to gain access to the hydrophobic midzone of biomembranes.

In the first set of experiments, the parameters chosen for testing were two membrane components, namely cholesterol and phospholipid fatty acids, both saturated and unsaturated. In addition, the ascorbic acid levels as discussed above were determined.

Cholesterol and fatty acids were measured by gas chromatography–mass spectroscopy, as previously described from this laboratory.[49]

Sodium methohexital (25 mg/kg/hr) was given intravenously to 18 cats for five hours following MCA occlusion. Blood pressure and ventilation were supported, as needed, to maintain normal arterial pressure and blood gases. In 12 cats, the same procedures were carried out, except no sodium methohexital was administered. At the end of five hours, animals were sacrificed and the brains were sectioned coronally. A symmetrical wedge of tissue was obtained from each side of a 6 mm thick slice taken through the middle cerebral artery territory, including cortex, white matter, and basal ganglia. Gray and white matter were used for ascorbic acid determinations, while only white matter was extracted for cholesterol. Symmetrical areas of cortex within this slice were used for determination of phospholipid fatty acids. Ascorbic acid was determined by measuring the amplitude of the ascorbyl radical signal by epr spectrometry after extracting the tissue in DMSO.[15] Cholesterol was determined by gas chromatography after extraction in ethyl acetate and complete silylation. The fatty acid profiles of the phospholipids of gray matter were studied by comparing the cortex of the ischemic area with comparable cortex in the contralateral hemisphere. The phospholipids were extracted selectively and then the fatty acids were hydrolyzed and simultaneously methylated. Measured aliquots were assayed by gas chromatography, using standards of pentadecanoate. The peaks were identified by comparison of the retention times of known fatty acid methyl ester standards, as well as by gas chromatography–mass spectroscopy. The areas of each peak were integrated and normalized to the pentadecanoate standard and to the weights of the tissue samples. The saturated fatty acids, palmitic (16:0) and stearic (18:0), and the unsaturated fatty acids, arachidonic (20:4) and docosahexaenoic (22:6), were compared in the ischemic versus the contralateral hemispheres. The effects of methohexital on these parameters were also evaluated.

Middle cerebral artery occlusion for five hours without the administration of the large doses of sodium methohexital resulted in the following changes, comparing the results from the ischemic area to the contralateral nonischemic middle cerebral artery territory. Ascorbic acid decreased 44%; cholesterol decreased 23%. The unsaturated fatty acids, docosahexaenoic and arachidonic, were decreased 27% and 37%, respectively, on the ischemic side. Minor changes were noted in the relative amount of the saturated fatty acids, palmitic and stearic, when comparing the two sides. Palmitic was reduced 9%, and stearic was reduced by 11%. In the animals treated with methohexital, no significant differences were noted between the ischemic and nonischemic sides in either ascorbic acid or cholesterol. The unsaturated, as well as the saturated, fatty acids showed no significant decreases on the right side following treatment with sodium methohexital. These results are summarized in Table 12-2.

In the second set of experiments, we

Table 12-2. Percent reductions in membrane lipids and antioxidants following MCAO for five hours

	Control (9%)	Treated*
Phospholipids		
Palmitic (16:0)	9	<3
Stearic (18:0)	11	<3
Arachidonic (20:4)	37	<5
Docosahexaenoic (22:6)	27	<5
Cholesterol	23	0
Ascorbic acid	44	4

*Treatment was methohexital, 25 mg/kg/hr, intravenously, starting at the time of occlusion and maintained for five hours.

studied the microcirculation within the parenchyma of the territory of the occluded MCA, compared to that of the contralateral MCA, with and without large doses of methohexital, at one and three hours, by SEM. The methods employed for fixation and tissue preparation have been previously detailed in our SEM work on impacted spinal cords.[17] Cats were sacrificed by intra-arterial perfusion with glutaraldehyde under conditions that assured optimum perfusion; coronal sections of the brain, 2 mm thick, were sliced. These were washed, dehydrated in graded ethanol, and critical point dried; coatings of gold-platinum 200 Å thick were applied, and entire coronal sections were mounted on stubs, making it possible to maintain landmarks and orientation in going from very low (×40) to high magnifications (×40,000). An AMR SEM was used for these studies at an accelerating voltage of 20 kV. A minimum of 100 vessels in the microcirculation of each MCA territory was examined. Ten cats were studied: two unoperated controls; two MCAO untreated and sacrificed at one hour; two MCAO untreated and sacrificed at three hours; two MCAO treated with methohexital and sacrificed at one hour; two MCAO treated with methohexital and sacrificed at three hours.

The results are depicted in Figs. 12-3 to 12-8. The low-power overview, topologically, is shown in Fig. 12-3, with successively

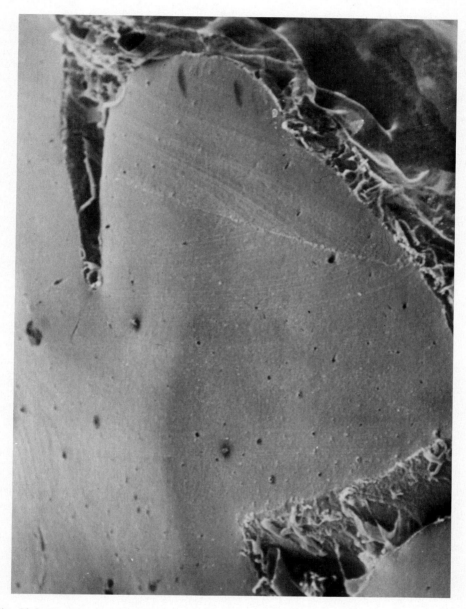

Fig. 12-3. Low-power, scanning electron micrograph of the cut surface of a coronal section through cat cerebrum in the territory of the middle cerebral artery (MCA). This is a nonoperated control, and the distinction between gray and white can be seen in the single gyrus and its bordering sulci. The leptomeninges are on the right. Blood vessels are seen as distinctively outlined black circles or ellipses, particularly in the gray matter of the gyrus toward the lower, left side. ($\times$ 30.)

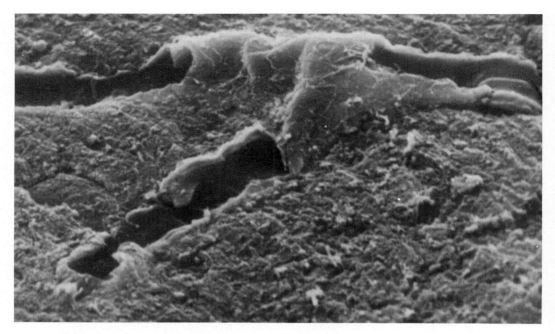

Fig. 12-4. A branching arteriole from the cut surface of a coronal section in the MCA territory of a nonoperated control. (×1000.)

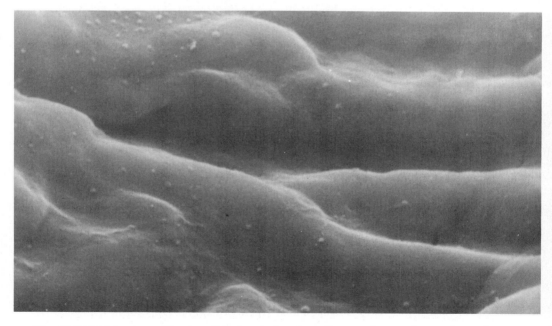

Fig. 12-5. A higher magnification of the luminal surface of a normal arteriole, similar to that in Fig. 12-4. The undulating surface is due to the contraction of elastic and muscle fibers, secondary to perfusion-fixation. Normal endothelial surface villi are present. (×20,000.)

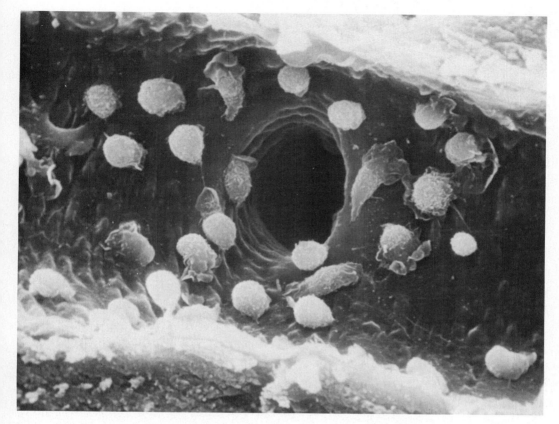

Fig. 12-6. An arteriole in the cortical territory of a three-hour occluded MCA. Numerous lymphocytoid, monocytoid cells adhere to the endothelium. The undulations of the luminal surface are due to the normal contraction of elastic and muscle fibers in the arteriolar wall. (×2300.)

greater magnifications to show an arteriole (Fig. 12-4) and its endothelial lining at still higher magnification (Fig. 12-5). The consequences of MCAO within the distal, parenchymal microcirculation are shown in Figs. 12-6 to 12-8; these include adherence of platelets and lymphocytoid-monocytoid cells to the damaged endothelium. Changes were progressively more severe at three hours than at one hour. Treatment with methohexital ameliorated but did not completely eliminate all of the changes in the microcirculation, as shown in Figs. 12-9 and 12-10.

The endothelium in untreated MCAO territories, in addition to having adherent blood cells, showed pathologic changes. Most notable was a loosening of the endothelium,

seen as a wrinkling of the surface. Loosening of the endothelial cells is a feature of decreased or absent oxygenation, as shown by the SEM work of others with hypoxic/anoxic perfusions of large vessels such as the carotid artery.[27] This change can be seen in our electron micrographs and appears to be absent in the methohexital-treated animals.

A possible correlation between the lipid free radical damage measured in MCAOs and the adherence of platelets and leukocytes seen by SEM in MCAOs lies in the reported effects of lipid peroxides on the synthesis of a specific blood vessel prostaglandin, PGI_2.[50] This substance, PGI_2, also known as prostacyclin, is produced by blood vessels from prostaglandin endoperoxides, which in turn

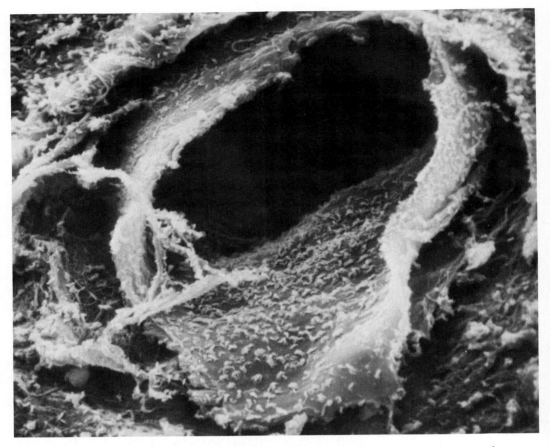

Fig. 12-7. A venule in the cortical territory of a three-hour occluded MCA. Numerous platelets adhere to the endothelial surface. (×6000.)

are synthesized by *normal, controlled* free radical oxidations of arachidonic acid (20:4)[54]; PGI_2 is the substance responsible for the normal nonadherent nature of endothelium.[28] The vessels actively keep their luminal surfaces free and clean by producing PGI_2, which is a potent disaggregator of platelets.[28] PGI_2 normally counterbalances the ever present thromboxane A_2 (TxA_2), which is a powerful aggregator of platelets and is produced by platelets.[18] PGI_2 and TxA_2 are normally in balanced production.[18] However, in the presence of lipid peroxides, PGI_2 synthesis is *selectively* inhibited and platelet/leukocyte adherence and aggregation begin immediately, under the influence of TxA_2.[50] If ischemia results in lipid free radical damage, as our results indicate, then lipid peroxides

are formed as radical products; these, in turn, could lead to decreased PGI_2 synthesis and cause the SEM changes that we have observed. The ability of methohexital to keep the microcirculation relatively free of adherent platelets and leukocytes and to maintain the endothelium as a flat, smooth lining, in MCAO territories is in keeping with the free radical hypothesis. Others have recently suggested that antioxidants be used to control adherence of platelets, atherosclerotic and other vascular occlusions in order to prevent the formation of lipid peroxides by pathologic free radical reactions.[18] Whether other substances with the antioxidant properties of barbiturates will protect against cerebral ischemia remains to be studied as a further test of the free radical hypothesis.

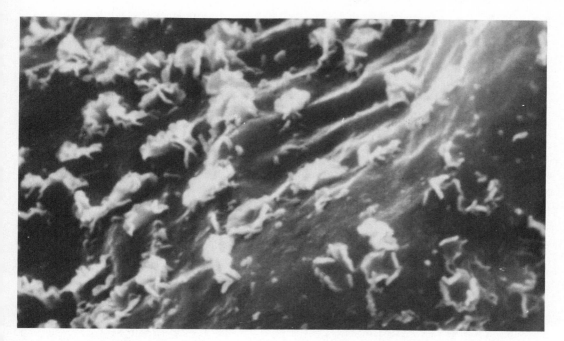

Fig. 12-8. A higher magnification of the luminal surfaces of Fig. 12-7. The platelets can be seen in greater detail. Some have multiple pseudopodal extensions, and others have complex surface folds. The endothelium has a wrinkled or loosened appearance. (×26,000.)

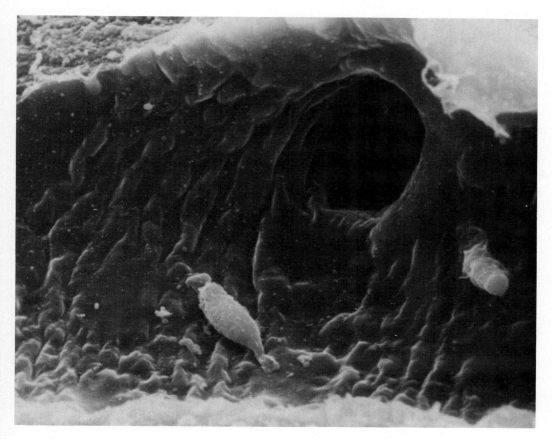

Fig. 12-9. An arteriole in the cortical territory of a three-hour occluded MCA, treated with methohexital, 25 mg/kg/hr. This is representative of decreased adherence of leukocytes as a result of barbiturate treatment. Compare with Fig. 12-6. (×2800.)

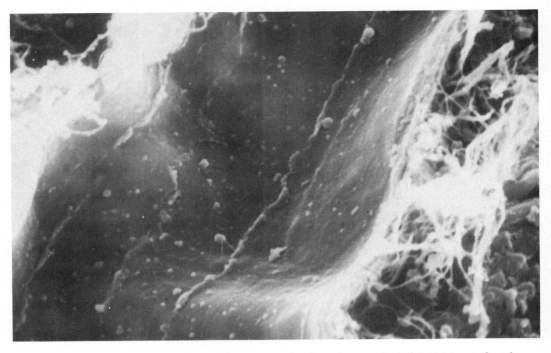

Fig. 12-10. A venule in the cortical territory of a three-hour occluded MCA treated with methohexital. An occasional platelet can be seen; however, the numbers are greatly decreased. Compare to Figs. 12-7 and 12-8. The endothelium appears tightly apposed to its substratum and is not loosened as it is in Fig. 12-8. ($\times$18,000.)

CONCLUSIONS

Four areas have been considered for possible explanations of the mechanism of action by which barbiturates protect against cerebral ischemia. Most frequently cited has been the reduction in $CMRO_2$. This is difficult to accept as a major mechanism of action for several reasons. Other agents, such as inhalation anesthetics, can produce a similar amount of reduction in oxygen utilization. Halothane anesthesia produces an almost equal reduction in $CMRO_2$, yet has been noted to potentiate ischemic lesions. As noted previously, the reduction seen in $CMRO_2$ following barbiturate anesthesia may be secondary to a reduction in neuronal function. This may represent a decrease in oxygen utilization but not in oxygen requirements of the cell. A further problem in accepting this as the mechanism of action is the observation by Hoff and Nemoto that doses far in excess of those required to re-

duce $CMRO_2$ are necessary to afford any degree of protection.[31,32,52] We conclude that none of these offers an adequate explanation for the mechanism of action. The observation that $CMRO_2$ is decreased is real enough, but we would suggest that this may be a secondary phenomenon.

The second area that has been discussed by Hanson and co-workers and Michenfelder concerns the increased flow produced by an inverse intracerebral steal.[30,46] Smith has discussed this, and the conclusions of these workers do not support this as a mechanism beyond a theoretical consideration.[73] When regional cerebral blood flow has been determined within ischemic areas of the brain in animals treated with barbiturates and inhalation anesthetics, no actual increase has been noted.[30] Our observations on the status of endothelial surfaces within the ischemic territory do suggest that at a capillary level perfusion may be improved by the administration of barbiturates. The involvement of barbiturates with platelet aggregating mechanisms will require further studies, but certainly this would be a fruitful area to pursue.

The reduction of cerebral edema by barbiturates has been demonstrated in models of cold injury but not as yet in cerebral ischemia. The failure of other agents, such as steroids and osmotic diuretics, to protect against cerebral ischemia would make control of edema in ischemia an unlikely mechanism for protection.

We have dealt at some length with the involvement of barbiturates with the electron transport chain. This offers some understanding at the molecular level of how reactions known to damage biomembranes can be inhibited. The evidence that barbiturates may prevent the formation of radical species within the mitochondrial membranes offers a possible explanation for their protective effect. Added to this is the observation that certain barbiturates have antioxidant properties. Thus, in addition to preventing the initiation of free radical reactions, barbiturates may be capable of quenching those reactions once started; in doing this, they assume some of the actions of normally occurring antioxidants, such as ascorbic acid, which may rapidly be depleted once ischemia occurs. Although we postulate that damage starts within mitochondrial membranes, it probably spreads rapidly to other cell membranes because of the proximities and continuities of mitochondrial membranes with other cell membranes.

Future work must define in more precise terms how this protection is brought about, and by which portion of the barbiturate molecule. One area that is currently under investigation in our laboratory is the development of a nonsedating analog of barbiturates. If the hypothesis that barbiturates are acting by controlling free radical reactions is accurate, it should be possible to design a barbiturate derivative that would retain those properties and yet not require the anesthetic sedative effects. An analogous situation is the use of saccharine and cyclamates as sweeteners without the caloric requirements of glucose. These agents have the molecular configuration to achieve the desired result, in this case, sweetening, without the other attributes of glucose. Similarly, one should be able to develop a protective agent that does not produce sedation as a side effect.

REFERENCES

1. Arnfred, I., and Secher, O.: Anoxia and barbiturates—tolerance to anoxia in mice influenced by barbiturates, Arch. Int. Pharmacodyn. Ther. **139:** 67, 1962.
2. Babior, B. M.: Oxygen-dependent microbial killing by phagocytes, N. Engl. J. Med. **298:**359, 1978.
3. Bleyaert, A. L., Nemoto, E. M., Safar, P., Stezoski, S. W., Moossy, J., Rao, G. R., and Michell, J.: Thiopental amelioration of postischemic encephalopathy in monkeys, Acta Neurol. Scand. **56**(suppl. 64):144, 1977.
4. Boveris, A., Cadenas, E., and Stoppani, A. O. M.: Role of ubiquinone in the mitochondrial generation of hydrogen peroxide, Biochem. J. **156:**435, 1976.
5. Boveris, A.: Mitochondrial production of superoxide radical and hydrogen peroxide. In Reivich, M., Coburn, R., Lahiri, S., and Chance, B., editors: Tissue hypoxia and ischemia, advances in experimental medicine and biology, New York, 1977, Plenum Publishing Corp., vol. 78, p. 67.
6. Caride, V. J., and Zoret, B. L.: Liposome accumulation in regions of experimental myocardial infarction, Science **198:**735, 1977.
7. Carlsson, C., Hägerdal, M., and Siesjö, B. K.: Protective effect of hypothermia in cerebral oxygen deficiency caused by arterial hypoxia, Anesthesiology **44:**27, 1976.
8. Chance, B., and Hallunger, G.: Inhibition of electron and energy transfer in mitochondria. I. Effects of amytal, thiopental, rotenone, progesterone and methylene glycol, J. Biol. Chem. **278:**418, 1963.
9. Clasen, R. A., Pandolfi, S., and Casey, D., Jr.: Furosemide and pentobarbital in cryogenic cerebral injury and edema, Neurology **24:**642, 1974.
10. Cohen, P. J.: Effect of anesthetics on mitochondrial function, Anesthesiology **39:**153, 1973.
11. Combs, G. R., Jr., Noguchi, T., and Scott, M. L.: Mechanisms of action of selenium and vitamin E in protection of biological membranes, Fed. Proc. **34:**2090, 1975.
12. Corkill, G., Chikovani, O. K., McLeish, I., McDonald, L. W., and Youmans, J. R.: Timing of pentobarbital administration for brain protection in experimental stroke, Surg. Neurol. **5:**147, 1976.
13. Demopoulos, H. B.: The basis of free radical pathology, Fed. Proc. **32:**1859, 1973.
14. Demopoulos, H. B.: Control of free radicals in biologic systems, Fed. Proc. **32:**1903, 1973.
15. Demopoulos, H., Flamm, E., Seligman, M., Poser,

R., Pietronigro, D., and Ransohoff, J.: Molecular pathology of lipids in CNS membranes. In Jöbsis, F. F., editor: Oxygen and physiological function, Dallas, 1976, Professional Information Library, p. 491.

16. Demopoulos, H. B., Flamm, E. S., Seligman, M. L., Jorgensen, E., and Ransohoff, J.: Antioxidant effects of barbiturates in model membranes undergoing free radical damage, Acta Neurol. Scand. **56** (suppl. 64):152, 1977.

17. Demopoulos, H. B., Yoder, M., Gutman, E. G., Seligman, M. L., Flamm, E. S., and Ransohoff, J.: The fine structure of endothelial surfaces in the microcirculation of experimentally injured feline spinal cords, Scanning Electron Microscopy/1978, vol. 2, p. 677.

18. Editorial: Prevention of thrombosis, The Lancet **1**: 127, 1977.

19. Ernster, L., Dallner, G., and Azzone, G. F.: Differential effects of rotenone and amytal on mitochondrial electron and energy transfer, J. Biol. Chem. **238**:1124, 1963.

20. Fields, W. S., Lemak, N. A., Frankowski, R. F., and Hardy, R. J.: Controlled trial of aspirin in cerebral ischemia, Stroke **8**:301, 1977.

21. Flamm, E. S., Demopoulos, H. B., Seligman, M. L., Tomasula, J. J., DeCrescito, V., and Ransohoff, J.: Ethanol potentiation of central nervous system trauma, J. Neurosurg. **46**:328, 1977.

22. Flamm, E. S., Demopoulos, H. B., Seligman, M. L., and Ransohoff, J.: Possible molecular mechanisms of barbiturate-mediated protection in regional cerebral ischemia, Acta Neurol. Scand. **56**(suppl. 64):150, 1977.

23. Flamm, E. S., Demopoulos, H. B., Seligman, M. L., Mitamura, J. A., and Ransohoff, J.: Barbiturates and free radicals. In Popp, A. J., Bourke, R. S., Nelson, L. R., and Kimelberg, H. K., editors: Neural trauma, New York, 1979, Raven Press, pp. 289-296.

24. Flamm, E. S., Demopoulos, H. B., Seligman, M. L., Poser, R. G., and Ransohoff, J.: Free radicals in cerebral ischemia, Stroke **9**:445, 1978.

25. Fong, K.-L., McCay, P. B., and Poyer, J. L.: Evidence that peroxidation of lysosomal membranes is initiated by hydroxyl free radicals produced during flavin enzyme activity, J. Biol. Chem. **248**:7792, 1973.

26. Garcia, J. H.: The cellular pathology of hypoxic, ischemic injuries: ultrastructure. In Jöbsis, F. F., editor: Oxygen and physiological function, Dallas, 1976, Professional Information Library, p. 277.

27. Gertz, S. D., Rennels, M. L., Forbes, M. S., Kawamura, J., Suraga, T., and Nelson, E.: Endothelial cell damage by temporary arterial occlusion with surgical clips: study of the clip site by scanning and transmission electron microscopy, J. Neurosurg. **45**:514, 1976.

28. Gryglewski, R. J., Bunting, S., Moncada, S.,

Flower, R. J., and Vane, J. R.: Arterial walls are protected against deposition of platelet thrombi by a substance (prostaglandin X) which they make from prostaglandin endoperoxide, Prostaglandins **12**:685, 1976.

29. Hakim, A. M., and Moss, G.: Cerebral effects of barbiturate: shift from "energy" to synthesis metabolism for cellular viability, Surg. Forum **27**:497, 1976.

30. Hanson, E. J., Jr., Anderson, R. E., and Sundt, T. M., Jr.: Influence of cerebral vasoconstricting and vasodilating agents on blood flow in regions of focal ischemia, Stroke **6**:642, 1975.

31. Hoff, J. T., Smith, A. L., Hankinson, H. L., and Nielsen, S. L.: Barbiturate protection from cerebral infarction in primates, Stroke **6**:28, 1975.

32. Hoff, J. T., Pitts, L. H., Spetzler, R., and Wilson, C. B.: Barbiturates for protection from cerebral ischemia in aneurysm surgery, Acta Neurol. Scand. **56**(suppl. 64):158, 1977.

33. Ingvar, D. H., and Lassen, N. A., editors: Cerebral function metabolism and circulation (Copenhagen 1977), Acta Neurol. Scand. **56**(suppl. 64): 1977.

34. Kellogg, E. W., III, and Fridovich, I.: Superoxide, hydrogen peroxide, and singlet oxygen in lipid peroxidation by a xanthine oxidase system, J. Biol. Chem. **250**:8812, 1975.

35. Lassen, N. A., and Tweed, W. A.: Anesthesia and cerebral blood flow. In Gordon, E., editor: A basis and practice of neuroanesthesia, Amsterdam, 1975, Excerpta Medica, p. 113.

36. Lawrence, J. H., Loomis, W. F., Tobias, C. A., and Turpin, F. H.: Preliminary observations on the narcotic effects of xenon with a review of values for solubilities of gases in water and oils, J. Physiol. **105**:197, 1946.

37. Lehninger, A. L.: Biochemistry, New York, 1975, Worth, p. 477.

38. Lucy, J. A.: Functional and structural aspects of biological membranes: a suggested structural role of vitamin E in the control of membrane permeability and stability, Ann. N.Y. Acad. Sci. **203**:4, 1972.

39. Macleish, D., Fishbein, M. C., Maroko, P. R., and Braunwald, E.: Hyaluronidase-induced reductions in myocardial infarct size, Science **194**:199, 1976.

40. Maroko, P. R., and Braunwald, E.: Effects of metabolic and pharmacologic interventions on myocardial infarct size following coronary occlusion, Circulation **53**(suppl I.I):162, 1976.

41. Marshall, L. F., and Shapiro, H. M.: Barbiturate control of intracranial hypertension in head injury and other conditions: iatrogenic coma, Acta Neurol. Scand. **56**(suppl. 64):156, 1977.

42. McGraw, C. P.: Experimental cerebral infarction: effects of pentobarbital in Mongolian gerbils, Arch Neurol. **34**:334, 1977.

43. Mellors, A., and Tappel, A. L.: The inhibition of mitochondrial peroxidation by ubiquinone and ubiquinol, J. Biol. Chem. **241**:4353, 1966.

44. Michenfelder, J. D., and Theye, R. A.: Cerebral protection by thiopental during hypoxia, Anesthesiology **39:**510, 1973.

45. Michenfelder, J. D.: The interdependency of cerebral functional and metabolic effects following massive doses of thiopental in the dog, Anesthesiology **41:**231, 1974.

46. Michenfelder, J. H., and Milde, J. H.: Influence of anesthetics on metabolic, functional and pathological responses to regional cerebral ischemia, Stroke **6:**405, 1975.

47. Michenfelder, J. D., Milde, J. H., and Sundt, T. M., Jr.: Cerebral protection by barbiturate anesthesia; use after middle cerebral artery occlusion in Java monkeys, Arch. Neurol. **33:**345, 1976.

48. Michenfelder, J. D., and Milde, J. H.: Failure of prolonged hypocapnia, hypothermia, or hypertension to favorably alter acute stroke in primates, Stroke **8:**87, 1977.

49. Mitamura, J. A., Seligman, M. L., Flamm, E. S., Ioppolo, A., and Demopoulos, H. B.: Loss of cholesterol and ascorbic acid in rat brain following cold trauma and protection by methylprednisolone, Brain Res. 1979 (submitted).

50. Moncada, S., Gryglewski, R. J., Bunting, S., and Vane, J. R.: A lipid peroxide inhibits the enzyme in blood vessel microsomes that generates from prostaglandin endoperoxides the substance (prostaglandin X) which prevents platelet aggregation, Prostaglandins **12:**715, 1976.

51. Moseley, J. I., Laurent, J. P., and Molinari, G. F.: Barbiturate attenuation of the clinical course and pathologic lesions in a primate stroke model, Neurology **25:**870, 1975.

52. Nemoto, E. M., Kofke, W. A., Kessler, P., Hossmann, K.-A., Stezoski, S. W., and Safar, P.: Studies on the pathogenesis of ischemic brain damage and the mechanism of its amelioration by thiopental, Acta Neurol. Scand. **56**(suppl 64):142, 1977.

53. Novak, R. F., and Swift, T. J.: Nuclear magnetic resonance studies of barbiturate-phospholipid interactions, Mol. Pharmacol. **12:**263, 1976.

54. Panganamala, R. V., Sharma, H. M., Sprecher, H., Geer, J. C., and Cornwell, D. G.: A suggested role for hydrogen peroxide in the biosynthesis of prostaglandins, Prostaglandins **8:**3, 1974.

55. Patten, B. M., Mendell, J., Bruun, B., Austin, W., and Carter, S.: Double blind study of the effects of dexamethasone on acute stroke. In Reulen, H. J., and Schürmann, K., editors: Steroids and brain edema, Berlin, 1972, Springer-Verlag, p. 259.

56. Petkau, A., Chelack, W. S., Pleskach, S. D., Meeker, B. E., and Brady, C. M.: Radioprotection of mice by superoxide dismutase, Biochem. Biophys. Res. Comm. **65:**886, 1975.

57. Petkau, A., and Chelack, W. S.: Radioprotective effect of superoxide dismutase on model phospholipid membranes, Biochim. Biophys. Acta **433:**45, 1976.

58. Pierce, E. C., Lambertson, C. J., Deutch, C., and others: Cerebral circulation and metabolism during thiopental anesthesia and hyperventilation in man, J. Clin. Invest. **41:**1664, 1962.

59. Pietronigro, D. D., Seligman, M. L., Jones, W. B. G., and Demopoulos, H. B.: Retarding effects of DNA on the autoxidation of liposome suspensions, Lipids **11:**808, 1976.

60. Plum, F., Alvord, E. C., and Posner, J. B.: Effects of steroids on experimental infarction, Arch. Neurol. **9:**571, 1963.

61. Rosomoff, H. L.: Protective effects of hypothermia against pathological processes in the nervous system, Ann. N.Y. Acad. Sci. **80:**475, 1959.

62. Ruzica, F. J., Beinert, H., Schepler, K. L., Dunham, W. R., and Sands, R. H.: Interaction of ubisemiquinone with a paramagnetic component in heart tissue, Proc. Nat. Acad. Sci. **72:**2886, 1975.

63. Schmiedek, P., editor: Microsurgery for stroke, New York, 1977, Springer-Verlag.

64. Seligman, M. L., and Demopoulos, H. B.: Spin-probe analysis of membrane perturbations produced by chemical and physical agents, Ann. N.Y. Acad. Sci. **222:**640, 1973.

65. Seligman, M. L., Flamm, E. S., Goldstein, B. D., Poser, R. G., Demopoulos, H. B., and Ransohoff, J.: Spectrofluorescent detection of malonaldehyde as a measure of lipid free radical damage in response to ethanol potentiation of spinal cord trauma, Lipids **12:**945, 1977.

66. Seligman, M. L., Mitamura, J., Shera, N., and Demopoulos, H. B.: Corticosteroid (methylprednisolone) modulation of photoperoxidation by ultraviolet light in liposomes, Photochem. Photobiol. **29:**549, 1979.

67. Sharpless, S. K.: The barbiturates. In Goodman, L., and Gilman, A., editors: The pharamcological basis of therapeutics. ed. 4, New York, 1970, Macmillan Publishing Co., Inc., p. 98.

68. Sheldon, P. W., Hill, S. A., and Moulder, J. E.: Radioprotection by pentobarbitone sodium of a murine tumor in vivo, Int. J. Radiat. Biol. **32:**571, 1977.

69. Siesjö, B. K., and Plum, F.: Pathophysiology of anoxic brain damage. In Gaull, G. E., editor: Biology of brain dysfunction, New York, 1973, Plenum Publishing Corp., vol. 1, p. 319.

70. Siesjö, B. K., Norberg, K., Ljunggren, B., and Salford, L. G.: Hypoxia and cerebral metabolism. In Gordon, E., editor: A basis and practice of neuroanesthesia, Amsterdam, 1975, Excerpta Medica, p. 47.

71. Smith, A. L., and Wollman, H.: Cerebral blood flow and metabolism; effects of anesthetic drugs and techniques, Anesthesiology **36:**378, 1972.

72. Smith, A. L., Hoff, J. T., Nielsen, S. L., and Larson, C. P.: Barbiturate protection in acute focal cerebral ischemia, Stroke **5:**1, 1974.

73. Smith, A. L.: Barbiturate protection in cerebral hypoxia, Anesthesiology **47:**285, 1977.

74. Spector, R.: Vitamin homeostasis in the central nervous system, N. Engl. J. Med. **296:**1393, 1977.

75. Trumpower, B. L.: Evidence for a protonmotive Q cycle mechanism of electron transfer through the cytochrome b-c complex, Biochem. Biophys. Res. Comm. **70:**73, 1976.

76. White, A., Handler, P., and Smith, E. L.: Principles of biochemistry, New York, 1973, McGraw-Hill Book Co., p. 356.

77. Wilhjelm, B. J., and Arnfred, S.: Protective action of some anesthetics against anoxia, Acta Pharmacol. Toxicol. **22:**93, 1965.

78. Willis, T.: The remaining medical works, London, 1681, Dring, Harper, Leigh and Martyn.

79. Yatsu, F. M., Diamond, I., Graziano, C., and Lindquist, P.: Experimental brain ischemia: protection from irreversible damage with a rapid-acting barbiturate (methohexital), Stroke **3:**726, 1972.

13

Altered consciousness and coma

BRYAN JENNETT

"Coma kills" would have been a fair slogan 20 years ago, before intensive care, as we now call it, began to reduce the mortality of unconscious patients. At best these rescued patients now recover completely; at worst they survive for a time without regaining mental function, a fate that awaits only a small minority. Recovery depends not only on combating the complications of the unconscious state, but also on reaching the right diagnosis and treating the cause of the coma appropriately.

Altered consciousness of some degree is a feature of many neurosurgical patients and is one of the most valuable neurologic signs. It may be a presenting feature in patients in whom the diagnosis has still to be made; the character and course of the conscious state may then provide useful diagnostic clues. Once the cause of the cerebral dysfunction is no longer in doubt, the course of the coma, its depth and duration, provide the most reliable sign of the severity of the brain damage, and so of the prognosis. Moreover, changes in the conscious state signal the efficacy of therapy and may herald the development of complications. So crucial is the continuous observation of conscious level in neurosurgical practice that long before the term intensive care was coined, neurosurgeons had developed a habit of collecting their unconscious patients, including all immediate postoperative intracranial cases, into one area of the ward where they could be observed by specially trained nurses.

Anesthetists increasingly take responsibility for the intensive care of comatose patients, and their therapeutic approach may handicap the surgeon who has still to establish a diagnosis or who has decisions still to make that depend on the changing state of consciousness. There is need therefore for constant review of the balance of benefits associated with various therapeutic interventions and their disadvantages; in the present context these drawbacks must include not only the actual hazards of therapy but the more subtle consequences of depriving the clinician of guidelines to further decision-making.

That is not, however, the purpose of this chapter, which is concerned with the definition of coma and its differentiation from other states of reduced responsiveness, with the causes of coma and their diagnosis, with the monitoring of coma, the description of its outcome, and with how to predict, while the patient is still in coma, what degree of recovery is probable.

PHENOMENOLOGY OF ALTERED CONSCIOUSNESS

Consciousness defies brief definition, but when it is altered, what is missing is readily

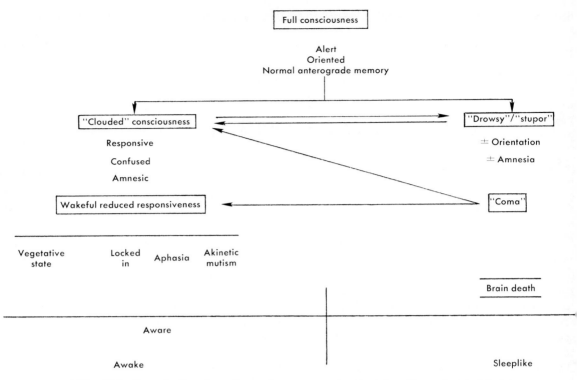

Fig. 13-1. Organic disorders of consciousness, contrasting sleeplike and wakeful states.

recognized. Two main kinds of abnormal conscious state are encountered in clinical practice. One is characterized by decreased arousal, varying from drowsiness and stupor from which the patient can be briefly aroused, to the unrousable states of coma and brain death. In the other, arousal or wakefulness is unimpaired, but the content of consciousness (as far as this can be judged) is altered. It is not possible to set all these separate states on a single hierarchical continuum; rather it is a branched tree, with a wakeful and a sleeplike side (Fig. 13-1).

Clouded consciousness

Clouded consciousness indicates confusion and disorientation but is compatible with wakefulness and alertness. Patients with focal lesions, such as tumor and abscess, commonly have a period during which this is the dominant disorder of consciousness before drowsiness and stupor develop; this represents a normal stage in recovery from coma-

producing insults such as head injury or vascular accident. Included in this category would also be the dementia of the elderly and some degenerating diseases in younger patients. Responsiveness is unimpaired, and the patient may indeed be hyperactive and unduly reactive to stimuli—characteristics that gave rise to the term delirium in the older literature. Patients who have recovered from these states are frequently amnesic for all that has happened during this period and during the state of altered consciousness can be shown to have a short-lived anterograde memory. For example, they frequently fail to remember what has happened earlier in the day, and they appear to start each day with the slate wiped clean, unable to remember their relatives sitting with them the day before or incidents in their day-to-day lives. They can usually be shown to be disoriented in time, if not in place, provided interrogation goes further than asking routine questions such as name and address, which can often be responded to almost reflexly as over-learned material.

Drowsiness and stupor

Drowsiness and stupor indicate a state of excessive and inappropriate sleepiness from which the patient can be aroused to speak, only to lapse back into sleep, even while the physician is completing the examination. These patients may be oriented and not overtly confused during such a period of forced wakefulness, and they will sometimes remember these episodes.

Coma

Coma is a widely used term, but its definition has tended to vary from one report to another. Most often it is taken to mean a patient who does not speak or one who does not obey commands. Yet such criteria are often blurred by qualifying clauses—not speaking more than occasional words or obeying only simple (or one-stage) commands. And definitions seldom make clear what is to be made of the patient who obeys but does not speak or (less commonly) the other way round. And neither do these descriptions require that the patient be in a sleeplike state with the eyes closed.

In recent years two definitions of coma have emerged, which are very similar and which are simple and practical to apply. The World Federation of Neurosurgical Societies' Committee on Head Injury suggested "an unrousable, unresponsive state, regardless of duration, with the eyes continuously closed." Considering the range of motor activity the limbs can show in response to pain even in deep coma and the preservation in most such patients of reflex eye movements and pupil reactions, it is misleading to describe coma as a state of unresponsiveness. Apart from this, the definition is a useful one. It corresponds closely with that used in a trans-Atlantic study of traumatic brain damage,[14] but the latter definition is more specific and more rigorous. It is "not obeying any commands, not uttering any words, and not opening the eyes." The inclusion of "eyes closed" ensures differentiation from wakeful forms of unresponsiveness (described below), while the requirement that the patients can neither obey nor speak excludes the 4% of patients who can do one but not the other and who would be regarded as still in coma by a less strict definition.

Wakeful states of reduced responsiveness

Wakeful states of reduced responsiveness are distinguished from coma by there being periods when the patient has his or her eyes open; these last for hours at a time and the patient is referred to as having a sleep/wake rhythm. But to be awake is not necessarily to be aware, and the most important distinction to make clinically in these patients is between the vegetative state, in which the patient is not sentient, and the other kinds of wakeful reduced responsiveness that are compatible with awareness and with remembered experience.

Vegetative state

The vegetative state is the term proposed in 1972 by Jennett and Plum[10] to describe patients who are left after an episode of acute brain damage without any behavioral evidence of a functioning cerebral cortex. These patients frequently follow a moving object (and, in particular, people) with their eyes, and their spastic arms show postural adjustments to various stimuli, including reflex grasping of the hand when something is put in the palm. These movements and the following with the eyes are often regarded by relatives as signs of sentient, responsive behavior and therefore as evidence of returning consciousness; even nurses and physicians unfamiliar with this state might likewise be deceived for a time and express optimism for the future. However, these behavioral activities have now been observed on many occasions in patients whose brains have subsequently been shown on dissection to have either widespread neocortical necrosis (from an ischemic episode such as cardiac arrest or carbon monoxide poisoning) or disconnection of an intact cortex by diffuse shearing lesions of white matter (from impact damage due to

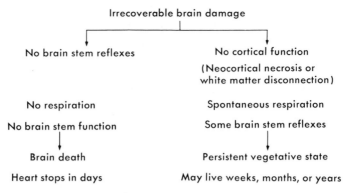

Fig. 13-2. Distinction between brain death and vegetative state.

head injury). Observation of the range of behavior possible during the brief period of survival of anencephalic monsters and in animals who have been subjected to varying degrees of decortication and decerebration provides further evidence of the wide range of behavioral responses possible at the subcortical level.

Although some patients with extensive progressive brain disease may eventually become vegetative, this state is most obviously recognized when a sudden episode of brain damage has been survived due to the application of intensive therapy during the acute stage. The availability of resuscitation procedures now ensures the continued existence of some patients with brains so badly damaged (from traumatic or nontraumatic insults) that they would previously have died during the acute stage. To this extent the vegetative state is an artifact of nature, produced and maintained by the exceptional efforts of modern medicine. The celebrated case of Karen Quinlan has brought this dilemma to public attention and has led to the expression of many opinions, by both physicians and the laity, about its ethical and economic implications.[2]

What that incident also brought to light was the possibility of confusing the vegetative state with brain death, in that it was predicted that Karen Quinlan could not survive without assisted ventilation. It must be emphasized that vegetative patients breathe normally and may live for years, given basic nursing care and adequate nutrition; brain-dead patients maintain a heartbeat only for days (Fig. 13-2).

Locked-in syndrome

The locked-in syndrome is the term coined by Plum and Posner[19] to describe the mute and tetraplegic patient who has suffered interruption of the motor pathways in the ventral pons, usually the result of infarction. This differentiation leaves the patient sentient and responsive but able to communicate only by evolving a code that uses the few muscles that are spared, namely those for eye and jaw movements and for blinking.

Akinetic mutism

Akinetic mutism describes a much higher level of activity than either of the two preceding states, but a rather less clear-cut one. These patients are inert but can move, and the tone of their limbs is usually normal. They do not speak much, but they may say an occasional word. This is a state associated with a variety of lesions, including recently ruptured anterior communicating artery aneurysm and some cases of extensive brain stem damage. Occasionally complete aphasia leaves the patient totally mute, but the relative normality of all other behavior distinguishes this state from the others described.

Rapid insults (such as head injury or intracranial hemorrhage) may produce coma almost immediately, but more gradually evolving cerebral conditions may cause a period of clouded consciousness before drowsiness and stupor supervenes due to the development of intracranial pressure and brain shift, or there may be a period of confused alertness. Recovery is usually by a different route, clouded consciousness being the stage before the return of full consciousness rather than drowsiness and stupor. Some patients recover from coma into a state of wakeful reduced responsiveness, and this often persists, rather than being a stage on the way to recovery. Some patients with sudden vascular disorders, particularly ischemia of the brain stem, may pass into one of the states of wakeful reduced responsiveness without more than a brief period in coma. On the other hand, after a severe head injury there is always a prolonged period of sleeplike coma.

DIAGNOSTIC PROBLEMS

The remainder of this chapter concerns various aspects of coma proper, as defined above. When coma presents a diagnostic problem, there are many possibilities, which are best categorized under four broad headings (see box below). The history will often make one kind of pathologic process more likely than another: head injury may be witnessed, or the patient may fall unconscious following a vascular accident; metabolic

causes will be suspected in a patient already systemically ill, and epilepsy when there is sudden unconsciousness associated with rapid recovery. Drugs cause a great deal of difficulty because they may be the primary cause of coma or only an aggravating factor. They include those taken by the patient prior to coming under medical care (including alcohol) and those given by physicians for various reasons, such as premedication for anesthesia, for the control of seizures, or to reduce agitation in patients with clouded consciousness, or to make it possible to institute ventilation in patients already in some degree of coma.

Biochemical and toxicologic tests may confirm a suspicion of metabolic or drug factors as a cause of coma. Focal neurologic signs will point to structural brain disease, confirmation of which is best sought by CT scanning. If this is not possible, isotope scanning or EEG provide poor substitutes, which may, however, point to the presence of a focal lesion, although seldom its nature. Further information can then be gained by angiography, although since the availability of CT scanning there are fewer physicians who are skilled in angiography; it is well recognized that complications following this procedure are not inconsiderable, especially when it is carried out by the occasional practitioner. Anesthesia may be required for CT scanning or for angiography, and if there is a strong suspicion that a structural lesion may be revealed, arrangements should be made to operate immediately under the same anesthetic if an operable lesion should be disclosed.

More than one cause may contribute to coma. Patients with vascular or drug-induced impairment of consciousness or those suffering an epileptic fit may fall and sustain a head injury; the most common example of this is when someone already drunk is assaulted or falls. Epilepsy may complicate structural brain disease, and the seizure may upset an already critical state of intracranial hemodynamics; the situation may be further confused by the giving of relatively large doses of depressant anticonvulsant drugs in

---

CAUSES OF COMA*

Structural	Traumatic
	Vascular
	Infective
Metabolic	Renal
	Hepatic
	Endocrine
	Hypothermia
Epilepsy	
Drugs	

*From Jennett, B.: In Baderman, H., editor: Management of Medical Emergencies, London, 1978, Pitman.

an attempt to prevent further seizures. Patients with metabolic disorders may be unduly sensitive to depressant drugs that are used therapeutically because of their inability to detoxify these. In patients with raised intracranial pressure or with impaired cerebral oxygenation or structural brain damage, the effect of drugs may be enhanced. As a consequence of these factors a normal dose of premedication may precipitate coma that lasts for many hours or even days; recovery from anesthesia may be delayed for the same reasons.

Monitoring changes in coma

Even when the diagnosis has been made it is vital to be able to recognize changes in the state of consciousness because these are usually the most sensitive index of the patient's response to treatment or of the development of new intracranial complications, some of which may call for urgent action. No laboratory investigation has been developed that can substitute for clinical observation of conscious level. In particular, routine EEG recordings are often unhelpful (apart from localizing focal brain damage during the diagnostic process). Indeed some patients with severe structural brain damage (e.g., after cardiac arrest) may be reported to have an improving EEG at a stage when it is becoming clear that they have suffered permanent and irreversible brain damage. Recent developments in the use of evoked cortical responses following somatic, auditory, and visual stimuli do show promise.[5] However, these require considerable expertise in their performance and interpretation and are time consuming. The significance of various findings has yet to be established.

There is therefore a premium on evolving a satisfactory method of monitoring the course of coma. A distinction should be made between what is appropriate for this purpose and what is needed to diagnose the cause of coma. For the latter, complete neurologic and general physical examinations are required. But monitoring calls for a simplified system, because repeated observations have to be made—and most of these will be done by nurses or junior medical staff. Such staff change frequently, even during a 24-hour period, and methods must therefore be reliable when used by different observers; moreover the findings of one member of staff must be readily communicated to another.

A practical scale that meets these needs and that provides both a useful bedside monitor and a means of categorizing the degree of coma in numerical terms has been evolved in Glasgow.[12] The numerical system facilitates comparison between groups of patients, and the scale has found application in a computerized data bank of patients with traumatic and with nontraumatic coma involving cases from several clinics in three countries.[14] It has been suggested by Langfitt[15] that this coma scale and the outcome scale described on p. 278 might usefully be adopted by neurosurgical units throughout the world for a trial period of, say, five years

---

GLASGOW COMA SCALE*

Eye opening

Spontaneous	4	
To speech	3	E
To pain	2	
Nil	1	

Best motor response

Obeys	6	
Localizes	5	
Withdraws (flexion)	4	M
Abnormal flexion	3	
Extensor response	2	
Nil	1	

Verbal response

Orientated	5	
Confused conversation	4	
Inappropriate *words*	3	V
Incomprehensible *sounds*	2	
Nil	1	

Coma score (responsiveness sum) = 3 to 15 (E + M + V)

---

*From Jennett, B., and Teasdale, G.: Aspects of coma after severe head injury, Lancet **1:**878-881, 1977.

in order to facilitate evaluation of head injuries and their management.

Three modalities of behavior (or responsiveness) are assessed, and each is recorded on a hierarchical scale that describes the response and allocates a number to it (high for normal, lower for progressively more abnormal responses). These numbers can be aggregated to give an overall responsiveness (or coma) score or sum, which ranges from 3 to 15 (see box, p. 272). The different responses and the terms used to describe these were evolved over a period of time during which formal observer/error trials were conducted in three countries; the resulting system has been shown to be reliable and reproducible in the hands of many different observers, including those with relatively little experience.[22]

Eye opening may occur spontaneously or only when the patient is spoken to (not necessarily the command to open his or her eyes) or when a painful stimuli is applied or not at all. Distinguishing coma from other unresponsive states already described depends crucially on eye opening.

Motor reactivity in the limbs depends, in patients not obeying commands (which is the normal response), on applying a painful stimulus—pressure on the nailbed using a pencil or supraorbital pressure. The response is recorded as *localizing* if the hands move above the chin toward the supraorbital stimulus; less directed flexion than this is recorded as normal flexion or flexor withdrawal. In some patients this flexor response is abnormal or spastic and is recorded as such if there is preceding extension movement in either arm or leg at the time of the examination or if there are two of the following responses: stereotyped flexion posture, extreme wrist flexion, abduction of the upper arm, or fingers flexed over the thumb. Observers not experienced in neurologic examination are often in doubt about recognizing abnormal flexion; if there is doubt it should be recorded as the next higher response (flexor withdrawal). For this reason our bedside chart for nurses does not include this particular response (Fig. 13-3). The next response is extension of the limb, and the lowest level is no motor movement at all in response to pain.

Different responses may be obtained from each of the four limbs, and even in one limb there may be a variation in the response during the course of a single examination. For assessing the depth of coma the rule is to take the best response during the examination of the best limb. The upper limbs usually show the greater range of responses and

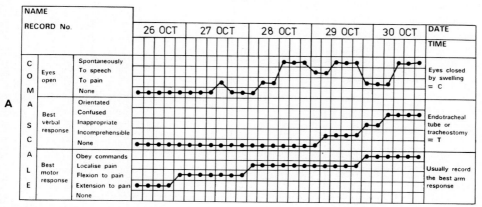

Fig. 13-3. A, Nurse's coma chart. Note that it does not include abnormal flexion from the Glasgow Coma Scale. This item is scored as flexion.

Continued.

are the basis for assessing the motor response. Variations in responsiveness over a period of hours or days is summarized by rating the best and the worst levels of the best motor response over a succession of periods of time; investigation reveals that it is the best responses that correlate more closely with outcome and are therefore the more reliable markers of severity of brain dysfunction as a whole. However, a focal lesion may cause hemiplegia and result in one limb having a consistently lower level of response; this indicates not the level of brain dysfunction as a whole but the localization of the brain damage. This is recorded elsewhere in our system, as the motor response pattern (see below). Notice that the system does not use the words decerebrate and decorticate or purposeful, all of which are subject to interpretation and are therefore less reliable.[22]

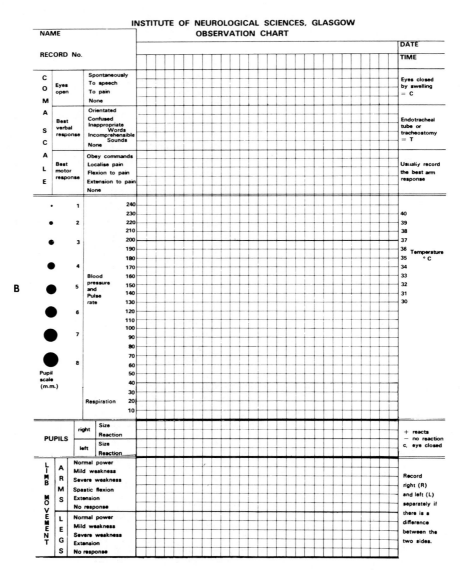

Fig. 13-3, cont'd. B, Nurse's observation chart incorporating coma chart, temperature, pulse, respiration, blood pressure, and reactivity of pupils and of all four limbs.

Speech is classified as normal if the patient is oriented, as confused if he or she can conduct a conversation but is disoriented, as inappropriate words if he or she utters only occasional expletives but does not carry on a conversation, as incomprehensible sounds if only grunts and groans are elicited, or there may be no vocalization at all.

A useful feature of this scale is that it still allows an assessment to be made if one component is untestable. For example, at the lower range of the motor responses a confident assessment can be made even if no verbal response is possible due to an endotracheal tube. However, as patients begin to emerge from coma, when the eyes open, the return of the verbal response becomes an important landmark, and assessment at this stage is very difficult if a patient is prevented from being able to show the level of verbal response. Some previous definitions of coma have, however, placed too much emphasis on speech and have sometimes depended on this alone. Although this is not, in our view, an appropriate definition, the significance of the return of speech as an indication of a certain level of brain functioning should not be underestimated.

Other aspects of coma

In addition to responsiveness on this simple scale it is useful to record other functions that are commonly affected in comatose patients; these include pupil reaction, eye movements, the pattern of motor responses in all four limbs, and cardiorespiratory features. These were all proposed by Plum and Posner in their classic text[19] as part of the phenomenology of coma, and there is indeed a close correlation between them and the level of responsiveness on the practical scale. However, there are exceptions to this relationship, usually when there is impairment of one or another of these functions due to local damage rather than as a reflection of brain dysfunction as a whole. For example, pupil reactions may be affected by damage to the globe or to the optic or oculomotor nerves intracranially or in the orbit; or they may be unreactive because of systemically or locally

administered drugs. The same caveats apply to the ocular movements, both spontaneous and reflex. Before eliciting the oculocephalic (doll's eye) reflex movements the examiner should be satisfied that there is no cervical spinal fracture before eliciting and the oculovestibular reflex—by irrigating cold water into the external auditory meatus—he or she should be certain there is clear access to the drum and that this is intact. If there is a recent perforation, cold water can be irrigated through a fine catheter. Eye movements should be recorded according to a hierarchical scale of responses, and we have also evolved a composite eye movement score to take account of missing data.

Autonomic abnormalities have long been recognized as a frequent manifestation of brain stem dysfunction and therefore as one of the phenomena observed in patients in coma. Respiration, in particular, is commonly regarded as of diagnostic and prognostic significance; systolic blood pressure and heart rate are also often referred to. However, the classic Cushing triad of bradycardia, hypertension, and abnormal breathing patterns is a late sign of brain stem distortion, and it is by no means a consistent constellation of signs even under these circumstances. Recent investigation of breathing patterns, using impedance pneumography, has shown that when there is acute brain damage, whether traumatic or due to other causes, there is great variation over a period of hours and sometimes even over minutes.[18] Furthermore, the association between certain patterns and either the location of the lesion or its prognosis is much less definite than was formally asserted.[17] Partly this is due to the fact that these functions are open to influence from extracranial factors such as hypoxia, hypovolemia or pulmonary complications, as well as being sensitive to the effect of depressant drugs. While respiratory abnormalities may not be a good index of the degree of coma, they may be important diagnostically or as an indication for therapeutic intervention.

Apart from the *best* motor response in *any* limb, which is used for the coma scale, the pattern of abnormality in all four limbs needs to be recorded. Asymmetry of response may indicate focal damage, due either to impact injury or to complications. This, together with the size and reactions of the pupils, the temperature, pulse, respiration, blood pressure, and coma scale, can be displayed on a single bedside chart.

RECOVERY FROM COMA

When a patient has been in coma for several hours or days, the first sign of recovery is usually eye opening. Soon after this, occasional words are usually uttered, commands are obeyed, or both. The delay between the return of these different functions varies somewhat, but if a patient has prolonged periods of spontaneous eye opening without either obeying commands or speaking, the possibility that he or she is passing into the vegetative state must be considered. Alternative explanations of failure to speak have been mentioned previously in this chapter.

In most patients eye opening is quickly followed by a period of clouded consciousness, the duration of which is usually related to the length of the coma preceding it. Some patients in this state after head injury go through a stage of disinhibited behavior, sometimes called traumatic delirium or cerebral irritation. This is sometimes aggravated by physical discomfort such as full bladder, headache, pain from extracranial injuries, or even thirst. Dealing with these may help to quiet the patient; it can also help to have the patient out of bed, unless associated injuries make this impossible. Such a patient is often less disturbed when among other patients than when shut up in a room alone. Sedation should be confined to night time if possible, because it can impede the mind that is trying to come to grips with reality again to have also to cope with depressant drugs. Occasionally the disturbance is so marked and persistent that temporary transfer to an acute psychiatric ward may be advisable, because the staff there are more used to coping with this kind of patient; however, psychiatric staff must be warned to resist the temptation to employ heavy sedation in dealing with this temporary disorder. The next

phase in recovery is a period of quiet confusion, and most patients pass directly from coma into this state. Behavior may seem almost normal to the casual observer but inquiry reveals persisting confusion. Patients are usually completely and permanently amnesic for this period of recovery (as they are also for any period of acutely disturbed behavior). This must be remembered when patients are asked to make statements to the police or others, because the statements may be subsequently denied. After head injury the duration of this posttraumatic amnesia is a good guide to the degree of diffuse brain damage, and it is probably equally useful after brain damage from other causes leading to coma. It must be distinguished from retrograde amnesia, which is loss of memory for a period immediately preceding the accident. The duration of this retrograde amnesia is very variable and indeed it often changes during the recovery period. By contrast, posttraumatic amnesia is usually quite constant, presumably because memory was never laid down during the period of recovery of the brain. Estimates of posttraumatic amnesia should be in fairly broad terms and the scale commonly used is as follows: less than five minutes, trivial injury; five minutes to one hour, mild; 1 to 24 hours, moderate, one to seven days, severe; more than seven days, very severe. There is a close correlation in the duration of disability after head injury and the duration of the posttraumatic amnesia.

Sequelae that may persist for months, and sometimes permanently, after acute brain damage are of two kinds, mental and physical. The former contribute more significantly to the overall disability and are more consistently found; however, they are more readily overlooked. These mental changes usually appear to reflect widespread or diffuse brain damage, while focal neurologic signs indicate local damage. Personality change is the most frequently reported, but even when it is marked, its recognition depends on the reports of relatives or previous associates of the patient; behavior that is quite within the normal limits for the population may represent a profound change in comparison with that patient's own previous personality. In the more severe cases, apathy, lack of drive, and a blunting of social restraint are the most common features. Specific loss of intellectual ability may be revealed by psychometric tests, and there are often persistent problems with memory on a day-to-day, hour-to-hour basis. But many patients who are markedly changed mentally after brain damage prove to have normal cognitive function, as routinely tested by psychologists. Physical sequelae include hemiplegia, aphasia, epilepsy, and disorders of the cranial nerves.

ASSESSMENT OF ULTIMATE OUTCOME

Concern with the demanding problems of the acutely ill patient in coma makes it difficult for those who work primarily in intensive care units to know much about the ultimate outcome of the patients whose lives they have saved. Even the neurosurgeon may lose track of these patients a few weeks later; at best his or her knowledge of further progress is often based on a brief follow-up visit, during which the degree of disability, particularly its mental component, may not declare itself.

Many of these patients make a satisfactory, even a complete recovery. Those who first reported, 20 years ago, that intensive respiratory care could greatly reduce mortality after severe head injury, hopefully asserted that serious sequelae would seldom be a problem.[6] This has proved to be overoptimistic, and a calculation ten years later indicated that some 1500 patients were leaving hospitals each year in Britain (population approximately 50 million) with permanent brain damage following head injury, an estimate later confirmed from different data. An epidemiologic report on the prevalence of vegetative survivors of acute brain damage in Japan indicated that there were rather more such patients following episodes of cerebral hypoxia of various kinds than following head injury.[6] Extrapolating from these reports it is probable that in the United States there are about 14,000 new patients each year with permanent brain damage following acute in-

cidents leading to coma; half of these are probably under 30 years of age and most of them will live for many years, because they have no progressive disease. This sizeable and accumulating population of disabled brain-damaged patients is the price paid for the patients who make a good recovery.

Whether that price is too high is a vexed and emotive issue, but some commentators are beginning to draw attention to the balance of benefits that accrue from intensive care when large numbers of patients are reviewed, and when their state a year later is considered rather than whether or not they are discharged alive from intensive care.[3,7] The figures are sobering, particularly when intensive therapy has rescued a patient from an incident in the course of a progressive disease (e.g., renal, respiratory or hepatic failure, malignant disease, or a stroke in the elderly). However, many incidents of brain damage occur in younger patients who are otherwise healthy (e.g., head injury or cardiac arrest associated with anesthesia for minor surgery).

The importance of assessing outcome critically is that it provides a measure of the effectiveness of therapeutic intervention, particularly when different methods have been used in patients whose initial severity was similar. Until recently outcome after brain damage has usually been described in terms that have not been clearly defined, and it has therefore been difficult to compare reports from different institutions or to form a clear view of the relative effectiveness of alternative methods of management. The international (Table 13-1) collaborative study of traumatic and nontraumatic coma has used a 5-point scale, which has been found to be practical and reliable in the hands of different observers.[11] In addition to patients who are dead and those who are in a vegetative state (p. 269) three other categories of survivor are recognized. The severely disabled are those who are conscious but dependent; the latter is defined as needing the attention of another person for some part of every 24 hours. While most of these severely disabled patients have a combination of mental and physical disability, some of them are physi-

Table 13-1. Outcome after severe brain damage*

Dead	Dead/vegetative	Dead/vegetative	Dead	Dead	Dead	
Survivors			Dependent	Vegetative	Vegetative	
	Conscious			Severely disabled	Degree of disability	5
		Severely disabled				4
						3
			Independent	Moderately disabled		
		Independent				2
				Good recovery		1
						0
	2	3		5	7	categories

*From Jennett, B., Snoek, J., Bond, M. R., and Brooks, D. N.: Assessment of disability in survivors after severe head injury (in press).

Table 13-2. Attainment of final outcome category*

Outcome one year after injury	n	Already in this category by	
		3 months	6 months
Moderate disability	118	62%	92%
Good recovery	236	69%	90%

*From Jennett, B., Teasdale, G., Galbraith, S., and others: Severe head injuries in three countries, J. Neurol. Neurosurg. Psychiatr. **40**:291-298, 1977.

GLASGOW OUTCOME SCALE*

Dead	—
Vegetative state	Nonsentient
Severe disability	Conscious but dependent
Moderate disability	Independent but disabled
Good recovery	May have minor deficits

*From Jennett, B., and Bond, M. R.: Assessment of outcome after severe brain damage, Lancet **1**:480-484, 1975.

---

cally intact but so mentally inadequate that they have to be in a mental hospital for their own care and attention. The moderately disabled are independent but disabled; they can live on their own, can organize their lives and are capable of work, although not necessarily that which they previously did. Those categorized as having made a good recovery may still have minor residual sequelae, but they are able to participate in all previous occupational and social activities. It is the capability to undertake activities rather than whether or not they are actually undertaken that matters; for example, some patients with moderate disability may be able to return to their jobs because they are compatible with even quite marked disabilities in some spheres. On the other hand many patients who have made a good recovery may not return to work for a variety of reasons. Similarly, whether the patient is in the hospital or at home is not a reliable measure of the degree of disability, because some severely disabled patients may by reason of exceptional family effort be at home.

The five outcome categories described on this scale can be reduced or expanded for particular purposes (Table 13-1) as de-

Table 13-3. Outcome of data bank head injuries*

	Survivors		
	3 months 534	6 months 515	12 months 376
Vegetative state	7%	5%	3%
Severe disability	29%	19%	16%
Moderate disability	33%	34%	31%
Good recovery	31%	42%	50%
Moderate/good	64%	76%	81%

*From Jennett, B., Teasdale, G., Galbraith, S., and others: Severe head injuries in three countries, J. Neurol. Neurosurg. Psychiatr. **40:**291-298, 1977.

scribed elsewhere.[9] Survivors may be categorized into those who are dependent or independent or into those who are conscious or not; patients in the upper three categories of survival may each be divided into a better and a worse class. This makes a more extended scale, which enables recovery to be described more accurately.

Outcome is sometimes assessed somewhat arbitrarily at the time of discharge from the acute hospital or even at the time of discharge from the intensive care unit. It is clear that this is too soon for an estimate of the ultimate outcome. On the other hand, the view that substantial improvement frequently occurs after a period of many months has not been borne out either for head injury or stroke. After head injury only 10% of patients improve from severe disability to moderate disability or from moderate disability to good recovery after six months; two-thirds of patients are already in their final outcome category within three months of injury (Table 13-2). When patients develop coma as a complication of systemic disease, such as hepatic or metabolic disorders, cardiac arrest in the course of some other major illness, or stroke in the background of progressive arterial disease, the long-term outcome may be difficult to assess because a further life-threatening incident may occur. For this reason the study of nontraumatic coma has contrasted the "best" outcome following the coma-producing incident as well as the "actual" outcome.[1] In the case of head injury this situation

does not arise and outcome at six months has been considered a useful time for assessment; there is relatively little change when the matter is reconsidered at one year (Table 13-3).

In patients left in a vegetative or a severely disabled state the question increasingly arises whether the quality of life is such that this should be regarded as a definitely better outcome than death. A consensus is emerging that the vegetative state is certainly worse than death, and there are many who would say that this is also the case for the more severely disabled of the next category. How long patients *can* survive in the vegetative state is not known and how long they *do* in fact commonly live are matters of some concern to families and their lawyers and to those providing continued health care. One patient is known to have died 18 years after a head injury sustained in 1959, which was about the time that intensive respiratory care began to become available; longer survivors than this can therefore now be expected. A Japanese survey[6] has revealed that two thirds of a series of more than 100 vegetative patients were still alive after more than three years, but this report included some patients with developmental and degenerative conditions. A factor that may influence the duration of survival is whether a decision has been made to withhold antibiotics or other active therapeutic intervention. Many physicians do now reach agreement with the family that this is the proper course to take, which reflects the growing acceptance of the view that continued survival in a vegetative state is regarded as an outcome worse than death.

PREDICTION OF OUTCOME

It is often asserted that the ultimate outcome after an episode of acute brain damage is difficult to predict; particularly after head injury it is common to hear of remarkable recoveries or of unexpected deterioration and death. However, formal statistical analysis of a relatively limited number of items of clinical data collected from patients in coma during the first few days after an episode of acute brain damage will enable the outcome to be predicted in broad terms in a substantial proportion of patients. These predictions are based on comparison with data banks of large numbers of patients who have coma of similar etiology and whose outcome in relation to early features is known. Different statistical methods can be used; that employed in the above studies was an independence model based on Bayes theorem.[13] It enables the probability of different outcomes to be predicted at the bedside, and this may be regarded by the clinician as another investigation to be taken into account when making his decision about further management. It provides another method of assessing the effectiveness of a new method of treatment, in that if this results in a better outcome than that predicted in a statistically significant proportion of patients, it would be judged to have influenced outcome. Another application of such predictions would be in the selection of patients for intensive therapy, either for initial treatment or for continuation of intensive therapy.

CONCLUSION

When coma complicates the course of any disease, whether systemic or primarily intracranial, there are problems for the patient and physician. For the patient the prognosis immediately becomes significantly worse, whatever the underlying cause, because coma reflects a severe degree of brain dysfunction and because of the hazards of the unconscious state per se. It is therefore important to have clear concepts and definitions of different states of altered consciousness and of how to recognize each of them and measure their severity. Only then can therapy be rationally based and the effects of treatment validly assessed.

REFERENCES

1. Bates, D., Caronna, J. J., Cartlidge, N. E. F., Knill-Jones, R. P., Levy, D. E., Shaw, D. A., and Plum, F.: A prospective study of nontraumatic coma: methods and results in 310 patients, Ann. Neurol. **2:**211-220, 1977.
2. Beresford, H. R.: The Quinlan decision: problem and legislative alternatives, Ann. Neurol. **2:**74-81, 1977.
3. Cullen, D. J., Ferrara, L. C., Briggs, B. A., Walker, P. F., and Gilbert, J.: Survival, hospitalization charges and follow-up results in initially ill patients, N. Engl. J. Med. **294:**982, 1976.
4. Frowein, R. A.: Classification of coma, Acta Neurochir. **34:**5-10, 1976.
5. Greenberg, R. P., Mayer, D. J., Becker, D. P., and Miller, J. D.: Evaluation of brain function in severe human head trauma with multimodality evoked potentials. I. Evoked brain-injury potentials, methods and analysis, J. Neurosurg. **47:**150-162, 1977.
6. Higashi, K., Sakata, Y., Hatano, M., Abiko, S., Ihara, K., Katayama, S., Wakuta, Y., Okamura, T., Ueda, H., Zenke, M. and Aoki, H.: Epidemiological studies on patients with a persistent vegetative state, J. Neurol. Neurosurg. Psychiatr. **40:**876-885, 1977.
7. Jennett, B.: The cost of rescue and the price of survival. In Phillips, C. I., and Wolfe, J. N., editors: Clinical practice and economics, London, 1977, Pitman Medical Publishing Co. Ltd.
8. Jennett, B.: Resource allocation for the severely brain damaged, Arch. Neurol. **33:**595-597, 1976.
9. Jennett, B., and Bond, M.: Assessment of outcome after severe brain damage, Lancet **1:**480, 1975.
10. Jennett, B., and Plum, F.: Persistent vegetative state after brain damage, Lancet **1:**734-737, 1972.
11. Jennett, B., Snoek, J., Bond, M. R., and Brooks, D. N.: Assessment of disability in survivors after severe head injury, (in press).
12. Jennett, B., and Teasdale, G.: Prognosis of neurosurgical patients requiring intensive care. In Ledingham, I. McA., editor: Recent advances in intensive therapy, London, 1977, Churchill-Livingston, pp. 33-45.
13. Jennett, B., Teasdale, G., Braakman, R., Minderhoud, J., and Knill-Jones, R.: Predicting outcome in individual patients after severe head injury, Lancet **1:**1031-1034, 1976.
14. Jennett, B., Teasdale, G., Galbraith, S., Pickard,

J., Grant, H., Braakman, R., Avezaat, C., Maas, A., Minderhoud, J., Vecht, C. J., Heiden, J., Small, R., Caton, W., and Kurze, T.: Severe head injuries in three countries, J. Neurol. Neurosurg. Psychiatr. **40:**291-298, 1977.

15. Langfitt, T. W.: Measuring the outcome from head injuries, J. Neurosurg. **48:**673-678, 1978.

16. MacIver, I. A., Frew, I. J. C., and Matheson, J. G.: The role of respiratory insufficiency in the mortality of severe head injuries, Lancet **1:**390-393, 1958.

17. North, J. B., and Jennett, S.: Abnormal breathing patterns associated with acute brain damage, Arch. Neurol. **31:**338-344, 1974.

18. North, J. B., and Jennett, S.: Impedance pneumog-

raphy for the detection of abnormal breathing patterns associated with brain damage, Lancet **2:**212-213, 1972.

19. Plum, F., and Posner, J. B.: Diagnosis of stupor and coma, ed. 2, Philadelphia, 1972, F. A. Davis Co.

20. Skillman, J. J.: Ethical dilemmas in the care of the critically ill, Lancet **2:**634-637, 1974.

21. Teasdale, G., and Jennett, B.: Assessment of coma and impaired consciousness, Lancet **2:**81-84, 1974.

22. Teasdale, G., Knill-Jones, R. P., and Van der Sande, J.: Observer variability in assessing impaired consciousness and coma, J. Neurol. Neurosurg. Psychiatr. **41:**603-610, 1978.

14

Brain death

JULIUS KOREIN

DEFINITION OF THE PROBLEM AND TERMINOLOGY

One of the major difficulties in dealing with the subject of brain death has been imprecise usage of terminology, as in the synonymous use of words such as cerebral death, irreversible coma, cortical death, and brain death. This has led to an inordinate amount of confusion.[47,49,50,52] The following list of standardized definitions is an attempt to clarify this situation:

death The classic usage defining the term relates to criteria used by a physician to ascertain the irreversible end-state of an individual. These criteria evaluate the cessation of vital functions. These vital functions have in the past included cessation of cardiac and respiratory activity and total unresponsiveness. These classic clinical criteria may be supplemented by observations relating to rigor mortis or even putrifaction. Implicit in the concept is *brain death*, which, however, was not included until the advent of modern resuscitative technology and life-support systems.

brain death Refers to irreversible dysfunction and/or destruction of the neuronal contents of the intracranial cavity. This includes both cerebral hemispheres (cortex and deep structures) as well as the brain stem and cerebellum. Total brain infarction to the first cervical level of the spinal cord is an equivalent term. The spinal cord may be, in fact, "alive." It should be noted that there is no inherent difference in the concepts of *death* and *brain death;* they are equivalent. Both are based on the destruction of the critical system of the human organism. Rather, they differ in the criteria utilized to diagnose death, since brain death is considered in the highly specified environment of an intensive care unit, where resuscitative techniques may be used to maintain respiration and other vital functions. Cardiac activity may persist independently without the presence of any brain function whatsoever. However, in adults who are brain dead, all vital functions cease within one week regardless of resuscitative attempts. In children and infants, resuscitative procedures may allow maintenance of "vital" functions for more prolonged periods. The criteria for brain death are detailed on pp. 288-291.

cerebral death Cerebral death, unfortunately, has been and is being used synonymously with brain death but anatomically gives no indication of the status of the structures in the posterior fossa. Therefore, in order to employ our terminology more precisely, we will *not* consider cerebral death as equivalent to brain death. Situations may arise where there is clinical evidence of cerebral death, but more refined techniques may indicate viability in the brain stem and even in portions of cerebral structures. One of the peculiarities of origin of this usage is a grammatical problem. Death of the cerebrum could be termed cerebral death, but death of

Support for this chapter derived in part from The Neurology Research Fund No. #8-0168-708, New York University Medical Center; NINCDS Contracts 71-2319 and 1-NS-2307, National Institutes of Health; and donations from Mrs. Renate Elias and Ms. Ann Weisenthal.

the brain has no equivalent such as "brainal death."

irreversible coma Initially, investigators used the term *irreversible coma* as equivalent to brain death and cerebral death. This was probably derived from translation of *coma dépassé* as irreversible coma rather than ultra coma or beyond coma. Such usage added to confusion with terminology, since strictly speaking irreversible coma may be considered as an umbrella that includes not only brain death and cerebral death but a large group of persistent vegetative or irreversible noncognitive states. It is therefore advocated that the term irreversible coma only be used with specific qualifications.

persistent vegetative or noncognitive states There are patients who may be described in a variety of ways and have diverse but well-circumscribed pathologic features who are, in fact, in an irreversible state. These include persistent vegetative state, irreversible noncognitive state, neocortical death, and apallic syndrome as well as others. The anatomic substrate of irreversible damage in these patients includes bilateral destruction of the cortex, the basal ganglia, the thalamus, or the central brain stem ascending reticular formation. Most often, these patients have combinations of lesions in these regions. They are *not* brain dead but reveal a variety of complex vegetative reflexes. In common, they show no cognitive behavior, and the state is irreversible. This group of patients must be clearly differentiated. Virtually all reports dealing with such patients who may survive from days to many years indicate that they do have some form of cephalic reflexes. They most often, but not always, have spontaneous respirations, EEG activity, and cerebral circulation. The prime example of such a patient is Karen Ann Quinlan.*

It should be noted that this chapter deals primarily with the problem of brain death and does not detail other complex problems that may be confused with brain death and that are tangentially related. These associated problems are discussed only to clearly differentiate them from brain death per se (i.e., persistent vegetative state) or to elucidate their relationship to brain death (i.e., organ transplantation).[47]

---

*References 10, 39, and 47, pp. 320-321.

The subject framework will be based on advances in the technology of resuscitation and maintenance of life support systems that are available in the modern intensive care units or recovery rooms. It is only within this environment that the classic criteria of death can be considered equivalent to the criteria of brain death. There is no inherent disparity in the concept of death; rather, under these highly specified conditions, two different sets of criteria may be used for diagnosing death. Conceptually, death of the brain is central to both sets of criteria and represents death of the human organism regardless of the function of other systems.

THE BRAIN AS THE CRITICAL SYSTEM

All living systems are members of a class of thermodynamically open systems that exchange energy and matter with the environment. They tend toward a steady (nonequilibrium, stationary) state by degrading matter and energy from the environment and thus increasing their own organization (i.e., they decrease their own entropy at the expense of the environment). This operation is performed by internal mechanisms specific to a given organism. Higher organisms have multiple levels of such mechanisms, which act on matter, energy, and information from the environment to perform these tasks.[51,75,100]

In approaching the problem of brain death, we must define death of cells, organ systems, components of the organism, and the organism itself. It is our thesis that death of the human organism may be equated with irreversible destruction and/or dysfunction of the critical system of that organism. The critical system is that system which is irreplaceable by an artifice, be it biological, chemical, or electromechanical. Further, the critical system subserves the essential behavioral characteristics of the individual. Virtually all organ systems are replaceable in humans, with the exception of the brain. The heart can be replaced by a pump, the kidneys by an appropriate dialysis unit, endocrine glands by hormonal replacement therapy, and so on. A limb may be artificial, but when it comes to the neuronal cells that comprise the central nervous system, an individual is born with a fixed number, which do not reproduce or regenerate. A neuron may grow by increasing its dendritic tree and interconnections with increased production of neurotransmitters. The soma may support growth of a crushed axon, but if the soma is destroyed, the process is irreversible. The brain depends on the neurons for its function, and the organism depends on the brain. If the brain is destroyed, or becomes irreversibly nonfunctional, the critical system is destroyed, and despite all other systems being maintained by any manner whatsoever, the organism as an individual functioning entity can no longer be considered to exist. If the brain in humans is destroyed, the human organism is no longer in a state of minimal entropy production; its state will progressively become more disorganized by spontaneous uncontrolled and irreversible fluctuations. Therefore, it will *never* return to its initial state as a sentient human being. The time course may be prolonged by artificial means, depending on the adequacy of functioning subsidiary control mechanisms, but the outcome of system dissolution is just as certain as that resulting from irreversible cardiac arrest. When brain death (that is, death of the cerebral hemispheres, brain stem, and cerebellum) occurs, irreversible cardiac arrest inevitably follows regardless of the maintenance of all resuscitative procedures. No currently available evidence has been presented that irreversible cardiac arrest may be postponed more than a week (exclusive of that in infants and children), and most often these final irreversible changes occur prior to 48 and even 24 hours after brain death.

This is clearly not the situation in which there may be an irreversible noncognitive state with persistence of brain stem structures, and although the argument may be raised that in such states the personality of the individual is destroyed, vegetative functions, including spontaneous cardiorespiratory activity, may persist for years with appropriate life support measures. There are several reasons for *not* considering patients in irreversible noncognitive or vegetative states as brain dead.[38,39,44,91,92] The determination of such irreversibility is still undergoing investigation and prognosis cannot always be sharply defined.[10,11,35,58] Furthermore, it is occasionally difficult to differentiate a patient in a purely noncognitive state from one who still has some semblance of cognition. Since communication is the key in making this determination (e.g., by means of eye movements in a patient with a locked-in syndrome), the possibility exists of situations in which the brain may respond to external stimuli in a manner that only can be observed by changes of electroencephalographic or cerebral blood flow activity. This may occur in a patient in whom the brain stem and cerebrum have been separated by a hemorrhage in the intracollicular region or in a patient with total motor paralysis due to muscle paralyzants or amyotrophic sclerosis. Such patients may have significant cerebral hemispheric function and brain stem function but be in an irreversible noncommunicative state.[47,48,71] In the majority of patients, appropriate clinical and laboratory evaluation allows the reliable diagnosis of persistent vegetative or noncognitive state, as in the case of Karen Ann Quinlan. Management of these patients is analogous to patients in other forms of irreversible chronic coma and anencephalic monsters who survive for prolonged periods. It is not unreasonable that many individuals would consider extending the definition of death of a person to such patients[92]; however, this must await guidelines based on more precise clinical research to prevent potential abuse and misdiagnosis. Currently, there is no significant degree of social acceptance for such a concept. For these reasons, we should not confuse patients in this group of persistent vegetative states with those who are brain dead as defined by current criteria, which will be further elaborated upon.

We reiterate that there are not two different concepts of death, rather that two different sets of criteria may be used to diagnose death. The conventional definition of death includes irreversible cessation of cardiorespiratory function that is rapidly followed by brain death within minutes if not seconds. Brain death is a situation arising as an outgrowth of resuscitative and life-support technology; it applies to the infrequent situation in which the brain dies while other systems are maintained artificially or are still viable. Both the classic definition of death and that of brain death are based on irreversible cessation of brain function. There is no inherent dichotomy of logic in this construct. Therefore, brain death is the essential equivalent of systemic death of an individual. This may be further illustrated both experimentally and clinically. If a dog's head is experimentally severed from the body and kept alive by an appropriate life support system and the same is done to the dog's body, the essence of the animal's "personality" is in the head, not the corpus. The head in such an experiment will eat, salivate, blink, sleep, and respond to stimuli to which it has previously been conditioned, for example, when its name is called. If a human is quadriplegic because of a cervical spinal cord transection but has a normal brain, he or she may be kept alive by a life support system; unquestionably he or she is a person who is aware and responds appropriately to external stimuli. However, if a person's cerebral hemispheres were destroyed by a shotgun blast, with subsequent deterioration of the brain stem, the temporary maintenance of the body by modern scientific methods does not mean that a human life is being maintained. To press the analogy to an extreme, we may culture skin cells from a person and keep them growing in artificial media for months. If we destroy these cultured cells, however, this does not constitute the killing of a person, although we are obliterating DNA molecules and tissues related to that person.

Structural substrate

We will consider in greater detail the structural and functional aspects of the cen-tral nervous system that are most significant in evaluation of brain death and distinguish them from other diagnostic entities. The CNS will be considered as three separate structural-functional entities: the cerebral hemispheres, the brain stem (and other posterior fossa structures), and the spinal cord.

Cerebral hemispheres. The cerebral hemispheres include all structures above the tentorium, that is, the cortex bilaterally, the basal ganglia, and thalamic nuclei as well as the limbic system. Functionally, the cerebrum subserves cognitive behavior such as awareness, learning, memory, purposeful voluntary movement patterns, speech, ideation, reasoning, mentation, and goal-directed activity. All aspects of sapient behavior are lost with the destruction of the cerebral hemispheres. However, as noted previously, such destruction of itself does not result in brain death, since vegetative behavior may persist.

Brain stem and posterior fossa structures. Brain stem and posterior fossa structures include the various nuclei and tracts and, most pertinent, the control mechanisms relating to complex stereotyped cephalic and other reflex patterns. In addition, the brain stem reticular formation may control aspects of consciousness.[40,42] Respiration is dependent on brain stem viability. Cardiac activity may continue without a brain stem, but modulation of such activity requires intact mechanisms within the stem. We may consider these as vegetative functions that may exist to varying degrees, depending on alterations elsewhere in the nervous system. Extraocular movements, pupillary reflexes, and a variety of fluctuating comalike states with eyes open or closed may persist with an intact brain stem. The issue is complicated by situations in which portions of the cerebrum are not totally destroyed.

Spinal cord. The spinal cord, that portion of the CNS below the stem from the foramen magnum down, may be viable despite total destruction of all neuronal elements above it (e.g., brain death). A variety of reflex and withdrawal phenomena may exist in these situations, and evidence of a living spinal cord does not preclude the diagnosis of brain death.[1]

Neurons do not reproduce and although axonal and dendritic regrowth may occur, destruction of the soma of a neuron is irreversible. Therefore, determination of irreversible destruction (or dysfunction) of neurons in the brain stem and the cerebrum (but not the spinal cord) is required to arrive at a diagnosis of brain death.

Critical factors in brain viability

The etiology of destruction or irreversible dysfunction of neurons within the intracranial cavity is based on several critical factors. These may not all be measurable in a simple manner, but they should be considered in terms of a particular patient in whom the question of brain death occurs. In these patients multiple etiologies are most often involved. Although it may not be possible to determine the exact mechanism leading to brain death, these factors must be considered in evaluating the patient. This allows the physician to use his or her judgment to determine what clinical and laboratory tests should be performed in order to establish the unequivocal diagnosis of brain death. It is permissible to err in considering a dead brain alive, but one must never diagnose a live brain as dead.

Intracranial pressure. Increase of intracranial pressure (ICP) to levels greater than the mean systemic blood pressure will exceed the perfusion pressure and thus stop intracranial circulation. If this persists for a sufficient period, irreversible neuronal changes will occur. Brain death from increased ICP is most commonly caused by intracranial hemorrhage, although other causes such as cerebral edema secondary to transient ischemia may also occur. Intracranial hematomas and neoplasms are less frequent causes of increased ICP in this group of patients. The duration of increased ICP above perfusion pressure that will produce irreversible total brain dysfunction may depend on such other factors as patient age, drugs, and hypothermia. Probably 20 minutes is sufficient, but in the adult human,

ICP above mean systolic blood pressure for one hour definitely results in death of intracranial neurons. There have been reports of increased ICP preventing angiographic filling that is reversible after the patient is treated surgically or with agents that reduce ICP, such as mannitol and steroids.[25,74] Monitoring of ICP may be a useful ancillary method in confirming the diagnosis of brain death.

Cerebral blood flow (CBF). Of great importance in maintenance of brain viability is adequate perfusion. If CBF decreases 20% of normal for one hour in the adult with an intact cerebrum, brain death will occur.[17,53,54] Values below 20% of normal CBF have been reported by Ingvar and co-workers in apallic syndrome.[38,39] In this situation, however, neuronal structures of the cerebral hemispheres have been destroyed, and the measurements represent blood flow requirements primarily of gliotic tissue.

Although most investigators consider the metabolic activity of neurons and their requirements for oxygen and glucose to be of primary importance, these requirements may decrease under many situations and not cause irreversible changes. In contrast, decrease of CBF or a substitute perfusate for a sufficient period of time is uniformly more disastrous. The example of iced saline exsanguination transfusion in the treatment of hepatic coma may be cited. In this situation, the patient's entire blood supply is drained and replaced by iced saline. There is a period during which nothing but iced saline is circulating in the patient. Then fresh whole blood is used to replace the iced saline. Since some patients survive this procedure without gross evidence of brain damage, we must assume that the maintenance of circulation prevents an irreversible state from occurring despite the lack of required metabolites.

Furthermore, there are diagnostic procedures available to evaluate cerebral circulation that are often more practical to perform in a clinical setting than is the evaluation of brain metabolites themselves.[19,41,78,82,87] The determination of cerebral and/or brain circulation becomes very significant from a clinical standpoint.

When intracranial blood flow is decreased below the critical level for a critical period, reestablishment of intracranial circulation is almost impossible. CBF values below 20% of normal for more than 20 minutes have been mentioned as approximations for this critical level and period. Although the mechanisms for this phenomena are not precisely known, some speculation is warranted. The concept of "no-reflow" phenomena with swelling of the perivascular glial cells has been considered but probably is not the major factor in humans.[3,24,55] The possibility of transient cerebral edema secondary to increased osmolarity of brain tissue occurs with critical decrease of CBF, and this may close off the intracranial vessels by exceeding the perfusion pressure. But the question that remains unanswered is why reestablishment of the circulation does not occur even under conditions of reestablishment of increased extracranial vascular pressure.

One may speculate on a hypothesis regarding the failure of reestablishment of CBF after transient cardiac arrest without invoking massive increase of ICP. The following sequence of events is suggested: After cardiac arrest intracranial blood flow drops markedly, with subsequent effects that are related to the period of time required to reestablish peripheral blood flow. If a critical deficit of CBF for a critical period occurs, there may be *relative* collapse of intracranial vascular structures whose volume may be replaced by minimal diffuse intracranial edema which does not markedly elevate ICP. However, this situation does lead to a set of factors that include marked increase of intracranial intravascular resistance (IVR). This results in diminution to obliteration of CBF. According to *Poiseuille's law*, resistance to laminar flow between the points is directly proportional to viscosity and length of the vascular structure and inversely proportional to the *fourth power* of the diameter of the vessel. Thus we may visualize diffuse transient collapse of the vascular tree including capillaries and significant decrease

of vascular diameter approaching zero. Both of these factors, especially the decrease in diameter, will cause a relatively huge rise in IVR that, along with other pathological changes, will be the major factor preventing the normal reestablished systemic circulation and blood pressure from also reestablishing intracranial flow.

Metabolism of oxygen ($CMRO_2$) and glucose. Neurons will die if they do not have sufficient oxygen and glucose. Anaerobic metabolism accounts for a very small part of the brain's energy reservoir. If neurons are deprived of oxygen and/or glucose for more than 10 minutes, irreversible changes occur. However, this may not be the case in children and infants, or if the patient is markedly hypothermic and/or is receiving large quantities of psychotropic drugs. The "housekeeping" energy to maintain viable neurons that are nonfunctioning but are still in a reversible state is above 20% of normal.[40,42] One can even lower this requirement by hypothermia and drugs that essentially place the neurons in a state of "suspended animation." They may require virtually no oxygen and glucose for a significant period and still be in a reversible state. It is for this reason that metabolic activity can be reduced and not necessarily result in brain death, in contrast to intracranial perfusion, which cannot be stopped for any prolonged period.

Temporal factors are clearly important, and the duration of the deficit must be judged in relation to the specific circumstances, especially those relating to the age of the patient, drug intoxication, and hypothermia. Additional factors include endogenous intoxication or encephalitis. The etiology of the basic process must always be considered as significant in the evaluation of the patient who may be brain dead. The relationship of the above-described factors and the clinical evaluation of the patient as well as studies on electrical activity in the brain and cerebral circulation that are used as criteria to determine brain death will become more apparent when these criteria are discussed in detail.

HISTORICAL DEVELOPMENT OF CRITERIA FOR BRAIN DEATH
Legal definition

The definition of death, while often made in a straightforward and simplistic manner, is in fact, a highly complex construct having many intricate facets and ramifications. Because of the limitations of knowledge surrounding the problem of death, the concepts and the criteria that developed were applied in a relatively direct and pragmatic manner in various societies. Death has been considered with reference to the state of the organism in an all-or-none manner; that is, that an individual organism is either dead or alive. This notion is both simplistic and naive, since death is not an event but a process. The controversy over the nature of this process was discussed in 1971 by Morison[62] and Kass.[46] The process of death occurs over a finite period. Since the process may be brief, the duration and means of evaluating the state of the organism are often limited. Practical requirements over the past several thousand years demanded a yes or no answer to the question of whether an individual was dead. Therefore, it was both reasonable and convenient to consider death as an event. Actually it is now known that death involves a complex series of changes which, if they occur rapidly enough, asymptotically approach the commonly used concept of an event. Before the advent of applications of modern science and technology to biology, the development of deeper understanding of the physiology of living systems, the utilization of intensive care units (ICU), and the therapeutic use of organs for transplantation, the distinction between death as a process and death as an event had limited significance. However, as the utilization of resuscitation and life-support systems increased, the necessity of defining the process of death has become essential. Although a statement of the moment of death is required by many agencies in our society, this "moment" may, in fact, be a period of long duration that cannot be precisely stated. The presumed end state of a multicellular organism, when all of its cells are dead, is not the moment of death nor is the time of pronouncement of death necessarily the moment of death, since many cellular components of the organism may still be alive. We must, therefore, consider the dynamic, organizational, and cellular aspects of the deteriorating human organism in order to redefine the process of death. Then we may obtain utilitarian criteria to define the moment of death.

Pius XII (1957)

The distinction between death of an organism and death of components of the organism was considered as a practical problem by a group of anesthesiologists who maintained patients on life-support systems although there was no evidence of brain viability. These patients had irreparable destruction of the brain. The question arose in the application of technical advances whether it was appropriate to keep the corpus or body "alive" in the absence of a brain, and the problem was presented in 1957 to Pope Pius XII. This resulted in a papal allocution entitled "The Prolongation of Life", which was published in the following year. Among the many significant statements contained in this document, two will be stressed. The first was that the pronouncement of death was not the province of the church but the responsibility of the physician: "It remains for the doctor . . . to give a clear and precise definition of 'death' and the 'moment of death' of a patient who passes away in a state of unconsciousness." The second point was that there came a time in the course of a patient's disease where the situation was hopeless and death should not be opposed by extraordinary means. The definitions of the words "hopeless" and "extraordinary" were not precisely stated in medical terminology, but it was clear that in hopeless cases resuscitative measures could be discontinued and death be unopposed. It was at this time that brain death and associated problems became the subject of increasing general interest. Historically, this proclamation initiated the surge in concept development, research, application, and controversy in use of the construct "brain death." Using the papal allocution as a point of departure, the history of the development of criteria for brain death will be reviewed.[70]

French neurophysiologists and coma dépassé (1959)

In 1959, several groups of French neurophysiologists were involved in salient research with patients who were in extremely deep coma. They coined the term "coma dépassé," which was literally translated as "beyond coma" or "ultra-coma," and by some authors, unfortunately, as "irreversible coma." The results of these studies were published by Fischgold and Mathis,[28] Jouvet,[45] and Mollaret and Goulon[61] in 1959. The patients they studied were in deep states of unresponsive coma, in which the absence of spontaneous respiration necessitated the use of a respirator. These patients, in addition, were areflexic. Studies performed included electroencephalography (EEG) as well as multiple electrophysiologic recordings from the surface of the cortex and deep structures of the cerebrum such as the thalamus. The finding of absent electrophysiologic activity was considered by these investigators as confirmation of irreversible dysfunction of the brain. Many other investigators published data relating to this problem and are referred to in general bibliographies by Smith and Penry (1972)[83] and Walker (1977).[97]

Harvard criteria (1968)

Most often quoted are the Harvard Criteria,[26] developed in 1968, which define cerebral death as irreversible coma (brain death) in terms of the following characteristics:

1. Absence of cerebral responsiveness
2. Absence of induced or spontaneous movement
3. Absence of spontaneous respirations (requiring the use of a respirator)
4. Absence of cephalic and deep-tendon reflexes
5. Absence of drug intoxication or hypothermia

6. Presence of a flat EEG
7. Persistence of these conditions for 24 hours

Although the Harvard Criteria may be and have been used effectively, they have within them a set of limitations that requires close scrutiny. The definition of coma is usually considered in terms of cerebral unresponsivity. There are, however, several manifestations that occur in patients who are in coma and cerebrally unresponsive who present with decerebrate phenomena, spontaneous seizures, and other forms of motor activity who are in a variety of chronic comas or in persistent vegetative states, as previously noted.[44,47] The common practice of considering brain death and cerebral death as equivalent terms leads to confusion. This is most evident when one considers the status of the brain stem; for example, the cerebrum may be destroyed and the brain stem remain intact, or the reverse may occur. Rarely, the cerebrum and brain stem may be completely separated from each other.[48]

Declaration of Sidney (1968)

In 1968, the Declaration of Sidney was made, which added two important statements to the problem of the diagnosis of brain death in relation to organ transplantation. The first was a reaffirmation that death is a process and that in a multicellular organism a large mass of cells might be alive but that this did not indicate that the organism as a whole was alive. Second, it declared that in situations related to organ transplantation, the pronouncement of death should involve two physicians unrelated to the transplant procedure itself.[30]

Minnesota criteria (1971)

In a clinical and pathologic study of brain death, Mohandas and Chou[60] reported that in patients with brain damage the nature of which is known, who show no spontaneous movement, and who are apneic with absent cephalic (brain stem) reflexes, all persistent for 12 hours, the outcome is invariably fatal. These criteria imply that the prediction of immanent death or a fatal prognosis is tantamount to brain death. The Minnesota Criteria are as follows:

1. Basic prerequisite: diagnosis of irreparable cerebral lesion
2. No spontaneous movements
3. No spontaneous respiration
4. Absence of brain stem reflexes
5. Persistence of condition unchanged for 12 hours

Notice the absence of the use of either EEG or a test for intracranial blood flow in these criteria.

Scandinavian criteria (1972)

In a symposium on brain death reported by Ingvar and Widen in 1972,[43] criteria were recommended for use in Scandinavia in patients with known primary or secondary brain lesions who were in unresponsive coma with apnea, absence of all cerebral functions including brain stem reflexes, and a single isoelectric EEG. Confirmation of absences in intracranial function was made by aortocranial angiography showing no circulation to the brain on two injections of contrast medium 25 minutes apart.

These criteria reduce the temporal delay to an absolute minimum (25 minutes). The circulatory criterion are not influenced by the presence of drugs that depress cerebral function, and since, collectively, clinical signs, EEG, and cerebral circulation are determined independently of one another, they are cross-confirmatory. While they imply total cerebral infarction as the definition of brain death, variations in the rate at which the circulation to the brain collapses would probably permit a variety of pathologic states to be observed at autopsy. The following summarizes the Scandinavian Criteria:

1. Unresponsive coma
2. Apnea
3. Absent brain stem reflexes
4. Isoelectric EEG
5. Nonfilling of cerebral vessels on two aortocranial injections (bilateral carotid and vertebral) of contrast media 25 minutes apart

Japanese criteria (1973)

From data derived from a Japanese study of brain death, Ueki and associates[90] reported that a diagnosed gross primary brain lesion, deep coma, bilateral dilated pupils with absent pupillary and corneal reflexes, and an isoelectric EEG predict brain death. In such patients, a fall in blood pressure of 40 mm Hg persistent for six hours signals that death is imminent. The Japanese Criteria are as follows:

1. Basic prerequisite: diagnosis of primary cerebral lesion
2. Deep coma
3. Respiratory arrest
4. Bilateral dilated pupils and absent pupillary and corneal reflexes
5. Flat EEG
6. Abrupt fall in blood pressure of 40 mm Hg with hypotension
7. Persistence of condition for at least six hours

Cerebral survival (CS) study criteria (1977)

A collaborative study was sponsored by the National Institutes of Health in order to establish more firm criteria for the diagnosis of brain death. The study involved 844 comatose apneic patients evaluated between 1970 and 1973.[4,47,97] The first set of 503 patients was statistically evaluated in order to develop more precise criteria. Other subsets of these patients were analyzed by Korein and co-workers,[53,54] Allen and co-workers,[1] and Bennett.[8] The conclusions may be summarized by the development of the criteria listed below*:

1. Prerequisite: all appropriate diagnostic and therapeutic procedures have been performed (diagnosis established)
2. Criteria (to be present for 30 minutes at least six hours after the onset of coma and apnea):
   a. Coma with cerebral unresponsivity
   b. Apnea
   c. Dilated fixed pupils

---

*See also G. Molinari.[47]

d. Absent cephalic reflexes
e. Electrocerebral silence
3. Confirmatory test: absence of cerebral circulation

CRITIQUE OF CRITERIA

Some of the difficulties encountered with all these criteria have been previously discussed. We will now attempt to expand on these problems and especially evaluate the Harvard Criteria.

Coma

The precise definition of unresponsive coma has been attempted by a variety of investigators, often using a grading scale; but coma is not linear and is multidimensional. The most severe state described considers clinical features such as total unresponsivity to stimuli, absence of spontaneous movements, fixed dilated pupils, absence of spontaneous respirations, and absence of all reflexes.[71] This clinical approach has several limitations, since it confounds cerebral, brain stem, and spinal cord function. If we consider coma in terms of absent cerebral responsivity, we still encounter the difficulty of seizures, decerebrate phenomena, complex brain stem reflexes, and the possible presence of respirations. We will, therefore, attend to those aspects of coma that relate to brain and brain stem dysfunction in order to accurately diagnose brain death. We will depend on ancillary studies to confirm the presence of a nonfunctioning cerebrum by such means as electroencephalography and alteration in cerebral blood flow in addition to clinical unresponsiveness and absence of spontaneous movement.

Apnea and test for respirator dependence

A most important dysfunction of the brain stem is that of failure to maintain respiration. Although a presumptive test for apnea was considered positive when the patient failed to override the respirator for 15 minutes,[99] more accurate tests for respirator dependence are described by Plum and Posner[71] and others.[59,77] They suggest, for example, that after the patient is ventilated for many minutes to half-an-hour with 100% pure oxygen, he be disconnected from the respirator. Arterial pH, P_{CO_2} and P_{O_2} are determined at that time and the patient is observed up to 10 minutes with 100% oxygen at six l/min administered passively via the tracheostomy. If no arrhythmia, cyanosis, or other untoward responses occur and the patient does not breathe spontaneously, a repeat sample of arterial blood for pH, P_{CO_2} and P_{O_2} is obtained, and the patient is placed back on the respirator. The period may be shortened depending on the clinical judgment of the physician, and the procedure should always be performed under the supervision of an inhalation therapist or an anesthesiologist. In practice, the usual period the patient is taken off the respirator is four to six minutes. The arterial blood values may be performed more frequently to determine whether the patient's P_{CO_2} has risen sufficiently to trigger respirations and to ensure that the P_{O_2} has not decreased to a detrimental level. Studies by Hass and co-workers[34] indicate the reservoir of oxygen in the lungs allows this test to be safely performed. A rather extreme version of this technique is used in France as reported by Milhaud and co-workers, during which the patient after being sufficiently primed with 100% oxygen is taken off the respirator for up to an hour.[59] It should be noted, as previously mentioned, that the inherent difficulty in these tests are that in no way do they evaluate the response of the patient to decreased P_{O_2} but only to increases of P_{CO_2} The level of P_{CO_2} in arterial blood should rise above 60 mm Hg. Occasionally a satisfactory test for apnea requires that the patient be off the respirator for a prolonged period.

Cephalic reflexes including pupillary activity

Other than respirations, there is a complex repertoire of cephalic reflexes and stereotyped patterns that are subserved by the brain stem. In situations such as the apallic syndrome, these are often obvious and since their presence excludes the diagnosis of brain death, they need not be discussed further. It is the absence of these reflexes that is significant in the diagnosis of brain death. The single most important cephalic reflex is the pupillary. The presence of a pupillary reflex indicates a degree of brain stem function that rules out the diagnosis of total brain death. Most often, fixed dilated pupils are seen. It is not uncommon, however, to have middilated pupils that are fixed.* In evaluating a series of some 50 cadavers, pupils are most often middilated and fixed, and inequalities in size are frequent (personal observations). Pinpoint pupils may occur with brain death but should alert the examiner to the possibility of stem function and possible drug intoxication. Rarely, fixed dilated pupils may occur in reversible situations, especially with drugs such as glutethimide (Doriden) or atropine. Fixed middilated pupils have been seen in a patient with tetanus who was being treated with muscle paralyzants and who met the clinical criteria of brain death.[9]

Other cephalic reflexes of importance include the oculocephalic reflex, response to caloric stimulation, and the pharyngeal reflex. Ouaknine advocates an atropine test using small dosages that will change the heart rate via the brain stem reflex arc without direct effect on the conduction system of the heart itself.[66,67] A frequent difficulty encountered in determination of brain stem viability is the presence of spontaneous electromyogram (EMG) activity in muscles of the head supplied by the cranial nerves that are observed during EEG recording. Several European investigators considered this in itself as evidence of meaningful brain stem function.[5] We have encountered some sporadic EMG activity frequently enough in patients who are unequivocally brain dead by all other criteria and do not accept this thesis.

*Greater than 5 mm.

Deep tendon reflexes (DTRs), induced and spontaneous movements

Presence of spinal reflexes as well as induced or spontaneous movements related to spinal cord activity alone do not preclude the diagnosis of brain death. This has been thoroughly verified by numerous investigators, as has been previously mentioned, and deserves no further comment. However, in contrast to withdrawal of a leg in response to a noxious stimulus, an arm movement may be a fragment of a brain stem reflex. One must carefully distinguish the substrate of the movement or reflex pattern, since if the response is derived from the brain stem, the patient is not totally brain dead.

Toxic agents

Reversible coma, including isoelectric activity in the EEG, has been well documented with a variety of central nervous system intoxicants, most notably barbiturates.* However, the concomitants of diagnosable brain death are not infrequently found in combination with intoxication and the significant drug levels in the blood. This is the primary reason for having an additional ancillary test for cerebral circulation. The absence or critical deficit of cerebral circulation in adults, even in the presence of intoxicants, allows such a diagnosis to be made with certitude. This situation may be less clear cut in infants and young children, and clinical judgment must be applied with acute awareness of the potential difficulties in these situations. In addition, the difficulty in ascertaining the drug involved is great, and if any doubt exists and adequate tests cannot be performed (i.e., for drugs or cerebral circulation), a therapeutic trial of renal dialysis may be indicated.

The problem with children and infants

Although criteria used for adults may be applied to older children, a serious dilemma may arise with infants and young children.[7,68] It is well documented that the immature

*References 4, 8, 9, 12, 26, 36, 73, 83, 97.

brain is far more resistant to anoxia and the transient decrease of cerebral blood flow. A case has been reported, for example, in which a child has been submerged in ice water for over 40 minutes with resultant complete recovery.[79] Other investigators, such as Ashwal and Schneider, have described situations in which "EEG activity" has been recorded for periods up to 30 days in the absence of detectable intracranial circulation.[6] This was demonstrated in children below the age of 30 months using a variety of techniques, including four-vessel angiography. Presumably the "EEG activity" was not artifactual. Although all these patients died, extreme caution must be used in diagnosing brain death, especially in patients below the age of 6 years. Perhaps modified criteria will be required for children and infants since the duration life support in this age group may continue for much longer periods than adults—for weeks to months rather than days.

LABORATORY AND OTHER ANCILLARY TESTS

It should be noted that more precise specification of the EEG criteria was developed during 1969 by Silverman and co-workers in conjunction with the American EEG Society (AEEG) and the statement of details relating to methodology has been published in 1976 by the AEEG.[2,80,81] These are detailed below. The emphasis on tests of the deficit in cerebral circulation were stressed primarily by European investigators in 1969.[19] The arrest of intracranial circulation was subsequently added to the definition of coma dépassé.

Electroencephalogram

The electroencephalogram is one of the most commonly used ancillary procedures in deriving the diagnosis of brain death in the United States. It should be clearly understood prior to any discussion of EEG itself that there are clear-cut restrictions and limitations in the use of EEG in confirming the diagnosis.[8,9,31,36] The EEG must only be used

in conjunction with appropriate clinical criteria, other laboratory tests, and the application of clinical judgment.

Recording techniques. One cannot use the routine recording techniques used in clinical EEG in an attempt to determine whether brain activity is absent. We will briefly define the purpose of the EEG as an ancillary test in the diagnosis of brain death and present modification of the recording procedures required.

If the EEG (with appropriately modified recording techniques) derived from scalp electrodes reveals no evidence of electro-cerebral activity above 2 μV. for a period of one-half hour, the record may be said to be isoelectric or indicate electrocerebral silence (ECS). The terms nul and flat and other subjective descriptions should be avoided. ECS indicates the absence of cortical and usually subcortical activity. This finding may be indicative of irreversible dysfunction of the cerebrum under specific conditions, since there are cases reported in which ECS has been present in a reversible condition (e.g., drug intoxication) and its application must be used with appropriate caution. Furthermore, there is a great variety of artifacts that may interfere with evaluation of the record, and these must be identified or eliminated to allow interpretation of a technically satisfactory EEG.

Further detail in recording technique and problems related to obtaining satisfactory records as well as artifact detection are described elsewhere.[2,9] Of paramount importance is that the interelectrode distance across the scalp should not be less than 10 cm, and the montage should include recordings from both hemispheres, preferably using the international 10-20 system. Electrodes would be placed on frontal, parasagittal, temporal, and occipital regions. Bipolar as well as unipolar recordings should be made, although the incidence of artifact in unipolar recordings is greater. Six to eight bilateral scalp electrodes with an ear lobe reference are suggested. The interelectrode

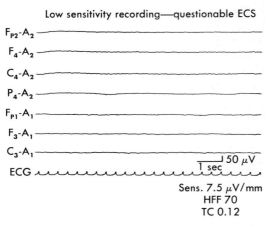

Fig. 14-1. EEG recorded at a sensitivity of 7.5 μV/mm contains some very low amplitude oscillations, which could be EEG activity but are not clearly recognizable as such. This type of record is frequently erroneously classified as "flat" or ECS. (Adapted from Bennett, D., Hughes, J., Korein, J., Merlis, J., and Suter, C.: An atlas of electroencephalography in coma and cerebral death, New York, 1976, Raven Press.)

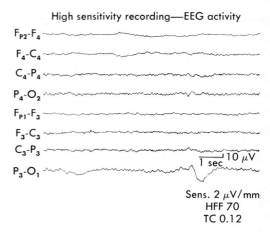

Fig. 14-2. EEG from same patient as in Fig. 14-1, but recorded at a sensitivity of 2 μV/mm, clearly contains mixed frequency EEG activity. Respirator artifacts are seen in channel 8. (Adapted from Bennett, D., Hughes, J., Korein, J., Merlis, J., and Suter, C.: An atlas of electroencephalography in coma and cerebral death, New York, 1976, Raven Press.)

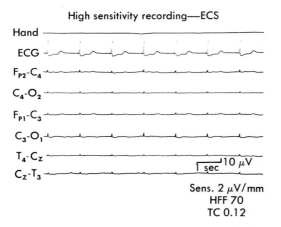

Fig. 14-3. Example of an ECS tracing recorded at the high gain required. ECG artifact is present but does not obscure the record. (Adapted from Bennett, D., Hughes, J., Korein, J., Merlis, J., and Suter, C.: An atlas of electroencephalography in coma and cerebral death, New York, 1976, Raven Press.)

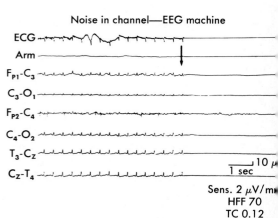

Fig. 14-4. Note the irregular sharp and fast activity in channel 5. At the arrow the machine was switched to the calibrate mode and the same kind of deflections was seen, indicating that these deflections represented noise arising within the amplifier of that channel. (Adapted from Bennett, D., Hughes, J., Korein, J., Merlis, J., and Suter, C.: An atlas of electroencephalography in coma and cerebral death, New York, 1976, Raven Press.)

impedance should range between 100 and 10,000 ohms. Autoclaved needle electrodes may be used, although surface electrodes are usually recommended. Maximal amplification of most commercially available electroencephalographs will allow a sensitivity of recording of 2 μV/mm, which is the minimal standard for evaluation of ECS. Appropriate calibration must be performed before and after the one-half hour recording, and all sensitivities must be utilized. High-frequency filters may be used to eliminate activity above 30 Hz; time constants of .3 to .4 seconds should be used during parts of the recording. An appropriate test for the integrity of the entire system should be run (i.e., touch each electrode gently with a swab to create an artifact potential in the record). Monitoring of ECG and other possible sources of artifact (such as EMG and respiration in two channels of the recording) is almost always necessary at high gain.

Further recommendations include test for EEG reactivity to stimuli such as pain, sound, and light as well as repetition of the entire procedure if there is any question as to the presence of ECS. With increased muscle artifact a muscle paralyzant may be used under the supervision of a qualified physician. Only a qualified experienced technician should perform the recordings, and the technician should have recourse to consult with the physician in charge if there are any problems in the recording.

It should be noted that if these recommendations are not followed, apparent ECS may be recorded (see Figs. 14-1 to 14-3). Further, in situations where artifact obscures the record, several techniques can be used to identify or eliminate them (Figs. 14-4 to 14-9).

Significance of electrocerebral silence. The significance of ECS depends primarily on the clinical state of the patient. Situations

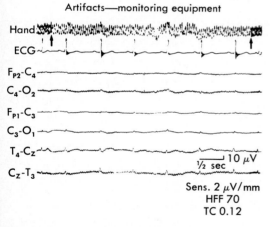

Fig. 14-5. Activity at 27 cycles/sec appears in all channels recording from the scalp but is especially prominent from the hand electrodes (channel 1). This artifact was introduced by monitoring equipment used in the intensive care unit. Paper speed has been changed to 60 mm/sec between the arrows. (Adapted from Bennett, D., Hughes, J., Korein, J., Merlis, J., and Suter, C.: An atlas of electroencephalography in coma and cerebral death, New York, 1976, Raven Press.)

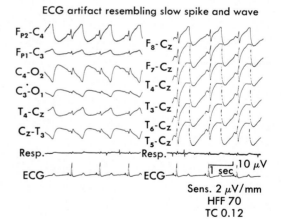

Fig. 14-6. *Left*, ECG artifacts may have the appearance of a slow "spike and wave complex," with the "spike" related to the QRS complex and the "wave" appearing at the time of the T wave. Note the different configurations of the artifact in the different scalp derivations. *Right*, with a common reference (C_z), the artifact is more prominent and is very similar in all channels. (Adapted from Bennett, D., Hughes, J., Korein, J., Merlis, J., and Suter, C.: An atlas of electroencephalography in coma and cerebral death, New York, 1976, Raven Press.)

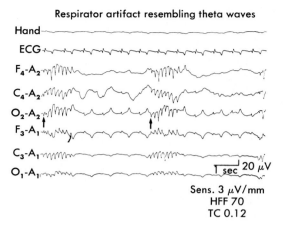

Respirator artifact resembling theta waves

Sens. 3 µV/mm
HFF 70
TC 0.12

Fig. 14-7. The bursts of 6 cycles/sec activity are synchronous with the respirator cycle (*arrows*). (Adapted from Bennett, D., Hughes, J., Korein, J., Merlis, J., and Suter, C.: An atlas of electroencephalography in coma and cerebral death, New York, 1976, Raven Press.)

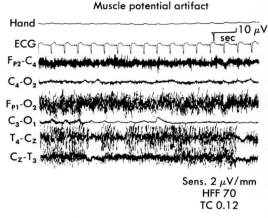

Muscle potential artifact

Sens. 2 µV/mm
HFF 70
TC 0.12

Fig. 14-8. High amplitude muscle potential artifact obscures the tracing so that cerebral activity cannot be assessed. (Adapted from Bennett, D., Hughes, J., Korein, J., Merlis, J., and Suter, C.: An atlas of electroencephalography in coma and cerebral death, New York, 1976, Raven Press.)

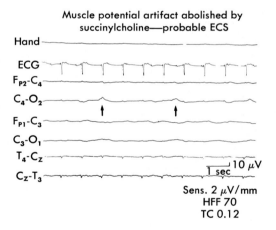

Muscle potential artifact abolished by
succinylcholine—probable ECS

Sens. 2 µV/mm
HFF 70
TC 0.12

Fig. 14-9. EEG from same patient recorded in Fig. 14-8. After succinylcholine the muscle activity disappears and the record can now be assessed, showing probable ECS. Some respirator artifact is seen, most prominently in channel 4 (*arrows*). (Adapted from Bennett, D., Hughes, J., Korein, J., Merlis, J., and Suter, C.: An atlas of electroencephalography in coma and cerebral death, New York, 1976, Raven Press.)

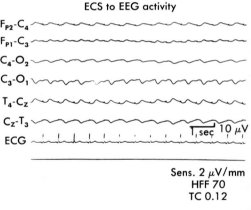

ECS to EEG activity

Sens. 2 µV/mm
HFF 70
TC 0.12

Fig. 14-10. Sample from a third EEG with ECS, performed approximately 24 hours after admission of a patient with apnea and coma due to barbiturate overdose in a run with increased interelectrode distances. This EEG revealed ECS throughout, as did the previous two recordings. All records were run for 30 min. ECG artifact is present throughout this montage. The patient at this time was still cerebrally unresponsive, apneic, and areflexic. The pupils were 2 mm, fixed and equal. (Adapted from Bennett, D., Hughes, J., Korein, J., Merlis, J., and Suter, C.: An atlas of electroencephalography in coma and cerebral death, New York, 1976, Raven Press.)

in which ECS does not confirm brain death include intoxications, metabolic disorders and encephalitis (rarely), the immediate aftermath of the intracranial insult (i.e., within six hours), and patients in whom brain stem viability alone is demonstrated by clinical examination (Figs. 14-10 to 14-14). If there is any uncertainty as to the significance of ECS reversibility, other studies such as determination of cerebral or intracranial circulation should be performed (see below). The problem of interpretation of ECS in young children and infants must be considered as a separate entity, as noted previously, although in many situations its significance is similar to that described in adults.[7,68,79]

Evoked potentials

Other electrophysiologic techniques have been used in evaluation of brain death and include the use of computer-averaged evoked potentials. Although these are recorded from scalp electrodes, the very early response is indicative of brain stem function. Visual and somatosensory stimuli are usually recorded as indicators of cerebral activity while the auditory evoked response has been studied somewhat more extensively in relation to the "far field" response by Starr and Achor[84,85] as an indicator of the functional integrity of the brain stem. Evidence has accumulated indicating that the evoked response is a more sensitive method of detecting residual cerebral function and may be present even when the EEG is isoelectric.[88] The advantage of having an electrophysiologic measure of brain stem function is also apparent. The limitations inherent in these techniques include specialized equipment and the requirement of experience

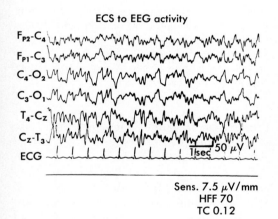

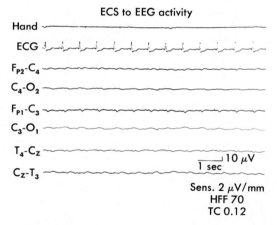

Fig. 14-11. EEG from same patient recorded in Fig. 14-10. Sample from the fourth EEG, performed on the second day, after nine hours of dialysis. The record contains predominantly theta activity with some delta and alpha frequencies. At this time the patient was stuporous, breathing spontaneously, and had normal cephalic reflexes, including pupillary responses. (Adapted from Bennett, D., Hughes, J., Korein, J., Merlis, J., and Suter, C.: An atlas of electroencephalography in coma and cerebral death, New York, 1976, Raven Press.)

Fig. 14-12. Sample from the first EEG, recorded from a patient four hours after the onset of coma due to transient cardiac arrest. Muscle artifact was present and eliminated with 60 mg of succinylcholine administered intravenously. The record was then considered to be one of ECS but was run for only 17 minutes. The patient was unresponsive, apneic, and areflexic except for sluggish pupillary responses. (Adapted from Bennett, D., Hughes, J., Korein, J., Merlis, J., and Suter, C.: An atlas of electroencephalography in coma and cerebral death, New York, 1976, Raven Press.)

ECS to EEG activity

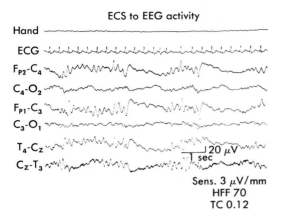

Sens. 3 μV/mm
HFF 70
TC 0.12

Generalized alpha
Hypertension—pontine hemorrhage—deep coma—dea

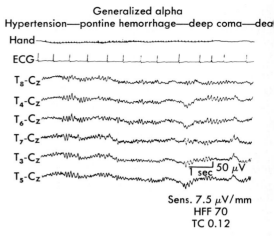

Sens. 7.5 μV/mm
HFF 70
TC 0.12

Fig. 14-13. Sample from the third EEG of the same patient as in Fig. 14-12, recorded two days after the arrest, shows more prominent 5-7/sec activity at 50 μV mixed with small amounts of delta posteriorly. Anteriorly, there are bursts at 80-100 μV and periods of relative suppression lasting 2-4 sec. The myoclonic seizures occurred intermittently. No further EEGs were performed. The patient died five days later. (Adapted from Bennett, D., Hughes, J., Korein, J., Merlis, J., and Suter, C.: An atlas of electroencephalography in coma and cerebral death, New York, 1976, Raven Press.)

Fig. 14-14. Example of diffuse activity, mostly in the alpha band, recorded from a 75-year-old hypertensive male one day after he was admitted. He was deeply comatose secondary to a hemorrhage in the pons. The rhythm at this time was nonreactive. The patient was on controlled ventilation. The pupils were pinpoint but reactive. Corneal and caloric reflexes were absent. Deep tendon reflexes were present, and bilateral Babinski signs were obtained. Minimal extremity withdrawal was noted to painful stimulation. (Adapted from Bennett, D., Hughes, J., Korein, J., Merlis, J., and Suter, C.: An atlas of electroencephalography in coma and cerebral death, New York, 1976, Raven Press.)

and interpretation. Artifacts related to these procedures are infrequent, and reproducibility results may be consistent. However, situations arise in which variability may occur. We would consider these tests as appropriate ancillary procedures for the diagnosis of brain death in those situations where other clinical and electroencephalographic criteria are fulfilled, but there is some doubt in relation to the patient's status because of drug intoxication. The possible use of this technique as an additional test in evaluation of brain death in infants and children might also be considered. Standardization of evoked potentials as an additional criteria for brain death is required.

Intracranial circulation

Angiography. The most accepted and direct method of determining absence of intracranial circulation is angiography. If the determination is required to test the critical deficit of circulation in both the cerebrum and posterior fossa, four-vessel angiography should be performed, usually by means of femoral catheterization. European investigators have stressed that the finding of absent intracranial circulation by this means is the sine qua non of brain death.[33] Ingvar and his co-workers, as already mentioned, include this procedure as a significant criterion to diagnose brain death.[43] Although there may be exceptions, as previously noted, such as transient lack of circulation with increased intracranial pressure, this method used in conjunction with clinical criteria is in fact a highly precise criterion that correlates with brain death[53,56] (Figs. 14-15 to 14-20). The definition of absent cerebral

Text continued on p. 305.

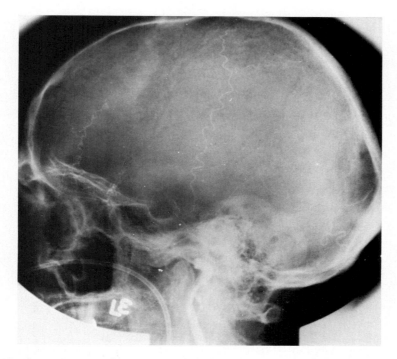

Fig. 14-15. This patient met the complete clinical and EEG criteria of brain death and underwent four-vessel angiography. This figure is a left common carotid angiogram showing the lateral projection after 6 sec. Note good visualization of the external carotid artery and its superficial branches over the scalp. (From Kricheff, I., Pinto, R., George, A., Braunstein, P., and Korein, J.: Angiographic findings in brain death. In Korein, J., editor: Brain death; interrelated medical and social issues, Ann. N.Y. Acad. Sci. **315:**168-183, 1978.)

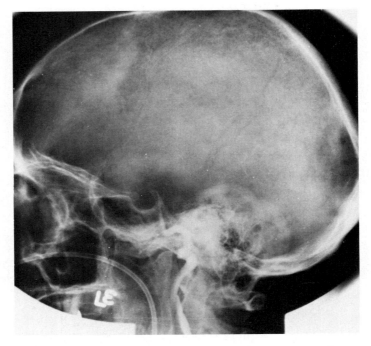

Fig. 14-16. Same angiogram as in Fig. 14-15 at 10 sec after injection. The internal carotid is opacified only as far as its precavernous portion. There is no intracranial filling whatsoever. (From Kricheff, I., Pinto, R., George, A., Braunstein, P., and Korein, J.: Angiographic findings in brain death. In Korein, J., editor: Brain death; interrelated medical and social issues, Ann. N.Y. Acad. Sci. **315:**168-183, 1978.)

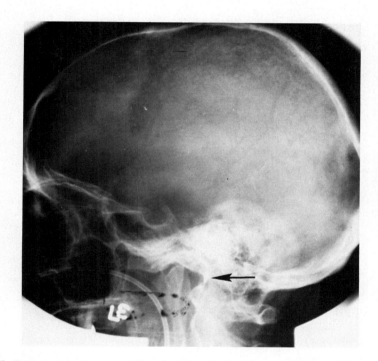

Fig. 14-17. Same angiogram as in Fig. 14-15 at 29 sec after injection. Note the continued absence of intracranial filling and the stasis of a droplet of radiopaque material in the extracranial internal carotid artery. This opacification persisted four minutes. (From Kricheff, I., Pinto, R., George, A., Braunstein, P., and Korein, J.: Angiographic findings in brain death. In Korein, J., editor: Brain death; interrelated medical and social issues, Ann. N.Y. Acad. Sci. **315:**168-183, 1978.)

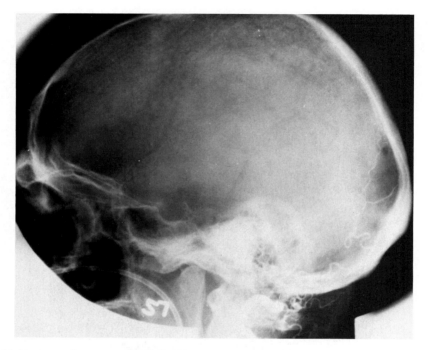

Fig. 14-18. Lateral projection of the left vertebral angiogram six seconds after injection in the patient described in Figs. 14-15 to 14-17. Note good visualization of extracranial muscular and scalp vessels arising from the vertebral arteries. The vertebral is opacified to the level of C1. (From Kricheff, I., Pinto, R., George, A., Braunstein, P., and Korein, J.: Angiographic findings in brain death. In Korein, J., editor: Brain death; interrelated medical and social issues, Ann. N.Y. Acad. Sci. **315:**168-183, 1978.)

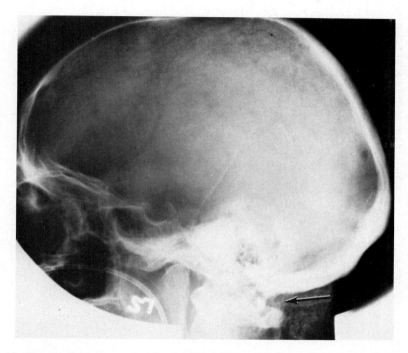

Fig. 14-19. Same angiogram as in Fig. 14-18 at 12 sec after injection. Note the persistent opacified droplet at the level of C1 in the vertebral arteries; this droplet also persisted over a prolonged period, similar to that seen in the extracranial portion of the internal carotid arteries, as seen in Fig. 14-17. There was no evidence of intracranial circulation in the posterior fossa. The findings illustrated in Figs. 14-15 to 14-19 are most common in all four vessels in those patients who meet the clinical and EEG criteria of brain death and represent the most extreme example of absence of intracranial circulation as demonstrated in angiography. (From Kricheff, I., Pinto, R., George, A., Braunstein, P., and Korein, J.: Angiographic findings in brain death. In Korein, J., editor: Brain death; interrelated medical and social issues, Ann. N.Y. Acad. Sci. **315:**168-183, 1978.)

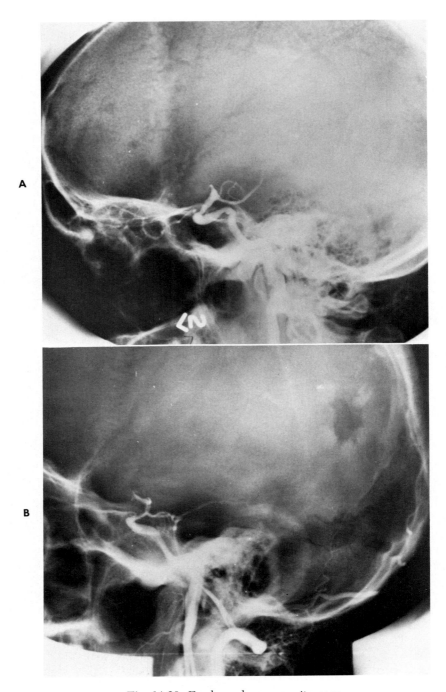

Fig. 14-20. For legend see opposite page.

circulation is based on absence of filling of the venous system. A difficulty with the technique is that it requires transport of the comatose apneic patient to the apparatus and cannot be done at the bedside. Currently, if there is any doubt in the diagnosis of brain death by other criteria, this remains the procedure of choice for confirmation of the diagnosis of brain death.

Results of studies using angiography to validate brain death often reveal a progressive set of changes with circulation first being impaired in the cerebral hemispheres. This then progresses to the posterior fossa structures, usually as a result of increased intracranial pressure.[96] Situations may arise where there is absent cerebral circulation in which posterior fossa circulation may be present.[17,53] The latter does not necessarily indicate a functional brain stem, since abnormalities may be so severe as to preclude reversible changes (see Fig. 14-21).

Gamma camera imaging. Another test of intracranial circulation is gamma camera imaging using isotopes as described by Goodman and co-workers[32] (Figs. 14-22 to 14-24).[47]

These techniques have recently improved in terms of resolution and equipment, which may be portable so that the procedure can be performed at the bedside. Although there are some disadvantages such as the high dose of IV radioisotope required, the difficulty in repeating the test within a short period and possible expertise required in interpretation, the method appears to be valid when used in conjunction with clinical and other criteria.[17]

Radioisotopic bolus technique. The radioisotopic bolus technique was developed as a portable radioisotopic technique to demonstrate cerebral circulatory deficit as part of a collaborative study to define and diagnose brain death[4] simply and rapidly in comatose apneic patients with electrocerebral silence. This technique involves an intravenous injection of 2 mCi of $^{99m}TcO_4$ and recording time/activity curves over the cranial cavity and a femoral artery simultaneously, using twin probe radioisotope detector equipment[14-17,53,54] (Figs. 14-25 to 14-27).

Its limitation includes the fact that it only assesses the critical deficit in circulation in

Text continued on p. 311.

Fig. 14-20. Other less frequent angiographic findings in patients who fulfill clinical and EEG criteria of brain death include stasis and retrograde flow. In both of these situations, although portions of the intracranial arteries are opacified, there is no evidence of intracranial circulation since the radiopaque material never reaches the venous system through the parenchyma of the brain: **A,** Lateral projection of the left internal carotid angiogram via femoral catheter in a patient who met all criteria for brain death. This radiograph was taken seven sec after the injection and shows minimal filling of the proximal middle cerebral artery, proximal portions of the left posterior cerebral artery, as well as portions of the anterior choroidal and posterior communicating arteries. There was no significant change 12 sec after injection, indicating stasis and, subsequently, there was retrograde washout of the opacified material. **B,** Lateral projection of the right vertebral angiogram in a patient meeting all criteria for brain death. The contrast material propelled by the force of the injection alone opacifies the right vertebral artery, the basilar artery, proximal portions of the posterior cerebral arteries, and both posterior communicating arteries. The circle of Willis is traversed with filling of both internal carotid arteries just beyond the level of the anterior clinoids; this represents retrograde flow. Subsequent radiographs revealed no intracranial circulation, although some stasis was present. Radiopaque material was drained through both carotid and vertebral arteries on the left side in a retrograde fashion. (**A** and **B** from Kricheff, I., Pinto, R., George, A., Braunstein, P., and Korein, J.: Angiographic findings in brain death. In Korein, J., editor: Brain death; interrelated medical and social issues, Ann. N.Y. Acad. Sci. **315:**168-183, 1978.)

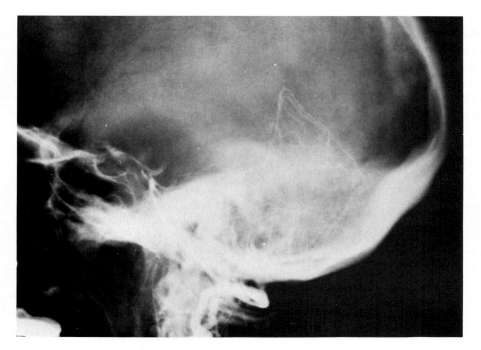

Fig. 14-21. Rarely, in patients who met the complete clinical and electroencephalographic criteria of brain death, in whom there was no angiographic demonstration of supratentorial intracranial circulation, evidence of severely abnormal posterior fossa circulation was present. This is illustrated by this left vertebral angiogram with slow (10 sec) posterior fossa circulation, including opacified arterial, intermediate and venous phases (the latter is not shown). Note the striking depression of the proximal portions of the superior cerebellar arteries and compression of the vermis as a result of massive transtentorial herniation. The basilar arteries are anteriorly displaced, and the tonsillar loop of the posterior inferior cerebellar arteries is anteriorly and inferiorly displaced, indicating tonsillar herniation. This patient had no evidence of spontaneous respirations or any cephalic reflexes. Clinically the posterior fossa was irreversibly dysfunctional. (From Kricheff, I., Pinto, R., George, A., Braunstein, P., and Korein, J.: Angiographic findings in brain death. In Korein, J., editor: Brain death; interrelated medical and social issues, Ann. N.Y. Acad. Sci. **315:**168-183, 1978.)

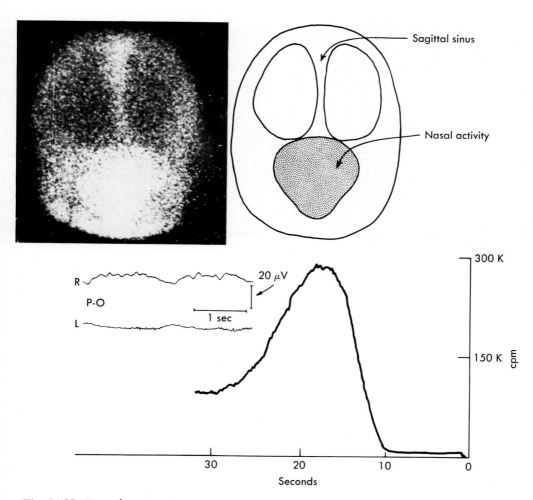

Fig. 14-22. Normal static gamma camera image, anterior projection, in an apneic, comatose patient following the administration of technetium 99m pertechnetate. The patient is not brain dead. Note the simultaneous presence of the parietal occipital EEG activity and the presence of a head bolus (see text). (From Korein, J., editor: Brain death; interrelated medical and social issues, Ann. N.Y. Acad. Sci. **315**:212-213, 1978.)

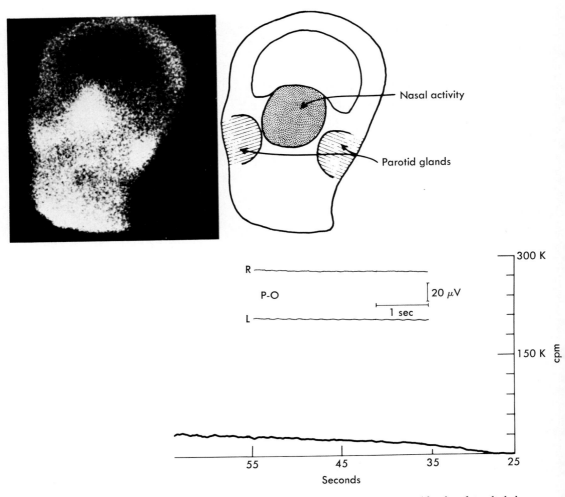

Fig. 14-23. Abnormal static gamma camera image, anterior projection (the head is slightly rotated), in a patient who fulfills all criteria of brain death, after injection of technetium 99m pertechnetate. There is no evidence of radioisotope activity in the brain area, in contrast to that in Fig. 14-22. Note the simultaneous absence of EEG activity in the parietal occipital leads and absence of a head bolus (see text). (From Korein, J., editor: Brain death; interrelated medical and social issues, Ann. N.Y. Acad. Sci. **315**:212-213, 1978.)

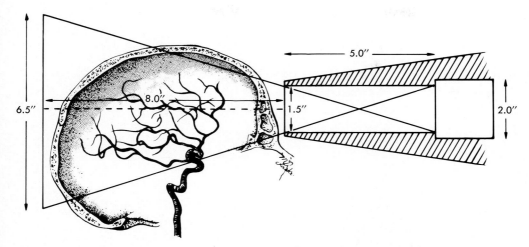

Fig. 14-24. Lateral view through skull showing placement of the head probe used to detect radioisotopic cerebral bolus. Note that all major cerebral vessels are included in the field of the collimator, which forms a truncated cone. The angle is such that the base of the skull and the posterior fossa are virtually excluded. (From Korein, J., Braunstein, P., George, A., Wichter, M., Kricheff, I., Lieberman, A., and Pearson, J.: Brain death. I. Angiographic correlation with the radioisotopic bolus technique for evaluation of critical deficit of cerebral blood flow, Ann. Neurol. **2:**195-205, 1977. By permission of Little, Brown and Co.)

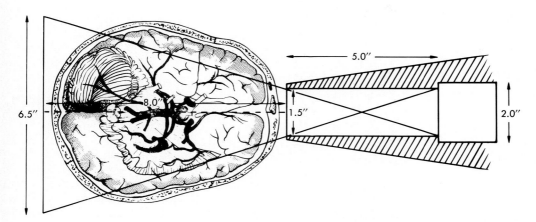

Fig. 14-25. Top view through skull showing brain and origins of the arterial tree. The position of the head probe is the same as in Fig. 14-24. A second probe (not illustrated) is used for a control and was most often placed over the femoral artery. (From Korein, J., Braunstein, P., George, A., Wichter, M., Kricheff, I., Lieberman, A., and Pearson, J.: Brain death. I. Angiographic correlation with the radioisotopic bolus technique for evaluation of critical deficit of cerebral blood flow, Ann. Neurol. **2:**195-205, 1977. By permission of Little, Brown and Co.)

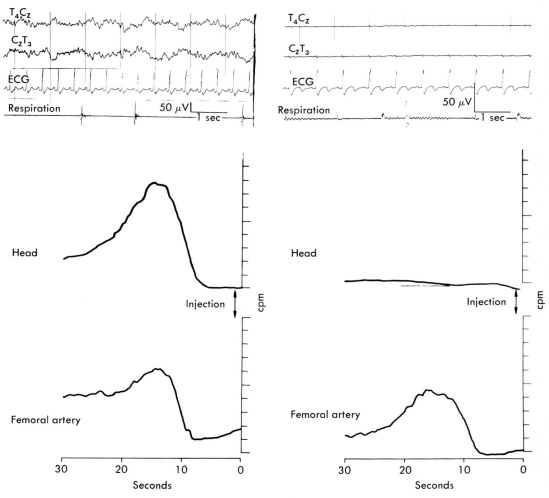

Fig. 14-26. EEG and bolus curves from head and femoral artery in a comatose, apneic patient who is not brain dead. Note the presence of EEG activity and large bolus from the head probe after injection of technetium 99m pertechnetate. (From Korein, J.: On cerebral, brain and systemic death; current concepts of cerebrovascular disease, Stroke **8:**9-14, 1973. By permission of the American Heart Association, Inc.)

Fig. 14-27. EEG and bolus curves from head and femoral artery in a patient who fulfills all criteria for brain death. Note absence of EEG activity at increased amplification and absence of head bolus despite the presence of a bolus in the femoral artery after injection of technetium 99m pertechnetate. (From Korein, J.: On cerebral, brain and systemic death; current concepts of cerebrovascular disease, Stroke **8:**9-14, 1973. By permission of the American Heart Association, Inc.)

the cerebral hemispheres, while brain stem dysfunction must be assessed by other means. This method has been used as an adjunct in successfully diagnosing brain death in children, but some discrepancies have been reported in relation to electrophysiologic activity in the absence of a bolus in children under the age of 30 months.[6,7] An additional problem is that the qualitative nature of the bolus technique may lead to an erroneous impression of the presence of cerebral circulation when in fact there is none. This type of error is acceptable. Evidence indicates that in those patients who may fulfill the clinical criteria of brain death, due to drug intoxication, for example, the decrease in CBF is not sufficient to result in the absence of a bolus. In those cases, such as apallic syndrome or neocortical death,[18,39] in which cerebral circulation may in fact be critically decreased and possibly result in an absent bolus, the clinical symptomatology fails to meet the criteria of brain death; that is, the patient has high stem reflexes and/or respirations. Although initially there was some controversy as to the significance of the radioisotopic bolus observed during the use of this technique, it has been subsequently clarified. There are fundamentally two different kinds of circulation involved. First, the cerebral circulation involves a rapid transit of a large amount of blood to a relatively small vascular reservoir. It has been calculated that CBF is normally above 750 ml/min and passes through a blood pool reservoir of 130 ml/min.[65,101] This very rapid transit through the relatively small cerebral blood reservoir causes a distinct registering of the arrival and departure of an intravenously injected bolus that remains reasonably coherent after emergence from the left ventricle. The appearance of such a tracing is essentially comparable to that which might be obtained over any large artery, for example, the femoral. Such a clear bolus effect appears to be absent in the dispersed peripheral type of extracerebral circulation. In contrast, in this second type of circulation, the extracerebral blood flow involves a relatively small amount of blood with a very slow

transit through a larger vascular reservoir in the scalp and skull.[13,29,101] This may be further illustrated by the studies of Ueda and co-workers[89] and Obrist and co-workers.[63,64,76] This problem is discussed in detail elsewhere.[53,54]

Bilateral retinal artery flow. "Laking" or visual observation of cessation of bilateral retinal artery flow by ophthalmoscope is highly correlated with absent cerebral circulation. However, often the lens is clouded and the retina cannot be visualized. It is possible, although highly unlikely, that this finding may be related to other causes.

Cerebral metabolic oxygen rate. Measurement of the cerebral metabolic oxygen rate ($CMRO_2$) may be considered useful as an experimental test for brain death. However, most of these measurements utilizing the Kety technique[78,82,97] are dependent on measures of CBF and are unreliable if CBF decreases critically.

Other techniques using isotopes with multiple probes have the difficulty of confounding intracranial and extracranial circulation. Finally, there are situations during which hypothermia and drugs are used in which the $CMRO_2$ may be reduced significantly and CBF maintained. This may be a reversible situation, as discussed previously, and therefore is not considered as a valuable test of irreversible dysfunction of the brain. Tests of energy utilization of the brain, such as the charge potential as described by Fein[27] are limited, since they can only be applied to specific small regions rather than to the brain itself and must also be considered to be experimental rather than have clinical utility.

Miscellaneous methods. Other indirect methods that pertain to evaluation of intracranial circulation include echoencephalography, rheoencephalography, and electroretinography.[66,97-99] Of these, echoencephalography would appear to have the greatest significance clinically, since it is a simple, nonevasive method for evaluation of pulsations related to intracranial circulation. Although it would appear that this ancillary technique may be of value in experienced hands, available evidence indicates that it should be used only in conjunction with other clinical and EEG criteria.

Other tests used for confirmation of brain death

There is a group of other laboratory or combined laboratory and clinical tests that may be used to confirm the diagnosis of brain death. These tests are less commonly used or may be recent developments with which further experience must be obtained. However, of a large variety of such confirmatory tests discussed in the literature, these appear to offer some promise in terms of their clinical significance and utilization.

1. Computerized axial tomography (CAT scan) of the head has been used to confirm the deterioration of structural integrity of the brain in patients who are brain dead. Although this is a nonportable technique, CAT scanning apparatus may be close to a neurologic or neurosurgical intensive care unit as described by Suter[86] and may be an effective, innocuous method of confirming the diagnosis.

2. In patients who have undergone neurosurgical intervention and who have a pressure transducer within the skull, persistent elevation for over one hour above mean systolic blood pressure is consistent with the diagnosis of brain death. Such elevation of intracranial pressure is compatible with inadequate perfusion of the brain.

3. Electronystagmography and calorics provide a more precise evaluation of absence of extraocular movements (EOMs), which is one of the necessary clinical criteria for the diagnosis of brain death. With total dysfunction of the brain stem there should be no eye movements in response to ice water calorics. This refinement has been considered useful by some investigators.[66]

4. The use of atropine in small doses (2 mg IV) has been advocated by Ouaknine[67] to test the integrity of the brain

stem. No tachycardia occurs in patients who lose the integrity of the brain stem after receiving this amount of the drug, which is too small to affect cardiac activity directly. It does, however, cause an indirect effect via the intracranial parasympathetic system (vagal dorsal nucleus), which affects cardiac rate. In brain death, the cardiac activity is influenced only by extracranial factors such as the sympathetic system and drugs acting directly on the heart. This test should be used while the ECG is being monitored.

5. Examination of the cerebrospinal fluid (CSF) may show fragments of cerebellar tissue and degenerated components of the brain stem and other portions of the intracranial contents. This finding is presumptive support for the diagnosing of brain death. Enzyme changes have also been reported to occur in brain death.[97] However, since these enzyme changes are not necessarily persistent, they do not definitely confirm brain death. Some investigators consider lumbar puncture to be a risk in a patient who is not brain dead but who has increased intracranial pressure. Therefore, CSF examination is usually not considered as part of the routine criteria in the diagnosis of brain death. Under special circumstances, it may be used, depending on the physician's clinical judgment and other findings.

6. Brain biopsy often shows grossly necrotic or swollen tissue with microscopic evidence of neuronal destruction. However, since this is only a regional sample, it cannot be considered sufficient to confirm brain death. Furthermore, the alterations seen with light microscopy in brain death may occur upwards of 20 hours after cessation of intracranial circulation.[69] Therefore, it may be doubly misleading in a patient whose cerebral circulation, for example, has ceased for only one hour.

In such circumstances, it is possible that the brain biopsy would show "normal cortical or cerebral tissue." This problem leads directly into the next subject, which is that of the respirator brain.

AUTOPSY FINDINGS IN BRAIN DEATH AND THE CONCEPT OF THE RESPIRATOR BRAIN

The gross and microscopic findings in brain death are as yet not unequivocally defined. Although the term respirator brain has been used to describe the stages of brain destruction associated with brain death, variability has been noted. The gross changes vary from the edematous, swollen, discolored early stage of deterioration to the fragmented, necrotic brain with portions in the spinal canal. Microscopic descriptions range from eosinophilic, anoxic, neuronal changes to pyknosis and absence of neurons. Absence of glial proliferation is the rule, although there is some debate on this. The blood vessels are usually empty with necrosis of the vascular walls. Unfortunately, the findings noted above are not uniformly observed, and this major difficulty is due to the lack of establishment of an appropriate "initial state" in order to calculate the period from which brain death begins. If, for example, clinical criteria or the isoelectric EEG is

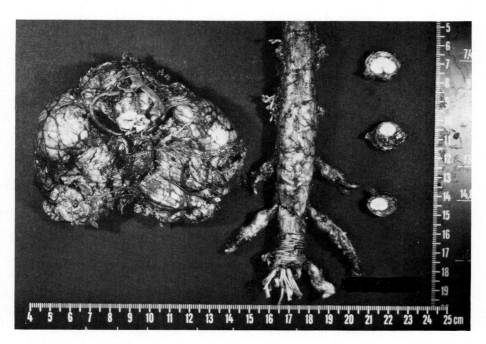

Fig. 14-28. Gross pathologic appearance of the brain and spinal cord in a patient who has met all clinical and electroencephalographic criteria of brain death with absent intracranial circulation for over 20 hours. The brain is markedly edematous, soft with dusky leptomeninges, herniation, and tissue disintegration. Portions of the posterior fossa structures have disintegrated and are present in the spinal subarachnoid space. The parenchyma of the spinal cord is preserved. A head bolus was not present. (From Pearson, J., Korein, J., and Braunstein, P.: Morphology of defectively perfused brains in patients with persistent extracranial circulation. In Korein, J., editor: Brain death; interrelated medical and social issues, Ann. N.Y. Acad. Sci. **315:**265-271, 1978.)

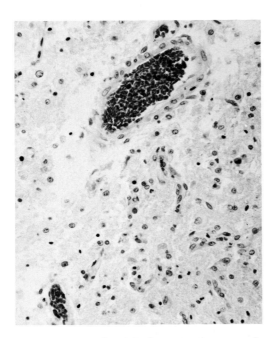

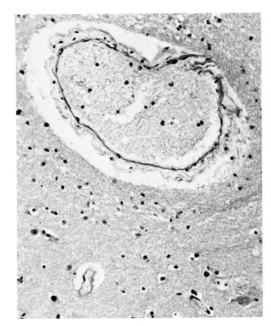

Fig. 14-29. Histologic findings in a patient who was apneic and comatose but did not have arrest of intracranial circulation for more than 20 hours prior to irreversible cardiac standstill. There was a head bolus present. Red cells in vessels are intact, and the vessel wall is reactive. There is a prominent macrophage response to tissue necrosis (×315 before 10% reduction). (From Pearson, J., Korein, J., Harris, J., Wichter, M., and Braunstein, P.: Brain death. II. Neuropathological correlation with the radioisotopic bolus technique for evaluation of critical deficit of cerebral blood flow, Ann. Neurol. **2:**206-210, 1977. By permission of Little, Brown and Co.)

Fig. 14-30. Histologic findings in a patient who met criteria of brain death and had evidence of arrest of intracranial circulation more than 20 hours after irreversible cardiac standstill. A head bolus was absent. Vascular contents are lysed. The vessel wall is necrotic. There is no macrophage response to the dead cells in the tissue (×315 before 10% reduction). (From Pearson, J., Korein, J., Harris, J., Wichter, M., and Braunstein, P.: Brain death. II. Neuropathological correlation with the radioisotopic bolus technique for evaluation of critical deficit of cerebral blood flow, Ann. Neurol. **2:**206-210, 1977. By permission of Little, Brown and Co.)

used, this may not unequivocally identify the specific time of total brain dysfunction. Since the pathologic changes result from cessation of cerebral circulation and/or complete anoxia and may not appear for up to 20 hours, we have chosen the absence of intracranial circulation as the indicator of the onset of brain death. If the pathologic examination is then made 20 hours after this time, the end result of a respirator brain then becomes more consistent and well defined.[50,69,97] Variations may occur relating to the initial pathologic process, but the lack of uniformity in observations of findings pre-

viously described in adults is no longer present. As noted previously, this avoids the problem of the pathologic description of a "normal" brain in a patient who is brain dead and has spontaneous cardiac arrest within two hours after arrest of cerebral circulation. A difficulty encountered in using this type of definition arises when all neurons are destroyed by a toxic-anoxic process and intracranial circulation remains intact. We have seen such a patient who met the clinical criteria of brain death but had evidence of intracranial circulation for approximately 24 hours followed by irreversible cardiac standstill.[54,69] On autopsy, all neurons in the central nervous system (brain and spinal cord) examined in sections from various regions showed severe eosinophilic changes that were considered incompatible with viability. The vascular structures, however, were intact.

Although there are several hypotheses relating to the cause of deterioration of the brain structure, we believe that the most reasonable one is that of autolysis and necrosis of dead tissue (Figs. 14-28 to 14-30).

DIFFERENTIAL DIAGNOSIS OF BRAIN DEATH

Many aspects of the differential diagnosis of brain death have already been considered. We will briefly list those conditions that must be clearly differentiated from brain death under existing criteria.[43,49,50,71,72]

Most significant are those situations in which clinical and certain laboratory criteria may be identical to those of brain death but which represent a reversible situation. Of these, drug intoxication is the most important. To evaluate this problem, two approaches may be used. The first, the most traditional, is evaluation of intoxicants in the blood or urine, but this approach has inherent limitations. The patient may be on medication for therapeutic purposes or facilities to evaluate drug levels may not be available; unless one has an idea of which drug or drugs the patient has been taking, screening tests may vary. Finally, the patient may be brain dead and still have significant drug levels as detected by laboratory tests.

Because of these factors, a second approach, which is to test the critical deficit in intracranial circulation, is deemed more appropriate. Should intracranial circulation be absent, the patient could be considered brain dead without resorting to any tests for drugs. If cerebral circulation is critically decreased and evidence of irreversible brain stem function is available, a similar conclusion may be reached.

Endogenous intoxications or other neurologic problems such as encephalitis may also, on rare occasions, appear to fulfill clinical and EEG criteria of brain death.[36] In these situations, if there is any doubt of the diagnosis, a test for the critical deficit of intracranial circulation would be indicated.

There are situations in the acute stage of intracranial insult within six hours in which clinical criteria of brain death may be present and one must either repeat the evaluations at a later time or consider utilizing a test for absence of intracranial circulation.[9]

Problems such as destruction of the cerebrum with brain stem viability or destruction of the brain stem with cerebral viability may occur, and these may be differentiated by clinical or laboratory tests as described previously. Rarely, an intracollicular cut caused by a hemorrhage may present a clinical picture that mimics brain death. Laboratory tests (i.e., the EEG) are usually sufficient to obtain the correct diagnosis in these situations. Fluctuations in the clinical picture also may occur.

Apallic syndrome[38,39,44] or neocortical death[18] usually can be differentiated from brain death by clinical findings alone. These patients often not only have spontaneous respirations and cephalic reflexes but most often have EEG activity as well. In those reported cases where EEG activity is absent and even when cerebral circulation was diminished, careful clinical evaluation allows the distinction between these persistent noncognitive or vegetative states from brain death.

The problem of anencephalic monsters is similar to the situation of apallic states, which are described above.[57] Utilizing current criteria, these monstrosities cannot be considered to be brain dead. The philosophical problem of considering individuals who are cerebrally dead might be mentioned in this light. Unless revised criteria that include patients in irreversible noncognitive states as dead are agreed upon and appropriate criteria established, we must consider such individuals in persistent vegetative states as alive (e.g., Karen Ann Quinlan[10,37,50]). Patients in locked-in syndromes with de-efferentation as well as those individuals with lack of total motor output such as may occur in amyotrophic lateral sclerosis or patients with combined effects of tetanus intoxication treated with muscle paralyzants[9] fall into the category of severe neurologic deficit and are neither brain dead nor in a persistent vegetative state.

The problem of young children and infants who fulfill the clinical criteria of brain death must be approached with even greater caution than that used in assessing adults with brain death. Clinical judgment must be used to a more significant degree in arriving at the diagnosis, since these children and infants, as mentioned, may persist in a state of brain death with full resuscitative support for prolonged periods, that is, as long as 30 days or more. A mitigating factor that also must be considered is that their resistance to anoxia and deficits in cerebral circulation is greater than that found in the adult.

DECISION-MAKING, RESPONSIBILITY, AND LEGAL ASPECTS

We will assume that all appropriate tests have been carried out and that in the clinical judgment of the anesthesiologist, neurologist, or neurosurgeon, the patient under question meets the current criteria of brain death. In this situation, what is the responsibility of the physicians involved and how do they proceed in the management? This will depend on the following factors:

1. What are the laws pertaining to brain death in a given state?
2. What is the common course of practice in the medical community and what are the regulations of the hospital facility?
3. Is the patient involved in a clear-cut medicolegal problem (i.e., victim of an assault where the actual charge would be changed to murder if the patient is pronounced brain dead)?
4. Is the patient a potential organ donor?

These factors must be considered even if we assume that the patient unequivocally meets the criteria of brain death.

State laws

If there are laws stating that if criteria for diagnosing brain death are fulfilled, they are equivalent to the classic criteria for diagnosing death, the patient may be pronounced dead at the time either criteria are fulfilled. The legal moment of death is, then, that time when the patient fulfills the appropriate criteria. A complete note should be written on the chart stating the criteria used, and all resuscitation procedures may be discontinued at that time. A difficulty that arises is that the patient may show sustained cardiac activity after this moment. The heart may beat or show signs of electrical activity for over 40 minutes after artificial ventilation is discontinued. This has been especially evident with prolonged physiologic monitoring. More rarely, there may be a transient return of spontaneous respirations[48] for up to eight hours. We may presume the latter occurs with the existence of survival of cells in the respiratory center of the brain stem despite virtual total destruction of other intracranial structures. Finally, in situations where organ transplantation is to be performed, maintenance of life-support systems is continued until the organs are removed, and there may be a significant time (hours) that elapses between the pronunciation of death and the removal of the organs.[23] In such a situation, where support has been maintained for 24 hours after the patient has been pronounced dead, should the hospital bill the patient's family for the extra day? What date should be used on the death certificate?

Hospital policy

Whether or not a state law is available defining death, one must consider the policy in the hospital. If no law is available, the practice of medicine in the area is of utmost importance. Complete uniformity of practice is not absolutely necessary, but guidelines should be available. It would be ideal if most centers with functioning intensive care units, emergency rooms, and recovery rooms essentially followed established procedures as in states where laws exist as described above. Interaction with the patient's family and hospital administration in the decision-making process may be required, although the actual pronunciation of death remains the province of the physician.

Medicolegal problems

In situations where the medicolegal aspect predominates, the medical examiner or appropriate authority should be consulted. For example, in some localities if organ transplantation is involved, the medical examiner must be informed before transplantation. These considerations are among those that should be established by the medical facility as a matter of policy. It is not advocated that the pronunciation of death, whether by classic or by brain death criteria, is a matter of consensus, since it is the physician who bears the ultimate responsibility for the pronunciation. Should the physician, however, apart from his or her clinical judgment recognize that the family does not wish such an action to be taken (i.e., using the criteria for brain death to pronounce an individual dead), he or she may simply wait. As noted, in adults there have been no reported cases of patients meeting the full criteria of brain death who did not have irreversible cardiac standstill within seven days (in contrast to infants and children).

Organ donors

If the patient is a potential organ donor and appropriate permission is obtained, the pronunciation of death should preferably be made by two physicians unrelated to the transplant procedure. The previous precaution should be adhered to, and both the family and transplant surgeon should have some precise understanding in relation to the time of the pronunciation of death, the time of the transplantation, and the availability of the body for burial or autopsy. In the latter situation, this may involve a medical examiner or appropriate administrative authority.

Capron discussed the form and substance of an appropriate statute for legislation equating brain death with death. After reviewing existing legislation, he points out the problem of using two different means (i.e., sets of criteria) of measuring the same single phenomena (i.e., death). The statute should clearly state that the concept of death is a single idea, based on either classic criteria or irreversible cardiopulmonary arrest and lack of spontaneous or induced activity or, with a patient who is artificially maintained by a life-support system, the criteria of irreversible cessation of total brain functions. The diagnosis will be made by a physician licensed to practice in a state and based on ordinary standards of medical practice. Death will have occurred at the time when the relevant functions cease. This formulation is a slightly modified version of Capron's model statute.[21,22] The relationship of the variety of problems in brain death and organ transplantation is discussed by Veith and co-workers[93-95] in greater detail.

The legal aspects as well as decision-making problems and moral-ethical-religious issues related to patients who are not brain dead but who are in persistent noncognitive or vegetative states is a far more complex issue and will not be discussed further. These problems and those related to the right to "die with dignity," cessation of life-support systems in terminal situations other than brain death, and writing of orders such as "do not resuscitate" as well as the problem of "extraordinary care" are discussed elsewhere.[47] The problem of brain death itself, although complex, is fundamentally resolved. A patient can be pronounced dead on the basis of appropriate criteria for brain death.

REFERENCES

1. Allen, N., Burkholder, J., and Comiscioni, J.: Clinical criteria of brain death. In Korein, J., editor: Brain death; interrelated medical and social issues, Ann. N.Y. Acad. Sci. **315:**70-96, 1978.
2. American Electroencephalographic Society: Guidelines in EEG; minimum technical standards for EEG recording in suspected cerebral death,

Willoughby, Ohio, 1970 (revised, 1976), The Society, pp. 21-27.

3. Ames, A., Wright, R. L., Kowada, M., Thurston, J. M., and Majno, G.: Cerebral ischemia. II. The no-reflow phenomenon, Am. J. Pathol. **52:** 437-453, 1968.

4. An appraisal of the criteria of cerebral death; a summary statement; a collaborative study. Sponsored by the National Institute of Neurological Diseases and Stroke (Contract NO1-NS-1-2316), J.A.M.A. **237:**982-986, 1977.

5. Arfel, G.: Altered states of consciousness; cerebral death, In Horner, R., and Nequet, R., editors: Handbook of electroencephalography and clinical neurophysiology, vol. 12, Clinical electroencephalography II, Amsterdam, 1975, Elsevier Scientific Publishing Co. pp. 5-23.

6. Ashwal, S., and Schneider, S.: Failure of electroencephalography to diagnose brain death in comatose children, Ann. Neurol. (accepted for publication, 1979).

7. Ashwal, S., Smith, A. J., Torres, F., Loken, M., and Chou, S.: Radionuclide bolus angiography: a technique for verification of brain death in infants and children, J. Pediatr. **91:**722-727, 1977.

8. Bennett, D.: The EEG in determination of brain death. In Korein, J., editor: Brain death; interrelated medical and social issues, Ann. N.Y. Acad. Sci. **315:**110-120, 1978.

9. Bennett, D., Hughes, J., Korein, J., Merlis, J., and Suter, C.: An atlas of electroencephalography in coma and cerebral death, New York, 1976, Raven Press, p. 244.

10. Beresford, R.: Cognitive death: differential problems and legal overtones. In Korein, J., editor: Brain death; interrelated medical and social issues, Ann. N.Y. Acad. Sci. **315:**339-348, 1978.

11. Beresford, R.: The Quinlan decision: problems and legislative alternatives. Ann. Neurol. **2:**74-81, 1977.

12. Bird, T. D., and Plum, F.: Recovery from barbiturate overdose coma with a prolonged isoelectric electroencephalogram, Neurology **18:**456-460, 1968.

13. Blinkov, S. M., and Glezer, II: The human brain in figures and tables, New York, 1968, Basic Books, Inc., Publishers.

14. Braunstein, P., Kricheff, I., Korein, J., and Corey, K.: Cerebral death: a rapid and reliable diagnostic adjunct using radioisotopes, J. Nucl. Med. **14:** 122-124, 1973.

15. Braunstein, P., Korein, J., and Kricheff, I.: Bedside assessment on cerebral circulation (letter), Lancet **1:**1291-1292, 1972.

16. Braunstein, P., Korein, J., Kricheff, I., Corey, K., and Chase, N.: A simple bedside evaluation of cerebral blood flow in the study of cerebral death: a prospective study on 34 deeply comatose patients, presented at the 73rd Annual Meeting of the American Roentgen Ray Society, Washington,

D.C., Oct., 1972; award paper of Soc. Neurol. Radiol., Am. J. Roentgenol. Radium Ther. Nucl. Med. **18:**757-767, 1973.

17. Braunstein, P., Korein, J., Kricheff, I., and Lieberman, A.: Evaluation of the critical deficit of cerebral circulation using radioactive tracers (bolus technique). In Korein, J., editor: Brain death; interrelated medical and social issues, Ann. N.Y. Acad. Sci. **315:**143-167, 1978.

18. Brierley, J. B., Graham, D. I., Adams, J. H., and Simpson, J. A.: Neocortical death after cardiac arrest; a clinical, neurophysiological and neuropathological report of two cases, Lancet **2:**560-565, 1971.

19. Brock, M., Fieschi, C., Ingvar, D. H., Lassen, N. A., and Schurmann, K., editors: Cerebral blood flow, Berlin, 1969, Springer-Verlag, p. 291.

20. Capron, A.: The development of law on human death. In Korein, J., editor: Brain death; interrelated medical and social issues, Ann. N.Y. Acad. Sci. **315:**45-61, 1978.

21. Capron, A.: Legal definition of death. In Korein, J., editor: Brain death; interrelated medical and social issues, Ann. N.Y. Acad. Sci. **315:**349-362, 1978.

22. Capron, A. M., and Kass, L. R.: A statutory definition of the standards for determining human death: an appraisal and a proposal, U. Pennsylvania Law Rev. **121:**87-118, 1972.

23. Chatterjee, S. N., Payne, J. E., and Berne, T. V.: Difficulties in obtaining kidneys from potential postmortem donors, J.A.M.A. **232:**822-824, 1975.

24. Chiang, J., Kowada, M., Ames, A., Wright, R. L., and Majno, G.: Cerebral ischemia. III. Vascular changes, Am. J. Pathol. **52:**455-476, 1968.

25. Clar, H. E., Agnoli, A., and Magnus, L.: Angiographische Befunde Bei Intracraniellem Kreislaufstillstand Infolge Erhohten Hirndrucks, Acta Radiologica **13:**312-317, 1972.

26. Definition of irreversible coma: Report of ad hoc committee (Chairman, H. K. Beecher) of Harvard Medical School to examine definition of brain death, J.A.M.A. **205:**85-88, 1968.

27. Fein, J.: Brain energetics and cerebral death. In Korein, J., editor: Brain death; interrelated medical and social issues, Ann. N.Y. Acad. Sci. **315:** 97-104, 1978.

28. Fischgold, H., and Mathis, P.: Obnubilations, comas et stupeurs, Electroenceph. Clin. Neurophysiol. vol. 11 (suppl.) Paris, 1959, Masson et Cie.

29. Folkow, B., and Neil, E.: Circulation, New York, 1971, Oxford University Press.

30. Gilder, S. S. B. (Twenty-second World Medical Assembly, Sydney, Australia): Death and the W.M.A., Br. Med. J. **3:**493-494, 1968.

31. Goldensohn, E.: Discussion of application and limitations of the EEG in brain death. In Korein, J., editor: Brain death; interrelated medical and

social issues, Ann. N.Y. Acad. Sci. **315**:137-142, 1978.

32. Goodman, J. M., Mishkin, F. S., and Dyken, M.: Determination of brain death by isotope angiography, J.A.M.A. **209**:1869-1872, 1969.

33. Hadjidimos, A. A., Brock, M., Baum, P., and Schurmann, K.: Cessation of cerebral blood flow in total irreversible loss of brain function. In Brock, M., Fieschi, C., Ingvar, D. H., Lassen, N. A., and Schurmann, K., editors: Cerebral blood flow: clinical and experimental results, New York, 1969, Springer-Verlag, pp. 209-212.

34. Hass, W., and others: In Korein, J., Braunstein, P., Kricheff, I., Lieberman, A., and Chase, N.: Measurement of cerebral blood flow by the bolus technique as an adjunct in the diagnosis of cerebral death; 142 studies on 80 patients of an innocuous IV procedure as an adjunct in the diagnosis of cerebral death, Circulation **51**:929-939, 1975.

35. Horan, D.: Euthanasia and brain death: ethical and legal considerations. In Korein, J., editor: Brain death; interrelated medical and social issues, Ann. N.Y. Acad. Sci. **315**:363-375, 1978.

36. Hughes, J.: Limitations of the EEG in the diagnosis of brain death. In Korein, J., editor: Brain death; interrelated medical and social issues, Ann. N.Y. Acad. Sci. **315**:121-136, 1978.

37. Hughes, C. J.: Supreme court decision of New Jersey, A-116, September term, 1975, in the matter of Karen Quinlan, an alleged incompetent, decided March 31, 1976.

38. Ingvar, D. H., and Braun, A.: Das Komplette Apallisch Syndrom, Arch. Psychiatr. Nervenkr. **215**:219, 1972.

39. Ingvar, D. H., Brun, A., Johansson, L., and Samuelsson, S. M.: Survival after severe cerebral anoxia with destruction of the cerebral cortex; the apallic syndrome. In Korein, J., editor: Brain death; interrelated medical and social issues, Ann. N.Y. Acad. Sci. **315**:184-214, 1978.

40. Ingvar, D. H., Haggendal, E., Neleson, N. J., Sourander, P., Wickhom, I., and Lassen, N. A.: Cerebral circulation and metabolism in a comatose patient, Arch. Neurol. **11**:13-21, 1964, and Ingvar, D. H.: Personal communication, 1967.

41. Ingvar, D. H., and Lassen, N. A., editors: Brain work; the coupling of function, metabolism and blood flow in the brain, Copenhagen, 1975, Munksgaard, p. 517.

42. Ingvar, D. H., and Sourander, P.: Destruction of the reticular core of the brain stem; a pathoanatomical follow-up of a case of coma of three years' duration, Arch. Neurol. **23**:1-8, 1970.

43. Ingvar, D. H., and Widen, L.: Brain death; summary of a symposium, Lakartidningen **34**:3804-3814, 1972.

44. Jennett, W. B., and Plum, F.: The persistent vegetative state: a syndrome in search of a name, Lancet **1**:734-737, 1972.

45. Jouvet, M.: Diagnostic electro-sous-cortico-graphie de la mort du systeme nerveux central au cours de certains comas, Electroenceph. Clin. Neurophysiol. **11**:805-808, 1959.

46. Kass, L. R.: Death as an event: a commentary on Robert Morison, Science **173**:698-702, 1971.

47. Korein, J., editor: Brain death; interrelated medical and social issues, Ann. N.Y. Acad. Sci. **315**: 1-454, 1978.

48. Korein, J.: Neurology and cerebral death—definitions and differential diagnosis; Transactions of The American Neurological Association **100**:61-63, 1975.

49. Korein, J.: On cerebral, brain and systemic death; current concepts of cerebrovascular disease, Stroke **8**:9-14, 1973.

50. Korein, J.: The problem of brain death: development and history. In Korein, J., editor: Brain death; interrelated medical and social issues. Ann. N.Y. Acad. Sci. **315**:19-38, 1978.

51. Korein, J.: Towards a general theory of living systems, presented in Naples, March, 1964. In Masturzo, A., editor: The 3rd International Conference of Cybernetic Medicine, Naples, 1966, Francesco Giannino and Figli, pp. 232-248.

52. Korein, J., and Maccario, M.: On the diagnosis of cerebral death: a prospective study on 55 patients to define irreversible coma, Clin EEG **2**:178-199, 1971.

53. Korein, J., Braunstein, P., George, A., Wichter, M., Kricheff, I., Lieberman, A., and Pearson, J.: Brain death. I. Angiographic correlation with the radioisotopic bolus technique for evaluation of critical deficit of cerebral blood flow, Ann. Neurol. **2**:195-205, 1977.

54. Korein, J., Braunstein, P., Kricheff, I., Lieberman, A., and Chase, N.: Measurement of cerebral blood flow by the bolus technique as an adjunct in the diagnosis of cerebral death; 142 studies on 80 patients of an innocuous IV procedure as an adjunct in the diagnosis of cerebral death, Circulation **51**:929-939, 1975.

55. Kowada, M., Ames, A., Majno, G., and Wright, R. L.: Cerebral ischemia. I. An improved experimental method for study; cardiovascular effects and demonstration of an early vascular lesion in the rabbit, J. Neurosurg. **28**:150-157, 1968.

56. Kricheff, I., Pinto, R., George, A., Braunstein, P., and Korein, J.: Angiographic findings in brain death. In Korein, J., editor: Brain death; interrelated medical and social issues, Ann. N.Y. Acad. Sci. **315**:168-183, 1978.

57. Lemire, R. J., Beckwith, J. B., and Warkany, J.: Anencephaly, New York, 1977, Raven Press, p. 270.

58. Levy, D. E., Knill-Jones, R. P., and Plum, F.: The vegetative state and its prognosis following nontraumatic coma. In Korein, J., editor: Brain death; interrelated medical and social issues, Ann. N.Y. Acad. Sci. **315**:293-306, 1978.

59. Milhaud, A.: Disconnecting test and oxygen up-

take in cerebral death diagnosis. In Korein, J., editor: Brain death; interrelated medical and social issues, Ann. N.Y. Acad. Sci. **315**:241-251, 1978.

60. Mohandas, A., and Chou, S. N.: Brain death; a clinical and pathological study, J. Neurosurg. **35**:211-218, 1971.

61. Mollaret, P., and Goulon, M.: Le coma dépassé, Rev. Neurol. **101**:3-15, 1959.

62. Morison, R. S.: Death: process or event? Science **173**:694-698, 1971.

63. Obrist, W. D., Thompson, H. K., King, C. H., and Wang, H. S.: Determination of regional cerebral blood flow by inhalation of 133-Xenon, Circ. Res. **20**:124, 1967.

64. Obrist, W. D., Thompson, H. K., Wang, H. S., and Cronquist, S.: A simplified procedure for determining fast compartment CBFs by ^{133}xenon inhalation. In Russell, R. W. R., editor: Brain and blood flow, London, 1971, Pitman, p. 11.

65. Oldendorf, W. H.: Absolute measurement of brain blood flow using non-diffuseable isotopes. In Brock, M., editor: Cerebral blood flow, Berlin, 1969, Springer-Verlag, p. 53.

66. Ouaknine, G. E.: Bedside procedures in the diagnosis of brain death, Resuscitation **4**:159-177, 1975.

67. Ouaknine, G. E.: Cardiac and metabolic alterations in brain death. In Korein, J., editor: Brain death; interrelated medical and social issues, Ann. N.Y. Acad. Sci. **315**:252-264, 1978.

68. Pampiglione, G., Chaloner, J., Harden, A., and O'Brien, J.: Transitory ischaemia/anoxia in young children and the prediction of quality of survival. In Korein, J., editor: Brain death; interrelated medical and social issues, Ann. N.Y. Acad. Sci. **315**:281-292, 1978.

69. Pearson, J., Korein, J., Harris, J., Wichter, M., and Braunstein, P.: Brain death II; neuropathological correlation with the radioisotopic bolus technique for evaluation of critical deficit of cerebral blood flow, Ann. Neurol. **2**:206-210, 1977.

70. Pius XII: The prolongation of life (an address of Pope Pius XII to an International Congress of Anesthesiologists, November 24, 1957), In the pope speaks, pp. 393-398, 1958.

71. Plum, F., and Posner, J. B.: The diagnosis of stupor and coma, ed. 2, Philadelphia, 1972, F. A. Davis, p. 286.

72. Posner, J.: Coma and other states of consciousness; the differential diagnosis of brain death. In Korein, J., editor: Brain death; interrelated medical and social issues, Ann. N.Y. Acad. Sci. **315**:215-227, 1978.

73. Powner, D.: Drug-associated isoelectric EEGs— a hazard in brain death certification, J.A.M.A. **236**:1123, 1976.

74. Pribram, H. F. W.: Angiographic appearance in acute intracranial hypertension, Neurology **11**:10-21, 1961.

75. Prigogine, I.: Thermodynamics of irreversible processes, Springfield, Ill. 1955, Charles C Thomas, Publisher.

76. Purves, M. J.: The physiology of the cerebral circulation, Cambridge, 1972, Cambridge University Press.

77. Schafer, J. A., and Caronna, J. J.: Duration of apnea needed to confirm brain death, Neurology **28**:661-666, 1978.

78. Shalit, M. H., Beller, A. J., Feinsod, M., Drapkin, A. J., and Cotev, S.: The blood flow and oxygen consumption of the dying brain, Neurology **20**:740-748, 1970.

79. Siebke, H., Breivik, H., Rod, T., and Lind, B.: Survival after 40 minutes submersion without cerebral sequelae, Lancet **1**:1275-1277, 1975.

80. Silverman, D., Saunders, M. G., Schwab, R. S., and Maslan, R. L.: Cerebral death and the electroencephalogram; report of the ad hoc committee of the American Electroencephalographic Society on EEG criteria for determination of cerebral death, J.A.M.A. **209**:1505-1510, 1969.

81. Silverman, D., Saunders, M. G., Schwab, R. S., and Masland, R. L.: Irreversible coma associated with electrocerebral silence, Neurology **20**:525-533, 1970.

82. Smith, A. J., and Walker, A. E.: Cerebral blood flow and brain metabolism as indicators of cerebral death, Johns Hopkins Med. J. **133**:107-109, 1973.

83. Smith, J. K. A., and Penry, J. K., editors: Brain death, NINDS Bibliography Sereis #1, PHS, HEW, NIH, NINDS, Bethesda, Md. 1972, Publication #(NIH) 73-347.

84. Starr, A.: Brain-stem responses in brain death, Brain **99**:543-545, 1976.

85. Starr, A., and Achor, L. J.: Auditory brain stem responses in neurological disease, Arch. Neurol. **32**:761-768, 1975.

86. Suter, C., and Brush, J.: Clinical problems of brain death and coma in intensive care units. In Korein, J., editor: Brain death; interrelated medical and social issues, Ann. N.Y. Acad. Sci. **315**:398-416, 1978.

87. Tabaddor, K., Gardner, T. J., and Walker, A. E.: Cerebral circulation and metabolism at deep hypothermia, Neurology **22**:1065-1070, 1972.

88. Trojaborg, W., and Jorgensen, E. O.: Evoked cortical potentials in patients with "isoelectric" EEGs, Electroenceph. Clin. Neurophysiol. **35**:301-305, 1973.

89. Ueda, H., Hatano, S., Molde, T., and Gondaira, T.: Discussion II on compartmental analysis of the human brain blood flow, regional cerebral blood flow, Acta Neurol. Scand. **41**:88, 1965.

90. Ueki, K., Takeuchi, K., and Katsurada, K.: Clinical study of brain death; presentation no. 286, Tokyo, 1973, Fifth International Congress of Neurological Surgery.

91. Veatch, R. M.: Death, dying, and the biological

revolution; our last quest for responsibility, New Haven, Conn., 1976, Yale University Press, p. 323.

92. Veatch, R. M.: Definition of death; ethical, philosophical and policy confusion. In Korein, J., editor: Brain death; interrelated medical and social issues, Ann. N.Y. Acad. Sci. **315**:307-321, 1978.

93. Veith, F.: Relationship of brain death to organ transplantation. In Korein, J., editor: Brain death; interrelated medical and social issues, Ann. N.Y. Acad. Sci. **315**:417-433, 1978.

94. Veith, F., Fein, J., Tendler, M., Veatch, R., Kleiman, M., and Kalkines, G.: Brain death II; a status report of legal considerations, J.A.M.A. **238**:1744-1748, 1977.

95. Veith, F., Fein, J., Tendler, M., Veatch, R., Kleiman, M., and Kalkines, G.: Brain death I; a status report of medical and ethical considerations, J.A.M.A. **238**:1651-1655, 1977.

96. von Bucheler, E., Kaufer, C., and Dux, A.: Zerebrale Angiographie zur Bestimmung des Hirntodes, Fortschr. Geb. Roentgenstr Nuklearmed **113**:278-296, 1970.

97. Walker, A. E.: Cerebral death, Dallas, Texas, 1977, Professional Information Library, p. 241.

98. Walker, A. E.: Cerebral death. In Tower, D. B., editor: The nervous system, (vol. II, New York, 1975, Raven Press, pp. 75-87.

99. Walker, A. E.: Pathology of brain death. In Korein, J., editor: Brain death; interrelated medical and social issues, Ann. N.Y. Acad. Sci. **315**: 272-280, 1978.

100. Wilson, J. A.: Principles of animal physiology, New York, 1972, Macmillan Publishing Co.

101. Wright, S.: Applied physiology, London, 1971, Oxford University Press, p. 143.

15

Neurologic intensive care

JAMES V. SNYDER
DAVID J. POWNER
AKE GRENVIK

Neurologic dysfunction from diverse central nervous system (CNS) insults (head injury, metabolic encephalopathy, post-ischemic encephalopathy) can be dramatically altered by aggressive application of current intensive care techniques.[10,14,129,130] Although intensive care of neurosurgical patients has become more complex, its basic therapeutic goal continues to be the provision of cerebral homeostasis for optimal neuronal survival and function. This homeostasis depends upon the supply of nutrients and oxygen in excess of cellular demand and upon the removal of metabolic wastes. Neurologic dysfunction and patient mortality as a reflection of neuronal cellular function are determined by the extent to which pathologic processes disrupt homeostasis or therapeutic modalities preserve it. This chapter focuses on those variables and mechanisms influencing the supply-demand relationship as outlined in Fig. 15-1. In addition, the limitations of various monitoring and diagnostic methods and the deleterious effects some forms of routine patient care can have on neuronal function are reviewed.

CEREBRAL CIRCULATION

The supply of nutrients to the brain as provided by cerebral blood flow (CBF) is directly related to cerebral perfusion pressure (CPP), that is, mean arterial pressure (MAP) minus intracranial pressure (ICP) or central venous pressure (CVP), whichever is higher, and is inversely related to cerebral vascular resistance (CVR) as shown in the following equation:

$$CBF = \frac{MAP - ICP \text{ or } CVP}{CVR}$$

CBF normally sustains neuronal function if mean CPP is maintained greater than 30 torr. However, normal values for total CBF may be misleading and actually insufficient for several reasons. First, in spite of its outwardly homogenous appearance, the normal brain is markedly inhomogenous anatomically with regard to cellular concentration and degree of vascularity and also physiologically in terms of blood flow and metabolism.[148] Second, total CBF may be "normal" at a time when regional maldistribution of blood flow, due to excessive perfusion in some areas and hypoperfusion in others, is occurring.

The major determinants of such regional cerebral blood flow (rCBF) are the patency of capillary lumina and the hydrostatic pressure gradient between the precapillary arterioles and the surrounding tissue. As arteriolar pressure may be only 30% to 40% of aortic pressure, slight elevations of tissue pressure might markedly reduce the regional transmural capillary pressure while having

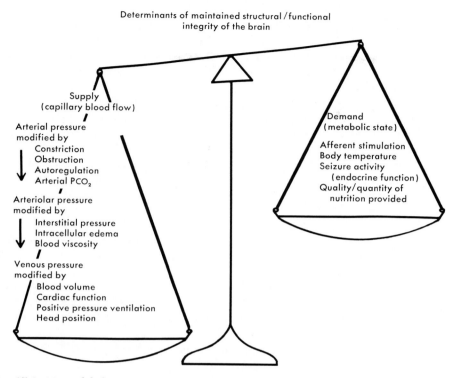

Supply/demand factors

Determinants of maintained structural/functional
integrity of the brain

Supply
(capillary blood flow)

Arterial pressure
modified by
  Constriction
  Obstruction
  Autoregulation
  Arterial PCO_2

Arteriolar pressure
modified by
  Interstitial pressure
  Intracellular edema
  Blood viscosity

Venous pressure
modified by
  Blood volume
  Cardiac function
  Positive pressure ventilation
  Head position

Demand
(metabolic state)

Afferent stimulation
Body temperature
Seizure activity
  (endocrine function)
Quality/quantity of
  nutrition provided

Fig. 15-1. Normal balance of factors required for neuronal survival: a supply of nutrients greater than demand.

little effect on total CPP.[19] In some pathologic states (e.g., trauma, tumor, metabolic, toxic or post-anoxic encephalopathy), therefore, it is the regional conditions and not the global measurements that determine neuronal survival. Factors that might disrupt the normal balance between regional CBF and metabolic needs[176] include:

1. Loss of CBF autoregulation (i.e., flow varies directly with perfusion pressure) due to extracellular accumulation of metabolites (e.g., hydrogen ion, adenosine, cyclic AMP, etc.) and potassium, resulting in complete loss of cerebral vascular tone.

2. Vasospasm, which occurs in head injury as well as subarachnoid hemorrhage, may reduce regional perfusion pressure.

3. Disruption of the blood-brain barrier as produced in trauma or as potentiated by hypertension and vasodilation of any cause may lead to local changes in tissue pressure and compromise rCBF.

4. Cellular edema results in compression of capillary lumina and impedance of flow.

5. Obstruction of normal pathways for CSF reabsorption compromises a major compensatory mechanism for ICP elevation.

6. Decreased brain compliance from any etiology limits adaptability of vascular lumina.

Disturbances of the normal coupling between CBF and CPP have been demonstrated clinically by the poor correlation between CBF and either CPP or ICP in patients following head injury.[51] Insignificant functional impairment is noted in the presence of an ICP of 100 torr in some patients while in others major neurologic changes occur at an ICP of only 15 torr.[121] Dramatic clinical improvement can sometimes be seen when the normally adequate CPP of 60 torr is increased by elevation of MAP in patients with vasospasm.[87] Therefore, although local tissue hypoperfusion might be improved by altering factors, which experimentally determine total perfusion such as MAP, ICP, and CVR, a healthy skepticism should be maintained in the extension of experimentally observed relations to current clinical practices. Particular features and potential therapeutic interventions to improve the relationship between brain perfusion and metabolism are considered below.

Arterial pressure

CBF is normally independent of CPP between 40 and 140 torr (so-called autoregulation). However, in chronically hypertensive patients, CBF autoregulation may be shifted to a higher CPP range of 80 to 200 torr. Likewise, an iatrogenic elevation of MAP above normal should theoretically be beneficial to those patients with brain insults who are normally hypertensive and in those patients who have developed partially occluded cerebral vessels where flow is dependent on a high MAP. However, increased MAP, especially in areas where autoregulation has been lost, can increase transudation of water from the intravascular to the extravascular space, increase local tissue pressure, and thereby decrease CPP and compromise rCBF.* Indeed, iatrogenic hypertension early after an insult may induce infarction in ischemic brain tissue or cause intracranial hemorrhage in infarcted brain.[102] However, hypertensive therapy several days after an ischemic insult has been found beneficial in relief of experimental cerebral edema[102] and in improving blood flow and brain function in patients following aneurysm surgery.[109]

Spontaneous arterial hypertension in brain injury probably results from excessive sympathetic discharge causing intensive systemic vasoconstriction. This can sometimes be

---
*References 6, 13, 58, 80, 102, 132, 180.

effectively reversed by chlorpromazine (11 in Fig. 15-7) as detailed on p. 333. Supplementary barbiturates may also be helpful in blood pressure reduction but usually induce CNS depression. Because of the potential for increasing cerebral blood volume (CBV), direct-acting vasodilators such as hydralazine and sodium nitroprusside are relatively contraindicated for blood pressure control when the cranium is closed unless ICP is monitored.[34,211] In addition to cerebral vasodilatation and an increased ICP, nitroprusside can result in harmful levels of thiocyanate and cyanide, especially in the presence of renal failure. Therefore, a maximum total dosage of 1.0 mg/kg has been recommended. However, these toxic effects of nitroprusside can be reduced by simultaneous administration of hydroxocobalamin[32] and thiosulfate.[140] Diazoxide has been used to decrease MAP in hypertensive patients who had no indications of cerebral vascular disease. MAP was effectively controlled without apparent clinical deterioration.[64] Unfortunately, the occasionally precipitous drop in MAP seen with diazoxide can be hazardous. Titrated infusion of trimethaphan may be the least dangerous of the rapidly acting potent antihypertensive drugs in patients with increased ICP. Titrated phentolamine warrants additional evaluation.[86]

The sometimes adverse effects of arterial hypertension early after cerebral insult as discussed above suggest that an arterial pressure below normal may prevent development of brain edema. However blood flow to those areas where vascular resistance is increased may then be compromised.[110]

Therefore, because of the potential harm from either increased or decreased arterial pressure and because present techniques for monitoring the effects of altered CBF are rather insensitive, arterial blood pressure should be maintained within the patient's normal range if there is no clear clinical indication to do otherwise.

Arterial hypotension in patients with intact brain stems is usually due to relative hypovolemia and is most appropriately treated by infusion of 5% or 25% solution

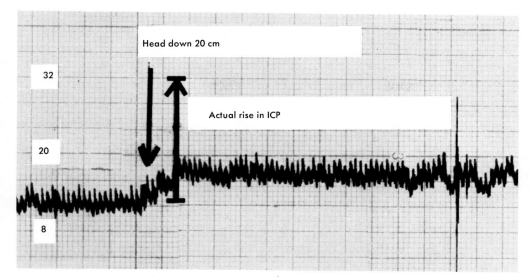

Fig. 15-2. Effect of moving the patient's head from an elevated to a supine position: ICP rose 19 torr when the patient's head was lowered 20 cm. Most of the ICP rise was obscured by failure to relevel the transducer with the center of the patient's head.

of albumin or other colloid. The higher albumin concentration is indicated when serum albumin concentration is less than 3 g/100 ml or if interstitial fluid volume has increased, as might be suggested by serial body weights or fluid intake and output measurements.

Venous pressure

In the minimally injured cat[38] and probably in normal humans[106] elevation of internal jugular venous pressure causes an increase in cerebral blood volume due to vascular dilatation but does not increase extracellular edema. Brain edema does occur, however, when venous pressure is elevated in areas where injured capillaries are present. This vasodilatation and edema tend to increase ICP and decrease CPP and CBF. Therefore, excessive jugular venous pressure should be treated by diuresis, dilatation of capacitance vessels (i.e., reduction in cardiac preload); and elevation of the patient's head (Fig. 15-2). Effects of the Valsalva maneuver are similar, causing concern about even mild coughing or straining (Fig. 15-7).[156]

Intracranial pressure

Factors increasing intracranial volume cause only a transient increase in ICP until the compensatory capacity of the calvarium by CSF displacement is exceeded. The magnitude of ICP elevation depends on the volume added, the time over which the increase occurs, and the intracranial volume-pressure (i.e., compliance) characteristics at that time.

The value of ICP monitoring is suggested by Becker's experience with head-injured patients,[10] in which all major deteriorations were accompanied or preceded by changes in the monitored ICP.[9]

Sensitivity to elevated ICP varies with etiology and with regional characteristics of the brain insult. For example, preliminary observations suggest that following head injury, CBF in patients with diffuse insult is less sensitive to increased ICP than in patients with mass lesions.[145,206,216] Similarly, CBF was not improved by reduction of ICP following subarachnoid hemorrhage (SAH) unless the initial value was greater than 35 torr.[82] However, the relation between mild-moderate elevation of ICP and CBF in communicating hydrocephalus was more equivocal,[82] and neurologic status can be quite sensitive to minimal changes in ICP in Reye syndrome.[142,143]

Without any elevation of ICP, regional perfusion may be severely compromised so that any further insult may markedly increase the extent of neuronal damage.[143,144] Therefore, rise in ICP should be recognized as a late development representing depletion of compensatory capabilities. Efforts to lower ICP are clearly warranted when the ICP rise is associated with a mass lesion or metabolic insult and probably in any patient with a related neurologic deficit. One exception is when ICP elevation is due to aneurysmal hemorrhage, when lowering of ICP might induce additional hemorrhage.

The dynamics of the form of brain interstitial edema that is due to pathologic alteration in permeability called vasogenic brain edema have recently been elucidated and are clinically relevant. The dynamics are at least superficially similar to those described for subcutaneous edema.[71] Differences include the following: the lymphatic system is absent in the brain, but circulation of CSF serves a similar purpose, and brain interstitial fluid pressure usually remains above atmospheric pressure.[125,180,181] Excessive interstitial fluid in the brain moves by bulk flow via an enlarged extracellular space in white matter to adjacent gyri, central white matter, and into the ventricular fluid. Maintaining ventricular fluid pressure low by aspiration of CSF or by inhibition of CSF formation (ethacrynate sodium, furosemide, acetazolamide) should augment drainage of this interstitial fluid. Experimentally, however, the movement of interstitial fluid can be blocked by prior hexachlorophene treatment via induction of intracellular edema.[180] The extracellular space cannot expand, and interstitial flow is impeded. Similarly, it can be postulated that interstitial obstruction occurring in the clin-

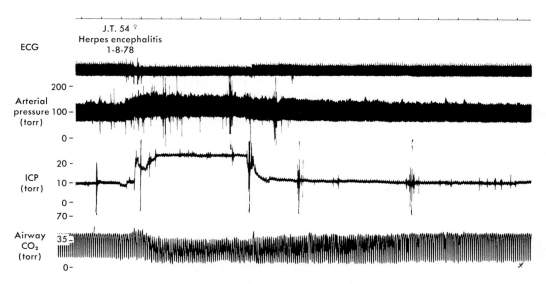

Fig. 15-3. Patient-regulated CO_2 control. An initial rise in arterial pressure was followed by an almost simultaneous change in ECG waveform (note change in height of ECG tracings) and increase in ICP due to a cough followed by a small plateau wave and a minimal rise in end tidal CO_2. The latter was promptly followed by the patient's increased spontaneous ventilatory efforts, which successfully lowered end tidal (and probably arterial) $P{CO_2}$ to 28 torr. The ECG waveform reverted to its prior height at the termination of the plateau wave, but spontaneous hyperventilation persisted for an additional period of nine minutes.

ical situation, as after ischemia, may adversely affect drainage of interstitial fluid and thereby further compromise local capillary flow.

Other common events in critically ill patients that threaten to compromise blood flow include arterial dilatation after minor increases in Pa_{CO_2} due to sedation or tracheal suction, postural drainage in the head-down position, increased interstitial fluid volume secondary to overhydration or low serum albumin concentration, fluid shifts associated with dialysis or therapy of hyperosmolar states, and the administration of many inhalational anesthetics.[196]

The detection of elevated ICP by routine

clinical examination is not always possible because of the unreliability of clinical signs often suggested as indicators of elevated ICP, such as hypertension, bradycardia, papilledema, vomiting, and a change in level of consciousness.* On the other hand, increased ICP is a potential cause of almost any CNS-related clinical sign, including changes in respiratory rate or rhythm and ECG waveform (Figs. 15-3 and 15-4, *B*).

In part because of clinical insensitivity to increased ICP, the risk of lumbar puncture is usually not warranted when an intracranial mass lesion is suspected, even in the absence

---

*References 100, 107, 114, 121, 144, 145, 207.

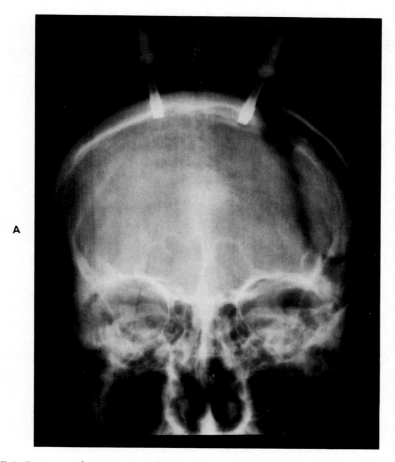

Fig. 15-4. Intracranial pressure gradient and patient regulation of Pa_{CO_2} and ICP. **A,** Unilateral decompression following head injury and craniotomy for removal of hematoma and lacerated left temporal lobe. Elevation of the unsecured bone flap is apparent.

Continued.

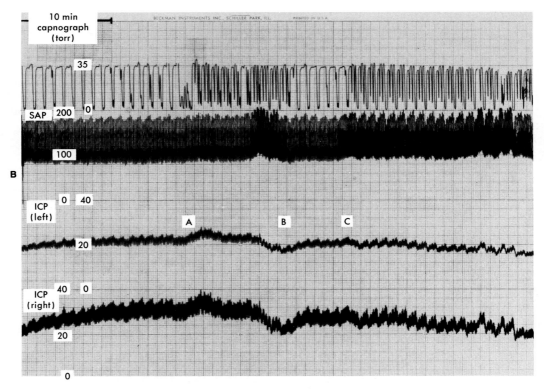

Fig. 15-4, cont'd. B, Simultaneous tracings of airway CO_2, MAP, and bilateral intracranial pressures from the same patient. The unilateral decompression was manifested by the persistently lower pressure on the injured left side. The resting exhaled CO_2 waveform (capnograph) indicates controlled mechanical ventilation at 10 breaths per minute. Arterial pressure remained stable, while ICP spontaneously rose more than 10 torr. Slight further elevation at *A* stimulated spontaneous ventilatory efforts by the patient, indicated by more frequent (30/min) downward deflections in the capnograph until ICP was controlled at *B*. The increased spontaneous breathing effort at *C* was less clearly induced by a recurrent elevation in ICP but did result in further lowering of ICP.

of clinical signs of increased ICP.[166] An exception is when infection is suspected.

Continuous direct monitoring of ICP in critically ill patients is the only reliable method of detecting changes in ICP. However, limitations of ICP monitoring must be emphasized. For instance, brain herniation is not necessarily related to increased ICP. Brain swelling and shifts may occur first, with the establishment of intracranial pressure gradients, which can occur even at low ICPs (Fig. 15-4).[104,123] ICP therefore may not reflect brain swelling or edema until these are advanced or very rapid in onset.

Monitoring of ICP may also be insensitive to dramatic changes in regional blood flow induced by osmotherapy.[21] These limitations may be overcome as the relationships of ICP (CSF pressure) to various kinds of change in volume are further investigated.[124,206,207]

The relationship between CSF volume change and the pressure response defines the CSF space elastance.[206] The pressure change resulting from injection of 1 ml of fluid into the ventricular catheter (volume-pressure response [VPR]) has been shown to be a more sensitive indicator than ICP alone of potential danger due to exhausted compen-

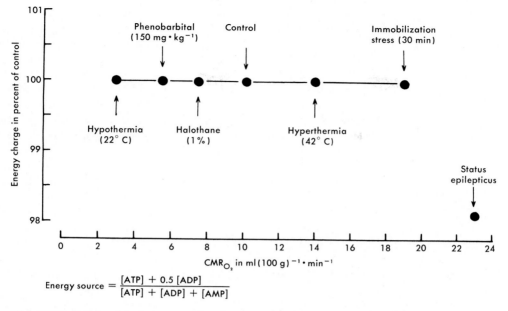

$$\text{Energy source} = \frac{[\text{ATP}] + 0.5\,[\text{ADP}]}{[\text{ATP}] + [\text{ADP}] + [\text{AMP}]}$$

Fig. 15-5. Relationship between adenylate energy charge (or energy state) and cerebral metabolic rate for oxygen (CMRO$_2$) in different conditions. Nitrous oxide anesthesia (70%) was used in the control animals. (Data from Siesjö, B. K., and others: Crit. Care Med. 4:283, 1976.)

satory mechanisms and of need for and response to osmotherapy and steroids.[145,206] A large change in pressure suggests that brain edema or other mass effect is already extensive and that minimal further insult may seriously compromise perfusion even if baseline ICP is close to normal.

Cerebrovascular resistance

Many of the determinants of cerebrovascular resistance are not readily measurable, such as vascular radius or length and blood viscosity.[156,158,159] When regional blood flow may be compromised, it is prudent to avoid the increased viscosity associated with high hematocrit values,[212] and hemodilution with infusion of dextran may be advantageous.[102] Vasospasm after head injury is well documented[127] and probably contributes to neurologic dysfunction, but no effective therapy has been documented. Iatrogenic hypertension in some patients with subarachnoid hemorrhage improves perfusion (see p. 324) but is likely to be associated with marked increases in brain edema following trau-

ma.[10,180] The influence of some direct-acting vasodilators is discussed above. For effects on hemodynamics of arterial Pco$_2$ manipulation, see p. 343.

DETERMINANTS OF METABOLIC RATE

Cerebral metabolic rate (CMR) as determined by oxygen consumption measurements may vary widely in the normal brain. For example, in the uninjured rat brain, fluctuations from 2.5 to 23 ml of O$_2$ per 100 g of tissue per minute have been observed in a wide variety of different conditions (Fig. 15-5).[198] In response to such demands, oxygen delivery can normally increase at least several-fold. However, when blood flow might be compromised, a reduction in metabolic demand and the prevention of those states producing an excessive oxygen need is therapeutically valuable. It is therefore implied that factors on the right side of Fig. 15-5 are likely to be detrimental to outcome when blood flow or oxygen delivery is compromised, and factors to the left may be protective. Variables influencing metabolic rate include temperature, seizures, and afferent stimulation.

Temperature

An elevation in body temperature increases the metabolic rate of neurons and experimentally has been shown to increase the severity of cryogenic brain edema under certain conditions by as much as 40%.[29] Therefore, suppression of hyperthermia is mandatory in patients with cerebral dysfunction. If active cooling is indicated, the esophageal or other core temperature should be monitored continuously. In addition, the application of cooling techniques to hyperthermic patients prior to suppression of the hypothalamus with antipyretics is misdirected, in that cooling may cause vasoconstriction and shivering. When this occurs, the desired decrease in metabolic rate is not achieved even though body temperature may drop because of the marked increase in metabolic rate associated with shivering.[178] Aspects of pharmacologic control of temperature regulation have been reviewed recently.[35,45] Chlorpromazine is often an effective antipyretic[45] through its vasodilatory effect, and may also decrease shivering via hypothalamic depression. Muscle relaxants may also be necessary to prevent shivering in some cases.

Seizures

Status epilepticus or intermittent but frequent seizures may adversely affect a large number of neurons and cause a permanent loss of cerebral function.[49] Mortality is closely related to the duration of seizure activity.[185,220] Injury results from transient breakdown of the blood-brain barrier due to the associated systemic hypertension[6,15,165] and possibly from an increase in metabolic rate far above the corresponding local increase in blood flow in previously injured brains. Continuous monitoring of the EEG for subclinical seizure activity[52,63] is warranted when possible (Fig. 15-6), and the administration of sufficiently large amounts of anticonvulsants must immediately be considered if seizure activity is detected. Agents producing muscle paralysis, while stopping the clinical manifestations of seizures, will not stop neuronal firing or relieve the marked increase in cerebral metabolic needs. In addition, hypocarbia, caused by overzealous mechanical or manual ventilation, may initiate seizures in susceptible individuals by inducing intracellular alkalosis.

Recurrent seizures may be rapidly treated with phenobarbital, 1 to 3 mg/kg intravenously, every 15 minutes (usually not more than 20 mg/kg) until seizures are controlled or hypotension or respiratory depression supervenes. However, there are no recognized permanent sequelae to larger doses of barbiturate, and a higher dosage as has been recommended for neonates may be useful in adults.[161] Diazepam, 2.5 to 10 mg or 40 to 200 mg sodium pentothal intravenously is effective transiently and may be repeated while therapeutic amounts of phenobarbital or phenytoin are being administered. Phenytoin up to 20 mg/kg, administered IV at less than 100 mg/min, has been advocated for acute control of status epilepticus without affecting CNS or cardiovascular function.[161,221] Other studies on depression of myocardial conduction and contractility suggest that the infusion be limited to 50 mg/min to adults.[222] In the first year of life, a total dose of *not less than* 30 mg/kg administered up to 3 mg/kg/min has been recommended.[2] Paraldehyde is sometimes effective when phenobarbitol is not, but it is irritating to veins and lungs and is offensive when exhaled. A titrated intravenous infusion typical of current intensive care practice was reported in 1949, in which seizure control was maintained by administration of 202 ml of paraldehyde over three days.[220] When necessary, paraldehyde can be infused slowly (1 ml over two minutes) through a central venous catheter.[188] A benzodiazepine (clonazepam) reportedly controlled 38 of 39 episodes of status epilepticus quickly and without side effects.[62]

For all the above, therapy should be titrated as necessary to control seizure ac-

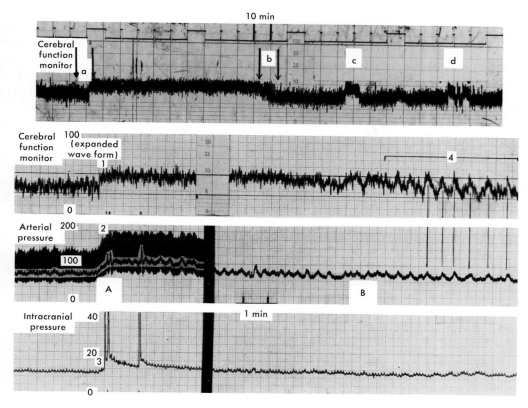

Fig. 15-6. Application of cerebral function monitor (CFM) and variable recording. Dramatic changes in cerebral activity (as at *a* and *b* in the CFM recording, top) were not accompanied by obvious motor activity in an adult patient following head injury. Because normal activity is usually between 10 and 40 units (μV on the recording), increases in activity similar to those shown had been considered to indicate improved perfusion associated with increased arterial pressure, or possibly an arousal phenomenon, but the rapidity of change suggested seizure activity. Simultaneous recording of the CFM tracing with intracranial and arterial pressures made it clear that the primary event was increased electrical activity and that the pressure changes were secondary. Focal seizure activity became clinically manifest within 24 hours. Detailed analysis: original CFM tracing (top strip marked *a* and *b*) and simultaneous higher speed recordings of CFM, ICP, and MAP (*A* and *B* on bottom) are displayed. In each section the mean arterial pressure tracing has been realigned as though it were made at the same moment as the other tracings. A sudden increase in cerebral activity (seen at *a*, and *1* in *A*) was followed by a 20 torr rise in mean arterial pressure (*2*). ICP increased slightly with arterial pressure and again with coughing 20 seconds later (*3*). Cerebral activity erratically dropped to previous levels 110 minutes later (*b*, and in *B*). Arterial pressure was stable by 30 minutes after *1*, but continued sensitive coupling of MAP with electrical activity is suggested by close correlation of those factors (*4* in *B*). Similar correlations persisted through later fluctuations (*c* and *d* in original CFM trace). The abrupt rise in cerebral activity that preceded changes in intracranial and arterial pressure strongly suggested that a functional event was primary, the most likely being subclinical seizure activity. If either the intracranial or arterial pressure had become elevated first, the interpretation would have differed greatly.

tivity in an area where cardiovascular, respiratory, and other parameters can be adequately monitored and supported when necessary.

Afferent stimulation

The mechanism for the deleterious effects of afferent stimulation has been suggested to be a catecholamine-mediated increase in cerebral oxygen uptake as identified during immobilization stress in rats, which can be prevented by the administration of nitrous oxide or propanolol or adrenalectomy.[26] Further neurologic recovery was

documented following 16 minutes global ischemia in monkeys if paralysis and controlled ventilation were continued for 48 hours post insult rather than allowing spontaneous hyperventilation.[14] Regional increases in CMR appear to occur with common forms of stimulation.[115]

The appropriate clinical application of these observations in the care of humans is not yet clear, but the avoidance of unnecessary stimulation and greater use of sedation are suggested. For instance, controlled, continuous IV infusions of barbiturate may be advantageous.[24]

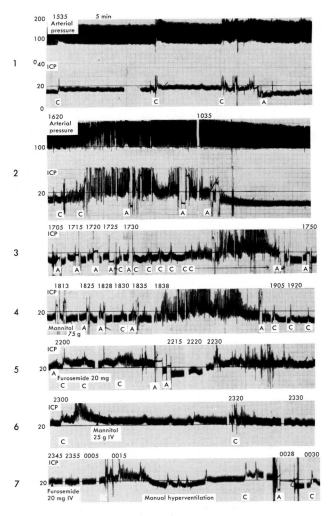

Fig. 15-7. For legend see opposite page.

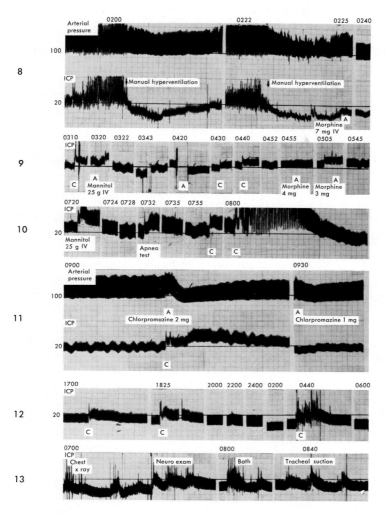

Fig. 15-7. An adult patient rapidly became less responsive eight hours following removal of a large arteriovenous malformation and subdural hematoma. CT showed no mass lesion. A ventricular catheter was inserted for decompression. This figure contains polygraphs from the first 42 hours after catheter insertion. In addition to other aspects of care, the goal was established to maintain ICP at less than 16 torr. Any minor stimulus, such as touching the patient's hand, provoked a cough response (indicated by *C*) and a prompt and often sustained increase in MAP (as in traces 1 and 2). The associated increase in ICP persisted abnormally each time, causing a progressive increase in ICP over the ensuing 18 hours, which responded poorly or was unresponsive to aspiration of CSF (indicated by *A*) or osmotherapy (traces 4, 6, 9, 10), morphine (traces 8, 9), or furosemide (traces 5, 7). Manual hyperventilation reduced MAP more than ICP (trace 8), causing a reduction in CPP and undeterminable changes in regional CBF. Chlorpromazine administration (trace 11) was followed by excellent ICP control without further depression of neurologic function. All other CNS-directed therapy except steroid administration was stopped. The ICP increases associated with coughing returned promptly to baseline (traces 12, 13), and there was no progressive increase in ICP during the ensuing 24 hours, despite tracheal or painful stimuli as necessitated by patient care (trace 13). Note that while chlorpromazine was helpful in the care of this patient, administration of only 2 mg IV promptly reduced arterial pressure 30 torr (trace 11). A small secondary increase in ICP, presumably due to cerebral vasodilation, followed the drop in MAP.

MONITORING

Because of the relative inaccessibility of the brain itself and our clinical inability to detect many pathophysiologic states in various regions, patient care must include frequent or perhaps even continuous monitoring of several variables. In such patients, drugs or therapy given commonly as part of routine patient care may produce profound effects on neuronal function. Likewise, treatment directed toward CNS changes may have an exaggerated or less than expected effect (Fig. 15-7). The unpredictable response to therapy, the relative insensitivity of clinical examination, and the desirability of detecting physiologic trends require that detailed and at times invasive monitoring methods should be considered. For convenience in this discussion, monitored parameters can be classified into functional, physical, and chemical categories, as grouped in Fig. 15-8.

Functional parameters

Neuronal function as reflected at the organ level by the patient's clinical examination correlates well with ultimate outcome following head injury[98,99] and is being evaluated for nontraumatic coma.[8] Obviously all medical personnel involved in the continu-

ing care of these patients must be familiar with the importance of proper examining techniques and changes in findings, both of which have been reviewed elsewhere.[170] Objective "neurologic score" forms have been helpful in following clinical changes (see pp. 336-337).[126] As has been noted previously, many intracranial processes may become advanced before a change is detected by a deterioration in cerebral function. In addition, the clinical evaluation is limited as a monitoring tool by the frequency with which it can be repeated.

Neuronal function can also be inferred from the electroencephalogram (EEG). Preliminary experimental and clinical data support the contention that diffuse and regional changes in the adequacy of nutrient blood flow, or at least the total supply-demand balance, can be detected by the EEG.[17,146,151] Alterations in seizure patterns were seen when oxygen or glucose availability became depressed,[12,150] and progressive EEG flattening was correlated with decreases in regional CBF.[215]

When computerized power spectrum analysis and voltage-frequency ratios are used, the EEG may be useful in following the depth of coma, identifying early adverse trends, predicting prognosis in head-

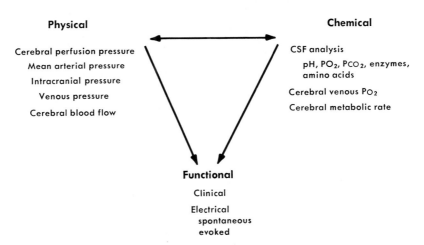

Fig. 15-8. Grouping of monitored variables as physical, chemical, and functional. Physical and chemical events tend to influence each other early and usually precede functional changes. Functional changes are late manifestations in a pathologic process but reflect a wider range of influences and are more directly indicative of clinical outcome.

injured patients, and detecting inadequate perfusion.[217] Continuous monitoring of the electrical manifestations of CNS function is possible using a modified EEG (cerebral function monitor [CFM])*[173] (Fig. 15-6). With this device, the amplitude and fre-

quency of cortical electrical activity are combined into a single slow trend recording, which has been useful in monitoring the effectiveness of therapy of seizures and in following adequacy of cerebral perfusion and oxygenation[17,189] and in early prediction of outcome following anoxic-ischemic insults. Of 14 patients monitored within two hours

---

*Applied Medical Research, Tampa, Fla.

GLASGOW-PITT COMA SCORE

Explanations

A. *Eye opening.* Do not decide whether a patient is attentive on the basis of eye movements. In the persistent vegetative state with decortication, patients have often been believed to be reacting visually to people around them, while these eye movements are probably primitive ocular following reflexes at the subcortical level. Eye opening in response to *sound* means response to any verbal approach, not necessarily the command to open the eyes. Eye opening in response to *pain* should be tested by a stimulus of the limbs; pressure on the face can cause grimacing and eye closure.

B. *Pupil response.* Direct bright light straight through the pupils.

C. *Best verbal response (understanding).* The stimulus for (C) is conversational questioning. *Oriented:* the patient should know who he is, where he is, and why he is there; and know the year, season, and month. *Confused* conversation means that the patient's attention can be held and he responds to questions in a conversational manner, but the responses indicate varying degrees of disorientation and confusion. If feasible, record verbatim what he says. *Inappropriate* verbal response describes intelligible articulation, but in an exclamatory or random way, usually by shouting and swearing; no sustained conversational exchange is possible. *Incomprehensible* speech refers to moaning and groaning, but without recognizable words.

D and E. *Motor responses.* The stimulus should first be a *verbal* one, and if there is no response to command, a *painful* stimulus should be applied. The significance of the response to pain is not easy to interpret unless the stimulus is applied in a standard way, and maintained until maximum response is obtained. Initially, pressure is applied to the fingernail bed with a pencil; this may result in either flexion or extension at the elbow. If flexion is observed, stimulation is then applied to the head and neck, and to the trunk to test for localization (appropriateness). In brain death, a spinal reflex may still cause the legs to flex in response to pain. For this reason, it is wise to test the upper extremities unless local trauma makes this impossible. *Obedience* means appropriate response to command. *Appropriate* means an appropriate response to pain. *Intermediate* response is unclear between appropriate and stereotyped. A *stereotyped* response is, for instance, an inappropriate flexor or extensor posturing. *No response* is usually associated with hypotonia to adequate painful stimulus, with spinal cord transsection ruled out as explanation for lack of response.

The best or highest response from any limb should be recorded. Some patients give variable responses during a single examination, improving as they become aroused. Responses from limbs on the same side may differ. When one limb responds differently from the other on the same side, this may indicate focal brain damage and for this purpose, the worst (most abnormal) response should be noted on the Special Care Flow Sheet. But *for the purpose of assessing the degree of altered consciousness it is the best response from the best limb that is recorded on this form.*

F. Test for lash, corneal, doll's eyes and carinal reflexes.

Continued.

Glasgow-Pitt Coma Score

Insult date: _____ / _____ / _____ Time: _____ _____ AM Pt. name: _____
 Day   Month   Year   Last   First
                                      _____ : _____ PM Hospital no.: _____

To be completed during the first half of each 8-hour shift or more often, as ordered. Fill in scores in numbers in opposite line. When in doubt, score observation with <u>highest</u> number (except seizures).

Worst (deep) coma score = 0.   Normal (best) score = 4 × 8 = 32

	Observation date:									
	Observation time:									
(A) Eye opening	Spontaneous	4								
	To sound	2								
	To pain	1								
	None	0								
(B) Pupil reaction to bright light	Normal	4								
	Constricted	3								
	Unequal, both react	2								
	Unequal, one reacts	1								
	None	0								
(C) Best verbal response (Understanding)	Oriented	4								
	Confused	3								
	Inappropriate	2								
	Incomprehensible	1								
	None	0								
	If trachea intubated, write "TI"									
(D) Best motor response right	Obedience	4								
	Appropriate*	3								
	Intermediate (unclear)	2								
	Stereotyped	1								
	None	0								
(E) Best motor response left	Obedience	4								
	Appropriate*	3								
	Intermediate (unclear)	2								
	Stereotyped	1								
	None	0								

*Any response to painful stimuli other than stereotyped flexion or extension of upper extremity.

		Glasgow-Pitt Coma Score—cont'd										
(F) **Cranial** **nerve** **response**	All present	4										
	Lash absent	3										
	Corneal absent	2										
	Doll's eye absent	1										
	Carinal (all) absent	0										
(G) **Score** **worst for** **seizures**	No seizure	4										
	Focal seizures	3										
	Generalized seizures	2										
	Status epilepticus myoclonus	1										
	Flaccidity	0										
(H) **Spont.** **breathing***	Normal	4										
	Cheyne-Stokes	3										
	Central hyperventilation	2										
	Irregular, hypoventilation, gasping	1										
	None (apnea)	0										
	TOTAL SCORE											
	Initials of observer:											

*If paralyzed, or ventilation controlled, score best guess.

of cardiac arrest and resuscitation, eight with tracings of 3 μV or less died, and one with activity greater than 10 μV recovered fully. Three patients with tracings between 3 and 10 μV died, and two survived.[66]

Cerebral evoked potentials (or responses) are neuronal electrical activity occurring in response to a distant stimulus; for example, the cortical activity specifically related to a peripheral somatosensory, auditory, or visual stimulus. As sensitive indicators of hypoxia, ischemia, compression, and other changes in the neuronal environment,[28] evoked response may prove a more reliable index of prognosis than has the clinical evaluation after brain[16,67,116] and spinal cord[133] injury. Even when spontaneous electrical activity is depressed by low CBF, metabolic factors, or drugs, the potential recovery of

some areas of the brain cortex can still be monitored by evoked responses.[67,126]

Physical factors

Those parameters that may mechanically affect nutrient blood supply such as ICP and arterial and venous pressures have already been discussed. Our monitoring techniques used for direct ICP measurement and oscilloscope display are similar to those described by Shapiro and co-workers[194] and are diagrammed in Fig. 15-9.

In addition, computerized tomography (CT) is particularly useful in localizing regional intracranial masses, and a more frequent use of this technique as part of neurointensive care has been proposed.[126] Computerized tomography has been modified both by incorporation of radionuclide studies[46,102] and with the use of a subtraction

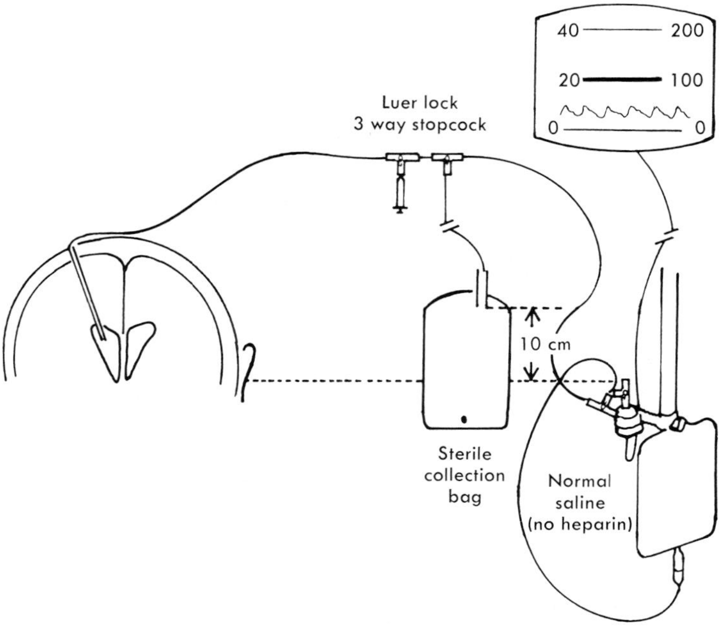

Fig. 15-9. Diagram of acceptable method of measuring ventricular fluid pressure with capability for CSF aspiration or drainage. Options: (1) monitor only, with Luer-lock stopcocks (Intralock LL3W, Sorenson Research Co.) *off* to syringe and collection bag; (2) measured aspiration of CSF via syringe into collection bag for therapy or for evaluation of compliance; (3) volume-pressure response (VPR) determination; (4) continuous pressure monitor and drainage of CSF with stopcock to collection bag open three ways. Note that because the connecting tubing functions as a siphon, the level at which ICP will be maintained is determined by the vertical distance between the entry port to the collection bag and the midcranium level (e.g., 10 cm). Note also that level of fluid in collection bag does not influence ICP. The system is never opened to air except for daily changes of tubing with sterile technique or if CSF samples are taken for analysis. The ICP waveform is displayed on a calibrated oscilloscope with gradicules for immediate evaluation. The saline bag is suspended at or below midcranium level to avoid accidental ventricular infusion.

technique that permits the detection of abnormalities in perfusion relative to changes in blood volume.[164]

The direct measurement of regional cerebral blood flow by repeated injections of indicator into the carotid artery has provided unique insight into intracranial dynamics and the effects of therapy.[21,51] Development of computer-based techniques utilizing either venous injection or inhalation of a radioactive indicator[155] has expanded investigation in this area.[94,95,139] Unfortunately, areas with no or very little blood flow may still not be represented. Determination of total cerebral blood flow has cor-

rectly predicted a poor outcome in some experimental models[102] and has also predicted the prognosis in some patients following stroke[85] and head injury[126] but in general has not proven very useful.

Chemical changes

Altered cellular function may be reflected by metabolic indicators measurable in the CSF as an extension of the extracellular environment and in cerebral venous blood. However, electrocerebral and clinical brain dysfunction can and does occur in the absence of any evidence of failure of brain metabolism during acute injury and during recovery, and metabolic monitoring has not been proven widely useful.

Cerebrospinal fluid (CSF) pH, P_{O_2}, and P_{CO_2} can occasionally support the diagnosis of CNS ischemia but are not reliable in establishing prognosis or in titrating care. Ischemia is associated with a lower P_{O_2} in the tissue and therefore CSF, but gas partial-pressure values in ventricular CSF can differ significantly from regional tissue levels.[193] CSF pH, P_{O_2}, and P_{CO_2} values obtained during a lumbar puncture vary considerably from ventricular and cisterna magna fluid and reflect intracranial status poorly.[101,171] Determination of the spinal fluid bicarbonate should provide a more reliable indicator of ischemia because it is less subject to equilibration with systemic blood and because it is less sensitive to sampling and measurement error. In the absence of metabolic acidemia, a decrease in CSF bicarbonate commonly reflects an equivalent increase in CSF lactate,[20,101,205] but this increase may also be due to local glycolysis, as in meningitis, carcinomatosis, and subarachnoid hemorrhage rather than ischemia.[169] CSF gas analysis is more sensitive to error induced by air bubbles in a sample than is blood analysis because of the lower gas content in CSF. If sampled during a lumbar puncture, a nonheparinized syringe is attached to a three-way stopcock and the stopcock inserted into the spinal needle. The syringe is held vertically with the tip up, and a small volume of CSF is aspirated and ejected together with the always present air bubble. Using "bubble free" technique, a 1 ml sample is then removed in the syringe and immediately injected into a blood gas analyzer that has been allowed to equilibrate with calibrating gas containing 5% CO_2. A pK and solubility coefficient calculated for CSF must be used in the determination of CSF bicarbonate.[191]

The significance of enzyme or amino acid levels within the CSF still remains investigational, awaiting correlation with other measurements of cellular or organ function.*

Cerebral venous P_{O_2} and oxygen content

---

*References 48, 57, 76, 84, 108, 138, 187, 218.

values may be elevated because of redistribution of perfusion to regions where resistance is low. Such areas generally receive blood flow in excess of demand while injured areas receiving less perfusion make a lesser contribution to the venous blood. The relative changes in cerebral venous P_{O_2} over time may be of value when continuous monitoring becomes available, but routine jugular bulb puncture and retrograde internal jugular catherization cannot be recommended at this time.

The determination of cerebral metabolic rate (CMR) as a means of evaluating oxygen consumption is affected as is CBF and cerebral venous O_2 measurements by the tendency to reflect well-perfused areas rather than those regions that receive poor flow. Presently, regional CMR measurements are dependent upon the availability of the short-lived $O_2{}^{15}$ molecule, which requires a cyclotron or similar generator.[177] Nonetheless, the use of radioactive oxygen, nitrogen, and carbon has been supported as economically feasible, especially when compared to the cost of CT scanning,[177] and initial studies have been presented.[4,176]

GENERAL ASPECTS OF SUPPORTIVE CARE

The delicate balance between neuronal metabolism and cerebral blood flow is also influenced by many general aspects of patient management, including pulmonary care, fluid and electrolyte therapy, nutrition, and the patient's acid-base balance.

Pulmonary care

Pulmonary care in the patient comatose from any cause is similar to that in any critically ill patient, except as modified by the following considerations. Activities such as postural drainage, chest physiotherapy, and tracheal suctioning, which may markedly increase intracranial pressure, should be timed so as to follow therapy directed at improving cerebral compliance, for example, osmotherapy (Fig. 15-17, *A*) or barbiturate administration[126] in patients with low brain compliance. In Fig. 15-17, *A*, glycerol was titrated to control ICP and was prophylactically given at an increased rate prior to tracheal suctioning to prevent the ICP elevation commonly associated with this procedure.[143] Suctioning is performed only as needed using a minimal trauma technique,[186] and cough induction by transtracheal catheter irrigation in the spontaneously breathing, nonintubated patient may be preferred to repeated nasotracheal suctioning. Secretions are kept thin by adequate systemic hydration, humidification of inspired gas, and intermittent ultrasonic nebulization of saline as indicated. Small doses of a bronchodilator may be used if the administration of nebulized particles induces bronchospasm.[50] A nonproductive cough should be promptly suppressed with intratracheal or intravenous xylocaine[202] and its occurrence minimized by the use of IV chlorpromazine or narcotics.

Hypoxemia may be especially harmful to the partially compromised brain, and its likely causes—atelectasis, aspiration, left ventricular failure, pneumonia, pulmonary contusion, or neurogenic pulmonary edema —must be prevented or treated. The decrease in functional residual capacity (FRC) in each of the pulmonary conditions above is also associated with an increased ventilatory drive attributed to the stimulation of stretch receptors in the lung. The physiologic abnormality in each of these pulmonary conditions, the reduced FRC, and the in-

creased respiratory drive may be normalized by the addition of positive end-expiratory pressure (PEEP) during spontaneous or mechanical ventilation. The level of PEEP used to ensure optimal respiratory and cardiac function is that amount associated with maximal mixed venous P_{O_2} or cardiac output.[106,210]

Any form of respiratory management, including the addition of PEEP, which might elevate peak or mean intrathoracic pressure, must be performed with caution so as to prevent a secondary decrease in venous return, left ventricular filling pressure, cardiac output, and systemic arterial pressure. As reviewed earlier, cerebral function may be exquisitely sensitive to such a hypotensive insult. Likewise, any increased intrathoracic pressure may be transmitted as an elevated central and jugular venous pressure and subsequently alter CPP adversely. Elevation of the patient's head relieves considerably the threat of increased ICP (Fig. 15-2)[1] from this mechanism. If mechanical ventilation or PEEP is discontinued abruptly during the weaning process, some authors[1] suggest that a sudden increase in venous return may occur and produce an abrupt increase in arterial and intracranial pressures. Therefore, care must be used both in the initiation and discontinuation of all forces of mechanical ventilation.

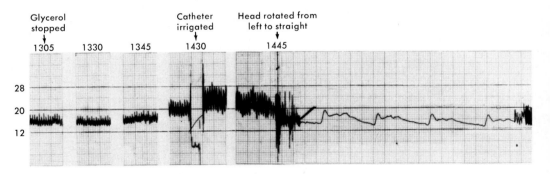

Fig. 15-10. An adult patient in coma from traumatic head injury was given a rapid infusion of glycerol to decrease ICP. A progressive rise in ICP over the subsequent hour caused concern that an ICP was "rebounding" because of increased brain osmolality until it was observed that the patient's head had become turned to the left. Returning the head to the neutral position apparently relieved compromised cerebral venous drainage and immediately decreased ICP.

Because optimal body positioning to avoid dependent edema in the brain and the lung bases are approximately opposite, there does not appear to be any ideal position for the comatose patient. Frequent changes in position, including semiprone but always with head elevated, are considered essential for the treatment and prophylaxis of pulmonary and cerebral congestion. The patient's head and neck should be maintained in a neutral position aligned with the trunk (Fig. 15-10). Caution should be used to avoid both orthostatic drops in arterial pressure and abrupt elevation of ICP precipitated by patient positioning.

The likelihood of deep vein thrombosis leading to pulmonary embolism remains high in the immobile patient. A recent study has suggested that minidose heparin prophylaxis is not contraindicated even in postoperative neurosurgery patients.[7] Other techniques to prevent formation of thrombosis, such as frequent, passive leg movements and compression devices,[199] should be considered.

Water, osmolality, and electrolytes

Excessive hydration may result from the administration of hypotonic fluid, hypoproteinemia, and increased secretion of antidiuretic hormone (ADH).[59] Although it should be appreciated that the optimal blood volume for a mechanically ventilated patient is higher than normal,[174] mechanical ventilation decreases free water clearance due to an increased secretion of ADH and to a shift in the distribution of renal blood flow from cortical to juxtamedullary glomeruli.[79,113] Humidification of inspired gas as a part of respiratory care decreases insensible water loss by about one-third and may further contribute to fluid retention. Decreases in hematocrit and serum sodium, increases in body weight, or other sequelae to overhydration such as decreased pulmonary compliance and increased pulmonary shunting are all reversible with water restriction and diuresis.[200]

CNS signs of primary or dilutional hyponatremia such as nausea, emesis, apathy, coarse muscular fibrillation, generalized muscle irritability, disorientation and convulsions occur at a serum sodium level of 115 to 127 mEq/l or at a somewhat higher value if the serum concentration is lowered rapidly.[103]

Dehydration resulting from an inadequate intake of water may occur in patients who neglect spontaneous fluid intake because of confusion or following a specific loss of the thirst response due to a hypothalamic lesion. Iatrogenic restriction of fluids for treatment of left ventricular dysfunction or to prevent overhydration may also be a contributing factor.[197] Excessive water loss as a cause of dehydration may be due to diabetes insipidus or to an osmotic diuresis. The latter, as associated with osmotherapy, administration of hyperosmolar carbohydrate infusions as parenteral nutrition, or after use of high osmolality contrast media for diagnostic studies, produces high losses of both salt and water. Dehydration is suspected and preferably prevented by a review of the patient's intake and output, changes in body weight, and the finding of hyperosmolality or hypernatremia.

Hypernatremia may occur with dehydration, excessive sodium administration including sodium bicarbonate and sodium penicillin,[90] or after large doses of glucocorticoids. The neurologic manifestations of hypernatremia include delirium, muscle twitching, hyperactive reflexes, and hemorrhagic encephalopathy in infants.[103]

Elevated blood urea and glucose levels are the principal clinical causes of the hyperosmolar syndrome. In a recent report of neurosurgical mortality, the incidence of nonketotic hyperglycemic hyperosmolar coma was 9% to 18%.[163] Hyperglycemia is more likely to occur in patients who are receiving high caloric, high carbohydrate diets, peritoneal dialysis, or corticosteroids and has been reported following administration of phenytoin.[103] Glucose intolerance was seen with toxic but not with therapeutic levels of phenytoin in a recent report.[23] CNS effects of hyperglycemia appear to be due to osmolality gradients and subsequent fluid shifts between the intracellular and extracellular fluid compartments of the brain.[30,54,60,65]

Intracellular dehydration may be a cause

of stupor in patients with ketoacidosis,[60] but cerebral depression may also occur during therapy and has been attributed to intracellular edema associated with rehydration,[54] reduction of elevated glucose levels, and to administration of excessive bicarbonate or inadequate phosphate and potassium.[54,111] Hyponatremia may also contribute to the encephalopathy in these patients,[47] and the $PaCO_2$ may rise during therapy of ketoacidosis and contribute to an increased ICP.[30] A brief review of these factors has recently been published.[105]

Salicylism has been associated with severe brain edema, which responded to osmotherapy and ventilatory support. Similar mechanisms to those in ketoacidosis could be involved, though uncoupling of oxidative phosphorylation has also been suggested.[18]

The association of uremia with electroencephalographic changes is well known. The dysequilibrium syndrome, which may occur during or up to 24 hours after dialysis, may include twitching, tremor, hyperreflexia, headache, emesis, grand mal seizures, and cardiac dysrhythmias. The mechanism for this syndrome might be an osmotically induced shift of water into the brain and CSF in response to either the delayed removal from brain of dialyzable substances or persistence of idiogenic intracellular molecules.[54] It is therefore prudent to reduce BUN levels more slowly in patients with cerebral insults or to minimize osmotic gradients by use of high concentrations of glucose in the dialysis fluid.[105]

Gastrointestinal/nutritional aspects

Nutritional imbalance with protein depletion as a cause of neurasthenic deterioration is seen in some patients following neurosurgical procedures.[22] The catabolic state that follows moderate and severe trauma[37] is further increased and prolonged after head trauma,[78] thus increasing the possibility of protein malnutrition. The administration of 100 g of glucose per day, as is routinely given in 2 liters of a 5% dextrose solution, has been shown to have a minimal protein sparing effect and, in addition, the

insulin stimulated by that glucose tends to decrease fat mobilization, resulting in accelerated breakdown of body protein. If the patient has previously been well nourished, such protein loss may be temporarily prevented by the infusion of essential amino acids without glucose during the recovery period.[92] Carefully administered total parenteral nutrition, ideally with all three main nutrients (carbohydrate, protein and fat), should be provided whenever tube feeding is impossible or contraindicated in patients who are unable to feed themselves.[5]

The increased incidence of gastrointestinal hemorrhage in critically ill patients, especially those with head injury, has led to the early therapeutic and sometimes prophylactic use of antacid titration or of the histamine II blocking agent cimetidine. Both approaches have been shown effective.[83] Although the antacid regimen is more costly in terms of effort, cimetidine has been incriminated as a cause of brain stem dysfunction and confusion.[36]

Serum protein

Serum protein as the principal determinant of plasma oncotic pressure may be decreased in patients receiving steroids[160] and in acute stress in brain-damaged patients because of a higher catabolic state.[37,78] A net loss of 30 to 60 g of protein per day is not uncommon.[37] Starling's concept[72] of the role of oncotic pressure as determining transcapillary fluid distribution suggests that hypoproteinemia is associated with either an intravascular hypovolemia or an increased interstitial volume, or both. The factors influencing this relationship should be monitored and any imbalances appreciated prior to the formation of clinically apparent edema, as an edematous state may represent the accumulation of 5 to 10 liters of excess fluid volume when first detected.[73] The validity of the Starling concept has been shown by Guyton[74] and Stein[204] in relation to the lung, and by Cervera and Moss[27] with regard to total body water. That the concept applies to the brain (cerebral edema) seems inevitable but has not been confirmed. It is our recommendation that hypoproteinemia should be prevented by enteral or parenteral nutrition when possible or treated more vigorously with concentrated (25%) albumin when the serum albumin is less that 3 g/100 ml or the colloid osmotic pressure is less than 20 torr.[40,175] Any excessive shift of interstitial fluid into the intravascular space can be appropriately treated with chemical diuresis. Relative contraindications to colloid therapy include gross hypervolemia, left ventricular failure, and the "capillary leak" syndrome.[182,183]

Metabolic acid base considerations

The systemic acidosis that may occur with renal failure and diabetes appears to stimulate central respiratory neurons and cause hyperventilation.[169] The spontaneous hyperventilation seen with hepatic encephalopathy has not been causally related to metabolic acidemia. Therapeutic "normalization" of the low Pa_{CO_2} in such conditions by various rebreathing techniques or with inspired CO_2 is ill advised, as it causes worsening of encephalopathy and cerebral depression.[172]

In metabolic alkalemia, as plasma bicarbonate accumulates, the CSF bicarbonate also increases and leads to a central respiratory depression. Often ventilatory drive becomes dependent upon the hypoxemia that evolves as a complication of the compensatory hypoventilation. Supplemental oxygen under such circumstances in patients with cerebral insults may remove the remaining ventilatory stimulus and induce further hypoventilation. Some of the contributing factors to metabolic alkalosis in this patient group may include hypovolemia, depletion of body stores of electrolytes, or the production of bicarbonate as a metabolic by-product of citrate after multiple blood transfusion. If the metabolic alkalemia requires treatment, electrolyte replacement may be sufficient or hydrochloric acid may be infused through a central vein.[81] Because of the potential for inducing an intracranial acidosis, acetazolamide, a carbonic anhydrase inhibitor, should not be used in patients with cerebral dysfunction.

ASPECTS OF SPECIFIC NEUROLOGIC THERAPY

Just as it is difficult to identify the particular regional pathologic mechanisms that may exist at a given time, the results of a given therapy may be impossible to precisely predict. Again it is assumed that a logical treatment program predicated upon an understanding of those principles previously discussed should produce the anticipated effect. However, when many such processes occur in areas "silent" to current monitoring techniques, the indications for therapy, and its effect, may go unrecognized. In general, treatment should be directed toward reestablishing or preserving the balance between neuronal nutritional needs and the available supply. By current concepts, therefore, it may be desirable at times to reduce the metabolic rate, increase blood flow to ischemic areas, avoid excessive flow and pressure, minimize factors that may enhance edema formation, and belatedly, reduce an elevated ICP to normal. Methods to accomplish one or more of these goals are discussed below, and examples of the variable effect on ICP are demonstrated in Fig. 15-7.

Cerebrospinal fluid drainage

Direct removal of CSF most consistently reduces ICP (Fig. 15-7) but only for a period of time, which is dependent upon brain tissue compliance, the reaccumulation of CSF, and subsequent increase in intracranial mass.[206] Reduction of the ventricular fluid pressure by inhibiting CSF formation with systemic diuretics improved CPP and secondarily decompressed the adjacent interstitium by permitting movement of that fluid into the ventricular system.[180]

Therapeutic hyperventilation

Cerebral vasoconstriction, as induced by lowering the Pa_{CO_2}, decreases the CBF and total CBV and hence ICP.[3,156] In clinical practice, hyperventilation lowered an elevated ICP in 9 of 15 trials in 11 patients following head trauma.[97] However, the ICP may decrease a variable amount and return to initial elevated levels in 15 to 80 minutes.[97] Hyperventilation may also decrease flow to borderline ischemic areas both by inducing vasoconstriction and by decreasing MAP (trace 8 in Fig. 15-7). It may also decrease the release of oxygen from oxyhemoglobin through the effect of alkalemia on the oxyhemoglobin dissociation curve. During prolonged hyperventilation in excess of patient demand, the total CBF has been shown to initially fall and then return toward normal levels as CSF bicarbonate decreases to compensate for the initial CSF alkalosis induced by hyperventilation.[156,192] Any subsequent change in ventilation that allows accumulation of CO_2 may induce a CSF acidosis as it rapidly equilibrates with a CSF that now has reduced buffering capacity. Posthyperventilation apnea may also occur in patients with cerebral dysfunction, so such patients should be carefully observed after hyperventilation and supplemental oxygen should always be administered to avoid hypoxia.[208]

Hypoventilation with elevation in Pa_{CO_2} causes vasodilatation of normal vascular beds and may direct blood away from vessels[156,213] perfusing ischemic areas—the "cerebral steal" phenomenon. Parenthetically, lowering of Pa_{CO_2} has also been shown to cause significant "steal," as in a patient with an arteriovenous malformation.[75] Hypercapnia may also increase ICP via increased CBV, which may likewise embarrass regional perfusion.

Because the effect of these complex mechanisms often cannot be predicted in the individual patient, the most prudent practice may be an attempt to allow the patient to "set" his or her own Pa_{CO_2} level and to support the patient at that level if respiratory assistance is required (Fig. 15-4, *B*). A higher Pa_{CO_2} than is normal for the patient is never indicated. Continuous monitoring of CO_2 concentration in exhaled gas is a useful measure of ventilation either in the spontaneously breathing patient or during mechanical ventilation (Figs. 15-3 and 15-4, *B*). In those situations such as paralysis, administration of sedatives or narcotics, or medullary dysfunction where the patient cannot determine his or her own optimal CO_2 levels, a Pa_{CO_2} of 25 to 35 torr is arbitrarily maintained by mechanical ventilation.

Corticosteroids and free radical ion formation

The widely used regimen of dexamethasone, 10 mg IV, followed by 4 mg every six hours is based principally on treatment of patients with CNS tumors.[61] A credible basis for efficacy of higher doses following head injury and for the "membrane stabilizing" action of steroids has been outlined by Demopoulous and others.[42,157] The inner, hydrophobic layer of cellular and intracellular membranes is made up of lipid side chains that are relatively unstable because of their dispersed physical arrangements and their degree of unsaturation. Highly reactive molecules with a single electron in the outer shell, so-called free radicals or radical ions, form spontaneously within this layer, especially in brain tissue. Such free radicals are catalyzed by heme and have the potential to propagate, especially in the presence of hypoxia, ethanol, and trauma.[55] It is likely that such propagation disrupts the function of membrane-bound enzymes and increases membrane permeability with resultant changes in electrolyte concentrations, membrane charge potentials, and opening of membrane interstices. That this mechanism plays a role in CNS pathophysiology is supported by the evidence for increased free radical ion formation in brain ischemia[56] and the observation that nonparalyzing impact injuries to the spinal cord result in paralysis when preceded by another free radical inducing agent, ethanol.[55] Because radical ion propagation contributes to CNS pathophysiology, it is of therapeutic interest that numerous drugs including barbiturates may act as scavengers to remove free radical ions.[41,56]

Molecules with a cholesterol base such as steroids are attracted to and fill the interstices of the lipid side chains, thus providing physicochemical stability. If this is the principal mechanism by which steroids function, their effect would be more in interrupting or preventing propagation of insult and promoting natural restorative processes than directly increasing reparative processes. The importance of early administration to decrease free radical propagation is also apparent. Clinically, steroids are most effective in therapy of patients with brain tumors, possibly because of the relatively slow rate of radical ion formation in such tumors, and have been shown to improve neurologic function in patients with primary and metastatic CNS tumors in doses up to 1,000 mg/day of methylprednisolone[119] and 96 mg/day of dexamethasone.[179] Improvement was seen within 24 to 48 hours, and the effect lasted three to six months.[118] Tumor inhibition and oncolysis are possible mechanisms of this action as well as steroid influence on the degree of peritumor inflammation and edema.[118] Even larger doses have been credited with improving survival after head trauma.[126] Although no convincing evidence of beneficial effect in stroke, cerebral hemorrhage, purulent meningitis, or anoxic-ischemic insult has been found, few reports exist that employed the early administration of steroid in doses comparable to those used for tumors. Acceleration of drug metabolism by concurrent phenytoin may require increased steroid dosage.[136] The incidence of peptic ulcer disease is not increased by steroid administration.[31]

Osmotherapy

Therapeutically induced osmotic gradients mobilize water from both normal and abnormal brain tissue.[102] Beneficial effects are via a subsequent decrease in ICP and at times, through improvement of CBF even when ICP is unchanged.[21] In the latter case, the removal of extravascular fluid presumably diminishes microcirculatory impedance and allows improved flow, which permits an expansion in blood volume to compensate for the osmotically removed fluid, thus maintaining the ICP.

Therapeutic dosages of mannitol have ranged from 0.2 to 4.0 g/kg given as a bolus or by infusion.[97,112] Boluses of up to 2.5 g/kg induced a decrease in ICP of more than 10% in 67 of 73 administrations to 44 neurosurgical patients with intracranial hypertension due to head trauma.[97] However, ICP returned to 80% or more of initial values 45 minutes to 11 hours later. Because the administration of 1 g/kg of mannitol as a bolus in some patients may markedly increase intravascular volume and produce detrimental effects on cardiopulmonary and central nervous system function, reports that a dramatic reduction of ICP could be obtained with smaller doses of 0.25 to 0.3 g/kg are therefore clinically useful.[112,131]

Advantages of long-term IV glycerol over IV mannitol may include a lower incidence of rebound phenomena, more sustained efficacy with prolonged or repeated administration, less diuresis with its consequent electrolyte disturbances, continuation of therapy in the presence of reduced or absent renal function, and its associated nutritional value (1 g/kg every six hours to a 70 kg patient provides about 1,000 calories per day).[214] However, these theoretical advantages have not yet been documented by carefully acquired data. Suggestive unpublished observations regarding glycerol therapy are exemplified and summarized below.

Glycerol concentration versus ICP. Fig. 15-11 shows the relationship of ICP to plasma glycerol concentration in 12 patients ages 19 months to 35 years with normal renal function and elevated ICP due to diverse insults. Glycerol caused a reduction of ICP at a plasma concentration of 1.5 to 3.0 mg/ml, which caused an increase in serum osmolality of about 15 to 30 mosmol/kg. It is unlikely that this correlation can be relied upon in the care of individual patients.

The close correlation between plasma glycerol concentration and idiogenic osmolality, that is, the osmolar gap shown in Fig. 15-12 suggests that the blood level of glycerol may be estimated in the absence of ethanol, lactate, and other osmotically significant plasma components by calculating the idiogenic osmolality. Idiogenic osmolality = measured osmolality − calculated osmolality, where calculated osmolality = $2(Na + mEq/l) + \dfrac{glucose \ mg/dl}{18} + \dfrac{BUN \ mg/dl}{2.8}$. The contribution of glycerol to plasma osmolality should approximately equal the idiogenic osmolality.

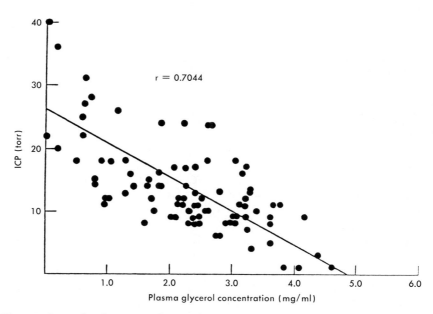

Fig. 15-11. Relationship between plasma glycerol concentration and intracranial pressure in 12 patients with elevated ICP. The relationship was statistically significant, with p < 0.001 and 95 degrees of freedom.[167]

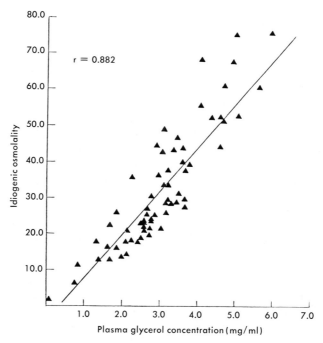

Fig. 15-12. Relationship between plasma glycerol concentration and idiogenic osmolality in 13 patients.[167] The relationship was significant, with p < 0.001 and 65 degrees of freedom.

Administration of glycerol to children

CLEARANCE. Total body clearance of a drug may be calculated by dividing the infusion rate by the steady-state plasma concentration. The relationship between a glycerol intravenous infusion rate ranging from 0.10 to 0.87 g/kg/hr and the steady-state plasma concentration was studied in 10 patients (weight ranging from 8 to 52 kg) with normal hepatic and renal function.[167] In these children the plasma levels of glycerol gradually rose to approach a constant level by approximately four hours, and the plateau or steady-state concentration was found to be directly proportional to the rate of infusion. The

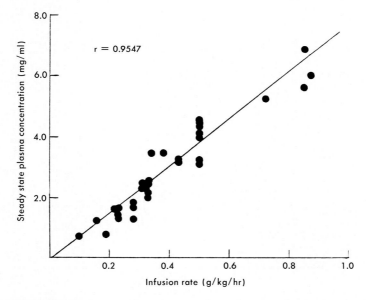

Fig. 15-13. Relationship between infusion rate and steady state plasma concentration in ten children treated with glycerol.[167]

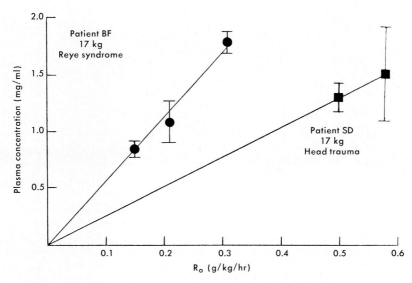

Fig. 15-14. Effect of liver function on clearance of glycerol (R_0) in two patients.[167]

clearance was 130 ml/kg/hr in this study. Fig. 15-13 is a plot of this relationship between infusion rate and steady-state plasma concentration indicating that the therapeutic level of 1.5 to 3.0 mg/ml plasma glycerol concentration was accomplished at an infusion rate of between 0.2 to 0.4 g/kg/hr.

EFFECT OF LIVER DISEASE. The effect of decreased liver function on glycerol clearance is suggested by Fig. 15-14 in which a patient with head trauma and normal liver function is shown to have had a clearance of approximately twice that of a patient with fulminant Reye syndrome. However, comparable variations in clearance in adults without significant liver dysfunction has also been noted.

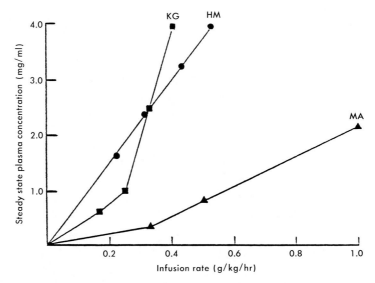

Fig. 15-15. Variable relationship between infusion rate and steady state plasma concentration of glycerol in three adults.[167]

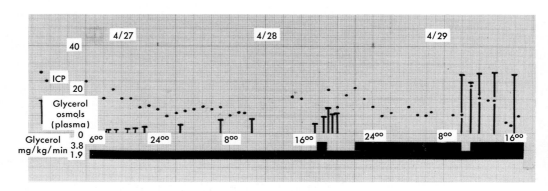

Fig. 15-16. Effect of constant rate infusion of glycerol on plasma glycerol concentration, indicated by ⊤, and on ICP, indicated by dots. Plasma glycerol continued to increase slowly over 16 hours of continuous administration at a rate of 0.7 g/kg infused over six hours. It remains unclear whether the corresponding decline in ICP was related to the therapy. Doubling the infusion rate of glycerol after 26 hours initially induced a sharper rise and finally a threefold increase in plasma concentration.

Administration of glycerol to adults

CLEARANCE. The relationship between infusion rate and steady-state plasma concentration in three head-injured adult patients with normal liver and renal function is shown in Fig. 15-15. There was a linear relationship between infusion rate and steady-state concentration in patient HM but not in patients KG and MA. The explanation for this variability is unexplained but emphasizes the need for periodic measurements of plasma osmolality at different infusion rates.

The optimal dose and rate of administration of any osmotic agent varies with the hepatic and renal function and intracranial circumstances in each patient and may not be predictable in critically ill patients without ICP monitoring. The effectiveness of each dosage change in lowering ICP is affected by the degree of rehydration in both injured and normal brain that has occurred since the previous dose[223] and upon the development of increasing brain or CSF osmolality.[184]

Fig. 15-16 shows the relationship of glycerol infusion rate, plasma concentration, and ICP in an adult patient with head trauma. A constant infusion rate of 1 g/kg over six hours (approximately 3 mg/kg/min) achieved a stable concentration but a minimal effect after several hours. Increasing the infusion rate resulted in increased plasma concentrations and a decrease in ICP. Multiple similar experiences have led to our practice of using a higher initial infusion rate of 5 mg/kg/min for 30 minutes followed by 3 mg/kg/min for 90 minutes in adults. Larger doses may be utilized in children.[142]

The need for titration of dosage according to ICP response is illustrated in Fig. 15-17, in which the sensitivity of intracranial dynamics to varying levels of osmotherapy is demonstrated.

Infusion rates can be varied according to the severity of tissue swelling as detected by CNS function, ICP, or brain compliance monitoring. Intravenous glycerol should usually be infused as a 10% solution in 5% dextrose in water, with or without 0.9%, 0.45%, or 0.25% saline. These solutions and a central venous catheter are used so as to minimize hemolysis[77,214] and any possible complications associated with extravasation.[88]

Observation of the plasma for pink color 20 and 60 minutes after the start of therapy or following an increased infusion rate is an effective and simple way to monitor for hemolysis as the primary adverse effect of glycerol. Discoloration of the urine is an insensitive sign of hemolysis and is usually due to other factors.[168]

Administration to children resulted in diuresis approximately equal to the volume infused.[143] Glycerol infusion may be associated with elevated blood glucose levels, especially in patients with a diabetic tendency.[190] A single case of metabolic intolerance of glycerol has been reported.[123]

Enteral administration of glycerol has also been found effective in a dose to adults of 1 g/kg every six hours.[184] However, clinical deterioration in ICP has been reported in one adult patient when glycerol was given as 1 gm/kg every four hours.[184] Improvement occurred with discontinuation of therapy. Variable gastrointestinal absorption in critically ill patients and gastric irritation with possible emesis and aspiration[214] may also limit the usefulness of this route.

REBOUND. All osmotherapeutic agents can cause a delayed increase in ICP, the so-called "rebound effect." A progressive decrease in responsiveness of an increased ICP to osmotherapy may be due to accumulation of the agent in brain tissue or CSF, thereby reversing osmotic gradients across the blood-brain interface (Fig. 15-17).[54,68,143,184] Such an accumulation may cause fluid to leave the plasma and enter the interstitial space as the serum concentration of the agent declines and may then yield a rise in ICP. In contrast to earlier impressions, a rebound effect can occur with glycerol (Fig. 15-17).[70] The apparent lower incidence with glycerol may be due to metabolism of the drug by the brain,[102] although this too has been questioned.[43]

Chronic hyperosmolality has also been associated with idiogenic molecules in the brain, which are osmotically active by-products of neuronal metabolism and which may

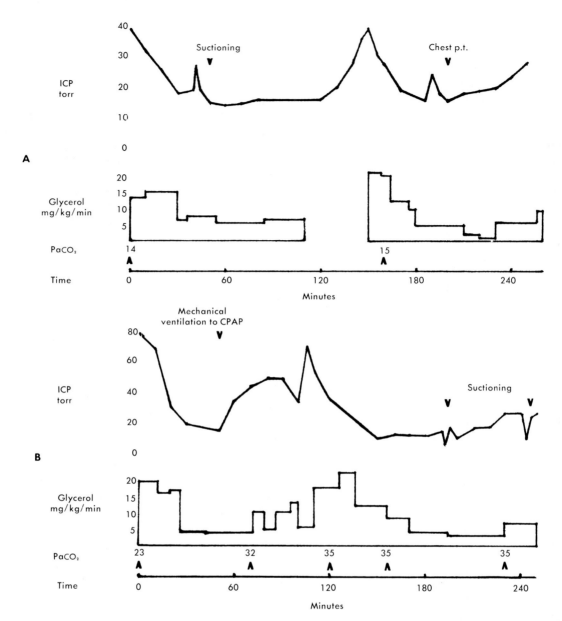

Fig. 15-17. A 2½-year-old girl sustained severe trauma in a car accident and on hospital admission was flaccid with 3-mm diameter equal unreactive pupils, absence of corneal and gag reflexes, doll's eyes, and response to cold caloric stimulation. A ventricular catheter was inserted on admission, and glycerol therapy was titrated according to ventricular pressure. At 55 hours after admission, the patient required dosages of 1 g/kg of 10% glycerol every two hours by continuous titrated infusion to maintain ventricular fluid pressure less than 40 torr. **A,** Coordinated osmotherapy and respiratory care. A high infusion rate of glycerol provided sufficient control of intracranial compliance so that an excessive rise in ICP during suctioning and later during chest physiotherapy was avoided. Steroids and hyperventilation were inadequate to control ICP. The inverse relationship between ICP and glycerol infusion rate clearly demonstrates control of ICP by this agent but is also compatible with high tissue concentrations of glycerol and a tendency for rebound effect on ICP. **B,** Relation of glycerol therapy to ICP control in the same patient as above during weaning from mechanical ventilation to spontaneous breathing with continuous positive airway pressure (CPAP).[143]

likewise decrease the plasma-brain osmotic gradient and tend to reduce the effectiveness of continuously administered osmotherapeutic agents. Therefore whether intermittent administration is more effective than continued infusion or how often subsequent doses are needed to control increased brain edema after earlier use of the same agent is not known.[69]

Chemical diuretics

Ethacrynic acid, furosemide, and acetazolamide have been shown to reduce interstitial (vasogenic) brain edema associated with tumors in humans and cryogenic lesions in cats and rhesus monkeys.[102,119,180] The mechanism appears to be through inhibition of CSF production, which secondarily allows improved drainage of interstitial edema fluid into the ventricles. In addition, a more rapid response in patients with increased jugular venous pressure may be through the expected decrease in systemic venous compliance associated with some chemical diuretics.[44] Diuretics also appear to supplement the effect of dexamethasone on peritumor edema in patients[137] on cryogenic edema in cats[119,120] and to control ICP with effect comparable to osmotherapy in operative patients.[33,181] Experimental data suggest chemical diuretics are less effective when edema is largely intracellular.[128,181]

Manipulation of metabolism and neurotransmission

Neurotransmitters as they influence neuronal metabolism and circulation are probably responsible for the normal "tight coupling" between normal brain circulation and metabolism, and uncoupling in pathologic states.[148]

Numerous drugs have been suggested to be useful in patient management to the extent that they decrease brain tissue metabolism or affect the product of metabolism in ischemia. The observed beneficial effects may be due to the direct depression of neuronal catecholamine release[96,147,224] or through depletion of neurotransmitter stores or by blocking afferent stimulation. Mem-

brane "stabilization" by physiochemical methods and through removal of free radical ions[41,42,56] has been proposed to prevent progressive neuronal damage. Depression of metabolic demands with induced hypothermia and some anesthetics may also be beneficial.[195] Most or all hypnotic drugs may depress catecholamine response and metabolic rate, but large doses are often required.[117,195] For example, diazepam has been shown to control increased CMR for oxygen in patients with head injury.[53] Narcotics affect specific central receptors and may have potent effects on neurotransmitter synthesis and metabolism but often cause pronounced neurologic depression as well as changes in pupillary signs in the dosage required to achieve sedation or to decrease ICP (Fig. 15-7).[162,203]

Barbiturates have been shown to improve neurologic recovery following stroke[141] and global brain ischemia[14] when given in large doses following experimental insults. Prompt and prolonged control of intracranial hypertension with barbiturates in patients with trauma and Reye syndrome, probably resulting in improvement of outcome, has been reported.[129,130] Barbiturate loading has also been used as prophylaxis against stroke in patients following surgery for cerebral aneurysm.[89] Possible mechanisms of barbiturate effect have been recently reviewed.[41,56,126,201] The depression of neurologic signs inherent in barbiturate loading increases the value of and the clinician's dependence upon monitoring devices, especially the evoked response[67,126] and ICP.[144]

Chlorpromazine and haloperidol may act by blocking catecholamine receptors[25,93] and prostaglandin synthesis.[45] Chlorpromazine specifically has been useful in control of hyperkinesis, central hyperthermia, shivering, and excessive systemic vasoconstriction and produces fewer changes in the functional level of response than other depressants. Whenever used, however, chlorpromazine may dramatically reveal the presence of intravascular hypovolemia as its mild vasodilatory effect produces hypotension (11 in Fig. 15-7). The drug is therefore injected intravenously in 1 to 5 mg increments at three to five minute intervals by a physician or nurse in constant attendance. Arterial pressure is monitored throughout the administration of the first 25 mg, and significant falls in pressure are treated with colloids. Chlorpromazine therapy is continued by 5 mg boluses as needed or by the infusion of 25 mg over 20 minutes every six hours. The same dose of 25 mg may also be given intramuscularly each six hours. Seizures and hypersensitivity to the drug are contraindications to its use.[91]

Neuromuscular paralysis can decrease ICP and edema formation due to decreased venous pressure by preventing excessive muscular activity and by allowing systemic venous pooling. No other specific advantages are recognized. Because CNS depressants may produce the same relaxation and benefit on ICP and also beneficially depress afferent stimulation, the use of barbiturates and phenothiazine-related drugs is preferred. Monitoring of ICP is often warranted when either drug class is used, as the value of clinical neurologic examination is minimal.

Hypothermia

Hypothermia decreases brain water and CBF, slows cerebral edema formation, decreases inflammatory reaction to injury, and may protect enzyme activity. The magnitude and frequency of plateau waves are decreased,[122] and ICP elevation resistant to other therapy often becomes responsive.[97,129,130] Therapeutic hypothermia has not been as widely studied as other modalities, although a recent survey is available.[11] While myocardial irritability is rare above 30° C in the absence of significant coronary or valvular disease, this potential complication and an increase in myocardial contractility during hypothermia are relative contraindications to this therapy in patients with myocardial ischemia. Venous thrombosis and subsequent embolism are potentiated by depression of cardiac output, blood hypercoagulability, and immobilization of the patient during hypothermia. Temperature suppression as well as steroid use make early diagnosis of sepsis more difficult.

Valuable preliminary observations have been made of the effect of hypothermia as a part of other current intensive therapy of comatose patients.[97,144,195] There is both clinical[144,195] and experimental[152] evidence that a combination of hypothermia with barbiturate administration is more effective in controlling ICP (clinical) and reducing CMR and CBF (experimental) than either technique alone.

SPECIAL CONSIDERATIONS

Management of patients with bleeding intracranial aneurysms has been recently reviewed.[87] Rebleeding has been noted to occur as ICP decreases toward normal and may be precipitated by a sudden reduction in ICP by lumbar puncture or intravenous hyperosmolar agents. Preoperatively, epsilon aminocaproic acid (EACA) may be given intravenously for one week, then orally, to retard fibrinolysis. The dose is 30 to 36 g/day. This therapy should be monitored with the streptokinase clot lysis time test. Bed rest and moderate hypotensive therapy is also commonly used. Aggressive efforts to lower ICP may precipitate further hemorrhage in some patients.[153] Two studies suggest that monitoring of ICP provides warning of impending aneurysm rupture and thereby might indicate earlier operation than would otherwise be considered.[135,154]

Neurologic deficits not attributable to other factors in a patient with subarachnoid hemorrhage or following surgery are often ascribed to vasospasm. Vasospasm has recently been shown to appear angiographically about three days following subarachnoid hemorrhage but usually to be resolved by the twelfth day.[219] A therapeutic regimen that appears successful in resolving neurologic deficit attributed to spasm combines plasma expansion and inotropic drugs, (e.g., dopamine or isoproterenol) to maintain an elevated mean arterial pressure. Xylocaine may be required to control ventricular dysrhythmias seen with isoproterenol administration.[209] Aminophylline has been given to dilate cerebral vessels, and oral kanamycin has been used to lower the blood level of serotonin to allow vasodilatation.[87]

SUMMARY

Much of the current therapy of intracranial pathologic processes is based upon empiric observations, both from the laboratory and bedside and is supported by reasonable explanations. However, it remains appropriate to question whether such gross observations can be correctly interpreted as few of the many clinically relevant physiologic or pathologic relationships have been sufficiently defined to allow secure inference of cause or effect. A certain mean arterial pressure, for example, may be necessary to perfuse ischemic brain tissue but simultaneously may augment edema formation in a different region of that patient's CNS. Likewise, manipulation of Pa_{CO_2} may improve or depress regional blood flow in the same or different areas. It is, then, the imprecision of some diagnoses and the unpredictability of therapy that have increasingly led to the application of more objective monitoring devices in an effort to confirm the presence of the suspected pathophysiology and to determine the effect of initial and subsequent therapy. As a result, physical factors such as ICP have been maintained closer to what was considered optimal. In several types of brain insults, evidence is accumulating that the outcome was clearly better than if therapy had not been directed by monitoring. Because instrumental monitoring invariably adds to the cost of patient care through more complex equipment, better trained personnel, and through an increased potential morbidity, the need for more controlled documentation of indications and benefits from various approaches is apparent. Morbidity may increase when personnel are inadequately trained to tend the devices and interpret their output. Therefore, if the balance between the supply for and the demands of neuronal metabolism is to be met and the meaningful integrated function of the brain preserved, continued objective exploration of those variables discussed here as well as others must proceed.

ACKNOWLEDGMENTS

It is our particular pleasure to acknowledge the following collaborators for their contributions to this text. The Department of Neurosurgery was continuously supportive in establishment of monitoring techniques; several individuals contributed to the concepts presented. Dr. Edwin Nemoto made valuable contributions to the chapter. Doctors John J. Mickell and William Pitlick reviewed and suggested revisions of portions of the text. Lois Bauer provided organization of data and text and graphic arts. Data collection by the ICU laboratory technicians with generous assistance by the nursing staff of the intensive care unit was supervised by Jeanne E. O'Malley. Linda Elliott and Janet Viaropulos provided skilled secretarial assistance through multiple revisions.

REFERENCES

1. Aidinis, S. J., Lafferty, J., and Shapiro, H. M.: Intracranial responses to PEEP, Anesthesiology **45:**275, 1976.
2. Albani, M.: An effective dose schedule for phenytoin treatment of status epilepticus in infancy and childhood, Neuropadiatrie **8:**286, 1977.
3. Alexander, S. D., and Lassen, N. A.: Cerebral circulatory response to acute brain disease: implications for anesthetic practice, Anesthesiology **32:**60, 1970.
4. Alpert, N. M., Ackerman, R. H., Correia, J. A., and others: Measurement of rCBF and $rCMRO_2$ by continuous inhalation of ^{15}O-labeled CO_2 and O_2. In Ingvar, D. H., and Lassen, N. A.: Cerebral function, metabolism and circulation, Copenhagen, 1977, Munksgaard, p. 186.
5. Ballinger, W. F.: Manual of surgical nutrition, Philadelphia, 1975, W. B. Saunders Co.
6. Barlow, C. F.: Physiology and pathophysiology of protein permeability in the central nervous system, In Reulen, H. J., and Schürmann, K.: Steroids and brain edema, New York, 1972, Springer-Verlag, p. 139.
7. Barnett, H. G., Clifford, J. R., and Llewellyn, R. C.: Safety of mini-dose heparin administration for neurosurgical patients, J. Neurosurg. **47:**27, 1977.
8. Bates, D., Caronna, J. J., Cartlidge, N. E. F., and others: A prospective study of nontraumatic coma: method and results in 310 patients, Ann. Neurol. **2:**211, 1977.
9. Becker, D.: Personal communication, 1978.
10. Becker, D. P., Miller, J. D., Ward, J. D., and others: The outcome from severe head injury with early diagnosis and intensive management, J. Neurosurg. **47:**491, 1977.
11. Black, P. R., Van De Vanter, S., and Cohn, L. H.: Current research review: effects of hypothermia on systemic and organ system metabolism and function, J. Surg. Res. **20:**49, 1976.
12. Blennow, G., Folbergrova, J., Nilsson, B., and Siesjö, B. K.: Cerebral blood flow and oxygen utilization in rats during bicuculline-induced sei-

zures; effect of substrate depletion, In Ingvar, D. H., and Lassen, N. A.: Cerebral function, metabolism and circulation, Copenhagen, 1977, Munksgaard, p. 224.

13. Bleyaert, A., Safar, P., Nemoto, R. M., and Stezoski, S. W.: Blood pressure control after cardiac arrest, Crit. Care Med. **6:**92, 1978.

14. Bleyaert, A. L., Nemoto, E. M., Safar, P., Stezoski, S. W., Moossy, J., Rao, G. R., and Mickell, J.: Thiopental amelioration of postischemic encephalopathy in monkeys, Anesthesiology **49:**390, 1978.

15. Bolwig, T. G., Hertz, H. M., and Westergaard, E.: Blood-brain barrier permeability to protein during epileptic seizures in the rat. In Ingvar, D. H., and Lassen, N. A.: Cerebral function, metabolism and circulation, Copenhagen, 1977, Munksgaard, p. 226.

16. Branston, N. M., Symon, L., Crockard, H. A., and Pasztor, E.: Relationship between the cortical evoked potential and local cortical blood flow following acute middle cerebral artery occlusion in the baboon, Exper. Neurol. **45:**195, 1974.

17. Branthwaite, M. A.: Prevention of neurological damage during open heart surgery, Thorax **30:**258, 1975.

18. Bray, P. F., and Gardiner, A. Y.: Salicylism and severe brain edema, N. Engl. J. Med. **297:**1235, 1977.

19. Brock, M.: Cerebral blood flow and intracranial pressure changes associated with brain hypoxia. In Brierly, J. B., and Meldrum, B. S.: Brain hypoxia, London, 1971, Heinemann, p. 14.

20. Brodersen, P., and Jorgensen, E. O.: Cerebral blood flow and oxygen uptake, and cerebrospinal fluid biochemistry in severe coma, J. Neurol. Neurosurg. Psychiatr. **37:**384, 1974.

21. Bruce, D. A., Langfitt, T. W., Miller, J. D., and others: Regional cerebral blood flow, intracranial pressure, and brain metabolism in comatose patients, J. Neurosurg. **38:**131, 1973.

22. Bryan-Brown, C. W., Savitz, M. H., Elwyn, D. H., and others: Cerebral edema unresponsive to conventional therapy in neurosurgical patients with unsuspected nutritional failure, Crit. Care Med. **1:**125, 1973.

23. Callaghan, N., Feely, M., O'Callaghan, M., and others: The effects of toxic and non-toxic serum phenytoin levels on carbohydrate tolerance and insulin levels, Acta Neurol. Scand. **56:**563, 1977.

24. Carlon, G. C., Kahn, R. C., Goldiner, P. L., and others: Long-term infusion of sodium thiopental, hemodynamic and respiratory effects, Crit. Care Med. **6:**311, 1978.

25. Carlsson, A., and Lindqvist, M.: Effect of chlorpromazine or haloperidol on formation of 3-methoxytyramine and normetanephrine in mouse brain, Acta Pharmacol. Toxicol. **20:**140, 1963.

26. Carlsson, C., Hagerdahl, M., Kassik, A. E., and others: A catecholamine mediated increase in

cerebral oxygen uptake during immobilization stress in rats, Brain Res. **119:**223, 1977.

27. Cervera, A. L., and Moss, G.: Crystalloid distribution following hemorrhage and hemodilution: mathematical model and prediction of optimal volumes for equilibration at normal volemia, J. Trauma **14:**506, 1974.

28. Chang, H. T.: The evoked potentials. In Magoien, H. W.: Handbook of physiology, neurophysiology, Washington, D.C., 1959, American Physiological Society, vol. 1.

29. Classen, R. A., Pandolfi, S., Laring, J., and others: Experimental study of relation of fever to cerebral edema, J. Neurosurg. **41:**576, 1974.

30. Clements, R. S., Jr., Blumenthal, S. A., Morrison, A. D., and others: Increased cerebral spinal fluid pressure during treatment of diabetic ketosis, Lancet **2:**671, 1971.

31. Conn, H. O., and Blitzer, B. L.: Nonassociation of adrenocorticosteroid therapy and peptic ulcer, N. Engl. J. Med. **294:**473, 1976.

32. Cottrell, J. E., Casthely, P., Brodie, J. D., and others: Prevention of nitroprusside-induced cyanide toxicity with hydroxocobalamin, N. Engl. J. Med. **298:**809, 1978.

33. Cottrell, J. E., Robustelli, A., Post, K., and Turndorf, H.: Furosemide- and mannitol-induced changes in intracranial pressure and serum osmolality and electrolytes, Anesthesiology **47:**28, 1977.

34. Cottrell, J. E., Patel, K., Turndorf, H., and Ransohoff, J.: Intracranial pressure changes induced by sodium nitroprusside in patients with intracranial mass lesions, J. Neurosurg. **48:**329, 1978.

35. Cox, B., and Lomas, P.: Pharmacologic control of temperature regulation, a Rev. Pharmacol. Toxicol. **17:**341, 1977.

36. Cumming, W. J. K., and Foster, J. B.: Cimetidine-induced brainstem dysfunction, Lancet **1:**1096, 1978.

37. Cuthbertson, D. P., and Tilstone, W. J.: Metabolism in the post-injury period. In Bodensky, O., and Stewart, C. P.: Advances in clinical chemistry, New York, 1969, Academic Press, vol. 12.

38. Cuypers, J., Matakas, F., and Potolicchio, S. J.: Effect of central venous pressure on brain tissue and brain volume, J. Neurosurg. **45:**89, 1976.

39. Davies, D. W., Greiss, L., Kadar, D., and Steward, D. J.: Sodium nitroprusside in children: observations on metabolism during normal and abnormal responses, Can. Anaesth. Soc. J. **22:**553, 1975.

40. de Luz, P. L., Shubin, H., Weil, M. H., and others: Pulmonary edema related to changes in colloid osmotic and pulmonary artery wedge pressure in patients after acute myocardial infarction, Circulation **51:**350, 1975.

41. Demopoulos, H. B., Flamm, E. S., Seligman, M. L., and others: Antioxidant effects of barbiturates in model membranes undergoing free radical damage. In Ingvar, D. H., and Lassen, N. A.: Cerebral

function, metabolism and circulation, Copenhagen, 1977, Munksgaard, p. 152.

42. Demopoulos, H. B., Milvy, P., Kakari, S., and Ransohoff, J.: Molecular aspects of membrane structure in cerebral edema. In Reulen, H. J., and Schurmann, K.: Steroids and brain edema, New York, 1972, Springer-Verlag.

43. DeSouza, S. W., Dobbing, J., and Adlard, B. P. F.: Glycerol in treatment of cerebral edema, Lancet 1:835, 1973.

44. Dikshit, K., Vyden, J., Forrester, J. S. and others: Renal and extrarenal hemodynamic effects of furosemide in congestive heart failure after acute myocardial infarction, N. Engl. J. Med. 288:1087, 1973.

45. Dinarello, C. A., and Wolff, S. M.: Pathogenesis of fever in man, N. Engl. J. Med. 298:607, 1978.

46. Drayer, B. P., Wolfson, S. K., Reinmuth, O. M., and others: Xenon enhanced CT for analysis of cerebral integrity, perfusion, and blood flow, Stroke 9:123, 1978.

47. Duck, S. C., Weldon, V. V., Pagliara, A. S., and Haymond, M. W.: Cerebral edema complicating therapy for diabetic ketoacidosis, Diabetes 25:111, 1976.

48. Duffy, T. E., Vergara, F., and Plum, F.: Ketoglutaramate in hepatic encephalopathy. In Plum, F.: Brain dysfunction in metabolic disorders, New York, 1974, Raven Press.

49. Dymond, A. M., and Crandall, P. H.: Oxygen availability and blood flow in the temporal lobes during spontaneous epileptic seizures in man, Brain Res. 102:191, 1976.

50. El-Naggar, M., Kintanar, D., Toyoma, T., and others: Saline, isoproterenol and racemic epinephrine aerosol therapy in patients on IPPV, Crit. Care Med. 2:129, 1974.

51. Enevoldsen, E. M., Cold, G., Jensen, F. T., and Malmros, R.: Dynamic changes in regional CBF, intraventricular pressure, CSF pH and lactate levels during the acute phase of head injury, J. Neurosurg. 44:191, 1976.

52. Escueta, A. V., Kunze, U., Waddell, G., Boxley, J., and Nadel, A.: Lapse of consciousness and automatisms in temporal lobe epilepsy: a videotape analysis, Neurology 27:144, 1977.

53. Escuret, E., Roquefeuil, B., Frerebeau, P., and Baldy-Moulinier, M.: Effect of hyperventilation associated with administration of central nervous depressants in brain injuries. In Ingvar, D. H., and Lassen, N. A.: Cerebral function, metabolism and circulation, Copenhagen, 1977, Munksgaard, p. 154.

54. Feig, P. U., and McCurdy, D. K.: The hypertonic state, N. Engl. J. Med. 297:1444, 1977.

55. Flamm, E. S., Demopoulos, H. B., Seligman, M. L., Tomasula, J. J., DeCrescito, V., and Ransohoff, J.: Ethanol potentiation of central nervous system trauma, J. Neurosurg. 46:328, 1977.

56. Flamm, E. S., Demopoulos, H. B., Seligman, M.

L., and Ransohoff, J.: Possible molecular mechanisms of barbiturate-mediated protection in regional cerebral ischemia. In Ingvar, D. H., and Lassen, N. A.: Cerebral function, metabolism and circulation, Copenhagen, 1977, Munksgaard, p. 150.

57. Fleischer, A. S., Rudman, D. R., Fresh, C. B., and Tindall, G. T.: Concentration of 3'5' cyclic adenosine monophosphate in ventricular CSF of patients following severe head trauma, J. Neurosurg. 47:517, 1977.

58. Forster, A., Van Horn, K., Marshall, L. F., and Shapiro, H. M.: Influence of anesthetic agents on blood-brain barrier function during acute hypertension. In Ingvar, D. H., and Lassen, N. A.: Cerebral function, metabolism and circulation, Copenhagen, 1977, Munksgaard, p. 60.

59. Fox, J. L., Falik, J. L., and Shalhoub, R. J.: Neurosurgical hyponatremia: the role of inappropriate antidiuresis, J. Neurosurg. 34:506, 1971.

60. Fulop, M., Tannenbaum, H., and Dreyer, M.: Ketotic hyperosmolar coma, Lancet 2:635, 1973.

61. Galicich, J. H., French, L. A., and Melby, J. C.: Use of dexamethasone in treatment of cerebral edema associated with brain tumors, Lancet 81:46, 1961.

62. Gastaut, H., Courjon, J., Poiré, R., and Weber, M.: Treatment of status epilepticus with a new benzodiazepine more active than diazepam, Epilepsia 12:197, 1971.

63. Geier, S., Bancaud, J., Talairach, J., and others: The seizures of frontal lobe epilepsy, Neurology 27:951, 1977.

64. Goldberg, H. I., Codario, R. A., Banka, R. S., and others: Patterns of cerebral dysautoregulation in severe hypertension to blood pressure reduction with diazoxide. In Ingvar, D. H., and Lassen, N. A.: Cerebral function, metabolism and circulation, Copenhagen, 1977, Munksgaard, p. 64.

65. Gottstein, U.: Diabetic and uremic coma. In Ingvar, D. H., and Lassen, N. A.: Brain work, Alfred Benzon Symposium VIII, Copenhagen, 1975, Munksgaard, p. 325.

66. Greenbaum, D. M., and Wagner, I.: Electroencephalographic trend recording as an indicator for survival in comatose patients (abstract), Crit. Care Med. 7:145, 1979.

67. Greenberg, R. P., Becker, D. P., Miller, J. D., and Mayer, D. J.: Evaluation of brain function in severe human head trauma with multimodality evoked potentials, J. Neurosurg. 47:163, 1977.

68. Guisado, R., Arieff, A. I., and Massry, S. G.: Effects of glycerol administration on experimental brain edema, Neurology 26:69, 1976.

69. Guisado, R., Arieff, A. I., and Massry, S. G.: Effects of glycerol infusions on brain water and electrolytes, Am. J. Physiol. 227:865, 1974.

70. Guisado, R., Tourtellotte, W. W., Arieff, A. I., Tomyasu, U., Mishra, S. K., and Scholtz, M. C.: Rebound phenomenon complicating cerebral de-

hydration with glycerol, J. Neurosurg. **42**:226, 1975.

71. Guyton, A. C., Taylor, A. E., and Granger, H. J.: Pressure-volume curves of the interstitial fluid spaces. In Circulatory physiology II: dynamics and control of the body fluids, Philadelphia, 1975, W. B. Saunders Co.

72. Guyton, A. C., Taylor, A. E., and Granger, H. J.: Equilibrium of pressures (Starling's equilibrium) at the capillary membrane. In Circulatory physiology II: dynamics and control of the body fluids, Philadelphia, 1975, W. B. Saunders Co.

73. Guyton, A. C.: Composite pressure-volume relationships between interstitial fluid pressure, interstitial total fluid volume, interstitial gel fluid volume and interstitial free fluid volume. In Circulatory physiology II: dynamics and control of the body fluids, Philadelphia, 1975, W. B. Saunders Co.

74. Guyton, A. C.: Effect of low plasma colloid osmotic pressure in causing pulmonary edema. In Circulatory physiology II: dynamics and control of the body fluids, Philadelphia, 1975, W. B. Saunders Co.

75. Hachinski, V., Norris, J. W., Cooper, P. W., and Marshall, J.: Symptomatic intracranial steal, Arch. Neurol. **34**:149, 1977.

76. Hagen, A. A., Gerber, J. N., Swelley, C. C., White, R. P., and Robertson, J. T.: Levels and disappearance of prostaglandin F_{2a} in cerebral spinal fluid; a clinical and experimental study, Stroke **8**:672, 1977.

77. Hägnevik, K., Gordon, E., Lins, L-E., and others: Glycerol-induced hemolysis with haemoglobinuria and acute renal failure, Lancet, p. 75, January 19, 1974.

78. Haider, W., Lackner, F., Schlick, W., and others: Metabolic changes in the course of severe acute brain damage, Eur. J. Intensive Care Med. **1**:19, 1975.

79. Hall, S. V., Johnson, E. E., and Hidley-Whyte, J.: Renal hemodynamics and function with continuous positive-pressure ventilation in dogs, Anesthesiology **41**:452, 1974.

80. Hamer, J., Alberti, E., Hoyer, S., and Wiedemann, K.: Influence of systemic and cerebral vascular factors on the cerebrospinal fluid pulse waves, J. Neurosurg. **46**:36, 1977.

81. Harken, A. H., Gabel, R. A., Fencl, V., and others: Hydrochloric acid in the correction of metabolic alkalosis, Arch. Surg. **110**:819, 1975.

82. Hartmann, A., Alberti, E., and Lange, D.: Effects of CSF drainage on CBF and CBF in subarachnoid hemorrhage and communicating hydrocephalus. In Ingvar, D. H., and Lassen, N. A.: Cerebral function, metabolism and circulation, Copenhagen, 1977, Munksgaard, p. 336.

83. Hastings, P. R., Skillman, J. J., Bushnell, L. S., and Silen, W.: Antacid titration in the prevention of acute gastrointestinal bleeding, N. Engl. J. Med. **298**:1042, 1978.

84. Heikkinen, E. R., Myllylä, V. V., Hokkanen, E., and Vapaatalo, H.: Cerebrospinal fluid concentration of cyclic AMP in cerebrovascular disease, Eur. Neurol. **14**:129, 1976.

85. Heiss, W. D., Zeiler, K., Havelec, L., Reisner, T., and Bruck, J.: Long-term prognosis in stroke related to cerebral blood flow, Arch. Neurol. **34**:671, 1977.

86. Henning, R. J., Shubin, H., and Weil, M. H.: Afterload reduction with phentolamine in patients with acute pulmonary edema, Am. J. Med. **63**:568, 1977.

87. Heros, R. C., and Zervos, N. T.: Intracranial aneurysms; recent advances in current neurology, Boston, 1978, Houghton Mifflin Co.

88. Hobbs, J. B., Chusilp, S., Kincaid-Smith, P., and McIver, M. A.: The mechanism of glycerol-induced acute renal failure, Lab. Clin. Med. **88**:44, 1976.

89. Hoff, J. T., Pitts, L. H., Spetzler, R., and Wilson, C. B.: Barbiturates for protection from cerebral ischemia in aneurysm surgery. In Ingvar, D. H., and Lassen, N. A.: Cerebral function, metabolism and circulation, Copenhagen, 1977, Munksgaard, p. 158.

90. Hoffman, T. A., and Bullock, W. E.: Carbenicillin therapy of pseudomonas and other gram-negative bacillary infections, Ann. Intern. Med. **73**:165, 1970.

91. Hooshmand, H.: Advances in the medical and surgical management of intractable partial complex seizures, MCV/Q **10**:208, 1974.

92. Hoover, H. C., Grant, J. P., Gorschboth, C., and others: Nitrogen-sparing intravenous fluids in postoperative patients, N. Engl. J. Med. **293**:172, 1975.

93. Horita, A., and Quock, R. M.: Dopaminergic mechanisms in drug-induced temperature effects. In Lomas, P., Schönbaum, E., and Jacob, J.: Temperature regulation and drug action, Basel, 1974, Karger, p. 75.

94. Ingvar, D. H., and Cirra, M. G.: Assessment of severe damage to the brain by multiregional measurements of cerebral blood flow. In Outcome of severe damage to the central nervous systems, Ciba Foundation Symposium 34, New York, 1975, Excerpta Medica, p. 97.

95. Ingvar, D. H., and Risberg, J.: Increase of regional cerebral blood flow during mental effort in normals and in patients with focal brain disorders, Exper. Brain Res. **3**:195, 1967.

96. Iversen, L. L., Rogawski, M. A., and Miller, R. J.: Comparison of the effects of neuroleptic drugs on pre- and postsynaptic dopaminergic mechanisms in the rat striatum, Mol. Pharmacol. **12**:251, 1976.

97. James, H. E., Langfitt, T. W., and Kumar, V. S.: Analysis of the response to therapeutic measures to reduce intracranial pressure in head injured patients, J. Trauma **16**:437, 1976.

98. Jennett, B., and Teasdale, G.: Predicting outcome in individual patients after severe head injury, Lancet 1:1031, 1976.

99. Jennett, B., Teasdale, G., Galbraith, S., and others: Severe head injuries in three countries, J. Neurol. Neurosurg. Psychiatr. **40**:291, 1977.

100. Johnston, I. H., Johnston, J. A., and Jennett, B.: Intracranial pressure changes following head injury, Lancet 2:433, 1970.

101. Kalin, E. M., Tweed, W. A., Lee, J., and MacKeen, W. L.: Cerebrospinal-fluid acid-base and electrolyte changes resulting from cerebral anoxia in man, N. Engl. J. Med. **293**:1013, 1975.

102. Katzman, R., Clasen, R., Klatzo, I., Meyer, J. S., Pappius, H. M., and Waltz, A. G.: Brain edema in stroke, Stroke **8**:512, 1977.

103. Katzman, R., and Pappius, H. M.: Brain electrolytes and fluid metabolism, Baltimore, 1973, The Williams & Wilkins Co.

104. Kaufmann, G. E., and Clark, K.: Continuous simultaneous monitoring of intraventricular and cervical subarachnoid cerebrospinal fluid pressure to indicate development of cerebral or tonsillar herniation, J. Neurosurg. **33**:145, 1970.

105. Kennedy, A. C., Linton, A. L., Luke, R. G., and others: The pathogenesis and prevention of cerebral dysfunction during dialysis, Lancet 2:790, 1964.

106. Kirby, R. R., Downs, J. B., Civetta, J. M., and others: High level positive end expiratory pressure (PEEP) in acute respiratory insufficiency, Chest **67**:156, 1975.

107. Kjallqvist, A., Lundberg, N., Pontén, U.: Respiratory and cardiovascular changes during spontaneous variations of ventricular fluid pressure in patients with intracranial hypertension, Acta Neurol. Scand. **40**:291, 1964.

108. Klun, B.: Spinal fluid and blood serum enzymes activity in brain injuries, J. Neurosurg. **41**:224, 1974.

109. Kosnik, E. J., and Hunt, W. E.: Postoperative hypertension in the management of patients with intracranial arterial aneurysms, J. Neurosurg. **45**:148, 1976.

110. Kovach, A. G. B., and Sandor, P.: Cerebral blood flow and brain function during hypotension and shock, Ann. Rev. Physiol. **38**:571, 1976.

111. Kreisberg, R. A.: Diabetic ketoacidosis: new concepts and trends in pathogenesis and treatment, Ann. Intern. Med. **88**:681, 1978.

112. Kuhner, A., Roquefeuil, B., Viguie, E., and others: Influence of high and low dosages of mannitol 25% in the therapy of cerebral edema. In Schürmann, K., Brock, M., Reulen, H. J., and Voth, D.: Brain edema: pathophysiology and therapy, New York, 1973, Springer-Verlag.

113. Kumar, A., Pontoppidan, H., Baratz, R. A., and others: Inappropriate response to increased plasma ADH during mechanical ventilation in acute respiratory failure, Anesthesiology **40**:215, 1974.

114. Langfitt, T. W.: Increased intracranial pressure. Youmans, J. R.: Neurological surgery, vol. I, Philadelphia, 1973, W. B. Saunders Co.

115. Larsen, B., Skinh j, E., Soh, K., and others: The pattern of cortical activity provoked by listening and speech revealed by rCBF measurements. In Ingvar, D. H., and Lassen, N. A.: Cerebral function, metabolism and circulation, Copenhagen, 1977, Munksgaard, p. 268.

116. Larsen, S. J., Sances, A., Ackmann, J. J., and Reigel, D. H.: Noninvasive evaluation of head trauma patients, Surgery **74**:34, 1973.

117. Lidbrink, P., Corrodi, H., Fuxe, K., and Olson, L.: Barbiturates and meprobamate: decreases in catecholamine turnover of central dopamine and noradrenaline neuronal systems and the influence of immobilization stress, Brain Res. **45**:507, 1972.

118. Lieberman, A., Brun, V. L., Glass, P., and others: Use of high dose corticosteroids in patients with inoperable brain tumors, J. Neurol. Neurosurg. Psychiatr. **40**:678, 1977.

119. Long, D. M., Maxwell, R., and Choi, K. S.: A new therapy regimen for brain edema. In Pappius, H. M., and Feindel, W.: Dynamics of brain edema, New York, 1976, Springer-Verlag, p. 293.

120. Long, D. M., Maxwell, R. E., Choi, K. S., Cole, H. O., and French, L. A.: Multiple therapeutic approaches in the treatment of brain edema induced by a standard cold lesion. In Reulen, H. J., and Schurmann, K.: Steroids and brain edema, New York, 1972, Springer-Verlag, p. 87.

121. Lundberg, N.: Continuous recording and control of ventricular fluid pressure in neurosurgical practice, Acta Psychiatr. Neurol. Scand. 38 (suppl. 149):1, 1960.

122. Lundberg, N., Troupp, H., and Lorin, H.: Continuous recording of the ventricular-fluid pressure in patients with severe acute traumatic brain injury, J. Neurosurg. **22**:581, 1965.

123. MacLaren, N. K., Cowles, C., Ozand, P. T., Shuttee, R., and Cornblath, M.: Glycerol intolerance in a child with intermittent hypoglycemia, J. Pediatr. **86**:43, 1975.

124. Marmarou, A., Shulman, K., and La Morgese, J.: Compartmental analysis of compliance and outflow resistance of the cerebrospinal fluid system, J. Neurosurg. **43**:523, 1975.

125. Marmarou, A., Shulman, K., Shapiro, K., and Poll, W.: The time course of brain tissue pressure and local CBF in vasogenic edema. In Pappius, H. M., and Feindel, W.: Dynamics of brain edema, New York, 1976, Springer-Verlag.

126. Marsh, M. L., Marshall, L. F., and Shapiro, H. M.: Neurosurgical intensive care, Anesthesiology **17**:149, 1977.

127. Marshall, L. F., Bruce, D. A., Bruno, L., and Langfitt, T. W.: Vertebrobasilar spasm: a significant cause of neurological deficit in head injury, J. Neurosurg. **48**:560, 1978.

128. Marshall, L. F., Bruce, D. A., Graham, D. I.,

and Langfitt, T. W.: Triethyl tin-induced cerebral edema: implications for determination of cerebral blood flow in edematous tissue. In Pappius, H. M., and Feindel, W.: Dynamics of brain edema, New York, 1976, Springer-Verlag, p. 83.

129. Marshall, L. F., Shapiro, H. M.: Barbiturate control of intracranial hypertension in head injury and other conditions; iatrogenic coma. In Ingvar, D. H., and Lassen, N. A.: Cerebral function, metabolism and circulation, Copenhagen, 1977, Munksgaard, p. 156.

130. Marshall, L. F., Shapiro, H. M., Rauscher, A., and Kaufman, N. M.: Pentobarbital therapy for intracranial hypertension in metabolic coma, Crit. Care Med. **6:**1, 1978.

131. Marshall, L. F., Smith, R. W., Rauscher, L. A., and Shapiro, H. M.: Mannitol dose requirements in brain-injured patients, J. Neurosurg. **48:**169, 1978.

132. Marshall, W. J. S., Jackson, J. L. F., and Langfitt, T. W.: Brain swelling caused by trauma and arterial hypertension, Arch. Neurol. **21:**545, 1969.

133. Martin, S. U., and Bloedel, J. R.: Evaluation of experimental spinal cord injury using cortical evoked potentials, J. Neurosurg. **39:**75, 1973.

134. Matz, R.: Hyperosmolar coma (letter), N. Engl. J. Med. **298:**855, 1978.

135. McGraw, C. P.: Intracerebral hemorrhage and intracranial pressure monitoring (abstract), Stroke **8:**137, 1977.

136. McLelland, J., and Jack, W.: Phenytoin/dexamethasone interaction: a clinical problem, Lancet **1:**1096, 1978.

137. Meinig, G., Aulich, A., Wende, S., and Reulen, H. J.: The effect of dexamethasone and diuretics on peritumor brain edema: comparative study of tissue water content and CT. In Pappius, H. M., and Feindel, W.: Dynamics of brain edema, New York, 1976, Springer-Verlag, p. 300.

138. Meyer, J. S., Stoica, E., Pascu, I., and others: Catecholamine concentrations in CSF and plasma of patients with cerebral infarction and hemorrhage, Brain **96:**277, 1973.

139. Meyer, J. S., Ishihara, N., Deshmukh, V., and others: Improved method for noninvasive measurement of regional cerebral blood flow by [133]xenon inhalation, Stroke **9:**195, 1978.

140. Michenfelder, J. D.: Cyanide toxicity and thiosulfate protection during chronic administration of sodium nitroprusside in the dog: correlation with a human case, Anesthesiology **47:**441, 1977.

141. Michenfelder, J. D., Milde, H. J., and Sundt, T. M.: Cerebral protection by barbiturate anesthesia; use after middle cerebral artery occlusion in Java monkeys, Arch. Neurol. **33:**345, 1976.

142. Mickell, J. J., Cook, D. R., Reigel, D. H., Painter, M. J., and Safar, P.: Intracranial pressure monitoring in Reye-Johnson syndrome, Crit. Care Med. **4:**1, 1976.

143. Mickell, J. J.: Personal communication, 1978.

144. Mickell, J. J., Reigel, D. H., Cook, D. R., Binda, R. E., and Safar, P.: Intracranial pressure: monitoring and normalization therapy in children, Pediatrics **59:**606, 1977.

145. Miller, J. D., Becker, D. P., Ward, J. D., and others: Significance of intracranial hypertension in severe head injury, J. Neurosurg. **47:**503, 1977.

146. Mosman, P. C. M.: Regional cerebral blood flow in neurological patients, Assen, The Netherlands, 1974, Van Gorcum & Co.

147. Nemoto, E. M., Kofke, W. A., Kessler, P., and others: Studies on the pathogenesis of ischemic brain damage and the mechanism of its amelioration by thiopental. In Ingvar, D. H., and Lassen, N. A.: Cerebral function, metabolism and circulation, Copenhagen, 1977, Munksgaard, p. 156.

148. Nemoto, E. M.: Pathogenesis of cerebral ischemia-anoxia, Crit. Care Med., Aug. 1978.

149. Nemoto, E. M., Snyder, J. V., Carroll, R. G., and Morita, H.: Global ischemia in dogs; cerebral vascular CO_2 reactivity and autoregulation, Stroke **6:**425, 1974.

150. Nilsson, B., Astrup, J., Blennow, G., and Siesjö, B. K.: Cerebral function and energy metabolism at critical threhholds of oxygen availability: a study in rats during status epilepticus induced by bicuculline. In Ingvar, D. H., and Lassen, N. A.: Cerebral function, metabolism and circulation, Copenhagen, 1977, Munksgaard, p. 112.

151. Norberg, K., Lunggren, B., and Siesjö, B. K.: Cerebral metabolism in relation to function in insulin-induced hypoglycemia. In Ingvar, D. H., and Lassen, N. A.: Brain work, Alfred Benzon Symposium VIII, Copenhagen, 1975, Munksgaard, p. 314.

152. Nordstrom, C-H., and Rehncrona, S.: Reduction of cerebral blood flow and oxygen consumption with a combination of barbiturate anesthesia and induced hypothermia in the rat, Acta Anesth. Scand. **22:**7, 1978.

153. Nornes, H.: The role of intracranial pressure in the arrest of hemorrhage in patients with intracranial hemorrhage, J. Neurosurg. **39:**226, 1973.

154. Nornes, H., and Magnaes, B.: Intracranial pressure in patients with ruptured saccular aneurysms, J. Neurosurg. **36:**537, 1972.

155. Obrist, W. D., Thompson, K. H., King, C. H., and Wang, H. S.: Determination of regional cerebral blood flow by inhalation of [133]Xenon, Circ. Res. **20:**124, 1967.

156. Olesen, J.: Cerebral blood flow, methods for measurement, regulation, effects of drugs, and changes in disease, Acta Neurol. Scand. **50** (suppl.):57, 1974.

157. Ortega, B. D., Demopoulos, H. B., and Ransohoff, J.: Effect of antioxidants on experimental cold-induced cerebral edema. In Reulen, H. J., and Schurmann, K.: Steroids and brain edema, New York, 1972, Springer-Verlag, p. 167.

158. Ott, E. O., Lechner, H., and Aranibar, A.: High blood viscosity syndrome in cerebral infarction, Stroke **5**:330, 1974.

159. Ott, E. O., Mathew, N. T., and Meyer, J. S.: Redistribution of regional cerebral blood flow after glycerol infusion in acute cerebral infarction, Neurology **24**:1117, 1974.

160. Owen, J. A.: Role of endocrine changes in the plasma protein response to injury. In Sobatka, H., and Stewart, C. P.: Advances in clinical chemistry, New York, 1969, Academic Press, vol. 12.

161. Painter, M. J., Pippenger, C., Mac Donald, H., and Pitlick, W.: Phenobarbital and diphenylhydantoin levels in neonates with seizures, J. Pediatr. **92**:315, 1978.

162. Papeschi, R., Thesis, P., and Herz, A.: Effects of morphine on the turnover of brain catecholamines and serotonin in rats—acute morphine administration, Eur. J. Pharmacol. **34**:253, 1975.

163. Park, B. E., Meacham, W. F., and Netsky, M. G.: Nonketotic hyperglycemic hyperosmolar coma, J. Neurosurg. **44**:409, 1976.

164. Penn, R. D., Walser, R., Kurtz, D., and Ackerman, L.: Tumor volume, luxury perfusion and regional blood volume changes in man visualized by subtraction computerized tomography, J. Neurosurg. **44**:449, 1976.

165. Petito, C. K., Schaefer, J. A., and Plum, F.: The blood-brain barrier in experimental seizures. In Pappius, H. M., and Feindel, W.: Dynamics of brain edema, New York, 1976, Springer-Verlag, p. 38.

166. Petito, F., and Plum, F.: The lumbar puncture, N. Engl. J. Med. **290**:225, 1974.

167. Pirakitikulr, P., and Pitlick, W.: Personal communication, 1978.

168. Pitlick, W. B.: Personal communication, 1978.

169. Plum, F., and Siesjö, B. K.: Recent advances in CSF physiology, Anesthesiology **42**:708, 1975.

170. Plum, F., and Posner, J. B.: The diagnosis of stupor and coma, ed. 3, Philadelphia, 1979, F. A. Davis Co. (in preparation).

171. Plum, F., and Price, R. W.: Acid-base of cisternal and lumbar CSF in hospital patients, N. Engl. J. Med. **289**:1346, 1973.

172. Posner, J. B., and Plum, F.: The toxic effects of carbon dioxide and acetazolamide in hepatic encephalopathy, J. Clin. Invest. **39**:1246, 1960.

173. Prior, P. F.: The EEG in acute cerebral anoxia, Amsterdam, 1973, Excerpta Medica.

174. Quist, J., Pontoppidan, H., Rilson, R. S., and others: Hemodynamic responses to mechanical ventilation with PEEP; the effect of hypervolemia, Anesthesiology **42**:45, 1975.

175. Rackow, E. C., Fein, I. A., and Leppo, J.: Colloid osmotic pressure as a prognostic indicator of pulmonary edema and mortality in the critically ill, Chest **72**:709, 1977.

176. Raichle, M. E.: Sensori-motor area increase of oxygen uptake and blood flow in the human brain during contralateral hand exercise; preliminary observations by the 0-15 methods. In Ingvar, D. H., and Lassen, N. A.: Brain work, Alfred Benzon Symposium VIII, Copenhagen, 1975, Munksgaard, p. 372.

177. Raichle, M. E.: Cerebral flow and metabolism. In Outcome of severe damage to the central nervous system, Ciba Foundation Symposium 34, New York, 1975, Excerpta Medica.

178. Raison, J. C. A., Chir, B., Osborn, J. J., and others: Oxygen consumption after open heart surgery measured by a digital computer system, Ann. Surg. **171**:471, 1970.

179. Renaudin, J., Fewer, D., Wilson, C. B., and others: Dose dependency of decadron in patients with partially excised brain tumors, J. Neurosurg. **39**:302, 1973.

180. Reulen, H. J., Graham, R., Fenske, A., and others: The role of tissue pressure and bulk flow in the formation and resolution of cold-induced edema. In Pappius, H. M., and Feindel, W.: Dynamics of brain edema, New York, 1976, Springer-Verlag, p. 103.

181. Reulen, H. J., Graham, R., Spatz, M., and Klatzo, I.: Role of pressure gradients and bulk flow in dynamics of vasogenic brain edema, J. Neurosurg. **46**:24, 1977.

182. Robin, E., Carey, L. C., Grenvik, A., and others: Capillary leak syndrome with pulmonary edema, Arch. Intern. Med. **130**:66, 1972.

183. Robin, E., Cross, C. E., and Zelis, R.: Pulmonary edema (Parts I and II), N. Engl. J. Med. **288**:239; 292, 1973.

184. Rottenberg, D. A., Hurwitz, B. J., and Posner, J. B.: The effect of oral glycerol on intraventricular pressure in man, Neurology **27**:600, 1977.

185. Rowan, A. J., and Scott, D. F.: Major status epilepticus, Acta Neurolog. Scand. **46**:573, 1970.

186. Sackner, M. A., Landa, J. F., Greeneltch, N., and Robinson, M. J.: Pathogenesis and prevention of tracheobronchial damage with suction procedures, Chest **64**:284, 1973.

187. Sambrook, M. A., Hutchinson, E. C., and Aber, G. M.: Metabolic studies in subarachnoid hemorrhage and strokes, Brain **96**:191, 1973.

188. Schmidt, R. P., and Wilder, B. T.: Epilepsy, Philadelphia, 1968, F. A. Davis Co.

189. Schwartz, M. S., Colvin, M. P., Prior, P. F., Strunin, L., Simpson, B. R., Weaver, J. M., and Scott, D. F.: The cerebral function monitor, Anesthesia **28**:611, 1973.

190. Sears, E. S.: Non-ketotic hyperosmolar hyperglycemia during glycerol therapy for cerebral edema, Neurology **26**:89, 1976.

191. Severinghaus, J. W.: Blood gas calculator, J. Appl. Physiol. **21**:1108, 1966.

192. Severinghaus, J. W.: Role of cerebrospinal fluid pH in normalization of cerebral blood flow in chronic hypocapnia, Acta Neurol. Scand. **14**:(suppl.):116, 1965.

193. Severinghaus, J. W., Nemoto, E., and Hoff, J.: The CO_2 shuttle in cerebral arteriolar ECF H^+ control. In Fieschi, C.: Cerebral blood flow and intracranial pressure, Basel, 1972, S. Karger AG, p. 56.

194. Shapiro, H. M., Wyte, S. R., Harris, A. B., and Galindo, A.: Disposable system for intraventricular pressure measurement and CSF drainage, J. Neurosurg. **36:**798, 1972.

195. Shapiro, H. M., Wyte, S. R., and Loeser, J.: Barbiturate-augmented hypothermia for reduction of persistent intracranial hypertension, J. Neurosurg. **40:**90, 1974.

196. Shapiro, H. M.: Intracranial hypertension: therapeutic and anesthetic considerations, Anesthesiology **43:**445, 1975.

197. Shenkin, H. A., Bezier, H. S., and Bouzarth, W. F.: Restricted fluid intake, J. Neurosurg. **45:**432, 1976.

198. Siesjö, B. K., Carlsson, C., Hagerdal, M., and Nordstrom, C-H.: Brain metabolism in the critically ill, Crit. Care Med. **4:**283, 1976.

199. Skillman, J. J., Collins, R. E. C., and Coe, N. P.: Prevention of deep vein thrombosis in neurosurgical patients: a controlled, randomized trial of external pneumatic compression boots, Surgery **83:**354, 1978.

200. Sladen, A., Laver, M. B., Pontoppidan, H.: Pulmonary complications in water retention in prolonged mechanical ventilation, N. Engl. J. Med. **279:**448, 1968.

201. Smith, A. L.: Barbiturate protection in cerebral hypoxia, Anesthesiology **47:**285, 1977.

202. Smith, F. R., and Kundahl, P. C.: Intravenously administered Lidocaine as cough depressant during general anesthesia for bronchography, Chest **63:**427, 1973.

203. Snyder, S. H.: Opiate receptors in the brain, N. Engl. J. Med. **296:**266, 1977.

204. Stein, L., Beraud, J-J., Morissette, M., and others: Pulmonary edema during volume infusion, Circulation **52:**483, 1975.

205. Sugi, T., Fujishima, M., and Omae, T.: Lactate and pyruvate concentrations, and acid-base balance of cerebrospinal fluid in experimentally induced intracerebral and subarachnoid hemorrhage in dogs, Stroke **6:**715, 1975.

206. Sullivan, H. G., and Becker, D. P.: ICP: monitoring and interpretation. In Cottrell, J., and Turndorf, H., editors: Anesthesia and neurosurgery, St. Louis, 1979, The C. V. Mosby Co.

207. Sullivan, H. G., Miller, J. D., Becker, D. P., and others: The physiological basis of intracranial pressure change with progressive epidural brain compression, J. Neurosurg. **47:**532, 1977.

208. Sullivan, S. F., and Patterson, R. W.: Posthyperventilation hypoxia: theoretical considerations in man, Anesthesiology **29:**981, 1968.

209. Sundt, T. M., Jr.: Management of ischemic complications after subarachnoid hemorrhage, J. Neurosurg. **43:**418, 1975.

210. Suter, P. M., Fairley, N. B., and Isenberg, M. D.: Optimum end-expiratory pressure in patients with acute pulmonary failure, N. Engl. J. Med. **292:**284, 1975.

211. Tabbador, K., Tavare, A., Marmarou, A., and others: Intracranial pressure and cerebral compliance during hypotension induced by sodium nitroprusside. In Ingvar, D. H., and Lassen, N. A.: Cerebral function, metabolism and circulation, Copenhagen, 1977, Munksgaard, p. 310.

212. Thomas, D. J., du Boulay, G. H., and Marshall, J.: Effect of haematocrit on cerebral blood flow in man, Lancet **2:**941, 1977.

213. Toole, J. F., and McGraw, C. P.: The steal syndromes, Ann. Rev. Med. **26:**321, 1975.

214. Tourtellotte, W. W., Reinglass, J. L., and Newkirk, T. A.: Cerebral dehydration action of glycerol, Clin. Pharmacol. Therapeut. **13:**159, 1972.

215. Trojaborg, W., and Boysen, G.: Relation between EEG, regional cerebral blood flow and internal carotid artery pressure during carotid endarterectomy, Electroencephal. Clin. Neurophysiol. **34:**61, 1973.

216. Tweed, W. A., and Overgard, J.: Brain edema after head injury. In Pappius, H. M., and Feindel, W.: Dynamics of brain edema, New York, 1976, Springer-Verlag, p. 323.

217. Uhl, R. R.: Monitoring: present concepts and future directions. In Current problems in anesthesia and crtical care medicine, vol. 1, Chicago, 1977, Year Book Medical Publishers, Inc.

218. Vapalahti, M., Hyyppä, M. T., Nieminen, V., and Rinne, U. K.: Brain monoamine metabolites and tryptophan in ventricular CSF of patients with spasm after aneurysm surgery, J. Neurosurg. **48:**58, 1978.

219. Weir, B., Grace, M., Hansen, J., and others: Time course of vasospasm in man, J. Neurosurg. **48:**173, 1978.

220. Whitty, C. W. M., and Taylor, M.: Treatment of status epilepticus, Lancet **2:**591, 1949.

221. Wilder, B. J., Ramsay, R. E., Willmore, L. J., Feussner, G. F., Perchalski, R. J., and Shumate, J. B.: Efficacy of intravenous phenytoin in the treatment of status epilepticus: kinetics of central nervous system penetration, Ann. Neurol. **1:**511, 1977.

222. Winkle, R. A., Glantz, S. A., and Harrison, D. C.: Pharmacologic therapy of ventricular arrythmias, Am. J. Cardiol. **36:**629, 1975.

223. Wise, B. L.: Effects of infusions of hypertonic mannitol on electrolyte balance and on osmolality of serum and cerebrospinal fluid, J. Neurosurg. **20:**961, 1963.

224. York, D. H.: Dopamine receptor blockade—a central action of chlorpromazine on striatal neurones, Brain Res. **37:**91, 1972.

16

Mechanisms of injury and treatment of acute spinal cord trauma

JOSEPH RANSOHOFF
EUGENE S. FLAMM
HARRY B. DEMOPOULOS

Surgical decompression of the spinal cord at the site of the compressive lesion, accompanied by appropriate measures for stabilization, provides the best chance of recovery from spinal cord trauma. Future care after trauma may include adjunctive pharmacologic therapy, because irreversible changes within long tracts that take several hours to occur[17,74] can be blocked by certain drugs.[16,28] Present and experimental approaches in the acute care following cord injury will be described.

There have been few well-organized efforts directed toward defining indications for early surgical treatment of the spinal cord in an attempt to preserve, improve, or restore cord function. Acutely done laminectomy without specific attention to stabilization has been condemned by some.[58,96,109] A number of patients with partial residual cord function developed permanent paralysis after early laminectomy.[58,96,109] Why laminectomy may aggravate injury, apart from operative bone or instrument damage, is not well understood. A recent study in cats after "clean" laminectomy showed a significant decrease in spinal cord blood flow[5] along the entire length of cord, suggesting that decreased spinal cord blood flow (SCBF) may be a ma-

jor cause of irreversible change after trauma.[8,108]

Operative or spontaneous surgical fusion months to years after injury may offer partial preservation of function in some patients.[77] Late surgical intervention may also prevent or correct spinal deformities that might diminish rehabilitation potential. This experience strongly suggests the need to attend to bony stabilization to prevent a resulting degree of increased instability of the spinal column and increase the likelihood of secondary injury.[50]

Immediate stabilization can be readily achieved with anterior cervical and thoracic surgical approaches with interbody fusion, external halo fixation for cervical injuries, Harrington rods with correction and stabilization of thoracic deformities, and acrylic wire mesh fusion in conjunction with endogenous bone graft for posterior stabilization.

The role and value of surgical decompression of the cord is still more controversial than the indications for stabilization. Early exploratory laminectomy[7] or no surgical treatment[52,58] has been recommended. Progressive loss of function, rare in our experience, is clearly an indication for immediate surgery,[11,102] and acute decompression combined with stabilization is recommended.[39,129]

The use of pharmacologic adjuvants stems from increased understanding of reactions occurring around injury induced in laboratory models using controlled impact injuries delivered by dropping a known weight a specified distance.[8,17,28,74,108] Decreased tissue perfusion,[8,31,108] physical/mechanical factors,[73] generation of biogenic amines,[87,92] and free radical-mediated membrane pathology acting alone or in concert may require polypharmaceutical approaches including perhaps some anesthetics or sedatives for control.

Important recent advances in the treatment of spinal cord injury have been related to early accident site recognition of injury, immediate and appropriate triage, and transfer to a spinal cord treatment center or major facility where neurosurgeons, anesthesiologists, neurologists, and orthopedists can collaborate in care. An ever increasing percentage of patients received with partial preservation of function attests to the importance of educational programs for all personnel involved in emergency medical services. During the first year of operation, the Spinal Cord Center at the New York University–Bellevue Medical Center received 12% of patients with partial injury, in contrast to 25% in the second and third years. This confirms the suspicion that without proper early care a large number of patients not totally paralyzed will become paralyzed from the additional trauma of poor handling or transportation with inadequate immobilization by ambulance at high speed on poor roads.

PRINCIPLES OF EARLY SURGICAL INTERVENTION

It is important to emphasize differences between cervical, thoracic, and lumbosacral regions of the spinal cord and column, which underlie the principles of management of spinal cord injury.

The critical cervical region, above the fourth cervical segment, includes control of respiration. Physiologic transection above C-3 is rarely associated with long-term survival. C-4 through C-7 encompasses anterior horn function of the upper extremities and long pathways serving the trunk, lower extremities, and sphincters. The cervical spinal column, characterized by maximal flexibility, is relatively fixed at the thoracic level and supports the entire weight of the skull and brain at the upper end. This arrangement makes the cervical spinal column vulnerable to fractures and fracture dislocations. Anterior osteoarthritic ridging in older individuals may compromise cord function after contusion by creating pressure against these ridges, even in the absence of a fracture or fracture dislocation.

The thoracic spinal column is relatively stabilized by bony structures of the thorax so that greater energy is required to produce fractures and fracture dislocations. The spinal cord to T-12–L-1 has the same important characteristics as the cervical spinal cord and, in addition, subserves the function of the thorax, lower extremities, and sphincters. The thoracic spinal cord rarely escapes injury with fractures or fracture dislocations because, unlike the cervical cord, the thoracic cord fits snugly into the thoracic canal.

The lumbar and lumbosacral spinal column is supported by heavy paraspinal musculature and heavily constructed, so a good deal of energy is required to produce fractures and fracture dislocations. Below L-1, the dural tube contains the cauda equina rather than spinal cord tissue. These nerve roots tolerate compression better than the spinal cord.

The four vectors of injury producing force applied to the spinal column are compression, extension, flexion, and rotation. Compression injuries produce explosion fractures of vertebral bodies and rupture sustaining ligaments. Extension injuries produce fractures of the posterior elements of the spinal column and disruption of anterior longitudinal ligaments. Flexion injuries are likely to compress vertebral bodies and disrupt posterior longitudinal ligaments and the intervertebral disc substance. Rotational injuries disrupt ligamentous structures, fracture or fracture dislocate facets, and damage vertebral bodies. Rotational and flexion or extension injuries are frequently combined, particularly in the cervical area, and produce extensive damage to the bony and ligamentous structures.

Immediate stabilization of the fracture site with rapid reduction of bony malalignment must be achieved. Initial x-ray examination should include tomography if no fracture is seen on routine anterioposterior and lateral films. The unwary clinician can be lulled into a false sense of security when a report of "no fracture" is received unless tomography is done and may be misled by a fracture classified as stable. There are probably very few fractures stable enough to allow the patient to ambulate or support the weight of the head in the immediate posttrauma period. Stability must be defined in terms of functional capacity. The fracture may be stable if the patient is kept at absolute bed rest, whereas weight bearing can produce progressive angulation and deformity. An unstable fracture requires immediate immobilization to protect the underlying spinal cord and to prevent eventual bony deformity.

In cervical and upper thoracic injury, early evaluation of pulmonary function is essential. A careful neurologic examination complemented with such electrophysiologic studies as somatosensory evoked cortical potentials (SEP) and the H-reflex may help assess the functional status of the cord. There appears to be considerable potential value in SEP as an acute monitoring system during laminectomy.[40,114] "Total" paraplegia or quadriplegia should be diagnosed only if (1) a 48-hour period has elapsed in which motor or sensory function can not be elicited, (2) total areflexia is present below the level of the lesion, and (3) SEP and H-reflex are absent.

Definitive neuroradiologic procedures should be done after large doses of steroids. Pantopaque myelography using a lumbar puncture is still probably the procedure of choice for definition of the status of the thoracic or lumbar cord, but if a cervical fracture is unstable, a C-1 study may be safer. Recently Metrizamide, a water-soluble contrast material (2-[3-acetamide-5-N-methyl acetamide-2, 4, 6-triiodobenzamide]-2-deoxy-d-glucose), has been released for clinical myelography by the Federal Drug Administration (FDA). Many studies of histologic, chemical, and physiologic responses to this material have been published.[9,117,121] While no studies to evaluate its effects on the previously traumatized spinal cord have been done, a complete cervical myelogram can be achieved via lateral C-1 puncture with the patient in the recumbent position while in skeletal traction, without manipulation and inherent risk to the cord. Evidence of external compression of the dural sac by bony fragments, extradural hematomas, or extruded disc material and ruptured ligaments distate an anterior, anterolateral, or posterior operative approach. Successful surgical intervention must provide immediate and absolute stabilization of bony elements involved at the site of injury. In the presence of a localized area of major spinal cord swelling the operative approach must be via laminectomy. Dural decompression, myelotomy for drainage of intramedullary hematoma and necrotic, hemorrhagic gray matter and insertion of a dural substitute may be necessary to provide adequate decompression. These procedures are probably applicable only in patients with total loss of function below C-6 within the first six hours after injury.

Injuries above C-3 are rarely associated with survival. These patients are respiratory dependent, and surgery on the spinal cord at that level in the acute state is not indicated. From C-4 through the remainder of the cervical spinal cord, the exact surgical procedure needs to be tailored specifically to the injury involved as defined by careful radiologic studies.

Intraoperative electrophysiologic monitoring of the spinal cord, particularly in patients with partial injuries, is of considerable assistance in evaluating immediate results. The technique of intraoperative somatosensory evoked potentials (SEP) is relatively similar to that used in the preoperative and postoperative evaluation of patients with spinal cord injuries.[40] We have seen immediate improvement in the SEPs from both anterior and posterior procedures in both cervical and thoracic spinal cord injuries. The technique for somatosensory evoked cortical potentials is described in several publications.[23,40,111,114]

PATIENT EXPERIENCE
Data base

During a 36-month period (1974 to 1977), 200 patients with acute spinal cord injuries were admitted to the New York University Spinal Cord Research Center for definitive treatment. One hundred fifty-four were referred from other institutions, and 46 were direct admissions via the Bellevue Hospital Center Ambulance Service. Twelve patients were not included in the research program for a variety of medical and sociologic reasons, leaving a data pool of 188 patients. An additional 45 patients admitted beyond a 10-day cut-off period served as a source of additional study material but are not included in the summary tables. The work-up and management regimens were basically according to the principles outlined below.

One hundred forty-four patients were totally paralyzed at the time of admission. Forty-four had partial function. There were three children between the ages of 9 and 10 and 49 adolescents from 11 to 20. One hundred and two patients were between 20 and 50 and the remainder, between 50 and 70. Three patients were between 70 and 80. Forty-nine patients sustained injury in falls and 46 in vehicular accidents. Thirty-four patients were injured during athletic activities, including 22 in water sports, the majority in diving accidents. Thirty-eight patients suffered gunshot wounds, nine were injured in miscellaneous accidents, including stabbings, bomb blasts, muggings, and so on. The time between injury and admission to the center was less than eight hours for 46 patients; an additional 57 patients were admitted within the first 24 hours, 39 within five days, and the remaining 23 within 6 to 10 days. Patients could be divided into three groups according to the level of the injury: 66 in the cervical area between C-4 and C-6; 23 between T-3 and T-6; and 34 between T-

Table 16-1. Age distribution of patients

Age	No. patients
1-10	3
11-20	49
21-30	50
31-40	33
41-50	19
51-60	19
61-70	12
71-80	3
TOTAL	188

Table 16-2. Mode of injury

Type	No. injured
Falls	49
Automobile accidents	46
Diving	22
Gunshot wounds	38
Motorcycle accidents	11
Sports injuries	13
Occupationally related	3
Other	6
TOTAL	188

Table 16-3. Time interval from injury to admission

Interval	No. patients
1-8 hours	55
9-24 hours	61
1-5 days	44
6-10 days	26
More than 11 days	2
TOTAL	188

Table 16-4. Level of spinal cord injury

Level	No. patients	Level	No. patients
C1-2	2	T1-2	5
2-3	3	3-4	15
3-4	5	5-6	10
4-5	24	6-7	3
5-6	52	7-8	9
6-7	16	8-9	4
7-8	1	9-10	6
		10-11	12
		11-12	22

10 and T-11. The remaining patients were evenly distributed at all other levels. Interestingly, nine patients sustained injuries from C-1 to C-3 and survived transfer to the center. These data are presented in tabular form (Tables 16-1 to 16-4).

Neurologic examination

Independent neurologic evaluations were performed within 12 hours after admission to the hospital and periodically thereafter. A late stage evaluation was performed on day 42 after initial spinal cord injury to ensure uniformity of neurologic reports during the entire period of six weeks. A total of 556 examinations was performed. The format for recording neurologic examination was developed by the National Collaborative Spinal Cord Study.

The superficial anal sphincter reflex was present in almost all spinal cord injury patients, an observation contradicting information usually presented. The anal sphincter reacted briskly on application of pin prick stimulation during the entire follow-up period in two patients with surgically verified total transection of the spinal cord at thoracolumbar level. An electromyogram (EMG) study is planned to further verify this phenomenon.

Electrophysiologic studies

We thought the SEP might detect residual sensory function not apparent on clinical examination and that this residual function might be the harbinger of potential improvement, but our experience has not borne out this expectation. We found no patient with an SEP who did not also have some clinical preservation. Conversely, some patients with clinical preservation did not have an SEP. Instead of being a sensitive indicator of residual function, the SEP appears rather to be a sensitive indicator of spinal cord damage. We did find that an SEP obtained from one or both lower extremities within 48 hours of injury correlated with return of clinical function. SEPs cannot be obtained from the lower extremities by stimulating only one peripheral nerve in 20% of normal patients.

Simultaneous stimulation of two nerves in one lower extremity did evoke SEPs and permits the lower extremities to be studied independently.

Three patients with clinically incomplete lesions were monitored during surgery; two patients had fractures of C-5 with fragments compressing the cord anteriorly, one had a T-12 fracture with ventral cord compression. The intraoperative SEPs improved immediately and dramatically during surgery in all three. Two of these three improved functionally over the next few weeks and are now ambulating. The third, however, with a C-5 fracture, is still severely quadriparetic, although her SEP amplitude almost doubled after decompression and fusion.

Pharmacologic therapy

Experimental evidence in our laboratory suggested in experimental models that epsilon-aminocaproic acid (EACA) added to steroid therapy significantly reduced the appearance and magnitude of central hemorrhagic necrosis[16] but no differences were seen in a randomized group of 100 patients given EACA 24 mg/day with 1 mg/kg methylprednisolone for 10 days or methylprednisolone alone.

After demonstrating that megadose corticosteroids (2 g/day for 15 to 151 days) are more effective than standard dose levels in treating brain edema, 1 g methylprednisolone per day is being evaluated as part of a study being conducted by the National Collaborative Spinal Cord Study. No complications attributed to the dosage levels have been identified in one acute spinal cord group, although sepsis occurred in three and steroid myopathy in two patients treated for brain edema.

Surgical therapy

We had programmed ourselves to early intervention in all patients in whom significant external cervical compression could be documented on myelography after maximum reduction with skeletal traction. Surgery was performed by the anterior or posterior approach, depending upon the site of external compression. In patients with no external compression and with evidence of spinal cord swelling to a near or total myelographic block, laminectomy, and dural decompression with the addition of midline dorsal myelotomy on a random basis was done. Operating jointly with orthopedists, immediate stabilization of the fractured site and long-term bony fusion for permanent stability was done. These guidelines were followed except where vasomotor or pulmonary instability, associated injuries, or medical problems contraindicated early surgical intervention.

One hundred and nine of 188 patients had cord decompression. Surgery was performed within the first 24 hours in 25% of cases, an additional 50% within the first five days, and the remaining 25% within 10 days of injury. The overall mortality rate within 30 days of injury was 9.5% (19/200). All deaths occurred in patients with high cervical injury from consequent pulmonary complications. No deaths occurred in patients with thoracic or lumbar injuries.

To evaluate the results of surgical intervention in acute spinal cord injury, one must pick a group in whom the risks of surgical intervention and increasing neurologic deficit can be weighed against the benefits accrued from early intervention. As many as 20% of patients with "total" paraplegia show some spontaneous recovery following conservative therapy. This statistical information is used by Guttman to justify his condemnation of any surgical procedure,[58] since improvement from surgery is difficult to separate in the first few hours after trauma from the natural course of the pathologic process.

We believe we have documented the safety of early surgical intervention by comparing outcome in 14 cervical, 5 thoracic, and 6 thoracolumbar fractures with incomplete paralysis and myelographic defect who were operated on between 12 hours and two weeks of injury, to 19 incompletes without myelographic compression who were not operated on, 13 anterior interbody fusions or vertebrectomy with fusion, 12 laminectomies with fusion and halo or Harrington rod stabilization were done.

No patient admitted for early surgery with spinal cord decompression was made worse by operation. Improvement in motor and sensory function at the level of the bony injury, although important to the patient, was not considered to be an indication of improvement in function of the spinal cord itself. One patient committed suicide. Of the remaining 24 patients, 16 are currently ambulating without the use of braces or any type of crutches (67%). Six utilize external aides to assist ambulation (25%), and two are nonambulatory (8%). Sensory function in five patients is entirely normal below the level of the lesion (21%), 16 showed significant improvement (67%), and 3 were unchanged following surgical intervention (13%). Four patients recovered full sphincteric and sexual functioning, and two have normal erections but without ejaculation.

Of the 19 nonoperated patients, nine can ambulate without braces (47%), six with braces (32%), and four cannot ambulate (21%). Two patients had no sensory loss on admission, five patients regained normal sensation, four showed improved sensation, and the remainder showed no change in the sensory status. Three patients recovered normal sphincteric and sexual function. While no definitively significant conclusions can be drawn from a comparison of these two small, nonrandomized groups, one might expect the prognosis following injury to be better in patients with near normal myelography than in patients with evidence of spinal cord compression or swelling. The two groups were almost identical in degree of recovery at six months, suggesting that surgical intervention may have been of benefit. We are continuing to investigate the role of acute surgical therapy in the treatment of spinal cord injuries to define more clearly where surgery may be of distinct benefit.

At present, the following clinical approaches are recommended:

1. Methylprednisolone administered for 10 days without a tapering schedule, starting at the time of initial phone contact with referring parties or possibly by paramedics in conjunction with tele-

communications with a neurosurgeon.

2. Neurologic evaluation by neurosurgeons and neurologists immediately on admission.

3. Radiologic studies immediately on admission; skeletal traction used and rapid reduction and alignment is attempted in cervical injuries without using manipulative techniques; myelography is done in all patients. In cervical and upper thoracic injuries, myelography is done immediately after early respiratory evaluation by an anesthesiologist. Emulsified Pantopaque or Metrizamide is done through a lateral C1-2 puncture except with C1-2 fractures. Thoracic and thoracolumbar injuries are studied via a lumbar instillation of Pantopaque, supplemented by a C1-2 puncture if necessary.

4. Electrophysiologic evaluation. The presence or absence of evoked somatosensory potentials should be determined as soon as possible after admission and periodically thereafter. Intraoperative SEPs may be a most valuable monitor of function during surgery.

5. Surgical therapy. In complete areflexic loss of neurologic function with compression, surgery can be undertaken up to 48 hours after injury for appropriate surgical decompression and stabilization or fusion. For complete lesions below C-5, surgery should be done only within 48 hours of injury. Patients operated on beyond 48 hours of a total lesion have no chance of neurologic recovery. Surgery for partial lesions can be performed up to 14 days after injury.

6. Monitor and follow respiratory function, use positive-pressure ventilation, humidity, airway and respiratory care, and chest physiotherapy as indicated.

PATHOGENETIC MECHANISMS OF SPINAL CORD DEGENERATION AFTER TRAUMA

The sequence of morphologic[17,31,73,74] and biochemical changes[27,28,83,87,92] resulting from impact injuries to the spinal cord in experimental models is similar to that seen after human cord injuries[123] and strongly suggests the use of animal models for study. The initial impacting force can be a minimal one and may directly cause few detectable structural changes; other organs and tissues injured in an identical manner usually show very few alterations and no permanent damage because postimpact alterations are responsible for permanent paraplegia. Reasons for the unusual sensitivity of the CNS and the irreparable tissue and cellular changes after impact injury are not known. A variety of possible causes relating to mechanical,[73] vascular,[8,108] biogenic amine,[87,92] and free radical chemical changes[27,28,31,83] have been described to occur over a period of hours after impact. It may be possible to intercede before irreversible injury if the exact mechanisms and chain of events are known. Presently, prevention of decreased perfusion and maintenance of membrane integrity are believed to be key goals of early chemical intervention.

The spinal cord and other nervous system components have strict requirements to maintain membrane integrity. The blood-CNS barrier maintains a unique environment for the CNS by excluding substances and enhancing the transport of such compounds as ascorbic acid,[113] but this requires that membrane lipids and proteins be structurally intact. The same is true for excitable membranes involved in conduction and transmission. Even minor perturbations in the configuration of strategic membrane molecules can have far-reaching consequences.[13,51,65,101] Altered fluidity of lipids that help to maintain the active shape of key enzymes like NaK-ATPase, adenylate cyclase, cytochrome oxidase, and prostaglandin synthetase will affect synaptosome formation. Disturbing the plasma endothelial membrane can lead to failure on part of endothelial cells to maintain a clear lumen.[31]

In experimental spinal cord trauma, ischemia and focal hemorrhage are the two major early pathologic components. Some scattered petechial hemorrhages seen in the central gray matter within the first 15 minutes after

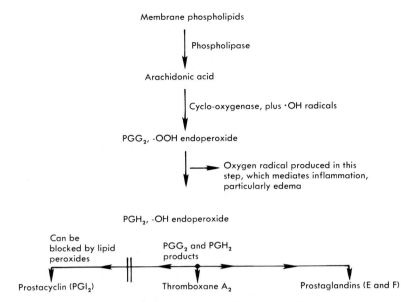

Membrane phospholipids

↓ Phospholipase

Arachidonic acid

↓ Cyclo-oxygenase, plus ·OH radicals

PGG_2, -OOH endoperoxide

↓ → Oxygen radical produced in this step, which mediates inflammation, particularly edema

PGH_2, -OH endoperoxide

Can be blocked by lipid peroxides ╫　PGG₂ and PGH₂ products

Prostacyclin (PGI_2)　　Thromboxane A_2　　Prostaglandins (E and F)

Fig. 16-1. A summary of the "arachidonic cascade" is depicted with the production of key substances.

injury enlarge and coalesce by 60 minutes.[17,74] Long tracts show no evidence of morphologic change ultrastructurally, except for enlargement of the periaxonal space in a small percentage of myelinated fibers.[34] The amount of blood extravasated into the gray reaches a maximum at three to four hours when petechial hemorrhages are seen in the long tract white matter.[17,74] Approximately 25% of myelinated fibers show enlargement of the periaxonal space and fraying of the myelin by four hours.[34] At 24 to 36 hours, the gray has undergone hemorrhagic necrosis, and the long tracts show extensive structural degeneration.[17,34,74]

Blood flow to the impacted segment of injured cord decreases markedly, suggesting that ischemia is also an important pathogenetic mechanism.[8,31,108] Except for petechial hemorrhages, studies of white matter by light and transmission electron microscopy have not revealed evidence of occlusion or vessel wall damage, particularly in the first one to two hours after injury. Diminished blood flow may be due to vasospasm, microvascular occlusions, or both.[31] There is no adequate explanation for the marked decrease in gray matter blood flow soon after

impact. There is a possibility that appropriately used vasoactive agents may interrupt these vascular perturbations and interrupt the cycle of self-perpetuating destruction.[46,49]

Presumably, mechanical deformation leads to membrane injury by free radical generation according to the following sequence of events: mechanical deformation → rupture of small vessels → extravasated blood → partial breakdown of extravasated blood → initiation and catalysis of free radical damage to membrane lipids by inorganic and organic iron and other blood-borne metals → further vascular pathology, including vasospasm, occlusion and rupture of components of the microcirculatory beds. Free radical reactions adversely affect lipid-dependent enzymes, disturb the endothelium, and cause a broad spectrum of cellular and tissue changes. The synthesis of prostacyclin (PGI_2), which is required to actively prevent platelet adherence and aggregation, can be inhibited by lipid peroxidases formed by free radical activity in endothelial cells. PGI_2 is generated in endothelial cells from arachidonate-derived prostaglandin endoperoxides in association with thromboxane A_2, another product of endoperoxides[36,57,86] (Fig. 16-1). Al-

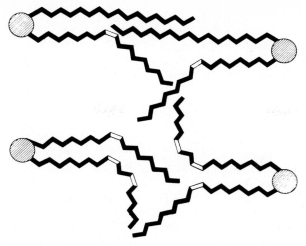

Fig. 16-2. Schematic representation of bimolecular leaflet of phospholipid molecules forming the skeleton of a plasma membrane. The circles are the glycerophosphate head groups, which are polar, while the fatty acid tails extend into the hydrophobic midzone. Unsaturated bonds are bent at an angle of 123 degrees, in the cisisomeric configuration in the fatty acid tails. In the normal membrane, there is a saturated carbon separating the two carbons that have unsaturated bonds. This saturated carbon is partly activated and can lose one of its hydrogens quite readily.

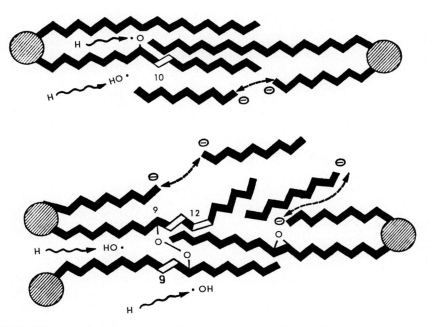

Fig. 16-3. Schematic representation of free radical peroxidative damage to fatty acids that formed the hydrophobic midzone seen in Fig. 16-2. The double bonds are now largely in the nonbent, trans configuration; a saturated carbon no longer separates the carbons with unsaturated bonds, and this is referred to as conjugation; alkoxy radicals, RO•, are present and react to form peroxides, ROOR, to join two adjacent fatty acids in an abnormal bond; mobile •OH radicals are shown as the result of hydroperoxide schism; hydrogens are shown being abstracted, possibly from adjacent lipid and protein molecules; abstracted hydrogens react with hydroxyls to form water in the hydrophobic midzone; fragmentation of fatty acid tails is shown with eventual production of negatively charged carboxylic acid groups, represented as a minus sign inside an oval mark. The numerals, 9, 10, 12, signify the carbon atom number in the carbon chain that makes up the fatty acid.

terations in vascular endothelium occur early and provide a link between lipid free radical damage and perturbations in spinal cord blood flow after impact injury.

Lipid free radical damage

Membrane phospholipids form the basic skeleton of cell membranes (Fig. 16-2). Fatty acid tails of phospholipids can be damaged by free radicals. Unsaturated fatty acids become progressively susceptible to radical attack as the number of double bonds increases.[24,29] Arachidonic acid (20 carbons long, with four unsaturations) undergoes radical reactions more readily than linolenic (18:3) and linoleic (18:2) acids. These reactions can be of graded severity and can proceed in irregular steps, depending on the strength of the initiating and catalyzing factors.[105] Figs. 16-2 and 16-3 summarize the consequences of pathologic, uncontrolled free radical damage to unsaturated membrane phospholipid fatty acids. Analogous changes take place in cholesterol, adjacent to the unsaturated site in the ring.[107] Radical reactions occur commonly but usually do not propagate because they are quenched by naturally occurring antioxidants (alpha-tocopherol, ascorbic acid, glutathione, and others) and enzyme defense systems (superoxide dismutase and glutathione peroxidase).[25,54,110] If antioxidants and protective enzymes are exhausted, there are natural free radical termination reactions that limit the degree of spread.[25] Propagation of irreversible destructive lipid free radical reac-

---

FREE RADICAL LIPID DAMAGE IN CNS

1. Spinal cord impact injury models in cats have shown
   Potentiation of trauma by ethanol[45]
   Appearance of increased levels of malonaldehyde[83]
   Appearance of increasing levels of lipid-soluble fluorescence, representing addition products of malonaldehyde[106]
   Destructive loss of extractable cholesterol[27]
   Consumption of a major CNS antioxidant, ascorbic acid[28]

2. Focal CNS cold trauma in cats and rats has shown
   Amelioration of cerebral edema with DPPD, an antioxidant[91]
   Destructive loss of polyunsaturated fatty acids from gray and white matter[84,85]
   Destructive loss of extractable cholesterol from gray and white matter[84,85]
   Consumption of a major CNS antioxidant, ascorbic acid, from gray and white matter[84,85]
   Amelioration of all free radical pathology parameters with synthetic corticosteroids, which have been shown to also have antioxidant properties in model membrane systems undergoing free radical damage[68,85,107]

Increased production of malonaldehyde[116]
Loss of thiols[97]

3. Regional CNS ischemia in cats has shown
   Destructive loss of polyunsaturated fatty acids from the gray matter[44,48]
   Destructive loss of extractable cholesterol from the white matter[44,48]
   Consumption of a major CNS antioxidant, ascorbic acid, from gray and white matter[43,44,48]
   Amelioration of all of the above with barbiturates, which were shown to have lipid antioxidant properties in model membrane systems undergoing free radical damage[26,44,48]

4. Hypoxia, brain
   Loss of thiols[130]

5. Biogenic amines
   6-OH dopamine is concentrated in sympathetic fibers and destroys them by free radical mechanisms[19]

6. Deficiency states
   Alpha-tocopherol deficiency leads to encephalomalacia[42]

tions requires catalysts that speed the reactions beyond the capacity of antioxidants and protective enzymes and beyond the normal reparability rate.

Initiation and catalysis of radical reactions by CNS trauma

CNS injury appears capable of initiating and catalyzing lipid free radical damage by virtue of ischemia and focal hemorrhages.

Ischemia initiates radical reactions in lipids because of sudden decrease in oxygen supply to mitochondrial electron transport chains. The mechanism of initiating and catalyzing free radical reactions is detailed in Chapter 12.[48]

Focal hemorrhage releases trace quantities of iron and copper, which catalyze lipid free radical reactions.[22, 9] Iron salts can also initiate and catalyze lipid radical reactions in liposomal model membranes, in vitro.[93,107] Citrate or high concentrations of phosphate inhibit destructive lipid radical reactions in liposomal membrane models by chelating catalyzing trace metals.[93]

Evidence for lipid radical damage in the central nervous system

In vivo, pathologic CNS free radical reactions occur after chemical or physical injury* (see box below). Lipid free radicals (e. g., alkyl, peroxy) are reactive transients without a high enough steady state concentration to permit physical detection, but

---

*References 10, 19, 28, 44, 48, 97, 116, 130.

PARAMETERS OF LIPID FREE RADICAL DAMAGE

1. Early, or moderate, free radical damage to membrane phospholipids
   Diene conjugation in fatty acids
   Cis isomerization or transisomerization in fatty acids
   Hindered rotation of nitroxide spin probes placed within liposome membrane systems composed of lipids from the damaged membrane system
   Minor losses in polyunsaturated acids such as arachidonic acid, 20:4, with quantitation by gas chromatography/mass spectrometry (GC/MS)
   Prevention of the above with lipophilic or amphipathic antioxidants
2. Late, or severe, free radical damage to membrane phospholipids
   Malonaldehyde production
   Lipid-soluble fluorescence due to malonaldehyde additions
   Production of short chain, and sometimes branched chain, fatty acids of lengths that are not normally present
   Decreased hindrance of rotation of nitroxide spin probes within liposome membrane systems composed of lipid from damaged membrane system

   Major losses in polyunsaturated fatty acids such as arachidonic acid, 20:4, *plus* minor losses in monounsaturated and saturated fatty acids
   Prevention of the above with lipophilic or amphipathic antioxidants
3. Free radical damage to cholesterol
   Decrease in extractable cholesterol measured by gas chromatography
   Appearance of several cholesterol oxidation products in polar solvents
4. Consumption of tissue antioxidants
   Ascorbic acid (reduced) by epr spectrometry
   Alpha-tocopherol
   Glutathione
   Cysteine
5. Alterations in protective enzymes
   Superoxide dismutase
   Glutathione peroxidase
6. Liposomes from CNS lipid extract from different animal models
   Rates of free radical damage under conditions of auto-oxidation
   Spin probe analyses of fluidity by epr spectrometry
   Permeability rates of solutes in aqueous channels

their presence can be inferred by such distinctive and characteristic changes as loss of susceptible molecules,[27,48] antioxidant consumption,[28,43,97,130] and the presence of metastable and final products.[83,106,116]

Radical reactions are initiated by low ascorbic acid concentrations, possibly by an indirect autooxidation of ascorbic acid to form O_2^- and then H_2O_2 and OH.[101] High ascorbic acid concentration normally found in the CNS does not initiate pathologic radical reactions.[101]

The earliest free radical changes involve consumption of the ascorbic acid, a CNS antioxidant, which decreases in concentration one hour after a 400 g-cm (20 g × 20 cm) impact injury of feline spinal cords[28] and at one hour following regional cerebral ischemia.[44]

Consequences of lipid free radical damage

A number of major proteins derive their active configurational shape from interactions between hydrophobic portions of proteins and fatty acid tails of specific membrane phospholipids.

Since phospholipid fatty acids are susceptible to free radical damage, these proteins are indirectly susceptible to free radical damage. Table 16-5 lists major phospholipid-dependent intrinsic membrane proteins.[51]

The protein enzyme NaK-ATPase is inhibited in rat brain microsomes by the chlorpromazine free radical and related free radicals.[13,101] Acetylcholinesterase, a membrane protein that is not intrinsic and not dependent on phospholipids, was not inhibited by lipid radical reactions that decreased NaK-ATPase activity.[101]

Cytochrome oxidase and succinic dehydrogenase, also phospholipid-dependent enzymes, can be inhibited by pathologic free radical reactions following trauma. Cytochrome oxidase activity is decreased 15 minutes after spinal cord impact injury,[65] resulting in decreased oxidative respiration and increased glycolysis.[62,65]

Membrane lipid free radical reactions involve endothelial cells. Arachidonic acid (four unsaturations), present in large quantities in platelets, is oxidized by platelet microsomes into prostaglandin (PG) endoperoxides, which are unstable intermediates. Ma-

Table 16-5. Phospholipid dependent proteins*

Microsomes	Plasma membrane	Mitochondria
Prostaglandin-synthetase system	NaK-ATPase	Cytochrome oxidase
Hydroxylase system with cytochrome P_{450}	Adenylate cyclase	Succinic dehydrogenase
NADH-cytochrome b5 reductase	Lectin binding glycoproteins and surface glycolipids	Monoamine oxidase
Steroid-glucuronyl transferase	5'-nucleotidase	NADH cytochrome c/NADH-ubiquinone reductase
UDP-glucuronyl transferase	RBC acetyl cholinesterase	Succinate-cytochrome reductase
Phosphatidic acid phosphatase		ATP synthetase system
Phosphoryl choline transferase		Hexokinase
Glucose-t-phospho-hydrolase		Citric acid cycle enzymes
		$NADPH_2'$:NAD oxidoreductase
		GTP-dependent acyl CoA synthetase
		Deoxycorticosterone 11-β-hydroxylase
		D-β-hydroxybutyrate dehydrogenase

*From Fourcans, B., and Jain, M. H.: Role of phospholipids in transport and enzymic reactions, Advances Lipid Res. **12:**147, 1974.

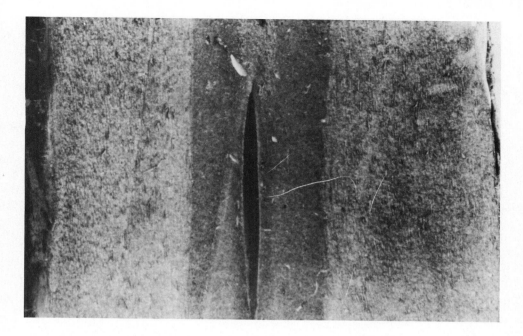

Fig. 16-4. Very low magnification of an obliquely cut, normal cat spinal cord showing the central canal (patent in cats) surrounding gray matter, and the long tracts in the white matter. (×40.)

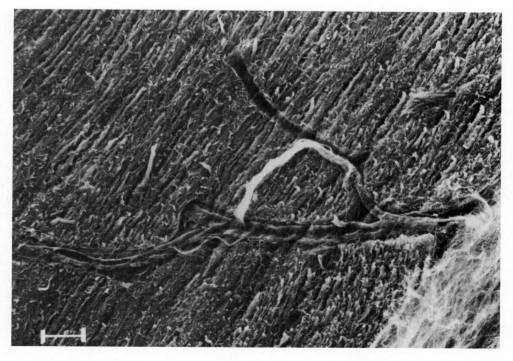

Fig. 16-5. Higher magnification of the white matter in Fig. 16-4. The meningeal surface is seen at one corner, displaying many collagen fibers. A small vessel, probably a venule, is seen in the long tracts; one branch has been artifactually detached from its neuroglial bed. Longitudinally oriented axons in large numbers are present. Openings made in the wall of the vessel by the section facilitate an intraluminal view of the endothelial lining. (×530.)

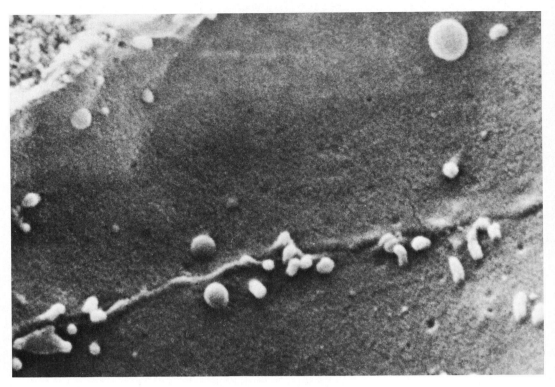

Fig. 16-6. Endothelial surface of a white matter capillary from a normal cat at very high magnification. The junction of two endothelial cells and many normally occurring microvilli are seen. Openings of pinocytic vesicles can also be seen in this topographic view of the plasma membrane of the endothelial cells. ($\times$45,000.)

jor classes of compounds produced from PG endoperoxides include prostaglandins E and F, thromboxane A_2 (TxA_2), prostacyclin (PGI_2). The latter two are directly antagonistic and far more powerful than the PGs.[36,57,86] Thromboxane A_2 is an extremely potent platelet aggregator, whereas prostacyclin prevents aggregation and disaggregates platelets.[36,57,86] The balance between TxA_2 and PGI_2 is critical for clotting homeostasis.[36] The absence of adherent material on normal endothelium is the result of incessant activity of endothelial cells to produce PGI_2.[36,57,86] Lipid peroxides selectively inhibit formation of PGI_2 and result in unopposed TxA_2 action.[36,86] Ischemia or trauma leads to lipid free radical damage and pro-

duction of lipid peroxides.[43,44,48] This may explain why ischemic or injured endothelium allows platelets and other coagulable material to adhere.[31,48] We used scanning electron microscopy to examine the endothelium of vessels within feline cord parenchyma at early periods following experimental injury using a low-angle, obliquely cut cord section[31] (Figs. 16-4 to 16-9).

The luminal surface shows significant pathologic change at one hour after impact injury. These ultrastructural changes are among the earliest seen in white matter after injury. The microcirculatory pathology progresses in severity over a one- to two-hour period and may explain evolving deficits in spinal cord blood flow following injury.[31]

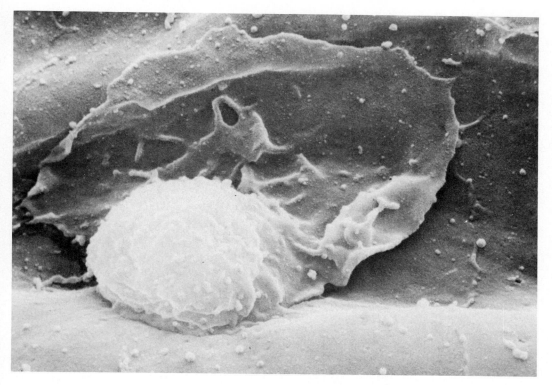

Fig. 16-7. High magnification of the lumen of an arteriole in the white matter of a cat injured one hour prior to fixation. A lymphocytoid/monocytoid cell is adherent to the endothelial surface via pseudopodallike extensions. A small crater is present in the endothelium in the right lower corner. The luminal surface is slightly undulated secondary to artifact caused by contraction of arteriolar muscle and elastic tissue when the fixative is perfused. (×16,900.)

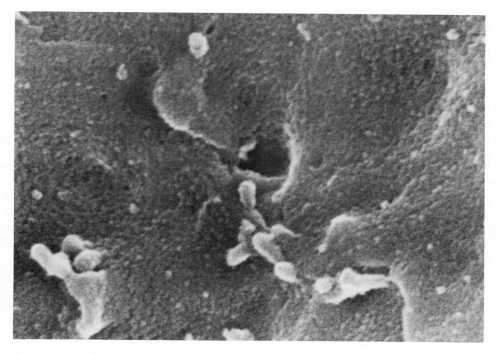

Fig. 16-8. One hour after impact injury, the junction of two endothelial cells in a white matter capillary shows overriding and a pathologic separation to form a hole. Compare with normal capillary endothelium in Fig. 16-6. (×87,000.)

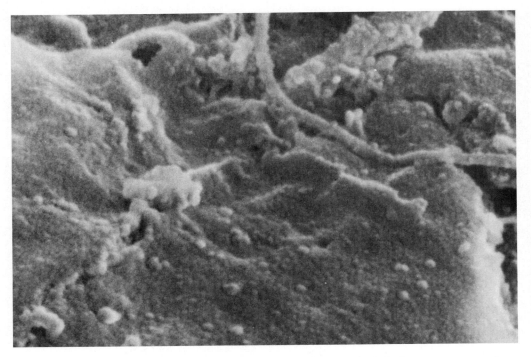

Fig. 16-9. One hour after injury, the endothelial lining of an occluded white matter arteriole shows marked pathologic changes. Compare to Fig. 16-6. The endothelial edges are thickened and have focal microglobular deposits; a curved strand of fibrin courses through the right upper corner of the figure. (×74,400.)

Spinal cord blood flow (SCBF)

Vasospasm and constriction of CNS arterial supply has been observed in head trauma, as well as in experimental spinal cord injury.[8,46,49,108] Spinal cord vessel caliber decreases following injury in a manner similar to cerebral vasospasm, following introduction of blood into the subarachnoid space and alterations in cyclic AMP.[35,46,49] The etiology of cerebral vasospasm following subarachnoid hemorrhage has not been defined fully, but serotonin, catecholamines, and prostaglandins have each been implicated as causal agents.[61,92] Reserpine and kanamycin, which decrease available serotonin, have been proposed to therapeutically prevent vasospasm following subarachnoid hemorrhage.[61,135] Various adrenergic blocks have been proposed to limit the vasoactive effects of catecholamines following CNS hemorrhage.[71,72,92] In addition to being potent vasoconstrictors, norepinephrine and serotonin potentiate platelet aggregation. These substances are known to be released following platelet aggregation, along with adenosine diphosphate and arachidonic acid derivatives, which further stimulate platelet aggregation.[127] Decreased cord perfusion after injury may occur from platelet aggregation coupled with chemically mediated large vessel vasoconstriction and thrombosis, a process initiated by endothelial injury.[88] Pharmacologic methods now available to control the synthesis and availability of each of these substances and the concentration of cyclic nucleotides and arachidonic oxidation products may be experimentally applied to treat cord injury.[46,49]

Vessels exhibiting cerebral vasospasm induced by experimental exposure to extravasated blood have a decreased cyclic AMP content.[46] Spasm can be ameliorated by agents that facilitate the formation of cyclic AMP or retard its degradation by stimulating adenylate cyclase or inhibiting phosphodiesterases. Cyclic AMP levels within ischemic brain tissue are reduced before the development of observable histologic change.[43,49] Thus, it seems appropriate to consider improving CNS perfusion following trauma by increasing cyclic AMP. Smooth muscle cyclic AMP can be increased by isoproterenol, PGE, and other beta-adrenergic agonists, and use of these agents is indeed associated with relaxation of vascular spasm.[46,49] Norepinephrine, epinephrine, and serotonin also potentiate platelet aggregation. Agents capable of increasing vessel cyclic AMP also inhibit platelet aggregation.[47] It may therefore be possible to improve cord perfusion by simultaneously inhibiting platelet aggregation and reversing CNS vasospasm using the same agents.

Loss of neurogenic control may be another mechanism resulting in blood flow change after trauma. Cerebral and spinal cord vessels are densely innervated with adrenergic and cholinergic fibers, and spinal cord blood flow (SCBF) autoregulation exists.[8,37,72,89,108] The adrenergic plexus in cerebral vessels is believed to originate mainly from cervical sympathetics with some contribution from central adrenergic neurons arising from the locus ceruleus.[60] The source of innervation of spinal cord vessels is not clear, but autoregulation and breakthrough may be under sympathetic control.[71] Spinal cord vessels may derive some adrenergic innervation from fibers within the thoracic spinal cord. Thoracic spinal cord injury may interfere with this innervation. Following injury, striking fluctuations in excitability of dorsal columns above and below the impact occur and persist from hours to days. If analogous fluctuations in adrenergic nerve fiber excitability occur after impact, autoregulation mediated by this innervation may be impaired and may account for alteration in control of SCBF.

In the first few hours after acute impact injury, SCBF is diminished in both gray (SCBFg) and white (SCBFw) matter.[8,99,100,108] Thirty minutes after a 400 g-cm impact at T-6, SCBFg was essentially obliterated and SCBFw decreased to 40% of control.[8] SCBF was reduced to 60% of control in cervical and lumbar cord segments. Decreases persisted at T-6 but returned to near normal in the cervical and lumbar segments after four hours.[8]

Hyperemia has been described in white matter immediately adjacent to the hemorrhagically infarcted central gray matter 24 hours after impact injury.[70,112] Intercellular potassium (Ke) is increased secondary to neuronal necrosis and red cell lysis. If Ke rises above its normal range of 2.5 to 3.0 mM, vascular dilatation occurs.[112,124] The extent and direction of change of other factors influencing blood flow is not known.

After injury with a 400 g-cm force in cats, vessels in the microcirculation of the long tracts develop progressively more endothelial pathology from one to two hours. The number of observable vessels decreases strikingly due to spasm and collapse of the microcirculation, and there is an increase in the number of occluded vessels.[31] These changes are seen distal to the injured segment but at two hours or later. The proximal segment endothelium is not normal after impact, but the changes appear minimal at two hours.

Potentiation of injury by ethanol

We have found that intravenous ethanol administered to barbiturate-anesthetized cats potentiates a nonparalyzing injury and causes permanent paraplegia.[45] An impacting force of 400 g-cm, induced by a 20 g weight falling 20 cm, results in permanent paraplegia in 95% of cats[17]; however, a force of 200 g-cm alone never causes permanent paralysis.[17,45] Ethanol converts the 200 g-cm impact injury into the equivalent of a 400 g-cm impact, structurally and functionally.[45]

The exact mechanism whereby ethanol produces this effect is not clearly understood. Ethanol increases membrane fluidity [104] and this might cause a variety of functional membrane perturbations. In the CNS where function depends upon the integrity of all membranes (e.g., neuronal, glial, and endothelium with tight junctions) this change may be critical.

All primary and secondary alcohols and the principal metabolite of ethanol, acetaldehyde, can add directly to the double bonds of unsaturated fatty acids in membrane phospholipids via free radical chemical reactions.[125] Acetaldehyde can be acted upon by xanthine oxidase, a ubiquitous enzyme, to produce the superoxide free radical $\cdot O_2^-$.[68] Superoxide radicals can spontaneously produce H_2O_2 and the hydroxyl radical, $\cdot OH$, in aqueous tissue compartments.[68] These substances, $\cdot O_2^- \cdot H_2O_2$, and $\cdot OH$, can initiate and catalyze lipid free radical reactions in cells.[68]

Ethanol injures liver cells by free radical reactions. Antioxidants have been used to ameliorate these changes.[32,33] Whether ethanol potentiates traumatic injuries in humans and whether the other toxic effects of alcohol in the myocardium and in the CNS are mediated by mechanisms that include free radical reactions remain to be investigated. The free radical reactions of ethanol are probably only one of several pathologic mechanisms operative in the potentiation of injury.[21,32]

EXPERIMENTAL APPROACHES FOR TREATMENT

Descriptions of the surgical, pharmacologic, and physical modes of treatment after injury produced in various experimental models[1,3,16] describe some degree of improvement in outcome, but no group of treatments has been found to be universally effective, and none consistently allows animals injured with threshold forces to regain the ability to walk. Further evidence of the inadequacies of treatment in spinal cord injury is the failure of experimental therapeutic modalities to be clinically useful. Specific therapeutic regimens have been used empirically without either laboratory evidence of efficacy or strong clinical evidence to support continued use. Corticosteroids,

for example, in ever increasing doses have become part of the usual neurosurgical armamentarium, but strong laboratory or clinical data to support these agents has yet to be obtained.

Efforts have been made to control hemorrhage within gray matter and edema in white matter. Myelotomy was introduced to remove blood clot and decompress the spinal cord internally.[2,3,53] Work in our laboratory confirmed that myelotomy and removal of the intraspinal cord clot is effective in allowing some animals to regain their ability to walk.[17]

The introduction of localized hypothermia to treat contused mammalian spinal cords served as a major stimulus to approach spinal cord injury as a problem with a potential solution.[1,12,120] Oxygen tension improves in contused spinal cords treated by local hypothermia.[69] The same type of improvement seen with hypothermia occurs when the injured spinal cord is irrigated with normothermic saline.[119] This raises the question of whether the improvement is a function of cooling or evacuation of some undetermined toxic product.[119]

Based on the presumption that steroids improve membrane stability and thereby decrease the capillary fluid leak, steroids in various dosages have been advocated to control cord edema following injury.[15,38,59]

We tried to control hemorrhage and edema using a combination of steroids and the antifibrinolytic agent EACA to reduce further bleeding within the central nervous system.[16] We were initially enthusiastic about this approach, since histologic changes following a 400 g-cm impact in cats were markedly reduced. No long-term improvement in the animals' ability to walk was seen in spite of the improved histologic appearance of the cords.[16]

Other attempts to treat spinal cord injury have included injection of proteolytic enzymes into the lesion,[81] immunosuppressive therapy,[41] and urea and dimethyl sulfoxide.[66] Levodopa ameliorates experimental paraplegia resulting from air emboli injected into the abdominal aorta, perhaps because of the levodopa metabolites in the CNS.[94] Crocetin is a water-soluble analog of beta carotene, a proven, specific free radical scavenger.[55,75] Beta carotene is used clinically to prevent pathologic lipid free radical reactions that occur in the rare disorder erythropoietic protoporphyria. Neurologic improvement in experimentally injured animals is seen after using Crocetin. If clinical improvement occurs after Crocetin, it may be due also to an enhancement of oxygen diffusivity,[55] although oxygen, which is seven times more soluble in nonpolar than polar substances, normally diffuses through the cord and brain.[78]

No early investigator has been able to reliably stop the development of permanent paraplegia following a 400 g-cm impact in experimental models. Significant amelioration of paraplegia in animal models and perhaps in patients probably requires a polypharmaceutic regimen aimed at increasing SCBF and preventing free radical damage.

We have treated eight cats with aminophylline, 1 to 3 mg/kg/hr, and isoproterenol, 1-3 μg/kg/hr (A and I), for five hours after a 400 g-cm impact to the thoracic cord. Three were used for histopathologic examination of short-term changes. Of five animals allowed to survive, three regained the ability to walk one to three weeks after injury. We demonstrated blood flow in the area of impaction in three animals treated and no flow in the impacted area of untreated animals using ^{14}C-antipyrine. Histopathologic examination of the impacted area of cats treated with aminophylline and isoproterenol (A and I) revealed somewhat less hemorrhage in the central gray matter compared to nontreated impacted animals at the same time period. Central hemorrhage is difficult to quantitate since it varies from animal to animal in the early time periods, but this study at least indicates that early treatment with A and I at this dosage does not increase central gray hemorrhage. If this data is substantiated, it may offer a clue about the pathologic hemodynamics involved in the development of central bleeding.

Agents acting directly on vascular smooth muscle, particularly nitroprusside, have been used to control spasm following subarachnoid hemorrhage.[4] Coupled with a pressor agent to avoid reduction in perfusion pressure this combination may warrant further study.

A self-perpetuating cycle may exist between physiologic changes and free radical damage. Free radical reactions can cycle back to produce detrimental change in physiology. Several links may exist between the two areas. Arachidonic acid oxidation to endoperoxides, PGs, thromboxanes, and lipid peroxides produced by free radical reactions block prostacyclin formation, increase platelet aggregation, and decrease blood flow. Blood flow and edema may be altered in response to cyclic AMP levels, which may be altered by adenylate cyclase activity, which in turn is dependent on intact membrane lipids.[46,49,51]

Table 16-6 lists pharmacologic agents that involve free radical reactions as a primary pharmacologic property or in the development of toxicity or injury. It may be essential to know whether an injured patient is taking a substance with antioxidant activity, since co-administration of one antioxidant may cancel the effect of the other.[30] Since many pro-oxidants can have additive and even synergistic effects,[45,126] it may be necessary to develop a list of pro-oxidant drugs and substances to avoid, once a better understanding of the mechanisms of spinal cord degeneration is achieved.

Anesthetics are preferentially soluble in lipids within lipid/aqueous systems.[59,104] Many anesthetics increase membrane fluidity and because of this, many substances may have anesthetic properties, including alkyl polyhalides, dimethyl sulfoxide (DMSO), ethanol, and the noble gases xenon and krypton.[78,98,103] Anesthetics are present in the hydrophobic membrane midzone in proximity to susceptible polyunsaturated fatty acids along with abundant oxygen.[78] Here free radical reactions may be stimulated and toxic effects produced, as possibly occurs with halothane,[14] or radical reactions may be aborted and tissue protection occur,

Table 16-6. Pharmacologic agents that involve free radical reactions

Anesthetics	Halothane[14]
	Chloroform[125]
	Trichlorethylene[125]
	Barbiturates[26,48]
	DMSO[6,82]
	Noble gases[78]
Tranquilizers	Chloral hydrate[125]
	Phenothiazines[13,90]
Chemotherapeutic agents	Adriamycin[18]
	Daunomycin[18]
	Mitomycin[18]
	Bleomycin[18]
Essential nutrient compounds	Alpha-tocopherol[79,134]
	Ascorbic acid[28,43,101]
	Retinol[55,75]
	β-carotene[55,75]
	Riboflavin[24]
	Flavinoids[24]
Essential metals	Selenium[20,63]
	Zinc[54,68,80]
	Iron[22,131]
	Copper[22,54,68,80,131]
	Manganese[54,68,80]
Anti-inflammatory	Corticosteroids and cholesterol[84,85,107]
	Salicylate analogs[36,57,86]
	Indomethacin[36,57,86]
	Superoxide dismutase[54,68,80]
Antimalarials	Chloroquine[30]
Hormones	Estrogen[122]
	Diethylstilbesterol[122]
Thiol compounds	Cysteine[97,130]
	Glutathione[97,110,130]
	β-β′ dimethyl cysteine[25,64]

as may be the case with some barbiturates[26,44] and DMSO.[6] Anesthetics may directly affect membrane proteins and other biochemical factors independently of any possible effects on the membrane lipids.

Alkyl polyhalides are a family of complex structures (including halothane, CCl_4, DDT, PCB, and PBB) which share the property of adding directly across the double bonds of polyunsaturated fatty acids by free radical addition reactions.[125] Free radical based toxins often act synergistically, for example, CCl_4 and C_2H_5OH.[126]

Barbiturates have a broad spectrum of biologic effects. These can be greatly modified by minor structural substitutions that alter lipid solubility or precise localization on membrane biomolecules.[95] The actions of barbiturates on free radical reactions are discussed in Chapter 12.

DMSO is an aprotic fluid that alters membrane structures,[133] scavenges •OH radicals,[6] stabilizes transient free radicals,[28] binds to water,[118] initiates oxidative reactions,[28] and acts as an excellent solvent for oxygen as well as many polar and nonpolar substances.[56] The cellular effects resulting from these actions include anesthesia, protection against radiation, other •OH radical–mediated pathology, and tissue dehydration. DMSO diminishes the periaxonal accumulation of fluid in myelinated fibers after spinal cord impact and has been used to ameliorate changes seen following spinal cord impact.[60] In our studies, using the 400 g-cm impact feline cord model, DMSO administered before as well as after impact decreased central hemorrhage and white matter edema seen on light microscopy. Seven of 20 cats impacted and treated with DMSO walked (35%), whereas only 1 out of 10 controls walked (10%).

Phenothiazines such as chlorpromazine (CPZ) also are membrane-active substances with many cellular effects.[90] Chlorpromazine readily assumes a free radical configuration that can inhibit NaK-ATPase in vitro.[13] There is evidence that the desired pharmacologic effects of CPZ are due to the nonradical configuration, not the free radical configuration. The cause of CPZ toxicity (tremors, melanosis) is not known.

Alpha-tocopherol is an essential nutrient compound found within cell membranes that may well serve as a general membrane antioxidant.[63,79] Many studies relate the administration of alpha-tocopherol to inhibition of free radical pathogenic mechanisms, but it is premature to suggest this be used clinically. Most antioxidants can also act as pro-oxidants, depending on the redox potential of the molecular environment, for example, ascorbic acid.[101] Free radicals occur normally in electron transport, prostaglandin synthesis, in leukocytes, and elsewhere. These systems may be interfered with by chronic, large doses of tocopherol and ascorbic acid, which some individuals advocate and many others take. The use of antioxidants will require careful and more specific research before wide use can be safely recommended.

Tocopherol is necessary for the integrity of vascular endothelium.[42,134] Slow cerebral and cerebellar endothelial cell degeneration leading to encephalomalacia occurs in tocopherol-deficient chicks given diet supplemented fatty acids. Ischemic endothelial changes and adherent platelets are seen in various sized vessels.[31,88] In capillaries and vessels within the injury site, platelet adherence might result in partial or complete occlusion. Tocopherol interferes with the synthesis of endoperoxides and prostaglandins and thereby prevents platelet aggregation onto ischemic or injured endothelial cells. The suggestion has been made that antioxidants be added to current clinical regimens that utilize acetylsalicylic acid or indomethacin.[36]

The essential metals also have major free radical implications. Selenium is necessary for activity of glutathione peroxidase, a major enzyme system involved in protection against pathologic free radical reactions that start in endoplasmic reticulum.[20] Exogenous selenium is not likely to have a role in ameliorating spinal cord trauma, since sufficient amounts are present in the normal diet of humans and laboratory animals to maintain glutathione peroxidase activity. Iron and copper may be major initiators and catalysts of radical damage in the impacted cord.[22,131] Auto-oxidation of lipids is catalyzed by five orders of magnitude in the presence of iron complexes and three orders of magnitude in the presence of copper.[22,131] Therapeutic chelation of iron and copper may become an important part of a care protocol. Many chelators, for example, β-β'-dimethyl cysteine, *d*-penicillamine, Cuprimine, are not entirely metal specific. β-β'-dimethyl cys-

teine, which can immediately quench free radicals,[25] removes as much iron from tissues as it does copper.[64] This drug enters the CNS and has been used in humans with Wilson disease. It may have use in CNS injuries because iron complexes from extravasated blood may initiate free radical lipid damage. It is effective in reversing coma induced by accidental pediatric ingestion of over-the-counter iron-containing mineral and vitamin preparations. β-β'-dimethyl cysteine is not inherently dangerous; its principal side effects include antigenicity and gastrointestinal irritation. It may be worthwhile to experiment with this material in laboratory models of spinal cord trauma.

The corticosteroids inhibit prostaglandin formation (PGE and PGF) by poorly understood mechanisms.[67] They may block arachidonic acid oxidation to endoperoxide, which would explain the observed decrease in synthesis of both PGEs and PGFs.[67] The result of decreased prostaglandin synthesis is a diminished inflammatory reaction. The mechanism by which corticosteroids block endoperoxide synthesis is not known; however, we have demonstrated[107] that corticosteroids exert an antioxidant effect and prevent free radical reactions; ovolecithin-prepared liposomes subjected to controlled free radical damage by ultraviolet light or iron catalysis are protected in a dose-dependent manner by methylprednisolone.[107] Not all steroids have this antioxidant property. Substitutions at different positions make a difference. The clinical effectiveness of corticosteroids as anti-inflammatory agents or antiarthritics suggests some type of antioxidant effect against $\cdot OH$ and $\cdot O_2^-$ radicals produced by granulocytic leukocytes and macrophages, in addition to the inhibition of PGs. An additional anti-inflammatory mechanism appears to depend on the amphipathic nature of the drug and its ability to pack into membranes. This results in so-called "membrane stabilization" and decreases the likelihood of freeing lysosomal hydrolases, which also participate in the inflammatory response.[128]

Polypharmaceutical regimens are likely

to be devised as critical adjuvants to the neurosurgical treatment of spinal cord trauma. Some agents will have to be used by anesthesiologists because some drugs might be anesthetics or anesthetic analogs, which may affect blood flow, blood pressure, and other vital parameters. The use of certain anesthetics and other pharmacologic agents may have to be reevaluated if they are shown to potentiate free radical damage or adversely perturb spinal cord blood flow.

REFERENCES

1. Albin, M. S., White, R. J., Acosta-Rua, G., and Yashon, D.: Study of functional recovery produced by delayed cooling after spinal cord injury in primates, J. Neurosurg. 29:113, 1969.
2. Allen, A. R.: Remarks on the histopathological changes in the spinal cord due to impact: an experimental study, J. Nerv. Ment. Dis. 41:141, 1915.
3. Allen, A. R.: Surgery of experimental lesion of spinal cord equivalent to crush injury of fracture dislocation of spinal column; a preliminary report, J.A.M.A. 57:878, 1911.
4. Allen, G. S., and Gross, C. J.: Cerebral arterial spasm, Surg. Neurol. 6:63, 1976.
5. Anderson, D. K., Nicolosi, G. R., Means, E. D., and Hartley, L. E.: Effects of laminectomy on spinal cord blood flow, J. Neurosurg. 48:232, 1978.
6. Ashwood-Smith, M. J.: Current concepts concerning radioprotective and cryo protectice properties of DMSO in cellular systems, Ann. N.Y. Acad. Sci. 243:246, 1975.
7. Benes, V.: Spinal cord injury, Baltimore, 1968, The Williams & Wilkins Co.
8. Bingham, W. G., Sirinek, L., Crutcher, L., and Mohnacky, C.: Effect of spinal cord injury on cord and cerebral blood flow in monkey, Acta Neurol. Scand. (suppl. 64) 56:132, 1977.
9. Block, B. B., and Ginocchio, A. V.: Local and systemic subarachnoid toxicity of metrizamide in mice and monkeys, Acta Radiol. (suppl.) 335:14, 1973.
10. Boehme, D. H.: Lipoperoxidation in human and rat brain tissue: developmental and regional studies, Brain Res. 136:11, 1977.
11. Braackman, R., and Penning, L.: Injuries of the cervical spine, Amsterdam, 1971, Excerpta Medica, p. 108.
12. Bricolo, A., Dalle Ore, G., Da Pian, R., and Facciolli, F.: Local cooling in spinal cord injury, Surg. Neurol. 6:101, 1976.
13. Brody, T. M., Akera, T., Baskin, S. L., Gubitz, R., and Lee, C. Y.: Interaction of NaKATPase with chlorpromazine free radical and related compounds, Ann. N.Y. Acad. Sci. 242:527, 1974.
14. Brown, B. R., Jr.: Hepatic microsomal lipoperoxidation and inhalation anesthetics: a biochemical and morphological study in the rat, Anesthesiology 36:458, 1972.
15. Bucy, P.: Emergency treatment of spinal cord injury, Surg. Neurol. 1:216, 1973.
16. Campbell, J. B., De Crescito, V., Tomasula, J., Demopoulos, H., Flamm, E., and Ortega, B.: Effects of antifibrinolytic and steroid therapy on the contused spinal cord of cats, J. Neurosurg. 40:726, 1974.
17. Campbell, J. B., De Crescito, V., Tomasula, J., Demopoulos, H., Flamm, E., and Ransohoff, J.: Experimental treatment of spinal cord contusion in the cat, Surg. Neurol. 1:102, 1973.
18. Chu, E. S.: Toxic effects of adriamycin on the ganglia of the peripheral nervous system, J. Neuropathol. Exp. Neurol. 36:907, 1977.
19. Cohen, G., and Heikkila, R. E.: The generation of hydrogen peroxide, superoxide radical, and hydroxyl radical by 6-hydroxydopamine, dialuric acid and related cytotoxic agents, J. Biol. Chem. 249:2447, 1974.
20. Combs, G. F., Jr., Noguchi, T., and Scott, M. L.: Mechanisms and action of selenium and Vitamin E in protection of biological membranes, Fed. Proc. 34:2090, 1975.
21. Comporti, M., Hartman, A. D., and Di Luzio, N. R.: Effect of in vivo, and in vitro ethanol administration on liver lipid peroxidation, Lab. Invest. 16:616, 1977.
22. Cowan, J. C., and Evans, C. D.: Flavor reversion and related forms of oxidative deterioration. In Lundberg, W. D., editor: Aut-oxidation and antioxidants, vol. 2, New York, 1962, Interscience, p. 593.
23. Cracco, R. Q., and Bickford, R. G.: Somatomotor and somatosensory evoked responses: peripheral nerve stimulation in man, Arch. Neurol. 18:52, 1968.
24. Demopoulos, H. B.: The basis of free radical pathology, Fed. Proc. 32:1859, 1973.
25. Demopoulos, H. B.: Control of free radicals in biologic systems, Fed. Proc. 32:1903, 1973.
26. Demopoulos, H. B., Flamm, E. S., Seligman, M. L., Jorgensen, E., and Ransohoff, J.: Antioxidant effect of barbiturates in model membranes undergoing free radical damage, Acta Neurol. Scand. (suppl. 64) 56:152, 1977.
27. Demopoulos, H. B., Flamm, E., Seligman, M., Mitamura, J., and Ransohoff, J.: Membrane perturbations in CNS injury: theoretical basis for free radical damage and a review of the experimental data. In Popp, A. J., Bourke, R. S., Nelson, L. R., and Kimelberg, H. K., editors: Neural trauma, New York, 1979, Raven Press, p. 75.
28. Demopoulos, H., Flamm, E., Seligman, M., Poser, R., Pietronigro, D., and Ransohoff, J.: Molecular pathology of lipids in CNS membranes. In Jobsis, F., editor: Oxygen and physiological

function, Dallas, 1976, Professional Information Library, p. 491.

29. Demopoulos, H. B., Milvy, P., Kakari, S., and Ransohoff, J.: Molecular aspects of membrane structure in cerebral edema. In Reulen, H. J., and Schurman, K., editors: Steroids and brain edema, Berlin, 1972, Springer-Verlag, p. 29.

30. Demopoulos, H. B., Poser, R. G., Jones, W. B. G., Lavietes, B. B., Coleman, P., and Seligman, M. L.: Manipulation of free radicals in pigmented melanomas. In Riley, V., editor: Pigment cell, vol. 2, Basel, 1976, Karger, p. 347.

31. Demopoulos, H. B., Yoder, M., Gutman, E., Seligman, M., Flamm, E. S., and Ransohoff, J.: The fine structure of endothelial surfaces in the microcirculation of experimentally injured feline spinal cords, Scanning Electron Microscopy 2: 677, 1978.

32. DiLuzio, N. R.: Antioxidants, lipid peroxidation, and chemical-induced liver injury, Fed. Proc. 32: 1875, 1973.

33. DiLuzio, N. R., Stege, T. E., and Hoffman, E. O.: Protective influence of diphenyl-p-phenylenediamine on hydrazine-induced lipid peroxidation and hepatic injury, Exp. Mol. Pathol. 19:284, 1973.

34. Dohrman, G. J., Wagner, F. C., and Bucy, P. C.: Transitory traumatic paraplegia: electron microscopy of early alterations in myelinated nerve fibers, J. Neurosurg. 36:407, 1972.

35. Dohrman, G. J., Wick, K. M., and Bucy, P. C.: Spinal cord blood flow patterns in experimental traumatic paraplegia, J. Neurosurg. 38:52, 1973.

36. Editorial: The prevention of thrombosis, Lancet 1:127, 1977.

37. Edvinsson, L.: Neurogenic mechanisms in the cerebrovascular bed. Acta Physiol. Scand. (suppl.) 427:35, 1975.

38. Eidelberg, E., Staten, E., Watkins, C. J., and Smith, J. S.: Treatment of experimental spinal cord injury in ferrets, Surg. Neurol. 6:243, 1976.

39. Erickson, D. L., Leider, L. L., and Brown, W. E.: One stage decompression-stabilization for thoracolumbar fractures, Spine 2:53, 1977.

40. Engler, G. H., Spielholz, N., Bernhard, W., and others: Somatosensory evoked potentials during Harrington instrumentation for scoliosis, J. Bone Joint Surg. 60A:528, 1978.

41. Feringer, E. R., Johnson, R. D., and Wendt, J. S.: Spinal cord regeneration in rats after immunosuppressive treatment, Arch. Neurol. 32: 676, 1975.

42. Fischer, V. W.: Cerebrovascular changes in tocopherol-depleted chicks, fed linoleic acid, J. Neuropathol. Exp. Neurol. 32:474, 1973.

43. Flamm, E. S., Demopoulos, H. B., Seligman, M. L., Poser, R. G., and Ransohoff, J.: Free radicals in cerebral ischemia, Stroke 9:445, 1978.

44. Flamm, E. S., Demopoulos, H. B., Seligman, M. L., and Ransohoff, J.: Possible molecular mechanisms of barbiturate-mediated protection in regional cerebral ischemia, Acta Neurol. Scand. (suppl. 64) 56:150, 1977.

45. Flamm, E. S., Demopoulos, H. B., Seligman, M. L., Tomasula, J. J., DeCrescito, V., and Ransohoff, J.: Ethanol potentiation of central nervous system trauma, J. Neurosurg. 46:328, 1977.

46. Flamm, E. S., Kim, J., Lin, J., and Ransohoff, J.: Phosphodiesterase inhibitors and cerebral vasospasm, Arch. Neurol. 32:569, 1975.

47. Flamm, E. S., and Ransohoff, J.: Treatment of cerebral vasospasm by control of cyclic adenosine monophosphate, Surg. Neurol. 6:223, 1976.

48. Flamm, E. S., Seligman, M. L., and Demopoulos, H. B.: Barbiturate protection of the ischemic brain. In Cottrell, J. E., and Turndorf, H., editors: Anesthesia and Neurology, St. Louis, 1979, The C. V. Mosby Co.

49. Flamm, E. S., Viau, A. T., Ransohoff, J., and Naftchi, N. E.: Experimental alterations in cyclic adenosine monophosphate concentrations in the cat basilar artery, Neurology 26:664, 1976.

50. Forsythe, H. F., Alexander, E., Jr., Davis, C., Jr., and Underal, R.: The advantages of early spine fusion in the treatment of fracture-dislocation of the cervical spine, J. Bone Joint Surg. 41-A:17, 1969.

51. Fourcans, B., and Jain, M. H.: Role of phospholipids in transport and enzymic reactions, Advances Lipid Res. 12:147, 1974.

52. Frankel, H. L., Hancock, D. O., Hyslop, G., and others: The value of postural reduction in the initial management of closed injuries of the spine with paraplegia and tetraplegia, Paraplegia 7:179, 1969.

53. Freeman, L. W., and Wright, T. W.: Experimental observations of concussion and contusion of the spinal cord, Am. Surg. 19:433, 1953.

54. Fried, R., and Mandel, P.: Superoxide dismutase of mammalian nervous system, J. Neurochem. 24:433, 1975.

55. Gainer, J. V.: Use of crocetin in experimental spinal cord injury, J. Neurosurg. 46:358, 1977.

56. Gorog, P.: Antiarthritic and antithrombotic effects of topically applied DMSO, Ann. N.Y. Acad. Sci. 243:91, 1975.

57. Gryglewski, R. J., Bunting, S., Moncada, S., Flower, R. J., and Vane, J. R.: Arterial walls are protected against deposition of platelet thrombi by a substance (prostaglandin X) which they make from prostaglandin endoperoxides, Prostaglandins 12:685, 1976.

58. Guttmann, L.: Spinal cord injuries, Oxford, 1976, Blackwell Scientific Publications.

59. Hansebout, R. R., Kuchner, E. F., and Romero-Sierra, C.: Effects of local hypothermia and of steroids upon recovery from experimental spinal cord compression injury, Surg. Neurol. 4:531, 1975.

60. Hartman, B. K., Zide, D., and Udenfriend, S.:

The use of dopamine-beta-hydroxylase as a marker for the central noradrenergic nervous system in rat brain, Proc. Nat. Acad. Sci. **69:**2722, 1972.

61. Heros, R. C., Zervas, N. J., Negoro, M.: Cerebral vasospasm, Surg. Neurol. **5:**354, 1976.

62. Heuser, D., Astrup, J., Lassen, N. A., Nilsson, B., Norberg, K., and Siesjo, B. K.: Are H^+ and K^+ factors for the adjustment of cerebral blood flow to changes in functional state: a microelectrode study, Acta Neurol. Scand. (suppl. 64) **56:**216, 1977.

63. Hoekstra, W. G.: Biochemical function of selenium and its relation to vitamin E, Fed. Proc. **34:**2083, 1975.

64. Hourani, B. T., and Demopoulos, H. B.: Inhibition of S-91 mouse melanoma metastases and growth by D-penicillamine, Lab. Invest. **21:**434, 1969.

65. Ito, T., Allen, N., and Yashon, D.: A mitochondrial lesion in experimental spinal cord trauma, J. Neurosurg. **48:**434, 1978.

66. Kajihara, K., Kawanga, H., de la Torre, J. C., and Mullan, S.: Dimethyl sulfoxide in the treatment of experimental acute spinal cord injury, Surg. Neurol. **1:**16, 1973.

67. Kantrowitz, F., Robinson, D. R., McGuire, M. B., and Levine, L.: Corticosteroids inhibit prostaglandin production by rheumatoid synovia, Nature **258:**737, 1975.

68. Kellogg, E. W., and Fridovich, I.: Liposome oxidation and erythrocyte lysis by enzymatically generated superoxide and hydrogen peroxide, J. Biol. Chem. **252:**672, 1977.

69. Kelly, D. L., Lassiter, K. R. L., Calogero, J. A., and Alexander, E.: Effects of local hypothermia and tissue oxygen studies in experimental paraplegia, J. Neurosurg. **33:**554, 1970.

70. Kobrine, A. I., and Doyle, T. F.: Role of histamine in posttraumatic spinal cord hyperemia and the luxury perfusion syndrome, J. Neurosurg. **44:**16, 1976.

71. Kobrine, A. I., Evans, D. E., and Rizzoli, H. V.: The effect of alpha adrenergic blockade on spinal cord auto-regulation in the monkey, J. Neurosurg. **46:**336, 1977.

72. Kobrine, A. I., Evans, D. E., and Rizzoli, H. V.: The effects of beta adrenergic blockade on spinal cord autoregulation in the monkey, J. Neurosurg. **47:**57, 1977.

73. Kobrine, A. I.: The neuronal theory of experimental traumatic spinal cord dysfunction, Surg. Neurol. **3:**261, 1975.

74. Koenig, G., and Dohrman, G. J.: Histopathological variability in "standardized" spinal cord trauma, J. Neurol. Neurosurg. Psychiatr. **40:**1203, 1977.

75. Krinsky, N. I.: Singlet excited oxygen as a mediator of the antibacterial action of leucocytes, Science **186:**363, 1974.

76. Kuchner, E. F., and Hansebout, R. R.: Combined steroid and hypothermia treatment of experimental spinal cord injury, Surg. Neurol. **6:**371, 1976.

77. Landau, B., and Ransohoff, J.: Late surgery for incomplete traumatic lesions of the conus medullaris and cauda equina, J. Neurosurg. **28:**256, 1968.

78. Lawrence, J. H., Loomis, W. F., Tobias, C. A., and Turpin, F. H.: Preliminary observation on the narcotic effects of xenon with a review of values for solubilities of gases in water and oils, J. Physiol. **105:**197, 1946.

79. Lucy, J. A.: Functional and structural aspects of biological membranes: a suggested structural role for vitamin E in the control of membrane permeability and stability, Ann. N.Y. Acad. Sci. **203:**4, 1972.

80. Lund-Oleson, K., and Memander, K. B.: Orgotein (SOD): a new anti-inflammatory metallo-protein drug: preliminary evaluation of clinical efficacy and safety in degenerative joint disease, Current Ther. Resp. **16:**706, 1974.

81. Matinian, L. A., and Andreasin, A. S.: Enzyme therapy in organic lesions of the spinal cord, Los Angeles, 1976, Brain Information Service, p. 156.

82. McGraw, C. P.: The effect of DMSO on cerebral infarction in the Mongolian gerbil, Acta Neurol. Scand. (suppl. 64) **56:**160, 1977.

83. Milvy, P., Kakari, S., Campbell, J. B., and Demopoulos, H. B.: Paramagnetic species and radical products in cat spinal cord, Ann. N.Y. Acad. Sci. **222:**1102, 1973.

84. Mitamura, J. A., Ioppolo, A., Seligman, M. L., Flamm, E. S., Ransohoff, J., and Demopoulos, H. B.: Loss of cholesterol and ascorbic acid in rat brain following cold trauma and protection by methylprednisolone (submitted for publication).

85. Mitamura, J. A., Shera, N., Seligman, M., Demopoulos, H. B., Flamm, E. S., and Ransohoff, J.: Membrane lipid loss with freeze lesion to rat brain and amelioration by methylprednisolone (submitted for publication).

86. Moncada, S., Gryglewski, R. J., Bunting, S., and Vane, J. R.: A lipid peroxide inhibits the enzyme in blood vessel microsomes that generates from prostaglandin endoperoxides the substance (prostaglandin X) which prevents platelet aggregation, Prostaglandins **12:**715, 1976.

87. Naftchi, N. E., Demeny, M., De Crescito, V., Tomasula, J., Flamm, E. S., and Campbell, J. B.: Biogenic amine concentrations in traumatized spinal cords of cats; effect of drug therapy, J. Neurosurg. **40:**52, 1974.

88. Nelson, E., Gertz, D. S., Rennels, M. L., Ducker, T. B., and Blaumanis, O. R.: Spinal cord injury: the role of vascular damage in the pathogenesis of central hemorrhagic necrosis, Arch. Neurol. **34:**332, 1977.

89. Nelson, E., and Rennels, M.: Innervation of intracranial arteries, Brain **93**:475, 1970.

90. O'Callaghan, M. A., and Duggan, P. F.: Differential effects of chlorpromazine and chlorpromazine free radical on calcium transport in sarcoplasmic reticulum vesicles, Biochem. Phramacol. **24**:563, 1975.

91. Ortega, B. D., Demopoulos, H. B., and Ransohoff, J.: Effect of antioxidants on experimental cold induced cerebral edema. Reulen, H. J., and Schurmann, K., editors: In Steroids and brain edema, New York, 1972, Springer-Verlag, p. 167.

92. Osterholm, J. L.: Noradrenergic mediation of traumatic spinal cord autodestruction, Life Sci. **14**:1363, 1974.

93. Pietronigro, D. D., Seligman, M. L., Jones, W. B. G., and Demopoulos, H. B.: Retarding effects of DNA on the aut-oxidation of liposome suspensions, Lipids **11**:808, 1976.

94. Popovic, P., Popovic, V., and Schaffer, R.: Levodopa-enhanced recovery from paralysis induced by air embolism, Surgery **79**:100, 1976.

95. Pulman, B., Coubeils, J. L., and Courriere, P.: A molecular orbital study of the conformation of barbiturates, J. Theor. Biol. **35**:375, 1972.

96. Ransohoff, J.: Lesions of the cauda equina, Clin. Neurosurg. **17**:331, 1970.

97. Rap, Z. M., and Wideman, J.: Changes in sulfhydryl group level and influence of exogenous glutathione on dynamics of vasogenic edema. In Pappius, H. M., and Feindel, W., editors: Dynamics of brain edema, 1976, Springer-Verlag, p. 164.

98. Rosenberg, P. H., Jansson, S. E., and Gripenberg, J.: Effects of halothane, thiopental, and lidocaine on fluidity of synaptic plasma membranes, Anesthesiology **46**:322, 1977.

99. Sandler, A. N., and Tator, C. H.: Effect of acute spinal cord compression injury on regional spinal cord blood flow in primates, J. Neurosurg. **45**:660, 1976.

100. Sandler, A. N., and Tator, C. H.: Review of the effect of spinal cord trauma on the vessels and blood flow in the spinal cord, J. Neurosurg. **45**:638, 1976.

101. Schaefer, A., Komlos, M., and Seregi, A.: Lipid peroxidation as the cause of the ascorbic acid induced decrease of ATPase activities of rat brain microsomes and its inhibition by biogenic amines and psychotropic drugs, Biochem. Pharmacol. **24**:1781, 1975.

102. Schneider, R. C.: Trauma to the spine and spinal cord. In Correlative neurosurgery. In Kahn, E. A., Crosby, E. C., Schneider, R. C., and Taren, J. A., editors: Springfield, Ill., 1969, Charles C Thomas, Publisher, p. 597.

103. Seeman, P.: The actions of nervous system drugs on cell membranes. In Weisman, G., and Clairborne, R., editors: Cell membranes, New York, 1975, HP Publishing Co., p. 239.

104. Seeman, P.: The membrane expansion theory of anesthesia. In Fink, B. R., editor: Molecular mechanisms of anesthesia, New York, 1975, Raven Press, p. 243.

105. Seligman, M. L., and Demopoulos, H. B.: Spin-probe analysis of membrane perturbations produced by chemical and physical agents, Ann. N.Y. Acad. Sci. **222**:640, 1973.

106. Seligman, M. L., Flamm, E. S., Goldstein, B., Demopoulos, H. B., and Ransohoff, J.: Spectro-fluorescent detection of malonaldehyde in response to ethanol potentiation of spinal cord trauma, Lipids **12**:945, 1977.

107. Seligman, M. L., Mitamura, J., Shera, N., and Demopoulos, H. B.: Corticosteroid (methylprednisolone) modulation of photoperoxidation by ultraviolet light in liposomes, Photochem. Photobiol. **29**:549, 1979.

108. Senter, H. J., and Venes, J. L.: Altered blood flow and secondary injury in experimental spinal cord trauma, New Orleans, 1978, American Association of Neurological Surgeons, p. 167.

109. Shields, C. L., and Stauffer, E. S.: Late instability in cervical spine fractures secondary to laminectomy, Clin. Orthop. **119**:144, 1976.

110. Sies, H., and Summer, K. H.: Hydroperoxide-metabolizing systems in rat liver, Eur. J. Biochem. **57**:503, 1975.

111. Singer, J. M., Russell, G. V., and Coe, J. E.: Changes in evoked potentials after experimental cervical spinal cord injury in the monkey, Exp. Neurol. **29**:449, 1970.

112. Smith, A. J. K., McCreery, D. B., Bloedel, J. R., and Chow, S. N.: Hyperemia, CO_2 responsiveness, and autoregulation in the white matter following experimental spinal cord injury, J. Neurosurg. **48**:239, 1978.

113. Spector, R.: Vitamin homeostasis in the central nervous system, N. Engl. J. Med. **296**:1393, 1977.

114. Spielholz, N., Benjamin, V., Engler, G., and Ransohoff, J.: Somatosensory evoked potentials and clinical outcome in spinal cord injury. In Popp, A. J., Bourke, R. S., Nelson, L. R., and Kimelberg, H. K., editors: Neural trauma, New York, 1979, Raven Press.

115. Steiner, M., and Anastasi, J.: Vitamin E, an inhibitor of the platelet release reaction, J. Clin. Invest. **57**:732, 1976.

116. Suzuki, O., and Yagi, K.: Formation of lipoperoxide in brain edema induced by cold injury, Experientia **30**:248, 1974.

117. Svare, A., and Talle, K.: Lumbar myelography with metrizamide; an evaluation of 15 cases, Acta Radiol. (suppl.) **335**:387, 1973.

118. Szmant, H. H.: Physical properties of DMSO and its functions in biological systems, Ann. N.Y. Acad. Sci. **243**:91, 1975.

119. Tator, C. H., and Deecke, L.: Value of normothermic perfusion, hypothermic perfusion and

acute durotomy in the treatment of experimental acute spinal cord trauma, J. Neurosurg. **39**:52, 1973.

120. Thienprasit, P., Bontli, H., Bloedel, J. R., and Chow, S. N.: Effect of delayed local cooling on experimental spinal cord injury, J. Neurosurg. **42**:150, 1975.

121. Tveten, L., and Salvesen, S.: Histology of the central nervous system of the rabbit after soboccipital injection of metrizamide, Acta Radiol. (suppl.) **335**:166, 1973.

122. Vladimirov, Y. A., Sergeev, P. V., Seifulla, R. D., and Rudnev, Y. N.: Effect of steroids on lipid peroxidation in liver mitochondrial membranes, Moleculyainaya Biologiya **7**:247, 1973 (translated by Consultants Bureau, Plenum Publishing Corp., New York).

123. Wagner, F. C., Van Gilder, J. C., and Dohrman, G. J.: Pathological changes from acute to chronic in experimental spinal cord trauma, J. Neurosurg. **48**:92, 1978.

124. Wahl, M., and Kuschinsky, W.: Dependency of the dilatory action of adenosine on the perivascular H$^+$ and K$^+$ at pial arteries of cats, Acta Neurol. Scand. (suppl. 64) **56**:218, 1977.

125. Walling, C., and Huyser, E. S.: Free radical additions to olefins to form carbon-carbon bonds. In Adams, R., Blatt, A. H., Boekelheide, V., Cairns, T. L., Cope, A. C., Curtin, D. Y., and Niemann, C., editors: Organic reactions, vol. 13, New York, 1963, John Wiley & Sons, p. 91.

126. Wei, E., Wong, L. C. K., and Hine, C. H.: Selective potentiation of carbon tetrachloride hepatotoxicity by ethanol, Arch. Int. Pharmacodyn. **189**:5, 1971.

127. Weiss, H. J.: Platelet physiology and abnormalities of platelet function, N. Engl. J. Med. **293**: 531, 1975.

128. Weissman, G.: Corticosteroids and membrane stabilization, Circulation (suppl. I) **53**:I-171, 1976.

129. Whitesides, T. E., and Shah, S. G. A.: On the management of unstable fractures of the thoracolumbar spine, Spine **1**:99, 1976.

130. Wideman, J., and Domanska-Janik, K.: Regulation of thiols in brain. I. Concentration of thiols and glutathione reductase activity in different parts of rat brain during hypoxia, Resuscitation **3**:27, 1974.

131. Williams, M. L., Shott, R. T., O'Neal, P. L., and Oski, F. A.: Role of dietary iron and fat on the vitamin E deficiency anemia of infancy, N. Engl. J. Med. **292**:887, 1975.

132. Windle, W. F., Smart, J. O., and Beers, J. J.: Residual function after subtotal spinal cord transection in adult cats, Neurology **8**:518, 1958.

133. Wood, D. C., and Wood, J.: Pharmacologic and biochemical considerations of DMSO, Ann. N.Y. Acad. Sci. **243**:7, 1975.

134. Yu, W. H. A., Yu, M. C., and Young, P. A.: Ultrastructural changes in the cerebrovascular endothelium induced by a diet high in linoleic acid and deficient in vitamin E, Exp. Mol. Pathol. **21**: 289, 1974.

135. Zervas, N. J., Hori, H., and Rosoff, C. B.: Experimental inhibition of serotonin by antibiotic: prevention of cerebral vasospasm, J. Neurosurg. **41**:59, 1974.

17

Induced hypotension

JAMES E. COTTRELL
BHAGWANDAS GUPTA
HERMAN TURNDORF

Deliberate hypotension to provide a bloodless field and better neurosurgical operative conditions was first proposed by Harvey Cushing in 1917.[14] When this technique is properly used, operative blood loss, operative time, morbidity, and mortality are decreased. Blood pressure is decreased chemically by direct or indirect arterial or venous dilators or by autonomic ganglion blocking agents. Perfusion pressure decreases proportionate to the decrease in vascular flow resistance, and within wide limits adequate tissue blood flow persists. Fine pressure adjustments, which may be needed to achieve the desired level of hypotension, can be attained by superimposing body position changes, altering airway pressure, control of heart rate, or the addition of other vasoactive drugs whose effects may complement the primary hypotensive agent. A safe hypotensive technique should be easily controllable, should not alter cerebral autoregulation or increase cerebral blood volume, should have a short plasma and biological half-life, should be nontoxic, and produce no toxic metabolites. The rational combination of combining drugs and mechanical maneuvers to induce hypotension are considered in this chapter.

PHARMACOLOGIC INDUCTION

Drugs presently used to induce hypotension include sodium nitroprusside (SNP),
glyceryl trinitrate (GTN), trimetaphan camsylate, pentolinium tartrate, and halothane (see box below). SNP directly dilates resistance vessels[23] and GTN predominantly dilates capacitance vessels.[22] Sympathetic ganglion transmission is blocked by trimetaphan and pentolinium, resulting in arteriolar and venular dilatation and usually decreased arterial pressure.[24] Increasing inspired halothane concentration progressively depresses myocardial contractility, stroke volume, and arterial pressure.[30]

Sodium nitroprusside (SNP)

SNP is presently the most widely used hypotensive agent in neurosurgical patients because plasma half-life is short and toxicity is relatively low if less than 1 mg/kg is infused in two to three hours or 0.5 mg/kg is infused in 24 hours.[39] Cerebral blood flow (CBF) can remain adequate even if mean cerebral perfusion pressure (CPP) is reduced

---

**COMMONLY USED DRUGS
FOR DELIBERATE HYPOTENSION**

Sodium nitroprusside
Glyceryl trinitrate
Trimetaphan camsylate
Pentolinium tartrate
Halothane

---

to 40 torr because cardiac output (CO) does not decrease proportionate to cerebrovascular resistance (CVR) decrease.[52] SNP-induced hemodynamic changes are due primarily to direct action on vessel walls and not to primary myocardial effects. Vessel wall relaxation results from nonspecific sulfhydryl receptor stimulation by SNP-relaxing contractile mechanisms, thereby producing vasodilation (Fig. 17-1).[41] Unless the rate of SNP infusion is controlled, blood cyanide (CN) and thiocyanate concentration may increase to dangerous (toxic) levels.[16] Tachyphylaxis may occur if high blood CN (>100 μg/100 ml) and metabolic acidosis occur.[2,12] Plasma renin activity (PRA) increases during SNP infusion, and this may result in rebound hypertension (RH).[10] Intracranial pressure (ICP) may be increased secondary to vasodilatation with decreased intracranial compli-

ance.[13,56] CN has been found in cerebrospinal fluid (CSF) during SNP infusion and may be a cause of cerebral hypoxemia.[11] Decreased platelet concentration and aggregation have been described.[37,44] Hypothyroidism after prolonged administration has been described as a result of thiocyanate blocking of thyroidal iodide uptake (see box, p. 389).[42]

Metabolism and toxicity. SNP is slowly decomposed to CN on contact with tissue and red blood cell (RBC) sulfhydryl groups.[43] SNP diffuses into RBCs rapidly. Cyanmethemoglobin and an unstable tetracyano compound believed to be $\{Fe(CN)_4 NO \cdot 2H_2O\}$[51] are formed when hemoglobin (Hgb) donates an electron to SNP. CN released by this unstable iron compound combines with thiosulfate to form thiocyanate (SCN) in a reaction catalyzed by liver and kidney rho-

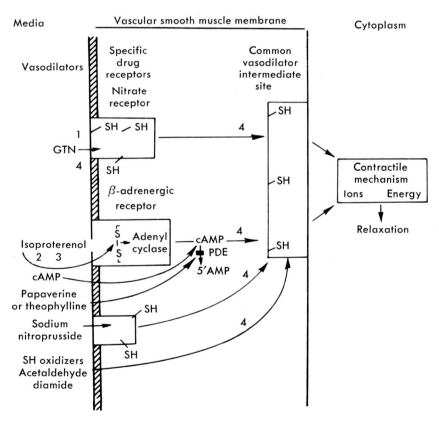

Fig. 17-1. Schematic diagram of the mechanism of action of vasodilators. (From Needleman, P., Jakschkik, B., and Johnson, E. M., Jr.: J. Pharmacol. Exp. Ther. **187:**324, 1973; © 1973 The Williams & Wilkins Co., Baltimore.)

SNP-INDUCED ABNORMALITIES

Cyanide and thiocyanate toxicity
Tachyphylaxis
Rebound hypertension
↑ Intracranial pressure
↑ Cerebrospinal fluid cyanide
↓ Platelet concentration and aggregation
Hypothyroidism

danese. Water-soluble cyanocobalamin results from CN combination with hydroxocobalamin, and both appear in the urine. Some hydrogen CN is exhaled (Fig. 17-2). CN reacts with the trivalent iron of mitochrondrial cytochrome to form a cytochrome oxidase–CN complex, which inhibits cellular respiration and results in cytotoxic hypoxia (Fig. 17-3). Fatalities have been reported when concentration of this complex is high.[27] Blood CN level is related to the total dose

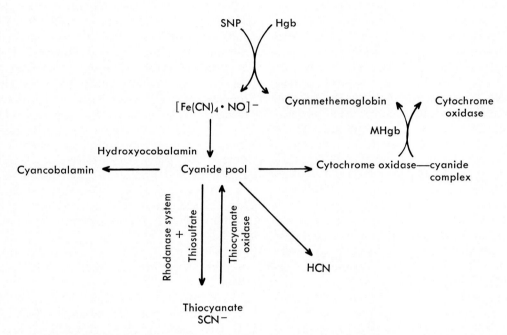

Fig. 17-2. Red blood cell biotransformation of sodium nitroprusside. (SNP, sodium nitroprusside; Hgb, hemoglobin; mHgb, methemoglobin; SCN⁻, thiocyanate; HCN, hydrogen cyanide.)

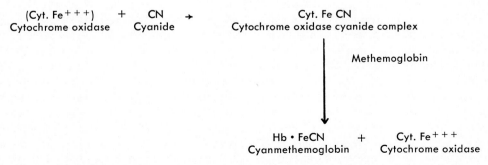

Fig. 17-3. Tissue cytochrome oxidase combines with cyanide to form cytochrome oxidase–cyanide complex. Methemoglobin frees cyanide from complex, forming cyanmethemoglobin.

Table 17-1. Nitroprusside safe dose

Date	Study	Dose (mg/kg/2-3 hrs)
1975	Davies	3.0
1976	Vesey	1.5
1977	Michenfelder	1.0-1.5
1979	Cottrell	0.5-0.7

of SNP administered per unit of time. If more than 0.7 mg/kg SNP is administered within three hours, CN level of 75 to 100 μg/100 ml may be seen in blood, and metabolic acidosis occurs as tissue oxygenation is impaired.[9] Four to 12 mg/kg of intravenous CN has been associated with death in humans.[18] One milligram of SNP contains .44 mg of CN. A total dose of 7.9 to 27.3 mg/kg of SNP can result in death. Of the fatalities attributed to SNP-induced CN toxicity, blood CN level in one patient was 400 μg/100 ml.[15] Signs of toxicity include tachycardia, metabolic acidosis, and eventual shock. Specific ion electrodes are now available to measure blood CN concentration in relatively simple fashion by reading millivolt electrode potentials of blood that can be referred to electrode potentials of standard CN solutions.[54] Lengthy biochemical methods are difficult and time consuming.[47] Correlation of blood CN level with subsequent metabolic acidosis has led to decreasing recommendations for safe limits of SNP dose (see Table 17-1). The diagnosis of impending CN toxicity should be made by measurement of blood CN level, since acidosis develops after CN transfer from blood and significant binding of CN to tissue.

Blood CN can be decreased chemically, but these methods in themselves are hazardous. Amyl nitrite and sodium nitrite can be given intravenously to facilitate methemoglobin (mHgb) formation.[6] CN combines preferentially with mHgb to form cyanmethemoglobin, preventing the cytochrome oxidase–CN tissue complex from forming (Fig. 17-3). Since mHgb does not readily give up oxygen to tissue, a cytotoxic hypoxia is converted to an anoxic hypoxia. Intravenous sodium thiosulfate acts as a sulfur

donor that facilitates conversion of CN to TCN through rhodanese systems.[40] TCN can be excreted in urine. TCN oxidase, however, can reconvert TCN to CN, increasing the likelihood of CN toxicity. Cobalamines are normally supplied in the diet and can combine with blood and tissue CN to form cyanocobalamin that is water soluble and rapidly excreted in the urine. In animals, hydroxocobalamin can decrease blood CN level after SNP.[45] Industrial CN poisoning has effectively been treated with intravenous hydroxocobalamin.[59] Intravenous hydroxocobalamin administered concomitantly with SNP results in lower blood CN level than SNP administered without hydroxocobalamin (Fig. 17-4).[9] The efficacy of hydroxocobalamin in reversing actual SNP-induced CN toxicity remains to be demonstrated. Hydroxocobalamin can be obtained after application for an Investigational New Drug Number from the Food and Drug Administration: Bureau of Drugs, Department of Health, Education and Welfare, Public Health Service, Rockville, MD 20857. Consent from Institutional Research Committees and patients are necessary prior to intravenous use.

SNP dose requirement and metabolism decrease in patients anesthetized with halothane.[5]

Tachyphylaxis. Increasing SNP dose requirements to maintain vascular effect has been described.[2,12] The pharmacologic mechanism of tachyphylaxis has not been satisfactorily explained, but high blood CN level may interfere with smooth muscle relaxation required to produce vasodilatation. SNP-induced vascular dilatation decreases as perfusion CN level increases in vitro. A similar failure to relax was seen as perfusate pH decreased.[55] This suggests that elevated CN prevents vasodilatation by interfering with vascular sulfhydryl receptor site oxidation, and this effect can be augmented by metabolic acidosis. Blood CN level is higher in patients who develop tachyphylaxis than in those who do not, and tachyphylaxis has been reported in patients without evidence of metabolic acidosis (Fig. 17-5).[12]

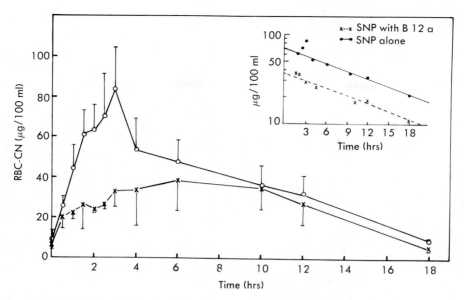

Fig. 17-4. Red cell cyanide (μg/100 ml) after sodium nitroprusside alone *(upper curve)* and after sodium nitroprusside and hydroxocobalamin *(lower curve).* (From Cottrell, J. E., Casthely, P., Brodie, J. D., and others: N. Engl. J. Med. **298**:809, 1978.)

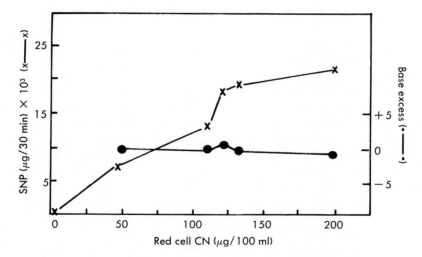

Fig. 17-5. Increasing sodium nitroprusside dose requirement and blood cyanide level with normal acid-base status in three tachyphylactic patients.

SNP should be promptly discontinued if tachyphylaxis develops, since high blood CN will result and may lead to CN toxicity.

Intracranial pressure (ICP). SNP dilates cerebral resistance vessels directly and may result in increased cerebral blood volume. If intracranial compliance is decreased, SNP in-fusion can increase ICP (Table 17-2).[13,56] The rapidity of cranial vessel dilatation and venous engorgement prevents accommodation by cerebrospinal fluid (CSF) transloca-tion from the cranium. Methods to im-prove intracranial compliance such as hy-perventilation and diuretic or barbiturate

Table 17-2. Cerebral perfusion pressure after hypotension induced by sodium nitroprusside (SNP)*

Measurement (torr)	Pre-SNP	Post-SNP
MAP	104 ± 2.55	70.9 ± 3.61
ICP	14.58 ± 1.76	27.61 ± 3.16
CPP	89.32 ± 3.57	43.23 ± 4.60

*From Cottrell, J. E., and others: J. Neurosurg. 48: 330, 1978. Mean arterial pressure (MAP) reduced by 33%; ICP, intracranial pressure; CPP, cerebral perfusion pressure.

Table 17-3. SNP-induced systolic blood pressure (SBP) changes

	Pre-SNP	During SNP	After SNP (30 min)
SBP (n = 12)	112 ± 3.92*	75 ± 3.08	144 ± 5.60†

*Mean ± S.E.M.
†Statistically significant (P < 0.001).

therapy may prevent or significantly reduce this increase. SNP should not be used in patients with low intracranial compliance until the cranium has been opened or until compliance has been improved by drugs or CSF drainage. If blood pressure reduction is necessary during anesthetic induction, intraoperatively before opening the cranium, in the postoperative period, or in the neurosurgical intensive care unit, other drugs that do not raise ICP like trimetaphan can be used.[56]

Rebound hypertension (RH). A 20 torr or greater systolic blood pressure (SBP) increase lasting 30 minutes has been described after abruptly discontinuing SNP[33] (Table 17-3). Plasma renin activity (PRA) increases after SNP in animals[31] and humans, possibly because of renal artery dilatation or renal ischemia (Fig. 17-6).[10] Renin has a plasma half-life (T½) of 30 minutes,[38] and SNP has a two-minute T½. Renin converts angiotensinogen to angiotensin I. Angiotensin II, a potent constrictor, is produced, and its activity continues for some

time after SNP vasodilation. RH may be particularly hazardous in the neurosurgical patient, since the upper limits of autoregulation can be exceeded and cerebral edema may form. To prevent RH, SNP infusion should be discontinued slowly over a period of 30 to 45 minutes. Propranolol decreases renin release and may be therapeutically useful. Saralysin (sarcosyl-1-alanine-8-angiotensin-II), if it becomes clinically available, may also be a useful agent to decrease RH.

Cerebrospinal fluid cyanide. Blood cyanide has been detected and measured in CSF after intravenous SNP in humans during craniotomy. CN increase in CSF follows blood CN level directly but in lesser amounts.[11] CN is a small molecule (MW 26) that can diffuse across membranes and transfers from plasma to CSF across the blood-brain barrier. Possible crossing sites include the choroid plexus, the arachnoid membrane overlying the subarachnoid space, and the tight junctional zones of epithelial cells. CN may also enter the CSF by a excretory "sink" action of CSF that extracts CN from the brain. CN encephalopathy with toxic edema may occur if significant diffusion of CN into the brain occurs. Patients with impaired autoregulation and reduced CBF may develop brain damage when exposed to minimal amounts of CN if significant quantities of cytochrome oxidase–CN complex form. Caution is advised when using SNP in patients with impaired autoregulation or with decreased intracerebral collateral circulation.

Platelet effects. Platelet disintegration and inhibition of human platelet aggregation in vitro has been reported.[37,44] Significant reduction in mean platelet count from 293,875 ± 31,336 to 200,125 ± 27,340 per cu mm one to six hours after SNP infusion, which returned to normal at 24 hours, has been reported in patients with congestive heart failure.[37] If SNP is to be given to patients with abnormal platelet activity or numbers or preexisting coagulopathies, laboratory tests should monitor the adequacy of coagulation.

Administration. SNP is supplied in a 5

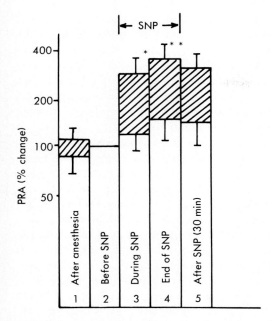

Fig. 17-6. Percentage change in plasma renin activity after SNP. Sample 2 equals 100% (log $\overline{X} \pm$ S.E.M.). *1,* After anesthesia. *2,* Before SNP. *3,* After SNP. *4,* End of SNP. *5,* 30 minutes after SNP. Asterisks indicate significant change; stippled area indicates study group.

ml amber rubber stoppered vial containing 50 mg of SNP dihydrate. SNP can be dissolved in 5% dextrose in water (D_5W) to the concentration desired. Fifty milligrams of SNP in 250, 500, or 1000 ml of D_5W makes a concentration of 200 μg, 100 μg, or 50 μg/ml, respectively. Once dissolved, SNP deteriorates in the presence of light. The container therefore should be wrapped in aluminum foil. An unstable SNP ion in aqueous solution reacts with a variety of substances within three to four hours to form highly colored salts. Other drugs should not be infused in same solution as SNP.

Since vascular response to SNP can be dramatic, SNP should be administered with an infusion pump (Sigmamotor's Volumet model 4200) or a Volutrol intravenous set. We prefer an infusion pump, since infusion rate remains more constant than with a microdrip regulator. When microdrip

techniques are used, a continuous increase in flow rate or increase height of the infusion may be required.

The usual dose of SNP is 0.5 to 10 μg/kg/min. Infusion is begun at 1 μg/kg/min and increased to achieve the desired MAP. If adequate reduction of blood pressure is not obtained with 10 μg/kg/min within 10 to 15 minutes, the infusion should be stopped to avoid CN toxicity. Direct arterial manometry should be used during SNP infusion.

Glyceryl trinitrate (nitroglycerin)

Glyceryl trinitrate (GTN) can be used intravenously to induce hypotension.[21] GTN has a short plasma half-life, is easy to control, and has no direct toxic effects or toxic metabolites. GTN dilates vessels directly by reacting with vascular smooth muscle sulfhydryl groups to form disulfide linkage and release of inorganic nitrite, which leads to relaxation (Fig. 17-1). GTN acts predominantly on capacitance vessels resulting in decreased venous return.[22] Progressive decrease in stroke volume reduces MAP.

GTN may not induce hypotension in younger patients, especially during narcotic-supplemented nitrous oxide–oxygen anesthesia. These patients may require other agents or techniques for significant blood pressure reduction.[21]

Metabolism and toxicity. GTN is rapidly metabolized in the liver by partial denitration catalyzed by gluthathione (GSH)-organic nitrate reductase to 1,3 and 1,2 glyceryl denitrate (GDH), glyceryl mononitrate (GMH), and inorganic nitrate. Most metabolites can be recovered in the urine within 24 hours. The half-life of GTN appears to be two minutes in rats and humans because of redistribution and rapid hepatic metabolism. The possibility of accumulating significant quantities of mHgb formation exists, since for each mole of GTN metabolized, one mole of nitrite (NO_2) is formed. We and others, however, have not detected measureable amounts of mHgb after 200 mg of intravenous GTN.

Intracranial pressure. Glyceryl trinitrate acts primarily on capacitance vessels with little arteriorlar dilatation. For this reason it has been suggested that ICP increase will not occur in patients with decreased compliance.[7] We and others, however, have found that ICP increase does occur after GTN-induced hypotension (Fig. 17-7).[25] This increase is attributed to increased cerebral blood volume from capacitance vessel dilatation. Cranial venous pressure increases from acute pooling of blood in the cranium before exit through rigid venous channels. CSF translocation from the cranium is slower than intracranial blood volume change. GTN, like SNP, should probably not be used intraoperatively until the dura is opened unless other methods to increase intracranial compliance or decrease ICP have been done. Prior to this, trimetaphan can be used to treat hypertension.

GTN may be preferable for induced hypotension in the neurosurgical patient, since toxic biotransformation products, tachyphylaxis, and RH have not been reported following its use.

GTN administration. GTN is supplied in 20 ml glass ampules containing 10 mg of GTN or 500 μg/ml. An investigational new drug number must be obtained from the Food and Drug Administration. Institutional Research Committee approval and patient consent must be obtained before intravenous use. GTN solution as obtained from the manufacturer is relatively stable when exposed to light and can be kept up to two years without refrigeration.

GTN is infused continuously for deliberate hypotension or to control increased blood pressure using a direct intravenous infusion without dilution. GTN is adsorbed by plastic bags and should be infused from glass bottles. An infusion pump is best for infusion at a beginning rate of 1 to 2 μg/kg/min with increases to achieve the desired blood pressure level. Good hypotensive response is usually seen at 2 μg/kg/min. Upper limits of infusion have not been set, since toxic effects have not been described.

Halothane

Halothane hypotension is produced by increasing inspired halothane concentration. Hypotension results primarily from myocardial depression. Vasodilatation occurs in the skin, brain, and splanchnic vessels, but

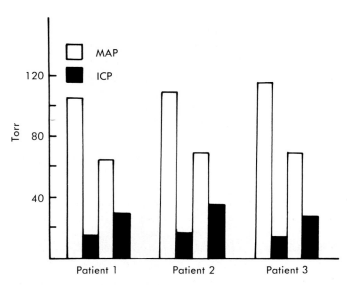

Fig. 17-7. Intracranial pressure increase in three patients after nitroglycerin-induced hypotension.

peripheral resistance does not decrease significantly because the tone of skeletal muscle and renal vessels increases.[30]

Halothane decreases cerebrovascular tone and will increase CBF in a dose-related manner provided that autoregulation limits are not exceeded.[32] ICP may be increased by the intracerebral blood volume increase that accompanies decreased vascular resistance. Cerebral autoregulation is lost as halothane concentration increases.[32] The combination of ICP increase and MAP decrease may result in a fall in CPP to less than 40 torr; if this is allowed to persist, brain ischemia may result. Hyperventilation can prevent cerebral halothane vasodilation;[1] but ICP increase has been reported in hyperventilated patients (Pa_{CO_2} 25 torr) with mass lesions after halothane.[28,29]

In the vasodilated state, cerebral edema is more likely to occur if systemic blood pressure is allowed to increase above 150 torr. The possibility of a secondary neurologic injury during halothane anesthesia therefore exists. In animals, greater neurologic deficits follow experimental focal ischemia if halothane anesthesia is used than if a barbiturate-based anesthetic sequence is used.[50]

We believe that halothane should not be used to induce neurosurgical hypotension because high concentration may be required, ICP increases before dural opening, and autoregulation loss, edema formation, and increased morbidity can occur. In addition, halothane biotransformation products may lead to organ toxicity.[57]

Ganglionic blocking agents

Of the numerous ganglionic blocking agents described since their accidental discovery in 1948, only trimetaphan is manufactured in the United States. Hypotension results from transmission blockade through autonomic ganglia as the result of receptor site occupancy and by postsynaptic membrane stabilization.[24] Because of their unselective nature on autonomic ganglia, parasympathetic as well as sympathetic activity is depressed. Parasympathetic depression leads to unwanted effects like tachycardia,

mydriasis, cycloplegia, reduced tone and gastrointestinal motility, and urinary retention.

Trimetaphan camsylate

Other than its ganglionic blocking properties, trimetaphan produces hypotension by histamine release and direct vasodilatation.[58] Trimetaphan has a half-life of one to two minutes because of rapid inactivation by plasma cholinesterase and renal excretion. This short half-life makes for easy control. Theoretical problems associated with trimetaphan include histamine release, which can dilate cerebral blood vessels and increase ICP. Histamine-induced bronchospasm, tachyphylaxis, and even myoneural blockade have been reported after trimetaphan.[27]

Direct cerebral toxic effects following trimetaphan have been reported. EEG burst suppression, slowing and high voltage waves,[36] and high brain lactate level suggesting increased glycolytic activity have been reported at MAP of 50 torr. This did not occur with other hypotensive drugs.[39] Trimetaphan may be the agent of choice for treating hypertension in the neurosurgical patient, since ICP increase has not been reported as MAP decreases.[56] This possibly can be explained by gradual reduction in MAP with autoregulation maintenance and little change in ICP. Trimetaphan probably should be avoided for induced hypotension to MAP of 50 torr because of evidence of direct cerebral toxicity.

Administration. Trimetaphan camsylate is obtained in 10 ml glass ampules containing 500 mg (50 mg/ml). Freshly prepared solutions should be used and excess discarded after 24 hours. A 0.2% solution (2 mg/ml) is prepared by dissolving 500 mg in 250 ml D_5W.

An infusion pump can be used to start the infusion at a rate of 2 to 4 mg/min (30 to 50 μg/kg/min) and titrated to achieve and maintain the desired level of hypotension. Desired hypotensive levels are usually obtained after 0.2 to 5 mg/min trimetaphan intravenously. Direct and continuous arterial blood pressure monitoring should be used. If resistance to high dosage occurs, head up tilt or increased airway pressure may be needed. If pressure still does not decrease, another hypotensive method should be chosen.

Pentolinium tartrate

Pentolinium is presently not manufactured in the United States. Pentolinium has a longer half-life than trimetaphan. It is given as a single intravenous dose of 2 mg and repeated every 15 minutes until the desired pressure level is attained. Peak action is 30 minutes and may last from one to four hours. MAP below 50 torr probably should not be induced with pentolinium because of its long duration of action. Pentolinium may have advantages for treating hypertension and inducing hypotension because intracranial compliance is not altered. Direct cerebral toxic effects have not been reported after pentolinium and histamine release is much less.

MECHANICAL MANEUVERS

Alterations in body position, mechanical ventilation, heart rate, and blood volume can be used in conjunction with the previously described drugs to obtain the desired hypotensive level. These mechanical maneuvers when used properly will decrease the total dose of potentially toxic drugs necessary for maintenance of hypotension.

Position

In the head-up position, gravitational forces produce venous pooling in the extremities, thereby effectively reducing venous return to the heart. This reduces cardiac output, stroke volume, and MAP. Position should be used cautiously in neurosurgical patients if autoregulation is altered, since flow will vary passively with perfusion pressure. For each 1 inch of head elevation above the heart, perfusion pressure decreases 2 torr.[20] If extreme head-up position is needed, MAP should be transduced at head level to minimize the likelihood of cerebral ischemia.

Positive airway pressure (PAWP)

PAWP increases mean intrathoracic pressure and decreases MAP by decreasing venous return to the heart.[8] Increase in respiratory dead space occurs when mean airway pressure increases effectively reducing pulmonary perfusion.[19]

PAWP by increasing intrathoracic pressure decreases venous outflow from the cranium. As cranial venous outflow pressure increases, cerebral blood volume increases and edema formation is facilitated. This increase in cerebral blood volume will increase ICP, especially in the supine position.[46] Head-up position will aid venous outflow by gravitational forces. The hazards of positive end expiratory pressure (PEEP) have been discussed in Chapter 11.

Pacemaker-induced hypotension

Increasing heart rate may progressively decrease ventricular diastolic filling time, stroke volume, cardiac output, and MAP.[17] Significant impairment of cardiac output produces tissue hypoperfusion and leads to metabolic acidosis. Mechanical hazards from pacemaker insertion and cardiac arrhythmias have prevented wide popularity of this technique.

MONITORING DURING DELIBERATE HYPOTENSION

Routine monitoring in the neurosurgical patient during induced hypotension should include electrocardiogram (ECG), blood pressure cuff, temperature probe, esophageal stethoscope, and Foley, central venous (CVP), and arterial catheters. Balloon-tipped flow directed thermodilution catheters for pulmonary artery pressure (PAP) measurement and CO calculation, subarachnoid screw for measurement of ICP, electroencephalogram (EEG) for neurophysiologic brain monitoring (Chapter 18), and Doppler (Chapter 9) for detection of air embolism are frequently necessary.

Electrocardiogram

Proper ECG monitoring is necessary during induced hypotension to detect rhythm disturbances. Myocardial ischemia can be detected with reasonable certainty by monitoring V_5. If ST segment changes occur, blood pressure level should be adjusted accordingly if arterial oxygenation and pH are normal.

Blood pressure cuff

A sphygmomanometer is helpful for determining the accuracy of indwelling arterial catheter transduced values when placed on the same arm or during periods of equipment malfunction.

Temperature

Temperature monitoring is especially important when hypotension is induced, since body heat dissipates more rapidly from dilated vessels. Lowered body temperature may decrease the effectiveness of vasodilators and increase dose requirements if compensatory vasoconstriction occurs. Rectal or midesophageal temperature measurement reflects core temperature.

Urine volume

Decreases in urinary output may indicate decreased renal perfusion and the need for higher blood pressure. Ionic and fluid replacement should be adequate prior to blood pressure level adjustment.

Central venous pressure (CVP)

CVP monitoring prior to induced hypotension aids in assessing adequacy of effective circulating blood volume. Greater hypotensive response will be seen in hypovolemic patients at the onset of deliberate hypotension. CVP catheters aid in treating air emboli (see Chapter 9).

Arterial catheters

Direct indwelling arterial catheters are accepted routine technique for all neurosurgical patients for continuous blood pressure monitoring and determination of arterial blood gas values. Radial, femoral, or brachial arteries are suitable for short-term cannulation. The temporal and dorsalis pedis arteries can be used, but cannulation may

be difficult to achieve and maintain because of their small diameter. After proper testing for patency of the palmar arch, radial artery cannulation is preferable over other arteries. Hazards have been described and include proximal arterial thrombosis and thrombotic and air emboli.[4] Arterial lines should be flushed continuously with heparin solution at 1 ml/min using an infuser. Manual flushing with blood pumps should be avoided, since damage to the intima occurs, enhancing thrombus formation.

Pulmonary artery catheters

Pulmonary artery pressures (PAPs) and calculation of CO have become easy with the introduction of balloon-tipped flow-directed thermodilution catheters. Techniques for catheter insertion have been described.[53] PAP is used to monitor fluid status, left heart function (especially in patients with ischemic or valvular heart disease), and to obtain mixed venous oxygen content (PV_{O_2}). Increase in PV_{O_2} at low MAP may indicate decreased tissue perfusion and oxygen extraction from hemoglobin.

An acute PAP increase in the sitting position suggests air embolus. Aspiration can be attempted through the CVP catheter if the catheter is perforated 30 cm proximal to the balloon tip where the superior vena cava joins the right atrium (Chapter 9).

Intracranial pressure monitoring

ICP monitoring (Chapter 4) is important during induction of hypotension because SNP, GTN, halothane, and PAWP increase cerebral blood volume and ICP. Significant increase can be treated appropriately and brain damage prevented.

CEREBRAL EFFECTS OF INDUCED HYPOTENSION

Induced hypotension ideally should decrease CPP without significantly decreasing CBF. This occurs when circulating blood volume and CO remain near normal as CVR decreases.

CBF will not support cerebral metabolism ($CMRO_2$) when mean CPP falls below 40 torr. CBF less than 18 ml/100 g/min occurs at 40 torr CPP.[49] Higher levels of CPP and CBF are required to maintain $CMRO_2$ in patients with chronic hypertension or altered autoregulation.[35] Compromised blood flow in vessels compressed by mass lesions will further decrease during deliberate hypotension. Lower CPP and CBF value may be permissible when anesthetic drugs suppress $CMRO_2$.

Lower limits of CPP and CBF necessary to maintain $CMRO_2$ have been determined in animals and humans by monitoring changes in jugular venous oxygen saturation, brain electrical activity (EEG), brain energy substances and metabolites, and regional CBF (rCBF) measurements.

Jugular venous oxygen saturation reflects the relationship between total CBF and $CMRO_2$. It is not a reliable method of determining regional cerebral ischemia. Jugular oxygen tension is normally 40 torr. During anesthesia with normotension increases to 55 torr have been documented with FI_{O_2} of 1. Increases in jugular venous oxygen above steady state may indicate decreases in cerebral perfusion with lack of brain tissue oxygen extraction from Hgb if FI_{O_2} remains constant.

Brain electrical activity can be monitored with a multichannel EEG, which is a reliable method of diagnosing regional ischemia (see Chapter 18). However, placement of electrodes would at best be difficult during craniotomy. Generally, EEG abnormalities occur when CBF falls below 18 ml/100 g/min or CPP falls below 40 torr.[3] Trimetaphan-induced hypotension, however, produces EEG abnormalities at MAPs of 50 torr.[36]

Brain energy substances—adenosine triphosphate, phosphocreatinine, glucose, glucose-6-phosphate and alpha-keto-gluterate—decrease when CBF is inadequate. Increasing concentration of brain lactate, pyruvate, and lactate/pyruvate ratio indicate brain ischemia and increased glycolysis. Decreases in brain energy substances and increases in glycolytic products occur when MAP reduction less than 50 torr is induced by SNP, trimetaphan, or halothane in animals.[39]

Regional CBF can be measured utilizing radioactive isotopes (Chapter 1). These measurements are difficult to achieve in the operating room with the cranium open. CBF normally varies from 18 to 80 ml/100 g/min.[34]

Maintenance of flow is critical when blood oxygen content is low.[48] Decreases in arterial oxygen tension (Pa_{O_2}) below 40 torr with normal CBF results in increased metabolites suggestive of ischemia but little change in brain energy substance. As CBF decreases with low Pa_{O_2}, evidence of brain energy substance depletion and progressive ischemia develop.

Alterations in arterial CO_2 affects cerebral metabolism, especially with induced hypotension (MAP 50 torr). As Pa_{CO_2} increases above 45 torr, brain energy substance concentration progressively decreases and lactate, pyruvate, and lactate/pyruvate ratios increase. Hypocarbia (Pa_{CO_2} less than 25 torr) with hypotension (MAP of 50 torr) produces metabolic changes consistent with depletion of brain energy supply and brain lactate acidosis.[26]

MAP can be reduced to 50 torr safely in most patients. Brain energy substances and metabolic breakdown products are not altered by the hypotensive drugs previously discussed except for trimetaphan at these pressures. Higher MAPs may be necessary in hypertensive patients with altered autoregulation in brain regions compressed by masses. CBF must be maintained during hypoxemia. Arterial CO_2 should be 35 to 45 torr during induced hypotension.

REFERENCES

1. Adams, R. W., Gronert, G. A., Sundt, T. M., and Michenfelder, J. D.: Halothane, hypocapnia and cerebrospinal fluid pressure in neurosurgery, Anesthesiology 37:510, 1972.
2. Amaranath, L., and Kellermeyer, W. F.: Tachyphylaxis to sodium nitroprusside, Anesthesiology 44:345, 1976.
3. Astrup, J., Symon, L., Brauston, N. M., and others: Cortical evoked potential and extracellular K^+ and H^+ at critical levels of brain ischemia, Stroke 8:51, 1977.

4. Bedford, R. F., and Wollman, H.: Complications on percutaneous radial artery cannulation; an objective propective study in man, Anesthesiology **38:** 228, 1973.

5. Behnia, R., Raymon, F., Cheng, S. C., and others: Metabolism of sodium nitroprusside in dogs awake and anesthetized with halothane, Anesthesiology **48:**260, 1978.

6. Chen, K., Rose, C. L., and Clowes, G. H.: Comparative values of several antidotes in cyanide poisoning, Am. J. Med. Sci. **188:**767, 1934.

7. Chestnut, J. S., Albin, M. S., Gonzalez-Abola, E., and others: Clinical evaluation of intravenous nitroglycerin for neurosurgery, J. Neurosurg. **48:** 704, 1978.

8. Cournand, M., Motley, J. L., Werko, L., and others: Physiological studies of the effects of intermittent positive pressure breathing on cardiac output in man, Am. J. Physiol. **152:**162, 1948.

9. Cottrell, J. E., Casthely, P., Brodie, J. D., and others: Prevention of nitroprusside-induced cyanide toxicity with hydroxocobalamin, N. Engl. J. Med. **298:**809, 1978.

10. Cottrell, J. E., Illner, P., Kittay, M. J., and others: Rebound hypertension after sodium nitroprusside-induced hypotension, Clin. Pharmacol. Ther. (In press.)

11. Cottrell, J. E., Patel, K., Casthely, P., and others: CSF cyanide after nitroprusside, Anesth. Analg. (Cleve.) (submitted for publication).

12. Cottrell, J. E., Patel, K., Casthely, P., and others: Nitroprusside tachyphylaxis without acidosis, Anesthesiology **49:**141, 1978.

13. Cottrell, J. E., Patel, K., Ransohoff, J. R., and others: intracranial pressure changes induced by sodium nitroprusside in patients with intracranial mass lesions, J. Neurosurg. **48:**329, 1978.

14. Cushing, H.: Tumors of the nervus acusticus and the syndrome of the cerebellopontine angle, Philadelphia, 1917, W. B. Saunders Co.

15. Davies, D. W., Greiss, L., Steward, D. T., and others: Sodium nitroprusside in children; observations on metabolism during normal and abnormal responses, Can. Anaesth. Soc. J. **22:**553, 1975.

16. Davies, D. W., Kadar, D., Steward, D. J., and others: A sudden death associated with the use of sodium nitroprusside for induction of hypotension during anesthesia, Can. Anaesth. Soc. J. **22:**547, 1975.

17. Dimant, S., Piper, C. A., and Murphy, T. O.: Pacemaker controlled hypotension in surgery, Surgery **62:**663, 1967.

18. Dreisbach, R. H.: Handbook of poisoning: diagnosis and treatment, Los Altos, Calif., 1971, Lange Medical Publications, p. 218.

19. Eckenhoff, J. E., Enderby, G. E. H., Larson, A., and others: Pulmonary gas exchange during deliberate hypotension, Br. J. Anaesth. **35:**750, 1963.

20. Enderby, G. E. H.: Postural ischemia and blood pressure, Lancet **1:**185, 1954.

21. Fahmy, N. R.: Nitroglycerin as a hypotensive drug during general anesthesia, Anesthesiology **49:**17, 1978.

22. Flaherty, J. T., Reid, P. R., Kelly, D. T., and others: Intravenous nitroglycerin in acute myocardial infarction, Circulation **51:**132, 1975.

23. Franciosa, J. A., Bieiha, M. H., Limas, C. I., and others: Improved left ventricular function during nitroprusside infusion in acute myocardial infarction, Lancet **1:**650, 1972.

24. Goodman, L. S., and Gilman, A.: The pharmacological basis of therapeutics, ed. 5, New York, 1975, MacMillan Publishing Co., Inc., p. 570.

25. Gupta, B., Cottrell, J. E., Rappaport, H., and others: Nitroglycerin raises intracranial pressure, J. Neurosurg. (submitted for publication).

26. Harp, J. R., and Wollman, H.: Cerebral metabolic effects of hyperventilation and deliberate hypotension, Br. J. Anaesth. **45:**256, 1973.

27. Ivankovich, A. D., Miletich, D. J., and Tinker, J. H.: Nitroprusside and other short acting hypotensive agents, Int. Anesth. Clin. **16** (2):14, 1978.

28. Jennett, W. B., Barker, J., Fitch, W., and others: Effects of anesthesia on intracranial pressure in patients with space occupying lesions, Lancet **1:**61, 1969.

29. Jennett, W. B., McDowall, D. G., and Barker, J.: The effect of halothane on intracranial pressure in cerebral tumors; report of two cases, J. Neurosurg. **26:**270, 1967.

30. Jordan, W. S., Graves, C. L., Boyd, W. A., and others: Cardiovascular effects of three techniques for inducing hypotension during anesthesia, Anesth. Analg. (Cleve.) **50:**1059, 1971.

31. Kaneko, Y., Ikeda, T., Takeda, T., and others: Renin release during acute release of arterial pressure in normotensive subjects and patients with renovascular hypertension, J. Clin. Invest. **46:** 705, 1967.

32. Keaney, N. P., Pickerodt, V. W. A., and McDowall, D. G.: CBF, autoregulation, CSF acid base parameters and deep halothane hypotension, Stroke **4:**324, 1973.

33. Khambatta, N. J., Stone, J. A., and Khan, L. U.: Hypertension following sodium nitroprusside, Physiologist **21:**64, 1978.

34. Lassen, N. A.: Cerebral blood flow and oxygen consumption in man, Physiol. Rev. **39:**183, 1959.

35. Lassen, M. A., and Tweed, W. A.: A basis and practice of neuroanesthesia. In Gordon, E., editor: New York, 1975, Excerpta Medica, p. 126.

36. Magness, A., Yashon, D., Locke, G., and others: Cerebral function during trimethaphan induced hypotension, Neurology **23:**506, 1973.

37. Mehta, P., Mehta, J., and Miale, T. D.: Nitroprusside lowers platelet count, N. Engl. J. Med. **299:**1134, 1978.

38. Michelakis, J. M., and Mizukoshi, M.: Distribution and disappearance rate of renin in man and dog, J. Clin. Endocrin. Metab. **32:**27, 1971.

39. Michenfelder, J. D., and Theye, R. A.: Canine systemic and cerebral effects of hypotension induced by hemorrhage, trimethaphan, halothane or nitroprusside, Anesthesiology **46**:188, 1977.

40. Michenfelder, J. D., and Tinkes, J. H.: Cyanide toxicity and thiosulfate protection during chronic administration of sodium nitroprusside in the dog, Anesthesiology **47**:441, 1977.

41. Needleman, P., Jakschik, B., and Johnson, E. M., Jr.: Sulfhydryl requirement for relaxation of vascular smooth muscle, J. Pharmacol. Exp. Ther. **187**:324, 1973.

42. Nourok, D. S., Glassock, R. J., Solomon, D. H., and others: Hypothyroidism following prolonged sodium nitroprusside therapy, Am. J. Med. Sci. **248**:129, 1964.

43. Page, I. H., Corcoran, A. C., Dustan, H. P., and others: Cardiovascular actions of sodium nitroprusside in animals and hypertensive patients, Circulation **11**:188, 1955.

44. Pfeiderer, T.: Sodium nitroprusside, a very potent platelet disaggregating substance, Acta Univ. Carol. (Med Monogr.) (Praha) **53**:247, 1972.

45. Posner, M. A., Tobey, R. E., and McElroy, H.: Hydroxocobalamine therapy of cyanide intoxication in guinea pigs, Anesthesiology **44**:157, 1976.

46. Raisis, J. E., Kindt, G. W., and McGillicuddy, J. E.: Effects of elevated cerebral venous pressure on intracranial pressure and cerebral blood flow, Scientific Program Manuscripts, Am. Assoc. Neurol. Surgeons, 1975, p. 26.

47. Shanahan, R.: The determination of sub-microgram quantities of cyanide in biological materials, J. Foren. Sci. Soc. **18**:25, 1973.

48. Siesjo, B. K., Norberg, K., Ljunggren, B., and others: A basis and practice of neuroanesthesia, Gordon, E., editor: New York, 1975, Excerpta Medica, p. 71.

49. Siesjo, B. K., and Zwetnow, N. N.: The effect of hypovolemic hypotension on extra and intracellular acid-base parameters and energy metabolites in the rat brain, Acta Physiol. Scan. **79**:114, 1970.

50. Smith, A. L., and Marque, J. J.: Anesthetics and cerebral edema, Anesthesiology **45**:64, 1976.

51. Smith, R. D., and Kruszyna, H.: Nitroprusside produces cyanide poisoning via a reaction with hemoglobin, J. Pharmacol. Exp. Ther. **191**:557, 1974.

52. Stoyka, W. W., and Schutz, H.: The cerebral response to sodium nitroprusside and trimethaphan controlled hypotension, Can. Anaesth. Soc. J. **22**:275, 1975.

53. Swan, H. J. C., Ganz, W., Forrester, J., and others: Catheterization of the heart in man with use of a flow directed balloon tipped catheter, N. Engl. J. Med. **283**:447, 1970.

54. Tark, M., Anderson, M. A., and Teat, D.: A simplified technique for measuring blood cyanide levels following nitroprusside infusion; scientific program abstracts, Int. Anesth. Res. Soc. p. 68, 1978.

55. Trembly, N. A. G., Davies, D. W., Volgyesi, G., and others: Sodium nitroprusside; factors which attenuate its action; studies with the isolated gracilis muscle of the dog, Can. Anaesth. Soc. J. **24**:644, 1977.

56. Turner, J. M., Powell, D., Gibson, R. M., and others: Intracranial pressure changes in neurosurgical patients during hypotension induced with sodium nitroprusside or trimethaphan, Br. J. Anaesth. **49**:419, 1977.

57. Van Dyke, R. A.: Anesthetic biotransformation; ASA annual refresher course lectures, 1978, p. 120.

58. Wang, H. H., Liu, L. M. P., and Katz, R. L.: A comparison of the cardiovascular effects of sodium nitroprusside and trimethaphan, Anesthesiology **46**:49, 1977.

59. Yacoub, M., Faure, J., Morina, H., and others: L'toxication dyanhydrique aigue; donnees actuelles sur le metabolisme du cyanura et le traitment par hydroxycobalamine, J. Eur. Toxicol. **7**:22, 1974.

18

Neurophysiologic evaluation and monitoring of brain function

RICHARD P. GREENBERG
RICHARD L. GRIFFITH

The clinical neurologic examination is the most widely performed and best method of assessing brain function. However, when used to evaluate patients whose level of consciousness has been altered, it has important limitations. In comatose patients, for example, the accuracy with which the neurologic examination can define location and extent of brain dysfunction or forecast patient outcome is compromised. Several different pathologic substrates, each requiring markedly different therapy and each with different outcomes, may produce the same clinical neurologic symptoms.

Improved evaluation of brain function in patients with altered levels of consciousness can be achieved by complementing the neurologic examination with other methods of evaluating brain function. It is important to realize that diagnostic studies commonly used to evaluate patients with altered levels of consciousness yield information concerning the anatomic condition, for example, the presence or absence of hematomas, brain displacements, and so on—not the functional condition of the brain. Brain electrical activity, on the other hand, like the patient's neurologic examination, depends upon neuronal

vitality for its realization and is therefore an important method of assessing the functional state of the brain irrespective of the presence or absence of anatomic alterations.

The study of brain electrical activity is particularly useful in confused or comatose patients because it offers an objective evaluation of central nervous system function that can be both complementary and supplementary to that obtained from the clinical examination. Computerized analysis of brain electrical activity enables diagnostic evaluations to be made that define areas of brain dysfunction that may not be obvious from the clinical examination alone. Studies of brain electrical activity can potentially make distinctions not always possible with the neurologic examination between dysfunction of the cerebral hemispheres or the brain stem and can help evaluate dysfunction of localized brain areas or individual neural systems and pathways (visual, auditory, motor, somesthetic). The techniques utilized clinically to record neuroelectrical potentials are noninvasive and allow frequent serial studies to be obtained at low risk to the patient. They provide a safe and simple method for indirectly evaluating the functional and metabolic state of the brain.

There are two techniques available with which to study neuroelectric phenomena in humans: spontaneous electrical activity (elec-

This work was supported in part by National Institutes of Health, NINCDS special projects grant No. 3 P50 NS12587 and Teacher Investigator Award No. 5 K07 NS00346 to Dr. Richard Greenberg.

troencephalogram [EEG]) and event-related computer averaged brain electrical potentials (evoked potentials). Much has been written elsewhere on the use of the electroencephalogram in clinical neurologic disease states; therefore, the following discussion on neurophysiologic evaluation and monitoring of brain function deals exclusively with evoked potential techniques.

BRAIN EVOKED POTENTIALS

While the electroencephalogram represents spontaneous or intrinsic brain electrical activity, event-related neuroelectric activity such as the sensory evoked potential represents the brain's response to the application of specific extrinsic stimuli.[8,9] Theoretically, any sensory stimulus sufficient to cause depolarization of a peripheral or cranial nerve can be used to evoke neuroelectric potentials in the central nervous system.[11,16] In practice the visual (flash of light), auditory (tone pip), and somesthetic (peripheral nerve depolarization) systems have been most often utilized for clinical evoked potential studies.*

Application of a brief sensory stimulus to a peripheral receptor can initiate a depolarization wave that travels toward the central ner-

---

*References 1, 2, 6, 15, 26, 30.

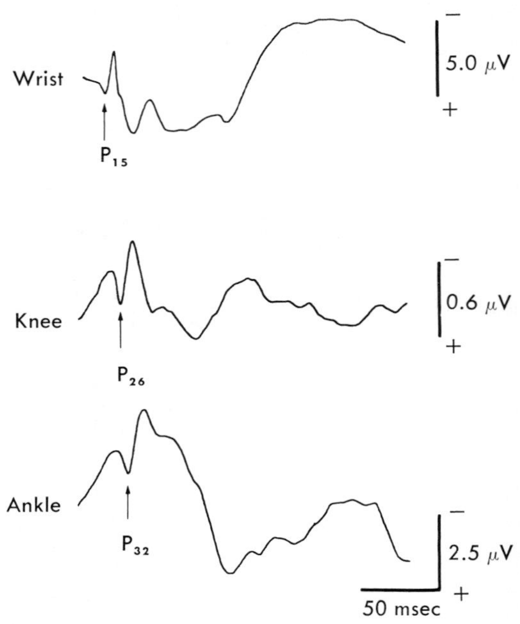

Fig. 18-1. Somatosensory evoked potentials recorded from parietal scalp after peripheral nerve stimulation at the wrist (median nerve), knee (common peroneal nerve), and ankle (posterior tibial nerve) in an adult. The initial positive wave (positivity down) can be recorded 15 msec after peripheral nerve stimulation at the wrist, but it requires 32 msec to arrive and be recorded when the posterior tibial nerve is stimulated at the ankle.

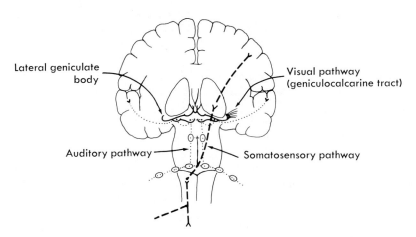

Fig. 18-2. Schematic view of sensory pathways involved in the generation of multimodality evoked potentials. The sensory input generating somatosensory and auditory evoked potentials traverses more caudal regions of brain stem than does sensory input for visual evoked potentials.

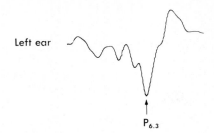

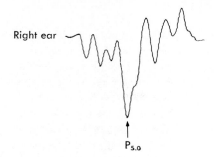

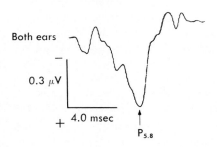

Fig. 18-3. Auditory brain stem potentials (far field) recorded after left, right, and then both ears were stimulated by 75 db tone pips in a patient with decreased hearing in the left ear subsequent to head trauma. The brain stem potentials generated by stimulating the right ear alone are normal with a 5.0 msec latency (normal) from time of stimulation to the fourth positive component (positivity down). Stimulation of the left ear alone, on the other hand, generated an abnormal brain stem response with a significant latency delay to the fourth positive component (P 6.3). Stimulation of both ears simultaneously produced an average of the potentials generated by each ear with a latency delay to the fourth positive component of 5.8 msec.

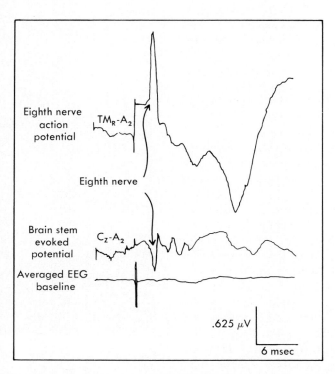

Fig. 18-4. Simultaneous eighth nerve action potential and brain stem evoked potential showing the normal appearance of the electrical wave produced by the eighth nerve. The eighth nerve action potential *(upper tracing)* was recorded from a cotton wick electrode near the tympanic membrane. The auditory brain stem evoked potential *(lower tracing)* was recorded at the vertex. Their electrical polarities are opposite because the electrical dipole is between the electrodes.

vous system at velocities determined by fiber diameter. The time interval from stimulation to arrival of the depolarization wave at the primary sensory receiving area in the cortex depends upon the patient's body size and site of stimulation, presence or absence of neuronal pathology, the conduction velocity of the axons, and the number of synapses in the respective neural pathways (Fig. 18-1). Groups of cortical neurons can then process this afferent impulse for variable time periods after its arrival, thereby generating potentials that may be recorded for seconds after stimulation.[11] Evoked potentials are recorded for variable epochs after stimulation, generally between 10 to 1000 msec as this time period allows the primary responses and the associated neural activity to be studied.[16]

For an evoked potential to be recorded from the scalp, both the neural pathway stimulated at the periphery and cortical neurons elaborating afferent information must be functional (Fig. 18-2).[27,33] It is sometimes possible to differentiate the location of structures in a neural pathway that generate components of complex evoked potentials by measuring the period of time elapsed from stimulation to the evoked potential component of interest. Evoked potentials arising from brain stem elements of the auditory and somesthetic system occur within the first 10 to 15 msec post stimulation, while the potentials that follow those early electrical events are generated by more rostral structures such as the cortex.[7,18,23,24,32]

Jewett and Williston introduced the concept of near field and far field (brain stem) recording of electrical potentials from the auditory system.[25] They demonstrated that electrical potentials seen in the first 6 to 7 msec post stimulation are generated by elements of the auditory system located in the brain stem. These were called auditory far field potentials (Fig. 18-3). They distinguished auditory far field potentials from the auditory near field potentials generated in more rostral elements of the auditory system located nearer to the recording scalp electrode in the cerebral cortex. It is thought that the first five early latency potentials (far

field) arise from the eighth nerve, cochlear nucleus, superior olivary complex, nucleus of the lateral lemniscus, and the inferior colliculus successively (Fig. 18-4).[32] Cracco demonstrated that early latency brain stem (far field) somatosensory evoked potentials could be recorded in humans, and these occur at approximately 10 msec and 12 msec post stimulation.[7]

EEG VERSUS EVOKED POTENTIALS

Central nervous system (CNS) neurons that respond to applied sensory stimuli and generate evoked potentials can also be responsible for the generation of the electroencephalogram.[8,9] Any mode of injury sufficient to cause neuronal dysfunction will stop or alter the EEG and evoked potential activ-

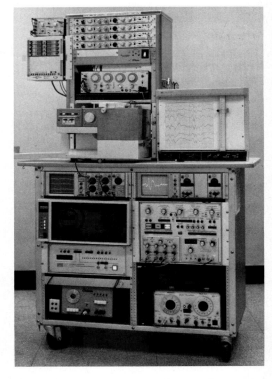

Fig. 18-5. A computer and evoked potential stimulating and recording equipment mounted on a single cart, which can be moved to a patient's intensive care unit bed or into the operating room. Data have been plotted on an x-y plotter as well as stored on magnetic tape.

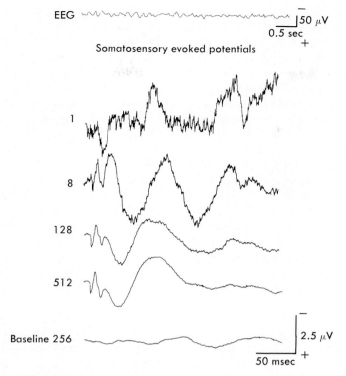

Fig. 18-6. An example of computerized signal averaging. The EEG *(top line)* has not been averaged. The somatosensory evoked potential is displayed after 1, 8, 125, and 512 epochs of time-locked EEG have been averaged.

ity as well.[4,29] Potentials generated following brain damage originate from surviving neurons. Since both EEG and evoked potentials depend upon neuronal functional integrity, what benefit can be derived from recording evoked potentials that cannot be gotten with the EEG alone? The technique of evoked potential recording offers diagnostic advantages that depend upon specificity in defining the location of functional loss in afferent neural pathways and cerebral cortex.[18,22,28,33]

EVOKED POTENTIAL GENERAL RECORDING TECHNIQUES

It is not feasible to record evoked potentials from scalp electrodes without signal averaging because the amplitude of an evoked potential is one to three orders of magnitude less than the amplitude of an EEG.[11,12,16] Various techniques have been used to extract the low amplitude evoked potential signal from the larger amplitude background electrical "noise" composed mainly of the EEG but also of nonneural electrical activity. Computers are now available at relatively low cost that can store and display the final average on an oscilloscope screen for photographic records of the evoked potential or plot the evoked potential on graph paper (Fig. 18-5). An example of computerized signal averaging is shown in Fig. 18-6 where the intrinsic, spontaneous EEG is progressively replaced by the completed evoked potential after 512 time-locked EEG epochs have been averaged.

Electrodes should be positioned on the scalp in a standardized, symmetrical manner, that is, the international 10-20 system, to assure consistent results within and between patients. Recordings employing linked ear electrodes as a common reference are often the most useful.

The electrical potentials generated by the

brain and measured by scalp electrodes are typically in the microvolt range. The operating room and the intensive care unit, both filled with a variety of electronic and electromechanical equipment, can be hostile environments for measuring such low energy signals. The alternating line current of the hospital's power system is the most persistent, though not the only electrical field able to distort and contaminate the scalp potentials. The ideal would be electrically shielded rooms in which to perform this type of monitoring, but the ideal is not always practical. Hospital electrical safety standards frequently require low resistance grounding systems to be connected to all metallic surfaces within reach of the patient. Such grounding reduces signal contamination, but the most effective method of reducing signal contamination is to make the wires connected to the scalp electrodes physically as short as possible. In other words, the amplifier should be brought to within a few inches of the patient's scalp. Differential voltage amplifiers that utilize low noise integrated circuit operational amplifiers are small enough to be placed close to the patient without inconveniencing the care of the patient.

A differential amplifier is designed to amplify the voltage difference between its two inputs without regard to the voltage difference between the inputs and the amplifier's power supply ground. The ability of the amplifier to perform this feat is termed "common mode rejection" and is measured in decibels. An amplifier for monitoring scalp potentials should have a common mode rejection of less than -60 db (a more negative number than -60 db) at the line frequency in use (commonly 60 hertz). The amplifier should track the slow and fast changes of the input signal with exactly the same voltage gain. This ability of the amplifier to boost fast changing signals by the same proportion that it boosts slow ones is reflected in its frequency response specifications. For monitoring spontaneous electrical activity an amplifier that has plus or minus 0.5 db from .15 Hz to 50 Hz is adequate. For certain modalities of averaged evoked potentials, the amplifier should have a frequency response of better than plus or minus 0.3 db from .15 Hz to 3,000 Hz. Additionally, the amplifier must have an input impedance of greater than 1,000,000 ohms to measure the scalp potential without drawing enough current to alter that potential.

The electrical diagram for a differential amplifier will normally have one amplifier input labeled with a plus sign and the other with a minus sign. These symbols indicate that the voltage on the minus input is the one subtracted to form the difference. Some amplifiers may have the plus input labeled G1 and the minus labeled G2. If the plus input is a larger voltage than the minus input, the amplifier's output will be a positive voltage. If the same inputs are reversed, the amplifier's output will become a negative voltage. Normally, the minus input of the differential amplifier is connected to the reference electrode. With this configuration, a positive output from the amplifier indicates that the brain's net electrical dipole moment is directed more toward than away from the active electrode.

Less than half a milliampere of alternating current passing through the upper torso of a human can induce fibrillation in the heart. Since scalp electrodes provide a low resistance path for current, the patient's electrical safety is a matter of concern during monitoring of the brain's electrical activity. Safety considerations make it desirable to electrically isolate the electronics attached to the patient from the hospital power system and its grounding. Powering the differential amplifiers with batteries and passing the signals to the processing and display portion of the monitoring system via light pulses and not electrical currents is the safest approach yet devised. Optical isolation and battery power is not only safe but can also be the solution to problems of line current signal distortion entering the amplifier through the grounding. Batteries can also shrink the amplifier's size and weight by eliminating the need for a transformer and rectifier circuit. Although optical isolation can be achieved in several ways, one simple method will illustrate the technique. A voltage-controlled oscillator connected to the amplifier can generate pulses at a rate proportional to the potential difference between two scalp electrodes. The pulses can then energize a light-emitting diode that flashes light down a small, flexible fiberoptic cable. At the end of the cable, many feet from the patient, a photo transistor detects the pulses and electronic circuits determine the pulse rate either for graphic display of the EEG or for further processing by other electronic circuits. Such optical transmission systems can transfer as many as 500,000 pulses of light per second so that a precision of 1 part in 500 can be achieved simply by electronically counting the number of pulses transmitted each millisecond. This straightforward technique would be quite satisfactory for monitoring spontaneous brain electrical activity and by slight modification also can be made to convey enough information for averaged evoked potential monitoring. It is very likely that optical isolation of physiologic signals, because of its safety for the patient, will eventually become the only acceptable method for electrically connecting to a patient.

EVOKED POTENTIAL SPECIFIC RECORDING TECHNIQUES
Visual evoked potentials

Visual evoked potentials are recorded from the left and right occipital scalp (O_1 and O_2), with a filter band-pass of 1 to 1000 Hz, in response to a 10 μsec strobe light flash located 10 inches from the nasion. The light flash may be delivered at 1 pulse per second to both eyes and then to each eye individually. Either 256 or 512 potentials should be averaged of the first 500 msec period of brain electrical activity after stimulation.

Somatosensory evoked potentials

Somatosensory evoked potentials can be recorded with a filter band-pass of 1 to 1000 Hz from the left and right parietal scalp electrodes (P_3 and P_4) in response to median nerve stimulation produced by a 0.5 msec constant-current square wave delivered at 1 pulse per second. The left and right median

nerves should be stimulated separately and the depolarizing pulse intensity clinically determined by observing the onset of thumb twitch and raising the stimulus intensity 2 mA above threshold. The ulnar nerves can also be used. An average of either 256 or 512 stimulations is needed to achieve adequate signal-to-noise ratios in the intensive care unit. The first 250 msec period of brain electrical activity post stimulus is averaged.

Somatosensory brain stem evoked potentials

Somatosensory brain stem evoked potentials are recorded with a filter band-pass of 30-3K Hz from a vertex scalp electrode referenced to the wrist opposite the median nerve depolarization. The initial 20 msec period is examined and 1024-2048 trails averaged. A 0.5 msec constant-current square wave delivered at 5 pps can be used for stimulation.

Auditory cortical evoked potentials

Auditory cortical evoked potentials are recorded from the vertex (C_z), with a filter band-pass of 1 to 600 Hz in response to a 0.5 msec 85 db tone pip with maximum energy of 2000 Hz. The sound is delivered to each ear individually at a rate of one stimulation every two seconds. Generally, 512 potentials of the first 400 msec are averaged to achieve an adequate signal-to-noise ratio. To reduce stimulation artifact, a stethoscopelike apparatus can be used allowing a microphone (Telephonics TDH-39) to be positioned away from the patient at the bell end of the stethoscope. Sound level calibration can be done with a sound level meter from the ear pieces of the stethoscope, and the delay caused by the microphone's distance from the tympanic membrane taken into account in the latency calculations.

Auditory far-field potentials recording

Auditory far-field potentials (brain stem potentials) recording is accomplished with the same auditory stimulation apparatus and sound level. Stimuli may be delivered eight

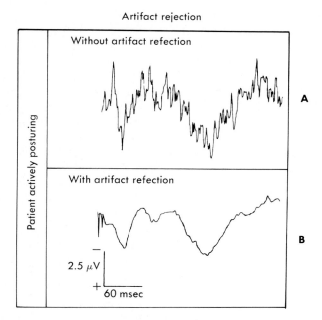

Fig. 18-7. A, Myogenic contamination of the auditory evoked potential from a decerebrate patient makes meaningful data analysis difficult. **B,** A clean auditory evoked potential was obtained after high frequency muscle potentials were eliminated (same patient) by artifact rejection techniques.

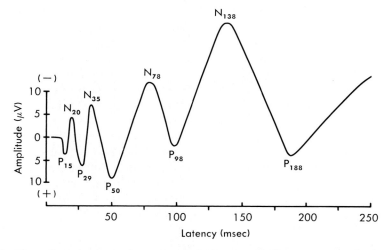

Fig. 18-8. This schematic somatosensory evoked potential illustrates a method of labeling waveforms. All waves, regardless of modality, are labeled as positive or negative (P or N) followed by the latency from time of stimulation to wave peak in msec. Positive waves are down by convention.

Table 18-1. Multimodality evoked potential normative data*

Somatosensory	P15 ± 1.1	N20 ± 1.4	P29 ± 3.7	N35 ± 3.0	P50 ± 4.2	N78 ± 6.6	P98 ± 9.2	N138 ± 9.8	P188 ± 10.2
Visual	P53 ± 5.4	N70 ± 7.8	P98 ± 9.6	N148 ± 14.0	P192 ± 14.0	N235 ± 18.0	P290 ± 26.0		
Auditory	P26 ± 2.2	N42 ± 3.8	P50 ± 5.6	N98 ± 9.6	P170 ± 12.6	N170 ± 18.0	P340 ± 21.0		
Brain stem	P1.5 ± .14	P2.5 ± .19	P3.6 ± .2	P4.7 ± .1	P5.6 ± .16	P6.7 ± .18	P7.2 ± .2	P10 ± .44	

*Latencies expressed as mean value msec ± standard deviation.

times a second to both ears and then to each ear individually. Vertex (C_z) recordings are made with a filter band-pass of 30 to 3000 Hz. The initial 20 msec period is examined, and about 2048 potentials averaged.

TECHNICAL PROBLEMS

Artifacts from potentials generated in muscle, 60 cycle alternating current, ECG, and so on are common and frustrating to deal with. Stimulating difficulties can occur from things such as blood and wax in the external auditory meatus, gaze preferences and eye movements, swollen eyelids, infiltrated IV fluid in the subcutaneous tissue over the nerve to be depolarized. These problems must be noted and corrected, but with attention to detail and careful technique, good quality evoked potentials can be recorded from most patients even in an active intensive care unit (Fig. 18-7).[20]

EVOKED POTENTIAL ANALYSIS

A suitable method with which to categorize the complex abnormal evoked responses produced by neuronal embarrassment is required.[16] Evoked potential wave latency, amplitude, duration, and morphology have been analyzed. Latency to each wave is the most commonly used clinical parameter. Typical latency data from 20 normal subjects is given in Table 18-1. By convention the waves, regardless of modality, can be labeled as either positive or negative (P or N) followed by the latency from time of stimulation to wave peak in milliseconds (Fig. 18-8). Computer programs that detect positive or negative evoked potential peaks and printout latency and amplitude data are available (Fig. 18-9). Greenberg and co-workers presented a system of grading sensory evoked potentials obtained from head injury patients that categorizes the abnormal evoked potentials by grouping them into four distinct patterns according to similarity of wave latencies and waveform.[20] The patterns that emerge are arranged into an ordered functional grading system I through IV (Fig. 18-10, Table 18-2). Grade I or II evoked potentials are mildly to moderately abnormal, whereas grade III or

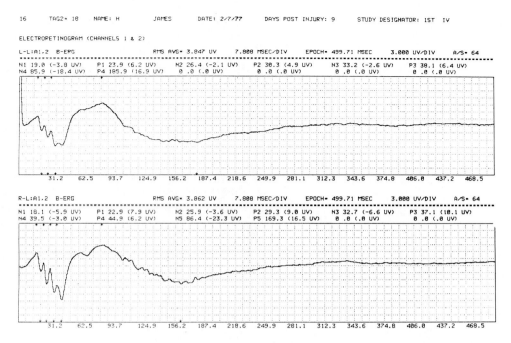

16   TAG2= 18   NAME: H   JAMES   DATE: 2/7/77   DAYS POST INJURY: 9   STUDY DESIGNATOR: 1ST IV

ELECTROPETINOGRAM (CHANNELS 1 & 2)

L-L:A1.2 B-EPG   RMS AVG= 3.847 UV   7.808 MSEC/DIV   EPOCH= 499.71 MSEC   3.000 UV/DIV   A/S= 64
N1 19.0 (-3.8 UV)   P1 23.9 (6.2 UV)   N2 26.4 (-2.1 UV)   P2 30.3 (4.9 UV)   N3 33.2 (-2.6 UV)   P3 38.1 (6.4 UV)
N4 85.9 (-18.4 UV)   P4 185.9 (16.9 UV)   0 .0 (.0 UV)   0 .0 (.0 UV)   0 .0 (.0 UV)   0 .0 (.0 UV)

31.2   62.5   93.7   124.9   156.2   187.4   218.6   249.9   281.1   312.3   343.6   374.8   406.0   437.2   468.5

R-L:A1.2 B-ERG   RMS AVG= 3.862 UV   7.808 MSEC/DIV   EPOCH= 499.71 MSEC   3.000 UV/DIV   A/S= 64
N1 18.1 (-5.9 UV)   P1 22.9 (7.9 UV)   N2 25.9 (-3.6 UV)   P2 29.3 (9.0 UV)   N3 32.7 (-6.6 UV)   P3 37.1 (10.1 UV)
N4 39.5 (-3.0 UV)   P4 44.9 (6.2 UV)   N5 86.4 (-23.3 UV)   P5 169.3 (16.5 UV)   0 .0 (.0 UV)   0 .0 (.0 UV)

31.2   62.5   93.7   124.9   156.2   187.4   218.6   249.9   281.1   312.3   343.6   374.8   406.0   437.2   468.5

Fig. 18-9. Electroretinograms printed by computer in analog form with the amplitudes and latencies of each positive or negative peak calculated automatically. This program allows a significant savings in time to be made by providing quick, accurate data analyses.

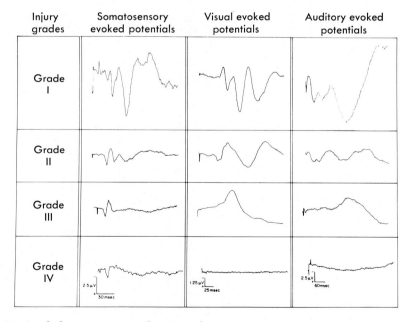

Fig. 18-10. Graded injury potentials. Four distinct injury patterns can be recognized in each modality and are arranged in a functional grading system I to IV according to increasing abnormality. Each evoked potential trace depicted above represents the grand average of at least 15 evoked potentials.

Table 18-2. Graded injury potentials*

Modality	Grade									No. studies
Somato- sensory	I	$^P15$	$^N20$	$^P29$	$^N35$	$^P50$	$^N78$	$^P98$		55
	II	$^P15$	$^N20$	$^P29$	$^N35$	$(^P50)*$	—†	—	—	27
	III	$^P15$	$^N23$	—	—	—	—	—	—	19
	IV	$^P15$	—	—	—	—	—	—	—	21
										122
Visual	I	$^P66$	$^N75$	$^P98$	$^N110$	$^P129$	$^N150$	$^P187$	$^N240$	62
	II	$(^P65)*$	—	$^N90$	—	—	$^P150$	—	$^N220$	29
	III	—	—	$^N95$	—	—	—	—	—	15
	IV	No activity		—	—	—	—	—		16
										122
Auditory	I	$^P45$	$^N63$	$^P87$	$^N143$	$^P232$	$^N370$			43
	II	$^P45$	$^N62$	$^P85$	$^N143$	$^P230$	$(^N260)*$			38
	III	—	—	—	—	—	$^N250$			17
	IV	No activity		—	—	—				24
										122
Brain stem potentials	I	$^P1.5$	$^P2.5$	$^P3.6$	$^P4.7$	$^P5.6$	$^P6.7$	$^P7.2$	$^P10$	65
	II	$^P1.5$	$^P2.5$	$^P3.6$	—	$^P6.1$	—	—		21
	III	$^P1.5$	—	—	—	$^P6.0$	—	—		5
	IV	$^P1.5$	—	—	—	—	—	—		6
										97

*Not always present, see p. 409.   †No activity.

IV evoked potentials are severely abnormal to absent.

EVOKED POTENTIAL EVALUATION OF BRAIN FUNCTION
Serial static studies

Two general methods can be employed to assess brain function with evoked potential techniques: serial static studies or continuous on-line studies. Static studies, recording sessions limited to a few minutes to several hours, are clinically the most common form of gathering data. The electrical data obtained in this manner can provide valuable insight into brain function, both with respect to the brain's condition during the recording session and also beyond that time (see below).

Recent work has suggested the hypothesis that evoked potentials may be capable of defining marginally functioning neurons that cannot be detected by the clinical neurologic examination.[18] Thus, a patient who at the time of evoked potential recording session is comatose and hemiparetic may have normal evoked potentials. This kind of dissociation of clinical and electrical data forecasts the complete recovery of the patient's level of consciousness and hemiparesis. Perhaps the evoked potentials are able to detect dysfunctional neurons, not dead neurons, and demonstrate their viability before they recover and function in a normal manner.

The obvious disadvantage of using serial static studies is the inability to obtain data at the moment an unexpected secondary insult occurs. For example, the reaccumulation of a subdural hematoma, or late developing significant hyponatremia with subsequent cerebral edema, elevated ICP, and brain herniation cannot usually be studied with static evoked potential techniques. Furthermore, monitoring brain function continuously in intensive care settings may provide early feedback concerning the efficacy of treatment regimens.

Continuous on-line studies

Systems of monitoring evoked potentials on-line in a continuous manner must be carefully planned to overcome technical and personnel difficulties. However, a good system will enable critical evoked potential data to be obtained during the occurrence of unpredictable secondary brain insults. Information concerning the mode of action of these events on brain function can thus be studied. For example, the level of elevated intracranial pressure sufficient to cause brain function compromise, the effect of steroids on neuronal function, and so on may be studied with continuously recorded evoked potentials. Moreover, with the advent of barbiturate coma as a treatment for specific head trauma patients, a new method of assessing brain function to replace the neurologic examination is needed.

It is possible to identify and overcome several problems in the implementation of a continuously recorded evoked potential ICU system. Stimulation equipment must be unobtrusive; therefore, strobe lights and bulky earphones could be detrimental to the success of the system. Electrodes must be few in number and placed and maintained to assure artifact-free recording. Perhaps the most difficult problems are data collection, reduction, storage, and analysis.

Continuous on-line evoked potential techniques

Visual. A visual stimulator composed of a series of light-emitting diodes (LED) placed in a small cup that is taped over a patient's closed eyelid can be used. This is a small unobtrusive device that can be maintained in place for days. The power supply is battery operated (9 volts) and can be triggered. Each patient should have one pair of these visual LED stimulators.

Somatosensory. Bipolar electrodes are placed over the left and right median nerve in the same manner as is in use for the serial studies. Stimulation is provided by a constant current stimulator present at each bedside.

Auditory. A TDH-49 microphone adapted to a stethoscope like hard rubber tubing is directed to the patient's external auditory canal. Each patient should have a sound pip generator at the bedside.

Therefore, one centrally located power supply will be used for each modality. This equipment must be triggered and temporarily sequenced by a dedicated computer and its peripherals.

Recording equipment. Electrodes should be placed at positions P_3 and P_4 as well as bilateral earlobes. We have chosen to use only two scalp electrodes and two earlobe reference electrodes because this is a practical solution to a major problem of electrode maintenance. All three modalities can be recorded from this placement even though evoked potential waveforms may be somewhat altered by electrode position. Nonetheless, each patient acts as his or her own control in this system, and thus change from baseline can be observed. We have successfully recorded all modalities from these electrode positions. The electrodes are held in place by inch-square collodion-soaked fine mesh gauze. This has been tested on our patients and found to maintain placement for 20 to 24 hours with adequate impedance levels to obtain clean evoked potentials.

Each bedside has one two-channel amplifier.

Sequence of data collection, reduction, analysis. Multimodality evoked potential baseline data is recorded. This data will provide the patient's baseline and be compared with the evoked potential study initially recorded by the on-line intensive care system. Computer programs are used to establish a range in which the evoked potentials may safely vary. Thereafter, the computer samples patient evoked potentials continuously in a sequential serial manner. Unlike the static study, data generated by the on-line system is stored and printed out only if it varies significantly from baseline; otherwise it can be discarded.

Correlations can, therefore, be made between the continuously recorded evoked potential data and significant changes in the patient's neurologic condition, intracranial pressure, CBF, and so on. Evoked potential data reduction grading system as described in general methods of analysis is used to perform the correlations with other studies.

EVOKED POTENTIAL DIAGNOSIS OF FOCAL NEUROLOGIC DEFICITS

Clinical evaluation of visual, auditory, or somesthetic system dysfunction in confused or comatose patients may sometimes be difficult. In the same patients, however, evaluation of these neural systems with evoked potential techniques can contribute much to the early diagnosis of neurologic deficits such as retrobulbar visual dysfunction, deafness, somesthetic deficits, or hemiparesis.*

_____
*References 6, 13, 14, 22, 31, 34.

Retrobulbar visual dysfunction

Electrophysiologic diagnosis of visual system dysfunction with evoked potentials requires first a careful consideration of retinal function, as the retina may be damaged by local trauma.[13,17,18] Electroretinograms assess retinal function and should be performed and analyzed prior to evaluation of visual evoked potential data.[3] For example, a patient's visual evoked potential study may appear isoelectric (grade IV), suggesting intracranial visual system dysfunction, when in fact the retina may be so severely traumatized that generation or transmission of visual information to the occipital lobes is inhibited. (Fig. 18-11). Stimulation of each eye separately can also enhance the diagnostic value of visu-

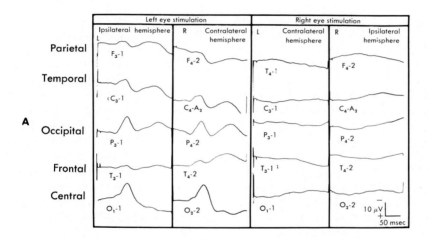

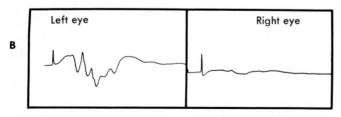

Fig. 18-11. The visual evoked potential study (**A**), recorded from scalp electrodes, had a different outcome depending on which eye was stimulated. Left eye photic stimulation (*upper left*) generated severely abnormal but detectable visual evoked potentials (grade III) while right eye photic stimulation produced apparent electrically silent visual evoked potentials (grade IV). The electroretinogram of each eye (**B**), however, revealed right eye retinal dysfunction that had caused the apparent grade IV (electrically silent) visual potentials.

Table 18-3. Electrophysiologic evaluation of focal deficits

Outcomes*	Grades		No. patients
	I-II	III-IV	
Hemiparesis	*Somatosensory evoked potential†*		
Acute (resolved)	6	0	6
Residual (permanent)	0	9	9
	(P < .001)§		15
Retrobulbar visual dysfunction‡	*Visual evoked potentials†*		
Visual dysfunction	1	9	10
No visual dysfunction	20	3	23
	(P < .001)§		33
Auditory dysfunction‡	*Auditory potentials†*		
Deafness	1	5	6
No deafness	24	3	27
	(P < .001)§		33

*Outcome determined from 3 to 30 months.
†Mean study performed on day 3.
‡18 of 51 patients died or could not be evaluated.
§Based on Fisher's exact test for 2-by-2 table.

al potentials because each optic nerve can be individually assessed in this manner.[34] Visual evoked potentials recorded a few days after ictus in comatose patients correlate well with dysfunction noted by neuro-ophthalmologic examination done months later when patients are responsive (Table 18-3). In one study, clinical evaluation alone of visual dysfunction performed in the early stages of the disease state correlated with the patient's final visual function in only 30% of cases, while the visual evoked potential data recorded a few days after ictus (mean day 3) correctly evaluated alternate visual function in 90% of cases.[18]

Auditory dysfunction

Deafness due to neurologic disease is difficult to clinically evaluate in children and in confused or comatose adult patients.[6] Auditory evoked potentials permit early diagnosis of deafness in these patients. It can be difficult to distinguish preexisting auditory disease from that due to the disease. Nevertheless, eighth nerve, brain stem, and hemispheric auditory dysfunction can be correctly evaluated electrically in most cases. Damage to the eighth nerve can be detected with brain stem auditory potentials.[31] The first po-

tential seen in these records reflects eighth nerve function and is delayed or absent with peripheral auditory system damage.[32] Each ear should be stimulated separately to distinguish unilateral auditory dysfunction. Binaural stimulation will often mask a unilateral deficit, as the evoked response obtained will be an average of the activity generated from each ear (see Fig. 18-3). Auditory dysfunction, defined by audiometric examination months after ictus, has been compared to auditory evoked potential data recorded early (Table 18-3). In the initial few days following the disease onset (mean day 3) clinical evaluation of auditory dysfunction was shown in this study to be accurate in 17% of cases when compared to the audiometric data gathered months later. Auditory evoked potential data obtained at the same time correctly diagnosed auditory dysfunction in 83% of cases.[18]

Hemiparesis or hemiplegia

Because of the close topographic association of the somesthetic and motor systems, associations between the presence or absence of hemiparesis and somatosensory evoked potential abnormalities have proven helpful in the diagnosis of motor deficits

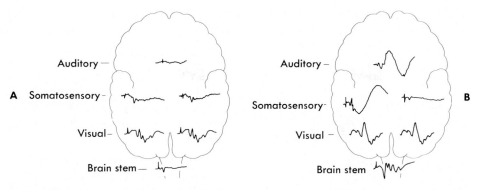

Fig. 18-12. Brain images with the approximate location of sites of generation of multimodality evoked potentials superimposed. In **A** the visual evoked potential is normal, while the somatosensory and auditory near and far field evoked potential in this comatose patient are absent, suggesting brain stem dysfunction. In **B** the right parietal lobe response to left median nerve depolarization is absent in a patient with dense left hemiparesis. All other multimodality evoked potentials were normal in this patient.

(Fig. 18-12, *B*). Abnormalities in somatosensory evoked potential data obtained in the first week after disease onset correlate well with the presence of residual lateralized motor deficits.[18] Mildly or moderately abnormal somatosensory evoked potentials (grades I or II) recorded in the acute disease period in patients with hemiparesis indicate the probable resolution of the hemiparesis some months later, while a severely abnormal or isoelectric somatosensory evoked potential indicates the likelihood of a persistent motor deficit (Table 18-3).[20]

LOCALIZATION OF FOCAL HEMISPHERIC NEUROANATOMIC LESIONS

Efforts to correlate evoked potential data with central nervous system anatomic lesions verified by either computerized axial tomograms, angiograms, intraoperative findings, or autopsy material have proven to be rewarding. The presence of a lesion such as a brain contusion does not necessarily imply a clinically detectable functional deficit; therefore the evoked potential will not reflect all anatomic lesions. However, when electrically detectable anatomic lesions are present, positive correlations with evoked potential data verify the accuracy with which this electrophysiologic technique can localize brain dysfunction. Although the data is scant, it appears possible to localize focal brain lesions in all but the frontal lobes.

Frontal lobe lesions

These lesions are poorly localized by present evoked potential techniques because of the lack of a technically suitable sensory stimulus with which to directly challenge them.[18] Direct cortical stimulation and response recording as applied by Grossman can provide some information about the frontal lobes; however, this technique requires the invasive placement of an electrode on the cortex.[21] Further refinements and the development of noninvasive means of stimulating the large frontal brain regions will help considerably.

Parietal lobe lesions

Somatosensory evoked potentials alone can accurately localize parietal lobe lesions.[18,33] The extent of a lesion necessary to alter the evoked response is not known. Damaged areas detected by abnormal somatosensory evoked potentials may include prerolandic frontal lobe as well as parietal lobe since clinical correlations with hemiparesis and aphasia have been made.[18,28] It can be seen in Fig. 18-12, *B*, that the right parietal lobe response to left median nerve depolarization is quite depressed in a patient with a left hemiparesis who had an acute subdural hematoma with severe right parietal lobe contusion noted intraoperatively. The left parietal lobe response to right median nerve stimulation as well as the visual and auditory near and far field responses are normal in this patient.

Temporal lobe lesions

Both the auditory and visual evoked potentials must be evaluated to determine temporal lobe lesions. Obtaining and evaluating one of these modalities alone is insufficient to detect the majority of temporal lobe lesions.[18] As can be seen in Fig. 18-13, both the right visual and auditory evoked responses were depressed in a patient who sustained a severe right temporal lobe hemorrhagic contusion, which was treated by surgical excision of the mass. The CT scan was

obtained postoperatively and was done on the same day as the evoked potential study.

Occipital lobe lesions

The visual evoked potentials correlate very well with occipital lobe lesions as long as electroretinograms are performed to avoid confusion with retinal dysfunction (Fig. 18-11).

DIAGNOSIS OF BRAIN STEM AND/OR HEMISPHERIC DYSFUNCTION

Localization of dysfunction in brain regions (differentiating brain stem from hemispheric dysfunction) is best accomplished by utilizing the wider scope afforded by multimodality evoked potentials (visual, auditory, and somatosensory) as opposed to one modality alone.[18,19,20] The sensory input producing somatosensory and auditory near field and far field evoked potentials traverses regions of the medulla, pons, midbrain, and part of the diencephalon located caudal to the lateral geniculate body, which is the most caudal

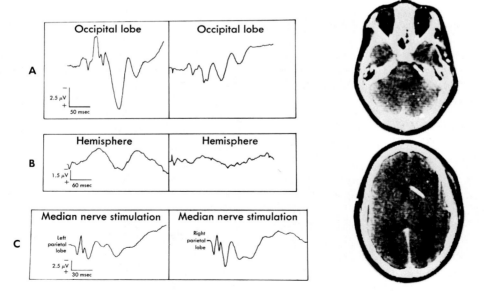

Fig. 18-13. The multimodality evoked potential study recorded postoperatively in a patient who required a partial right temporal lobectomy. **A**, Visual response. **B**, Auditory response. **C**, Somatosensory response. The CT scan *(right)* was done postoperatively on the same day as the evoked potential study.

region traversed by sensory input producing visual evoked potentials (see Fig. 18-2).[7,14,30,32-34] Visual sensory input leaves its caudal position in the lateral geniculate body and turns rostrally into the cerebrum, passing through the temporal and parietal lobes into the occipital lobe. Therefore, abnormal somatosensory and auditory near and far field (brain stem) evoked potentials recorded from comatose head trauma patients with normal visual evoked potentials (Figs. 18-12, A, and 18-14) implicate dysfunctional brain stem more than dysfunctional cerebral hemispheres.[18,19,35] On the other hand, an electrophysiologic cerebral hemispheric dysfunction may exist if the data indicate normal auditory and somatosensory brain stem potentials (far field) and abnormal auditory near field evoked potentials coupled with abnormal visual and somatosensory near field potentials.[5,18,19]

Brain stem dysfunction

Brain stem lesions are difficult to verify except at autopsy; therefore, relatively few cases are available with which to correlate human evoked potential data. Starr and Hamilton compared auditory brain stem potentials with autopsy material and intraoperative observations in 10 patients to determine the brain stem structural correlates of far field and auditory response. They concluded that lesions of different regions of the brain stem can be associated with abnormalities of the auditory brain stem response.[32] Wilkus and co-workers could not obtain auditory evoked potentials in a patient with an extensive infarct of the pons. They were able to obtain, however, normal visual evoked responses and EEG.[35]

Greenberg and co-workers correlated multimodality evoked potentials with three patients who had autopsy-confirmed brain stem lesions secondary to head injury.[18] The gross autopsy examination of one patient, who expired 10 days after head trauma, revealed a cerebrum that was moderately edematous, especially on the side of a partial left temporal lobectomy that had been done on the day of admission. The brain stem was grossly

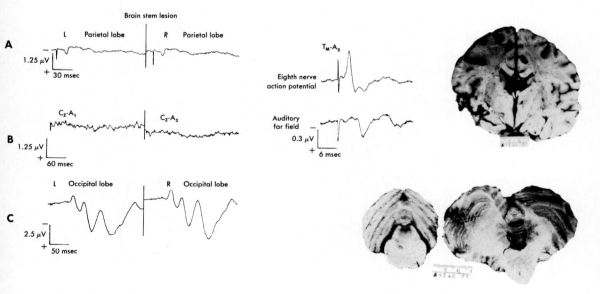

Fig. 18-14. The multimodality evoked potential study recorded in vivo in a patient who subsequently died and whose autopsy *(right)* revealed in the brain stem many small hemorrhages and clusters of microglial cells on the microscopic examination. **A,** Somatosensory evoked potential median nerve stimulation. **B,** Auditory evoked potential. **C,** Visual evoked potential.

normal except for two small agonal hemorrhages, but microscopically, clusters of microglial cells (del Rio Hortega silver carbo-
nate stain) were seen to be scattered
throughout the midbrain, pons, and medulla.
Somatosensory and auditory near field potentials were severely depressed (grade IV) in
this patient, and the auditory brain stem potentials were grade III (Fig. 18-14). A normal simultaneous eighth nerve action potential ruled out eighth nerve focal damage as a
cause of the severely abnormal auditory responses (Fig. 18-14, *D*).[10] Visual evoked potentials were near normal bilaterally (grade I)
(Fig. 18-14, *C*). Thus, the results of both
modalities whose pathways traverse the
medulla, pons, midbrain, and part of the diencephalon, that is, somatosensory, and
auditory near and far field potentials, were
severely abnormal. The visual evoked brain
injury potentials were unaffected by the
brain stem lesion because the optic pathways
did not traverse the damaged caudal regions
of the brain stem.[18]

PROGNOSIS AND OUTCOME WITH EVOKED POTENTIALS

Evoked potential data can be correlated
with patient prognosis perhaps more closely
than it can with patient diagnosis.[18,19] Utilizing a functional grading system to analyze
evoked potential abnormal data, encouraging
results have been obtained associating the
data recorded in the first few days following
disease onset with the patient's neurologic
condition at subsequent time periods.
Whether used to evaluate single neural pathways or areas of brain traversed by many
neural systems, severe evoked potential abnormalities (grade III or IV) correlated well
with residual or permanent neuronal dysfunction, while mild evoked potential abnormalities (grade I or II) bespoke eventual
functional recovery. It is possible, in certain
instances, to predict in the first few days following ictus when the patient may still be in
coma the chance of functional recovery of
specific areas of compromised brain.[18]

Focal neurologic deficits

A severely depressed or absent evoked potential of any modality (visual, auditory, or
somatosensory) recorded early indicated permanent dysfunction of the specific neural
system tested.[18] Moreover, correlations of
evoked potential data with intraoperative and
autopsy findings demonstrated that severely
abnormal evoked potentials are usually obtained only in the most profoundly lesioned
brains.[37] Mild-to-moderate evoked potential
abnormalities predicted functional recovery
assuming the absence of secondary insults.

The capacity of evoked potential data to
forecast functional recovery of a neural system, even when the data was recorded in the
first week following trauma and the functional recovery took place months later, may be
related to the number of compromised neurons, their location, or the reversibility of
cellular dysfunction. It would appear that
evoked potential waveforms became profoundly altered only if the neuronal substrate was irreversibly damaged. Milder
evoked potential abnormalities result perhaps from neurons with reversible dysfunction or from areas of injury that are small
and whose function can be assumed by surrounding undamaged cells.

Coma

Duration of coma has been studied with
multimodality evoked potentials (visual,
somatosensory, auditory) by Greenberg and
co-workers (1977), because of the more extensive areas of brain that can be sampled
with multimodality evoked potentials as compared to one modality alone.[18] It was found
that at least 80% of comatose patients who
had mildly abnormal visual, somatosensory,
and auditory evoked potentials (grades I or
II) obtained within the first week after ictus
(mean day 3) became responsive within 30
days. Interestingly, those patients whose
multimodality evoked potential study was
mildly abnormal and who did not regain consciousness within 30 days were commonly
over 55 years old. Furthermore, using multimodality evoked potential data, the duration

of coma following head injury was found to be dependent on cerebral hemispheric dysfunction while brain stem dysfunction did not correlate with prolonged coma.

Outcome

Multimodality evoked potentials recorded early (mean day 3) and later (mean day 14) in the hospital course of patients have been correlated with the patients' final outcome.[18] Outcome categories were divided into two groups so that good recovery and moderate disability were in one group and severe disability, vegetative, and dead were in the other group. In the early period studied, only the somatosensory evoked potential could be clearly associated with the patients' final outcome three months or more later. By the second time period, auditory as well as somatosensory evoked potentials were able to prognosticate patient outcome. If somatosensory evoked potentials performed in the first week were only mildly abnormal (grade II or III), 90% of patients could be expected to have a good recovery or to be only moderately disabled assuming no secondary insult occurred after the first week. Therefore, graded somatosensory evoked potentials appear to be powerful prognostic tools for evaluating outcome within days of the onset of neurologic disease states.

It is clear that evoked potentials, especially in comatose patients, can provide better localization of central nervous system dysfunction than has heretofore been possible. This sensitive measure of brain function can be particularly useful in improving diagnosis and thus management in patients with neurologic disorders.

REFERENCES

1. Allison, T.: Recovery functions of somatosensory evoked responses in man, Electroenceph. Clin. Neurophysiol. **14**:331, 1962.
2. Allison, T., Matsumiya, Y., Goff, G. D., and Goff, W. R.: The scalp topography of human visual evoked potentials, Electroenceph. Clin. Neurophysiol. **42**:185, 1977.
3. Armington, J. C.: The electroretinogram, New York, 1974, Academic Press.
4. Astrup, J., Symon, L., Branston, N. M., and Lassen, N. A.: Cortical evoked potential and extracellular K^+ and H^+ at critical levels of brain ischemia, Stroke **8**:52, 1977.
5. Brierley, J. B., Graham, D. I., Adams, J. H., and Simpson, J. A.: Neocortical death after cardiac arrest: a clinical, neurophysiological and neuropathological report of two cases, Lancet **2**:560, 1971.
6. Cody, D. T. R.: Cortical evoked responses in neuro-otologic diagnosis, Arch. Otolaryngol. **97**:96, 1973.
7. Cracco, R. Q., and Cracco, J. B.: Somatosensory evoked potential in man: far field potentials, Electroenceph. Clin. Neurophysiol. **41**:460, 1976.
8. Creutzfeldt, O. D., Watanabe, S., and Lux, H. D.: Relations between EEG phenomena and potentials of single cortical cells. I. Evoked responses after thalamic and epicortical stimulation, Electroenceph. Clin. Neurophysiol. **20**:1, 1966.
9. Creutzfeldt, O. D., Watanabe, S., and Lux, H. D.: Relations between EEG phenomena and potentials of single cortical cells. II. Spontaneous and convulsoid activity, Electroenceph. Clin. Neurophysiol. **20**:19, 1966.
10. Cullen, K. K., Jr., Ellis, M. S., Berlin, C. I., and Lousteau, R. J.: Human acoustic nerve action potential recordings from the tympanic membrane without anesthesia, Acta Otolaryngol. **74**:15, 1972.
11. Donchin, E., and Lindsley, D. B.: Diagnostic uses of the average evoked potentials, Washington, D.C., 1969, NASA, SP-101, pp. 311-332.
12. Elul, R.: Brain waves: intracellular recording and statistical analysis help clarify their physiological significance, Data Acquisition Processing Biol. Med. **5**:93, 1966.
13. Feinsod, M., and Auerbach, E.: Electrophysiological examinations of the visual system in the acute phase after head injury, Eur. Neurol. **9**:56, 1973.
14. Giblin, D. R.: Somatosensory evoked potentials in healthy subjects and in patients with lesions of the nervous system, Ann. N.Y. Acad. Sci. **112**:93, 1964.
15. Goff, W. R., Matsumiya, Y., Allison, T., and Goff, G. D.: The scalp topography of human somatosensory and auditory evoked potentials, Electroenceph. Clin. Neurophysiol. **43**:57, 1977.
16. Goff, W. R., Matsumiya, Y., Allison, T., and Goff, G. D.: Cross-modality comparisons of average evoked potentials. In Donchin, E., and Lindsley, D. B., editors: Average evoked potentials: methods, results and evaluations, Washington, D.C., 1969, NASA, SP-191, pp. 95-141.
17. Greenberg, R. P., and Becker, D. P.: Clinical applications of evoked potential data in severe head injury patients, Surg. Forum **26**:484, 1975.
18. Greenberg, R. P., Becker, D. P., Miller, J. D., and others: Evaluation of brain function in severe human head trauma with multimodality evoked potentials. II. Localization of brain dysfunction and correla-

tion with post-traumatic neurological conditions, J. Neurosurg. **47:**163, 1977.

19. Greenberg, R. P., Mayer, D. J., and Becker, D. P.: The prognostic value of evoked potentials in human mechanical head injury. In McLaurin, R. L., editor: Head injuries: second Chicago symposium on neural trauma, New York, 1976, Grune & Stratton.

20. Greenberg, R. P., Mayer, D. J., Becker, D. P., and others: Evaluation of brain function in severe human head trauma with multimodality evoked potentials. I. Evoked brain injury potentials, methods, analysis, J. Neurosurg. **47:**150, 1977.

21. Grossman, R. G., Turner, J. W., Miller, J. D., and Rowan, J. O.: The relation between cortical electrical activity, cerebral perfusion pressure, and CBF during increased ICP, In Langfitt, T. W., editor: Cerebral circulation and metabolism, New York, 1975, Springer-Verlag, pp. 232-234.

22. Halliday, A. M.: Changes in the form of cerebral evoked responses in man associated with various lesions of the nervous system, Electroenceph. Clin. Neurophysiol. **25:**178, 1967.

23. Jewett, D. L.: Volume-conducted potentials in response to auditory stimuli as detected by averaging in the cat, Electroenceph. Clin. Neurophysiol. **28:**609, 1970.

24. Jewett, D. L., Romano, M. A., and Williston, J. S.: Human auditory evoked potentials: possible brain stem components detected on the scalp, Science **167:**1517, 1970.

25. Jewett, D. L., and Williston, J. S.: Auditory evoked far fields averaged from the scalp of humans, Brain **94:**681, 1971.

26. Kooi, K. A., and Bagchi, B. K.: Visual evoked re-

sponses in man: normative data, Ann. N.Y. Acad. Sci. **112:**254, 1964.

27. Larson, S. J., Sances, A., Jr., and Christenson, P. C.: Evoked somatosensory potentials in man, Arch. Neurol. **15:**88-93, 1966.

28. Liberson, W. T.: Study of evoked potentials in aphasics, Am. J. Phys. Med. **45:**135, 1966.

29. Meldrum, B. S., and Brierley, J. B.: Brain damage in the Rhesus monkey resulting from profound arterial hypotension. II. Changes in the spontaneous and evoked electrical activity of the neocortex, Brain Res. **13:**101, 1969.

30. Picton, T. W., Hillyard, S. A., Krausz, H. I., and Galambos, R.: Human auditory evoked potentials. I. Evaluation of components, Electroenceph. Clin. Neurophysiol. **36:**179, 1974.

31. Starr, A., and Achor, L. J.: Auditory brain stem responses in neurological disease, Arch. Neurol. **32:**761, 1975.

32. Starr, A., and Hamilton, A. E.: Correlation between confirmed sites of neurological lesions and abnormalities of far field auditory brain stem responses, Electroenceph. Clin. Neurophysiol. **41:**595, 1976.

33. Stohr, P. E., and Goldring, S.: Origin of somatosensory evoked scalp responses in man, J. Neurosurg. **31:**117, 1969.

34. Vaughan, H. C., Jr., and Katzman, R.: Evoked response in visual disorders, Ann. N.Y. Acad. Sci. **112:**305, 1964.

35. Wilkus, R. J., Harvey, F., Ojemann, L. M., and Lettich, E.: Electroencephalogram and sensory evoked potentials, Arch. Neurol. **24:**538, 1971.

Index

A

Abrodil, 127
Absorption coefficients and EMI CT head scanner, 132
Acetazolamide, 12, 14, 343, 351
    cerebrospinal fluid secretion and, 46, 48
    hypertension, intracranial, and, 106-107
Acetylcholine, 10
Acetylcholinesterase, 372
Acid base balance, 343
Acidosis, lactic, 11-12
Acromegaly, 160-161
Actinomycin D, 49
Adrenal failure, secondary, 160
Adriamycin, 380
Adult respiratory distress syndrome, 213-217
    treatment of, 214
Air, instillation of, in pneumoencephalography, 122-123
Air embolism; *see* Embolism, air
Akinetic mutism, 178, 270-271
Aldactone; *see* Spironolactone
Alkalosis, metabolic, 31, 343
Alkyl polyhalides, 379, 380
N-allynormorphine, 16
Alpha-tocopherol, 380-381
Alphaprodine, 143
Althesin, 3-4, 17
    brain oxygen consumption and, 29
    for supratentorial tumor, 156
Amiloride, 49
Aminophylline, 11, 352, 379
Amipaque; *see* Metrizamide
Amnesia
    posttraumatic, 276
    retrograde, 276
Amplifier, differential, 406
Anal sphincter reflex and spinal cord injury, 365
Analgesics, narcotic, 16-17
Anaphylaxis from contrast media, 147-148
Anemia, 9
Anencephalic monsters, 315
Anesthesia
    cerebral metabolic oxygen rate and, 27-30
    induction of, 161-163
    maintenance of, 163

Anesthesia—cont'd
    for neuroradiology, 138-149
    for posterior fossa procedures, 168-182
    principles of, 161
    recovery from, 163
    for supratentorial tumor, 150-167
Anesthetics
    energy balance and, 30-31
    free radical reactions and, 379, 380
Aneurysms, bleeding intracranial, 352
Angiogram, retrograde brachial, 130
Angiography, 143-145
    anesthesia for
        general, 144-145
        local, 145
    brain death and, 298-305, 306
    cerebral, 129-131
        catheter, 130-131
        technique for, 144
    complications of, 143
    diagnosis by, 271
    selective, 143
    spinal cord, 128-129
        hazards of, 145
Angiotensin, 5, 14, 225
Anticonvulsants, 330
Antidepressants, tricyclic, 225
Antihistamines for anaphylaxis, 147-148
Antimycin A, 253
Antioxidants, barbiturates as, 253
Anxiety and cerebral blood flow, 4
Apallic syndrome, 291-292, 315
Apnea
    brain death and, 291
    after head injury, 188, 212-213
    neuroradiology and, 120
Apoplexy, 12
Arachidonic acid, 256, 372
Arachidonic cascade, 368
ARDS; *see* Adult respiratory distress syndrome
Arfonad; *see* Trimethaphan camphorsulfonate
Arrhythmias, cardiac, and posterior fossa procedures, 168
Arteriography, indications for, 192